HUMAN RESPIRATORY VIRAL INFECTIONS

HUMAN RESPIRATORY VIRAL INFECTIONS

EDITED BY

SUNIT K. SINGH, PhD
Molecular Biology Unit
Faculty of Medicine
Institute of Medical Sciences
Banaras Hindu University (BHU)
Varanasi, India

CRC Press
Taylor & Francis Group
Boca Raton London New York

CRC Press is an imprint of the
Taylor & Francis Group, an **informa** business

Boca Raton, FL 33487-2742

First issued in paperback 2020

ISBN [illegible]
ISBN [illegible]

Visit the Taylor & Francis Web site at
http://www.taylorandfrancis.com

and the CRC Press Web site at
http://www.crcpress.com

Contents

Foreword

Respiratory infections are a major cause of morbidity and mortality in humans worldwide, and most acute upper and lower respiratory infectious conditions are primarily caused by viruses. Many of these viruses cause the highest burden of disease in specific risk groups such as young infants, the elderly, and immune-compromised individuals. While most of the respiratory viruses of humans have been identified during the course of the last century, a dozen "new" highly relevant respiratory viruses have been discovered in the last decade. These do not only include viruses that have been circulating in humans for many decades or even centuries, such as human metapneumovirus, human bocavirus, and human coronaviruses NL63 and HKU1, but also viruses that have recently emerged as a result of interspecies transmissions from animal reservoirs.

This book on human respiratory virus infections edited by Dr. Sunit K. Singh first gives a state-of-the-art overview of the knowledge of the anatomy and physiology of the human respiratory tract and its defense mechanism against virus infections. Factors that are crucial for the spread of respiratory virus infections such as environmental factors, cough formation, and aerosol development are addressed. A description of the tools to diagnose these respiratory infections and general measures for their management at the level of individual patients and the population at large, as well as an overview of animal models to test such intervention strategies, conclude Section I of this book.

Section II gives a detailed description of established and well-known respiratory viruses as well as more recently emerged viruses of the human respiratory tract and the way in which either of these may cause disease in individuals with different preexisting conditions or risk factors. The commonly known viruses that infect the respiratory tract, and either alone or in combination with other viruses or bacteria cause more or less severe upper and lower respiratory tract conditions such as the plethora of rhino-, Rota- and paramyxoviruses, or cause more systemic disease, like adeno- or measles viruses, are described in great detail. Of the more recently identified human respiratory viruses originating from animal reservoirs, such as influenza viruses from birds, and Hendra- and Nipah viruses as well as SARS- and MERS-coronaviruses from bats, their etiologic role, and burden of disease and development of intervention strategies are also covered in great detail.

Collectively, the data presented in this book provide an extensive and timely overview of the current knowledge of long known and newly emerged respiratory viruses of humans and the ways to diagnose and combat them efficiently with state-of-the-art intervention tools.

Professor Ab D.M.E. Osterhaus
Department of Viroscience
Erasmus MC Rotterdam
Erasmus University Rotterdam
The Netherlands

Preface

Respiratory virus infections have a major impact on human health. Acute human respiratory viral infections are the most common infections worldwide. Upper respiratory tract viral infections such as the common cold are exceedingly prevalent in infants, young children, and adults. These respiratory viral infections can also lead to complications such as acute otitis media and asthma exacerbation. However, lower respiratory tract infections such as pneumonia, bronchitis, and bronchiolitis occur less frequently.

Clinical presentations of respiratory viral infections overlap among those caused by various viruses and even bacteria. Accurate diagnosis of respiratory viral infections helps in patient management and prevention of secondary spread. Our understanding of human respiratory viral infections has increased exponentially over the past few decades. The diagnosis of respiratory viral infections has evolved substantially in recent years, with the development of novel molecular detection methods as well as a better understanding of virus structures and functional relationships with their hosts, better recognition of the true correlates of protection in many viral infections, and progress in vaccine development. On the one hand, we are equipped with better diagnostic tools and therapeutic strategies, and on the other hand, we are challenged by different viruses every day. This book describes up-to-date information on specific respiratory viral infections, diagnostic methods, and the newer technology platforms for the detection of respiratory viruses.

The book is divided into two sections. The first section addresses general aspects such as the anatomy of the human respiratory system, immunological interactions in lungs during infection, aerosol spread and communicability of viruses infecting the respiratory system, environmental variables affecting the transmission of viruses, infection control and prevention, and clinical and laboratory diagnosis of respiratory viral infections. The second section of this book covers the specific viruses infecting the respiratory system such as adenoviruses, rhinovirus, respiratory syncytial virus, human influenza virus, swine and avian influenza viruses affecting human population, parainfluenza virus, coronavirus, metapneumovirus, henipavirus, bocavirus, and mixed respiratory viral infections. Overall, this book deals with the basic and applied aspects of virology, focusing on the human respiratory viral infection mechanisms of the pathogenesis of specific viruses, diagnosis, treatment, epidemiology, and vaccine-related research.

This book has been written in order to provide an overview of human respiratory viral infections to basic scientists, biomedical researchers, medical and basic science students and scholars, physicians, pediatricians, pulmonologists, epidemiologists, virologists, molecular biologists, immunologists, vaccinologists, and microbiologists.

I have greatly enjoyed my interaction with the large panel of internationally renowned virologists, biomedical scientists, and infectious disease experts whose enthusiasm and commitment have led to the production of great chapters for this book. The professional support provided by Taylor & Francis Group/CRC Press greatly contributed to the final presentation of the book. I am highly thankful to my family and parents for their understanding and continuous support during the compilation of this book.

Sunit K. Singh

Acknowledgments

I highly acknowledge the support of virologists, immunologists, and infectious disease experts whose willingness to share their expertise has made this extensive overview on human respiratory viral infections possible.

Acknowledgments

I highly acknowledge the support of virologists, immunologists, and infectious disease experts whose willingness to share their expertise has made this extensive overview on human respiratory viral infections possible.

Editor

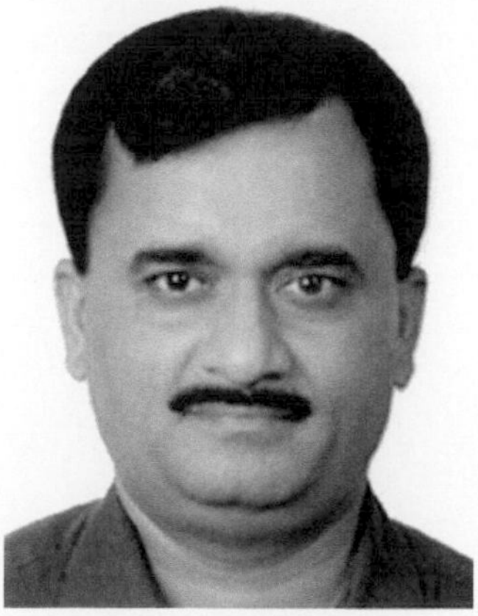

Dr. Sunit K. Singh earned his bachelor's degree from GB Pant University of Agriculture and Technology, Pantnagar, India, and his master's degree from the CIFE, Mumbai, India. After receiving his master's, Dr. Singh joined the Department of Pediatric Rheumatology, Immunology, and Infectious Diseases, Children's Hospital, University of Wuerzburg, Wuerzburg, Germany, as a biologist. Dr. Singh completed his PhD at the University of Wuerzburg in the area of molecular infection biology.

Dr. Singh completed his postdoctoral training at the Department of Internal Medicine, Yale University, School of Medicine, New Haven, Connecticut, and the Department of Neurology, University of California, Davis, Medical Center, Sacramento, California, in the areas of vector-borne infectious diseases and neuroinflammation, respectively. He has also worked as a visiting scientist at the Department of Pathology, Albert Einstein College of Medicine, New York; the Department of Microbiology, College of Veterinary Medicine, Chonbuk National University, Republic of Korea; the Department of Arbovirology, Institute of Parasitology, Ceske Budejovice, Czech Republic; and the Department of Genetics and Laboratory Medicine, University of Geneva, Switzerland. He has extensive experience in the area of virology and immunology. He served as a scientist and led a research group in the area of molecular neurovirology and inflammation biology at the prestigious Centre for Cellular and Molecular Biology, Hyderabad, India. Presently, he is serving as an Associate Professor (Molecular Immunology) at Molecular Biology Unit, Faculty of Medicine, Institute of Medical Sciences, Banaras Hindu University (BHU), Varanasi, India.

His main areas of research interest are neurovirology and immunology. There are several awards to his credit, including the Skinner Memorial Award, Travel Grant Award, NIH-Fogarty Fellowship, and Young Scientist Award. Dr. Singh is associated with several international journals of repute as an associate editor and an editorial board member.

Contributors

Faezeh Fathi Aghdam
Priority Research Centre for Asthma and Respiratory Diseases
Hunter Medical Research Institute and the University of Newcastle
New South Wales, Australia

Eric T. Beck
Microbiology Department
Dynacare Laboratories
Milwaukee, Wisconsin

Viktoriya Borisevich
Department of Pathology
University of Texas Medical Branch
Galveston, Texas

Nicole M. Bouvier
Department of Medicine—Infectious Diseases
and
Department of Microbiology
Mount Sinai School of Medicine
New York, New York

Rossana Cavallo
Azienda Ospedaliera Città della Salute e della Scienza di Torino
University of Turin
Turin, Italy

Thomas Edward Cecere
Department of Biomedical Sciences and Pathobiology
Virginia-Maryland Regional College of Veterinary Medicine
Virginia Tech
Blacksburg, Virginia

Anne B. Chang
Queensland Children's Medical Research Institute
Queensland University of Technology
and
Department of Respiratory Medicine
The Royal Children's Hospital
Brisbane, Queensland, Australia

and

Menzies School of Health Research Charles Darwin University
Tiwi, Northern Territory, Australia

Allison F. Christiaansen
Department of Microbiology
University of Iowa
Iowa City, Iowa

Cristina Costa
Azienda Ospedaliera Città della Salute e della Scienza di Torino
University of Turin
Turin, Italy

Rik L. de Swart
Department of Viroscience
Erasmus Medical Center
Rotterdam, the Netherlands

Rory D. de Vries
Department of Viroscience
Erasmus Medical Center
Rotterdam, the Netherlands

Marcela Echavarria
Centro de Educacion Medica e Investigaciones Clinicas (CEMIC) University Hospital
Buenos Aires, Argentina

Daniel P. Eiras
Department of Medicine
Weill Cornell Medical College
New York, New York

Olivier Escaffre
Department of Pathology
University of Texas Medical Branch
Galveston, Texas

Giacomo Faldella
S.Orsola-Malpighi Hospital
Bologna, Italy

Judith M. Fontana
Department of Public Health
Weill Cornell Medical College
New York, New York

Pieter L. A. Fraaij
Department of Viroscience
Erasmus Medical Center–Sophia Children's Hospital
Rotterdam, the Netherlands

Frantzeska Frantzeskaki
Second Department of Critical Care
University of Athens Medical School
Attikon Hospital
Haidari, Athens, Greece

Stephen B. Greenberg
Department of Medicine
Baylor College of Medicine
Houston, Texas

Philip M. Hansbro
Priority Research Centre for Asthma and Respiratory Diseases
Hunter Medical Research Institute and the University of Newcastle
New South Wales, Australia

Kevin S. Harrod
Infectious Diseases Program
Lovelace Respiratory Research Institute
Albuquerque, New Mexico

Kelly J. Henrickson
Department of Pediatrics
Medical College of Wisconsin and Children's Hospital of Wisconsin
Milwaukee, Wisconsin

Jonathan Hoffmann
Emerging Pathogens Laboratory (LPE)
Foundation Mérieux
Lyon, France

Robert J. Hogan
Department of Veterinary Biosciences and Diagnostic Imaging
and
Department of Infectious Diseases
University of Georgia
Athens, Georgia

Alan Chen-Yu Hsu
Priority Research Centre for Asthma and Respiratory Diseases
Hunter Medical Research Institute and the University of Newcastle
New South Wales, Australia

Michael G. Ison
Divisions of Infectious Diseases and Organ Transplantation
Northwestern University Feinberg School of Medicine
Chicago, Illinois

Adriana E. Kajon
Lovelace Respiratory Research Institute
Albuquerque, New Mexico

Cory J. Knudson
University of Iowa
Iowa City, Iowa

Matti Korppi
Tampere Center for Child Health Research
University of Tampere and Tampere University Hospital
Tampere, Finland

Frederick T. Koster
Department of Preclinical Microbiology and Immunotoxicology
Lovelace Respiratory Research Institute
and
Departments of Internal Medicine (Emeritus) and Computer Science
University of New Mexico
Albuquerque, New Mexico

Anastasia Kotanidou
First Department of Critical Care
and Pulmonary Services
University of Athens Medical School
Evangelismos Hospital
Athens, Greece

Marcello Lanari
Pediatrics and Neonatology Unit
Imola General Hospital
Imola, Italy

Ruisi Hazel Lin
Department of Microbiology
National University of Singapore
Singapore

Anthony W.I. Lo
Department of Anatomical and Cellular
Pathology
The Chinese University of Hong Kong
Hong Kong

Su-Ling Loo
Priority Research Centre for Asthma
and Respiratory Diseases
Hunter Medical Research Institute
and the University of Newcastle
New South Wales, Australia

Joseph P. Lynch III
Department of Internal Medicine
University of California
Los Angeles, California

Ian M. Mackay
Queensland Children's Medical Research
Institute
University of Queensland
Brisbane, Queensland, Australia

Tze-Minn Mak
NUS Graduate School for Integrative Sciences
and Engineering
National University of Singapore
Singapore

Nikolaos Manitsopoulos
First Department of Critical Care
and Pulmonary Services
University of Athens Medical School
Evangelismos Hospital
Athens, Greece

Fleur M. Moesker
Department of Viroscience
Erasmus Medical Center
Rotterdam, the Netherlands

Samira Mubareka
Sunnybrook Health Sciences Centre
Toronto, Ontario, Canada

Laurent P. Nicod
Service de Pneumologie
Centre Hospitalier Universitaire
Vaudois
Lausanne, Switzerland

Hubert G.M. Niesters
Department of Medical Microbiology
University of Groningen
Groningen, the Netherlands

Kerry-Ann F. O'Grady
Queensland Children's Medical Research
Institute
Queensland University of
Technology
Brisbane, Queensland, Australia

Stylianos E. Orfanos
First Department of Critical Care
and Pulmonary Services
Evangelismos Hospital
and
Second Department of Critical Care
University of Athens Medical School
Attikon Hospital
Athens, Greece

Ab D.M.E. Osterhaus
Department of Viroscience
Erasmus Medical Center
Rotterdam, the Netherlands

Gláucia Paranhos-Baccalà
Emerging Pathogens Laboratory (LPE)
Foundation Mérieux
Lyon, France

Kristy Parsons
Priority Research Centre for Asthma
and Respiratory Diseases
Hunter Medical Research Institute
and the University of Newcastle
New South Wales, Australia

Carl Persson
Department of Clinical Chemistry and
Pharmacology
Lund University Hospital
Lund, Sweden

Jennifer R. Plourde
Lovelace Respiratory Research Institute
and
Department of Pathology
University of New Mexico Health Science
Center
Albuquerque, New Mexico

Janette C. Rahamat-Langendoen
Department of Medical Microbiology,
University of Groningen
Groningen, the Netherlands

Owen Benjamin Richmond
Department of Biomedical
Sciences and Pathobiology
Virginia-Maryland Regional
College of Veterinary Medicine
Virginia Tech
Blacksburg, Virginia

Andrew Riordan
Alder Hey Children's Hospital
and
Department of Clinical Microbiology Infection
and Immunology
University of Liverpool
Liverpool, United Kingdom

Barry Rockx
Department of Pathology and Department of
Microbiology and Immunology
University of Texas Medical Branch
Galveston, Texas

Chad J. Roy
Tulane National Primate Research
Center
Covington, Louisiana

and

Department of Microbiology and
Immunology
Tulane School of Medicine
New Orleans, Louisiana

Mirella Salvatore
Department of Public Health
and Department of Medicine
Weill Cornell Medical College
New York, New York

Oliver Schildgen
Kliniken der Stadt Köln
Institut für Pathologie
Klinikum der Privaten Universität
Witten-Herdecke
Cologne, Germany

Verena Schildgen
Kliniken der Stadt Köln
Institut für Pathologie
Klinikum der Privaten Universität
Witten-Herdecke
Cologne, Germany

Jennifer Elana Schuster
Vanderbilt University Medical Center
Nashville, Tennessee

W.H. Seto
Department of Microbiology
Queen Mary Hospital
Hong Kong

Francesca Sidoti
Azienda Ospedaliera Città della
Salute e della Scienza di Torino
University of Turin
Turin, Italy

Sunit K. Singh
Institute of Medical Sciences (IMS)
Banaras Hindu University (BHU)
Varanasi, India

Anoop Kumar Sinha
Department of Biology
Colvin Taluqdars College
Lucknow, India

Jennifer L. Smith
Department of Preclinical Microbiology and Immunotoxicology
Lovelace Respiratory Research Institute
Albuquerque, New Mexico

Sheree Smith
University of Western Sydney
Sydney, Australia

and

Imperial College
London, United Kingdom

Yee-Joo Tan
Department of Microbiology
National University of Singapore
Singapore

Kentigern Thorburn
Alder Hey Children's Hospital
and
Department of Clinical Microbiology
Infection and Immunology
University of Liverpool
Liverpool, United Kingdom

K.F. To
Department of Anatomical and Cellular Pathology
The Chinese University of Hong Kong
Hong Kong

Stephanie Michelle Todd
Department of Biomedical Sciences and Pathobiology
Virginia-Maryland Regional College of Veterinary Medicine
Virginia Tech
Blacksburg, Virginia

Lena Uller
Department of Experimental Medical Science
Lund University
Lund, Sweden

Silvia Vandini
S.Orsola-Malpighi Hospital
Bologna, Italy

Steven M. Varga
Department of Microbiology and Department of Pathology
University of Iowa
Iowa City, Iowa

Daniel Verreault
Tulane National Primate Research Center
Covington, Louisiana

Thomas G. Voss
SRI International
Harrisonburg, Virginia

Ellie Walker
Northwestern University Feinberg School of Medicine
Chicago, Illinois

Peter A.B. Wark
Hunter Medical Research Institute and the University of Newcastle
and
Department of Respiratory and Sleep Medicine
John Hunter Hospital
New South Wales, Australia

Grant Waterer
University of Western Australia
Perth, Western Australia, Australia

Kayla A. Weiss
University of Iowa
Iowa City, Iowa

John V. Williams
Vanderbilt University Medical Center
Nashville, Tennessee

Section I

Human Respiratory System and Disease Management

1 Overview on Anatomy of Human Respiratory System

Anoop Kumar Sinha and Sunit K. Singh

CONTENTS

1.1 INTRODUCTION

The respiratory system is composed of a conducting portion that brings oxygen to the lungs and the respiratory portion that exchanges oxygen and carbon dioxide gases with the blood stream. Air contains many microbes and viruses carried on dust and droplet nuclei; therefore, respiratory system is the most common portal of entry for these infectious agents. Considering the challenges faced by respiratory system through respiratory pathogens, the respiratory system evolved effective defense mechanisms.

Over a lifetime, an individual gets exposed to many infectious agents; however, in most situations, the individual does not develop a disease. If a pathogen is able to breach the first lines of defense, a highly specialized and specific protection in the form of adaptive immune response will be activated. Furthermore, this process will initiate the generation of the immunological memory, enabling the individual with a more quickly and effectively response at the next contact with the same agent.

On the contrary, if the foreign agent can overcome both defenses, the result is disease. In certain cases, the line of defense, when triggered, can also cooperate with the damage instead of healing, making the disease more severe. Thus, the immunopathology of viral respiratory infection is a frequent consequence of the immune response against the viruses infecting respiratory system.

The primary aim of this chapter is to summarize the important features of the anatomy of respiratory system, which will help readers understand the host and viral interaction in respiratory infection.

Respiration is defined as exchange of gases between alveolar air and blood in lungs and between blood and body cells. It is a sum of three processes:

- Breathing or pulmonary ventilation is carrying air through external nostrils into the lungs (inspiration) and expelling out used air (expiration) from lungs through the same passage.
- External respiration is exchange of gases between the alveolar air and blood; oxygen diffuses into blood and carbon dioxide leaving out blood into alveolar air.
- Internal respiration or tissue respiration is gaseous exchange between blood and body cells.

The cellular respiration is the process by which cells produce energy for smooth running of cellular processes and storage in energy-rich compounds. It may (aerobic respiration) or may not require oxygen (anaerobic respiration).

The respiratory system starting from the nose up to lungs can be differentiated into an upper and a lower respiratory tract. The former includes nose, pharynx, and associated structures while the latter refers to larynx, trachea, bronchi, and lungs. The part of the system that transports air into the lungs and where no exchange of gases takes place constitutes the conducting portion that includes nose, pharynx, trachea, bronchi, and their branches. The remaining portion includes respiratory bronchioles, alveolar ducts, alveolar sacs, and alveoli where gaseous exchange takes place in the respiratory system. However, the respiratory bronchioles and alveolar ducts perform both conducting and respiratory functions, and hence are called transitional airways [1]. The bronchi and their branches along with associated blood and lymph vessels, nerves, pleural membranes, and interlobular septa form the nonparenchymatous part of lung. The alveoli where gaseous exchange takes place constitute the parenchyma, about 87% of the total lung volume [2].

1.2 UPPER RESPIRATORY TRACT

1.2.1 Nose

The nose opens out through a pair of external nares or nostrils (Figure 1.1). The nose can be divided into the external portion, which is in fact termed as the nose, and the internal portions, being the nasal cavities (*nasal fossae; cavum nasi*). The nose is the only visible part of the respiratory system, protruding from the face, and lying in between the forehead and the upper lip. The external portion of the nose is partly supported by the bone and partly hyaline cartilage covered with muscles and skin and has an inner lining of mucous membrane. The superior attachment of nose to forehead between eyes is the root and the tip of nose at the inferior end is the apex. The anterior border between root and apex is the dorsum nasi. It is supported by elastic cartilage; hence, it is flexible. The superior part of dorsum nasi forms the bridge and is supported by the bone [3].

The internal part of nose has a large cavity in the skull below the cranium that posteriorly connects with the pharynx through a pair of internal nares (choanae). The nasolachrymal duct and the ducts of paranasal sinuses also open into the internal nose. The roof of internal nose is formed by ethmoid bone and the floor is formed by palatine bones and palatal processes of maxillae; the two together form the hard palate. The lateral walls of internal nose are formed by ethmoid, maxilla, lachrymal, palatine, and inferior nasal bones. The space inside external and internal nose, the nasal cavity, is divided into right and left halves by a vertical partition called nasal septum. The anterior part of nasal cavity just inside the nostril is the vestibule. The vestibular lining has hair to filter

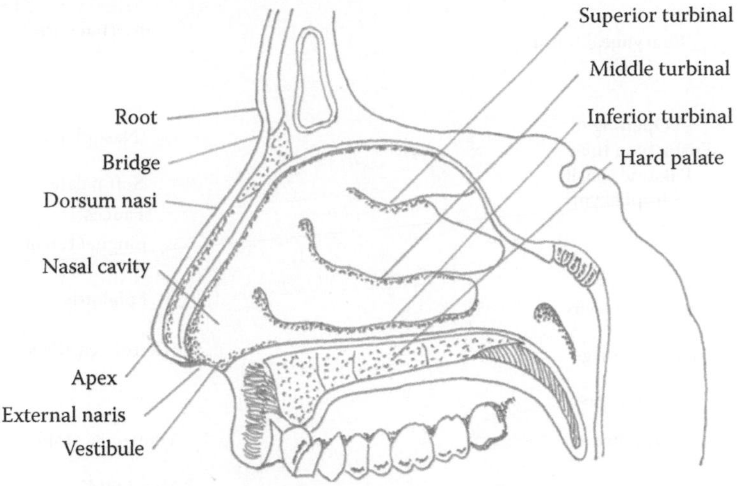

FIGURE 1.1 Structure of nose and nasal cavity.

out large dust particles of air. The upper nasal cavity has extensions of superior, middle, and inferior nasal conchae or turbinals forming three shelves that divide each side of the nasal cavity into groove-like passages, the superior, middle, and inferior meatuses. The shelves and meatuses are lined with mucous membranes. Olfactory receptors are present in the membrane lining the superior conchae and the adjacent septum, and hence are called the olfactory epithelium [3].

The mucous membrane below the olfactory epithelium contains capillaries, pseudostratified columnar epithelial cells, and many goblet cells. The blood in capillaries helps in warming the air passing through the conchae and meatuses. The mucous from goblet cells traps dust particles of air. The fluid drains down from nasolachrymal ducts, and secretions from paranasal sinuses and mucous from goblet cells moisten the air. The cilia move down the dust-laden mucous toward the pharynx for elimination from respiratory tract either by swallowing or spitting.

1.2.2 Pharynx

The pharynx (Figure 1.2), about 13 cm in length, is funnel shaped starting from internal nares and extends up to the cricoid cartilages of larynx.

The pharyngeal wall is composed of skeletal muscles and lined with mucous membranes. The pharynx serves as the passage for food and air and a resonating chamber for sound. It can be differentiated into three divisions—nasopharynx (epipharynx), oropharynx (mesopharynx), and laryngopharynx (hypopharynx).

1.2.2.1 Nasopharynx

The uppermost part of pharynx starting from internal nares up to the level of soft palate is the nasopharynx. The nasopharyngeal wall has four openings, two internal nares and two of Eustachian or pharyngo-tympanic tubes. The Eustachian tubes help in equalizing air pressure on both sides of the tympanic membrane. The nasopharynx is lined with pseudostratified ciliated columnar epithelium; the cilia move the mucous toward the inferior part of pharynx. A pair of pharyngeal tonsils or adenoids is located in the posterior wall of the nasopharynx.

1.2.2.2 Oropharynx

It is posterior to oral cavity from uvula up to the level of hyoid bone. The opening of the oral cavity in the oropharynx is known as the fauces. A pair each of palatine tonsils and lingual tonsils are located in the oropharynx. The lining of the oropharynx is formed by stratified squamous

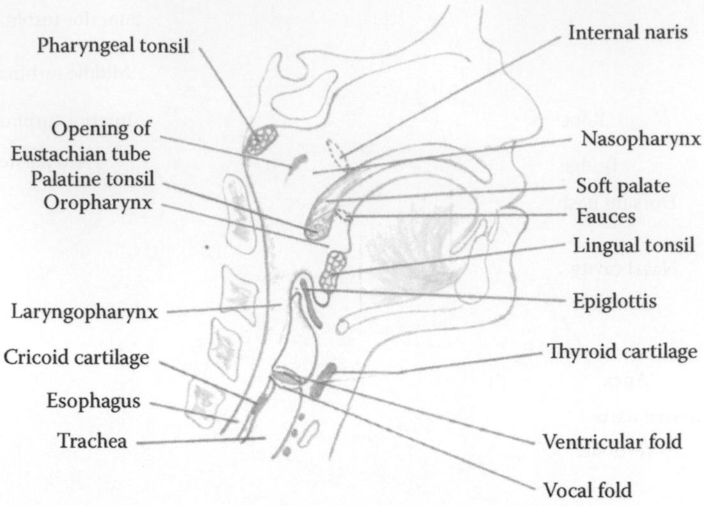

FIGURE 1.2 Structure of pharynx.

epithelium. The oropharynx is a common passage for air, food, and drinks; so, it serves both respiratory and digestive functions.

1.2.2.3 Laryngopharynx

The third and lowest part of pharynx is laryngopharynx or hypopharynx, which extends from hyoid bone downward up to the beginning of the esophagus and larynx. It is lined with stratified squamous epithelium and, like oropharynx, serves respiratory and digestive functions.

1.3 LOWER RESPIRATORY TRACT

1.3.1 Larynx

The larynx or sound box or voice box in the neck is an organ for sound production, breathing, and preventing entry of ingested food into trachea (Figure 1.3). The larynx is commonly known as the voice box as it houses the vocal folds that are responsible for sound production (*phonation*). It serves as a sphincter in transmitting air from the oropharynx to the trachea and also in creating sounds for speech.

It is a tubular structure about 10.4 cm long and connects the pharynx with trachea. The larynx in newborn infants is at the level of the second and third cervical (C_2–C_3) vertebrae, gradually descending down as the child grows [2–4]. The larynx in adults is somewhere near the level of the C_3–C_6 vertebrae and is supported by cartilages. The laryngeal skeleton has nine cartilages, three unpaired and three paired. The three unpaired cartilages are epiglottis, thyroid, and cricoids and the three paired cartilages are arytenoids, corniculate, and cuneiform.

The epiglottis is a flat, leaf-shaped elastic cartilage; the base or stem is attached to thyroid cartilage and the free portion or leaf remains unattached. It moves up and down to open or close the glottis. When the glottis is closed, the food and liquids are kept out of the larynx and enter the esophagus; if it fails to close, these enter the larynx instead of the esophagus and we say we have "swallowed down our Sunday throat." A cough reflex follows to expel any solid or liquid material if it happens to enter the larynx.

The thyroid cartilage (Adam's apple) in the anterior wall of larynx is the largest cartilage formed by two fused plates of hyaline cartilage. It is larger in men than in women. The cricoid cartilage is a ring of hyaline cartilage forming the inferior wall of larynx and is attached to the first cartilaginous tracheal ring.

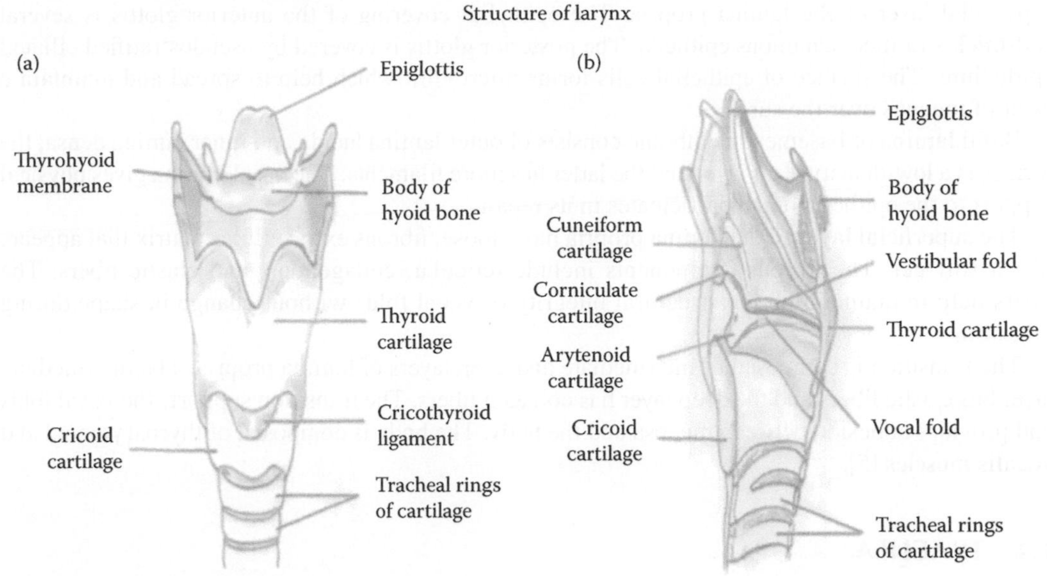

FIGURE 1.3 Larynx and laryngeal cartilages. (a) Anterior view and (b) posterior view.

Paired arytenoid cartilages are triangular and hyaline in nature. They attach to vocal folds and intrinsic pharyngeal muscles. Arytenoids are the most important cartilages as they move the vocal folds or true vocal cords and influence their position and tension. Corniculates are small, paired elastic cartilages at the apex of each arytenoid cartilage. Cuneiform cartilages are also paired, elastic, and anterior to the corniculate cartilages.

The mucous membrane of the larynx forms two pairs of vocal folds, a pair of upper or false vocal folds or ventricular folds and a lower pair of true vocal folds. The false vocal folds are nonmuscular, covered with respiratory epithelium and responsible for resonance. The true vocal folds are covered with stratified squamous epithelium and have skeletal (voluntary) muscles. The vocal folds in men are thicker and longer than in women due to the influence of androgens and hence, vibrate more slowly. The only muscle to separate the vocal folds for normal breathing is the posterior cricoarytenoid.

Glottis consists of true vocal folds and the space between them is called the rima glottidis. It can be differentiated into an anterior glottis or intermembranous space covered with several cell-thick, stratified squamous epithelium and a posterior glottis or intercartilaginous region lined with pseudostratified ciliated epithelium. The vocal folds vibrate in anterior glottis to produce sound. The posterior glottis has a wider opening between vocal folds for inspiration and expiration.

When the skeletal muscles of the larynx, known as intrinsic muscles, contract, the vocal folds are stretched into the airway and the rima glottidis is narrowed. The larynx generates the sound of a specific frequency that is altered when it travels through the vocal tract. The vocal folds vibrate when air is directed against them setting up sound waves in the air column in pharynx, nose, and mouth. The loudness of sound depends on the pressure of air and the pitch is controlled by tension on vocal folds. The force of expiration also contributes to loudness. A higher-pitch sound is produced when vocal folds are pulled by muscles and vibrate more rapidly. A low-pitch sound is produced by decreasing muscular tension. Although sound originates from vibration of vocal folds, certain other structures are important for converting sound into recognizable speech. The pharynx, mouth, nasal cavity, and paranasal sinus all function as resonating chambers.

1.3.1.1 Histology of Vocal Folds

The vocal folds can be differentiated into three main layers, the cover, transition, and body. The cover consists of an outer epithelium or mucosa, basement membrane or basal lamina, and the superficial layer of the lamina propria. The epithelial covering of the anterior glottis is several cell-thick stratified squamous epithelia. The posterior glottis is covered by pseudostratified ciliated epithelium. The surface of epithelial cells forms microvilli, which help to spread and maintain a layer of mucous over the surface.

Basal lamina or basement membrane consists of outer lamina lucida and inner lamina densa; the former is a low-density clear layer and the latter has more filaments. The basal lamina gives physical support to the epithelium and participates in its repair.

The superficial layer of the lamina propria has a loose, fibrous extracellular matrix that appears like a soft gel. The fibrous components include reticular, collagenous, and elastic fibers. The fibers help in maintaining the structural integrity of vocal folds without change in shape during vibration.

The transition is composed of intermediate and deep layers of lamina propria. The intermediate layer has elastic fibers and the deep layer has collagen fibers. The transition supports the vocal folds and provides adhesion between mucosa and the body. The body is composed of thyroarytenoid and vocalis muscles [5].

1.4 TRACHEA

The trachea (Figure 1.4a) or windpipe is about 12 cm long and 2.5 cm in diameter. It begins below the larynx near the sixth cervical vertebra and bifurcates into right and left primary bronchi at the level of the fifth thoracic vertebra. The trachea is supported on the anterior and lateral sides by about 16–20 incomplete C-shaped rings of hyaline cartilage. The dorsal wall of trachea facing the esophagus is membranous and has an incomplete portion of a cartilage ring. The rings prevent collapsing of tracheal wall inward. The free ends of incomplete tracheal rings are interconnected by trachealis muscle; it contracts to reduce the lumen of trachea to increase the force of airflow, as in coughing. The last tracheal ring projects inward to form a small internal ridge called the carina. The mucous membrane covering of carina is a very sensitive part of the respiratory system and is associated with the cough reflex.

The tracheal wall consists of four layers, mucosa, submucosa, hyaline cartilage, and adventitia (Figure 1.4b). The mucosa has pseudostratified ciliated columnar epithelial cells, goblet cells secreting mucous, and smaller basal cells not reaching up to the luminal surface.

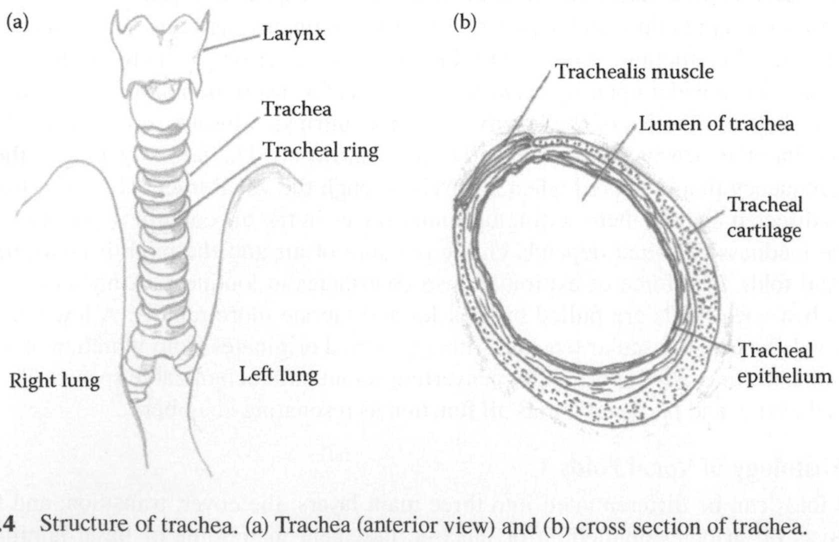

FIGURE 1.4 Structure of trachea. (a) Trachea (anterior view) and (b) cross section of trachea.

1.5 BRONCHI

The right and left primary bronchi connect with the respective lungs, the right primary bronchi being shorter and wider than the left primary bronchi. The right bronchus is 2.5 cm long and supported by 6–8 cartilage rings; the left bronchus is 5 cm long and has 9–12 rings. The primary bronchi, such as trachea, are also supported by incomplete cartilage rings and lined with pseudostratified ciliated columnar epithelium. Each primary bronchus after entering the lung divides into smaller bronchi known as secondary bronchi, one to each lobe of the lung, three in the right, and two in the left lung.

The secondary bronchi divide into still smaller branches, the tertiary or segmental bronchi, and finally the bronchioles. The branching pattern continues further, eventually forming terminal bronchioles. The branching from the trachea up to the terminal bronchioles is known as the bronchial tree.

Some structural changes can be noted as the branching pattern becomes more extensive. The pseudostratified columnar epithelium slowly changes into nonciliated cuboidal epithelium in terminal bronchioles. The incomplete rings of cartilage are gradually replaced by small cartilage plates that also disappear in bronchioles. A decrease in the cartilage increases smooth muscle content of bronchioles, which form spiral bands and their contraction is affected by autonomic nervous system (ANS) and various chemicals. The parasympathetic nervous system (PSNS) and histamine cause constriction of bronchioles; sympathetic nervous system (SNS) and epinephrine dilate them.

1.5.1 Morphology of Conducting Airways

A conducting airway consists of surface epithelium of mainly ciliated and secretory cells, subepithelial tissue, and glands. Tall columnar ciliated cells, goblet cells, and smaller basal cells are characteristic of tracheal and proximal bronchial epithelium [6]. The ciliated cells have thinner bases, firmly attached to basal lamina and 200–300 cilia arise from the surface. The neighboring cells are also attached to each other through tight junctions [7] near their apices to put up a barrier to prevent entry of substances in intercellular spaces [8]. The adjacent ciliated cells are connected to each other and to basal cells by desmosomes.

Goblet cells, about 20–30% of cells in proximal bronchi [9] that gradually decrease in number distally to very few in respiratory bronchioles [10], have secretory granules containing mucin near the apices.

Basal cells attached to basement membrane are roughly triangular in shape, abundant in proximal airways, and decrease in number distally to almost absent in bronchioles [11]. They can give rise to new epithelial cells and also attach them to basement membrane.

Clara cells, cuboidal or columnar in shape, are mainly found in membranous bronchioles. Their cytoplasm has many vesicles containing lipid and protein [12], including a Clara cell-specific protein (CC10, CC16, and protein I) and surfactant apoprotein [13]. Clara cell-specific protein may have some role in the immune response [14]. They can also form new bronchiolar epithelium to replace the damaged cells [15].

Neuroendocrine cells are very few, only 0.5% of bronchial epithelium in adults. The neurosecretory granules in their cytoplasm contain various peptides with local effects— gastrin-releasing peptide, somatostatin, substance P, endothelin, and enkephalin [16]. These peptides are mostly secreted at the bases, but some laterally diffuse to adjacent epithelial cells or into the lumen of the airway.

Dendritic and Langerhans cells have long cytoplasmic extensions and elicit immune response. The Langerhans cells are believed to function as antigen-processing and antigen-presenting cells and also stimulate proliferation of T-cells [17]. Lymphocytes are present throughout the conducting airways and involved in processing and reacting to the antigen. Some mast cells are also found in airway epithelium [18].

The basement membrane attaches the epithelium to the underlying connective tissue by means of hemidesmosomes and adhesion molecules. Fibroblasts are located just beneath the basement membrane. The subepithelial tissue can be differentiated into lamina propria and submucosa. Lamina propria has a network of capillaries and reticulin fibers and also bundles of elastic and nerve fibers. Submucosa has cartilage and muscles and the major portion of tracheobronchial glands. The tracheal cartilage plates are 16–20, U-shaped structures and their open ends are noncartilaginous and membranous. The spaces between successive tracheal plates contain smooth muscles, tracheal glands, collagen, and elastic fibers.

The tracheal muscle is mainly found in the membranous portion and forms longitudinal and transverse bundles.

The tracheobronchial glands are extensions of surface epithelium into the submucosa. Their size and number are greater in a proximal portion of airways [19], but absent in small bronchi and bronchioles. The glands open over the surface through ducts. Several branched secretory tubules arise from the collecting duct, which are lined by mucous-secreting cells and serous cells. The serous cells contain several substances including lysozyme, lactoferrin, and transferrin, which play a significant role in airway defense. Other cells taking part in airway defense—lymphocytes, plasma cells, macrophages, and mast cells—are found in lamina propria and submucosa.

1.6 LUNGS

Each lung is enclosed in a pleural cavity lined by two membranes, outer parietal pleura and inner visceral pleura separated by a space, the pleural cavity. Parietal pleura lines the chest wall, mediastinum, and diaphragm. The visceral pleura is a thin layer of connective tissue that at certain places extends into each lung to divide it into lobes, three in the right and two in the left lung.

A pair of lungs (Figure 1.5) is lodged in the thoracic cavity superiorly extending above the clavicles. The broad inferior base of each lung is concave and fits over the convex area of diaphragm. The superior portion of each lung is narrow, forming the apex or cupula. The anterior or costal surface lying against the ribs is rounded. The medial or mediastinal surface has a hilus through which primary bronchi, pulmonary blood vessels, lymphatic vessels, and nerves enter and exit. The left lung medially has a concavity, the cardiac notch to accommodate the heart.

The right lung is thicker and broader than the left lung, and also a bit shorter as the diaphragm is shifted up on the right side to accommodate the liver behind. Each lung is divided into lobes

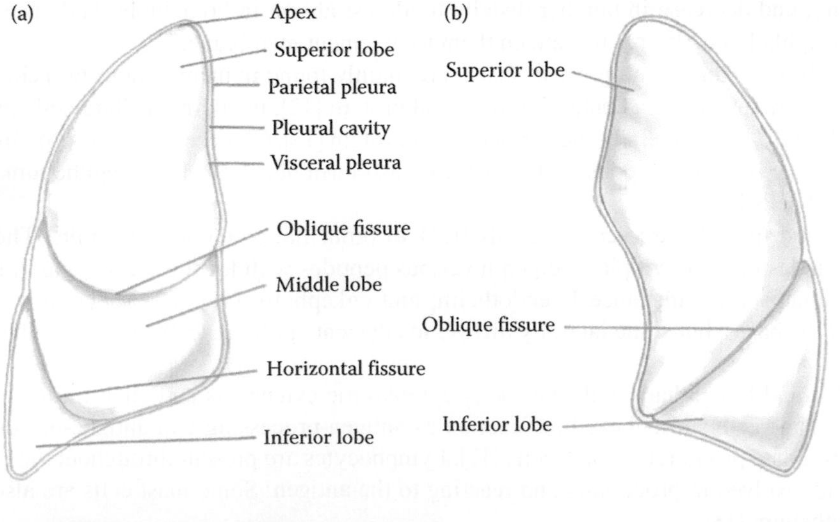

FIGURE 1.5 (a) Right and (b) left lung.

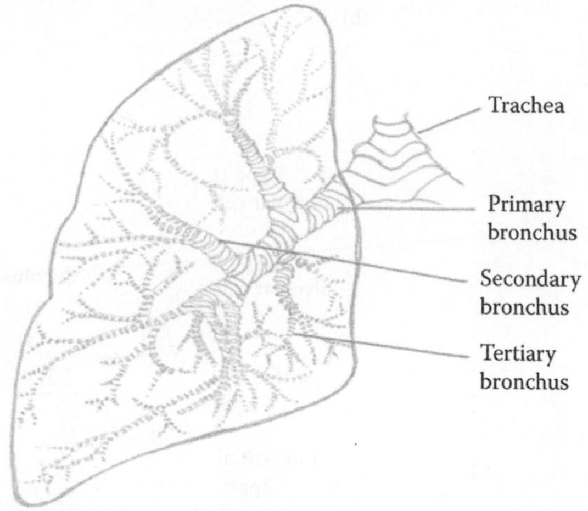

FIGURE 1.6 Bronchial tree in right lung.

by fissures. The left lung has an oblique fissure to separate the superior lobe from the inferior lobe. The right lung has two fissures, a horizontal fissure and an oblique fissure. The upper part of an oblique fissure separates the superior lobe from the inferior lobe and the lower part separates the inferior lobe from the middle lobe. The horizontal fissure divides the superior lobc forming a middle lobe.

The right primary bronchus divides to form three secondary or lobar bronchi—superior, middle, and inferior—one to each lobe of the right lung (Figure 1.6). The left primary bronchus forms a superior and an inferior secondary, or lobar, branch for the two lobes of the left lung. The secondary bronchi further divide to form tertiary or segmental bronchi, 10 in each lung. The portion of lung tissue supplied by each tertiary bronchus is called the bronchopulmonary segment that is further divided into many small lobules, each enclosed in elastic connective tissue and supplied by arterioles, venules, lymphatic vessels, and a branch of terminal bronchiole. The terminal bronchiole divides into very fine respiratory bronchioles and each bronchiole subdivides forming several alveolar ducts. An alveolar duct connects with an alveolar sac into which open several minute chambers, the alveoli. The pulmonary alveoli are the terminal ends of the respiratory tree and the sites of gaseous exchange between alveolar air and blood.

A pair of human lungs contains about 700 million alveoli and the alveolar membrane has surface area of about 70 m^2 [20]. The average diameter of an alveolus is about 200 μm with a slight increase during inhalation [21]. A network of capillaries is wrapped around each alveolus covering about 70% of its surface area.

1.6.1 Alveolar Membrane

The alveoli are lined with an epithelial layer overlaid by the extracellular matrix and surrounded by capillaries (Figure 1.7). The alveolar wall may have pores between alveoli called the pores of Kohn. Three major types of cells or pneumocytes [22] can be recognized in the alveolar wall: (1) type I or squamous alveolar cells form the lining of the alveolar wall; (2) type II or granular pneumocytes are cuboidal and secrete surfactant (phospholipid and protein mixture) to lower the surface tension of water; and (3) macrophages or dust cells are phagocytic and destroy foreign materials such as bacteria.

Type I pneumocytes are squamous epithelial cells covering about 95% of the alveolar surface and are responsible for the exchange of gases in alveoli. They cannot form new cells to replace the dead cells; hence, new type I cells are formed by type II cells [23].

The extracellular matrix contains both collagen and elastic fibers. The elastic fibers permit an increase and decrease in alveolar space during inhalation and exhalation.

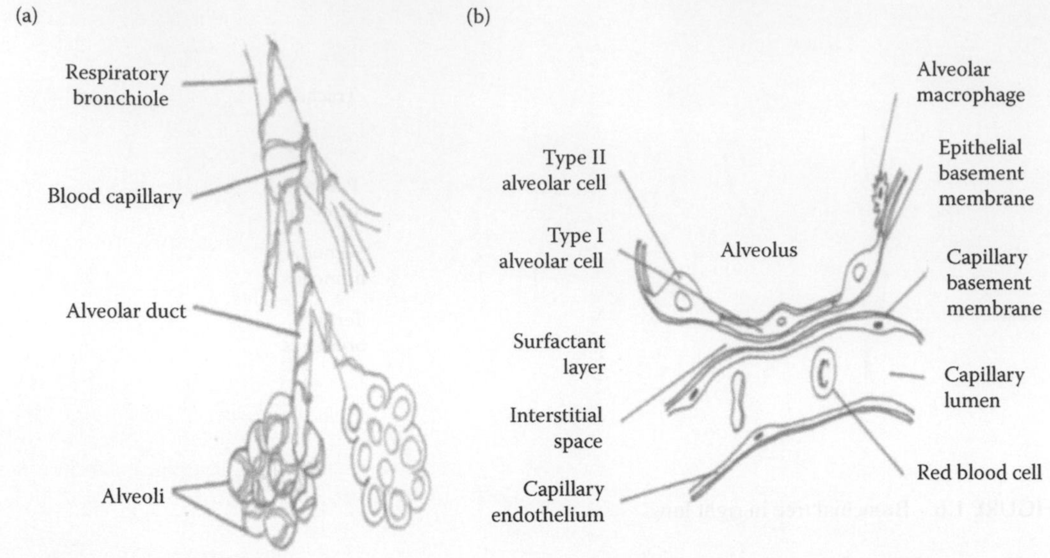

FIGURE 1.7 (a) Lung alveoli and (b) histology of alveolar membrane.

1.6.1.1 Macrophages

Macrophages destroy pathogens and dead cells in the alveolar membrane [23]. The pathogens enter into macrophages and are enclosed by the membrane to form a phagosome. The phagosome is fused with primary lysosomes to form phagolysosomes [24]. The pathogen inside the macrophage is killed by both oxidative and nonoxidative processes.

The oxidative process involves enzyme activation leading to oxygen uptake (respiratory burst) and reduction of oxygen to reactive oxygen intermediates, which have toxic effects upon microorganisms [24].

The oxygen-independent mechanism includes secretion of bactericidal enzyme lysozyme, production of acid, iron-binding protein, and synthesis of cationic polypeptides [24].

The lysosomes contain a variety of hydrolytic enzymes and antimicrobial peptides, for example, proteases, nucleases, phosphatase, esterase, and lipase.

Certain microorganisms can escape digestion by macrophages. Some can even grow and replicate inside them [24]. Mycobacteria escape digestion by preventing fusion of the lysosome with the phagosome. Some leave the phagosome to enter the cytoplasm. The phagocyte in such cases produces several toxic molecules to induce starvation of a pathogen by deprivational mechanisms [24].

Alveolar macrophages in the lower respiratory tract protect and prevent inflammation by secreting nitric oxide, prostaglandin, interleukin-4 and interleukin-10 (IL-4 and IL-10), and transforming growth factor-β [25–27].

1.6.2 Respiratory or Alveolar–Capillary Membrane

The exchange of gases between alveolar air and blood occurs by diffusion through the walls of the alveolus and capillary; both together form the alveolar–capillary membrane or respiratory membrane. It consists of (i) an alveolar epithelial layer of type I and II alveolar cells and free macrophages, (ii) a basement membrane supporting the alveolar epithelial layer, (iii) a capillary basement membrane often fused or closely applied to epithelial basement membrane, and (iv) an endothelial lining of the capillary. The total thickness of the membrane is only 0.5 μm.

1.6.2.1 Surfactant

The surfactant is a lipoprotein formed by type II alveolar cells. The lipid and protein components of lipoprotein or phospholipoprotein have both hydrophilic and hydrophobic regions; the former faces toward water and the latter faces toward air at air–water interface of alveoli. The surface tension arises at air–water interface because polar water molecules are more attracted toward each other than to gas molecules in air. This attractive force in lungs causes collapse of the alveoli. The surfactant reduces this collapsing force or surface tension.

The normal surface tension of water is 70 dyn/cm and in lungs, it is 25 dyn/cm. The surfactant phospholipid molecules decrease surface tension to a very low level, almost to zero toward the end of expiration. This decrease in pulmonary surface tension increases compliance, which is defined as the ability of lungs to expand. The lungs can inflate more easily and reduce the work of breathing or energy required to inflate the lungs and the possibility of alveolar collapse during expiration.

The functions of surfactant include compliance of lungs and prevent collapse of lungs (atelectasis). Surface tension forces draw fluid from capillaries into alveolar spaces. The surfactant reduces fluid accumulation and keeps the air passages dry by reducing surface tension [28].

The surfactant proteins, especially SP-A and SP-D bind to sugars over the surface of pathogens, opsonise them, and are then phagocytosed by macrophages; hence, they play an important role in immunity. If surfactant is destroyed or inactivated, there is greater possibility of reduction in immune response, lung inflammation, and infection [29].

During inspiration, the alveoli increase in size and the surfactant is more spread out over the surface. This spreading of surfactant increases surface tension and slows the rate of alveolar expansion, which helps other alveoli to expand. An alveolus expanding more quickly has to overcome rise in surface tension, which slows its rate of expansion. If reduction in size is quicker, the surface tension will reduce further making room for other alveoli to expand easily.

1.6.2.2 Surfactant Composition

The main components of surfactant include about 40% dipalmitoylphosphatidyl choline (DPCC), 40% other phospholipids, 5% surfactant-associated proteins (SP-A, B, C, and D), and the rest is formed by cholesterol and other substances.

DPCC is a phospholipid with two 16 carbon-saturated fatty acids, a phosphate group, and an amine group. It is the strongest surfactant in comparison to other phospholipids. The temperature at which pure DPPC changes from gel state to liquid is 41°C that is higher than the normal body temperature; hence, its absorption kinetics is low. Phosphatidyl choline forms about 85% of surfactant lipid and has saturated fatty acid chains. Phosphatidyl glycerol (PG) is about 11% of surfactant lipid and has unsaturated fatty acids to make it more fluid. Neutral lipids and cholesterol are also constituents of surfactant lipid but their surfactant properties are much lower than DPPC.

The raw materials for synthesis of lipid components of surfactant diffuse from blood into type II alveolar cells where assembly, packaging, and secretion takes place. Alveolar surfactant has a half-life of 8–10 h after which it may be either degraded by macrophages or reabsorbed into type II pneumocytes through clathrin-mediated endocytosis where about 90% of DPPC is recycled and only 10% is digested by macrophages.

Proteins constitute only about 10% of surfactant, half of which are plasma proteins and the rest is formed by apolipoproteins SP-A, B, C, and D. Apolipoproteins are formed in type II alveolar cells and form lamellar bodies in cytoplasm that have concentric rings of lipid and proteins. SP-A and SP-D have carbohydrate-binding sites that allow them to coat bacteria and viruses and promote phagocytosis. SP-A may be involved in controlling production of surfactant through a negative feedback mechanism.

SP-B and SP-C are hydrophobic membrane proteins and help in spreading of surfactant over the surface. SP proteins also reduce the phase-transition temperature of DPPC from 41°C to below

37°C [30] that improves its adsorption and interface-spreading speed [31]. The faster adsorption velocity is important in maintaining the integrity of gas-exchange membrane of lungs. SP proteins also fasten the DPPC to the interface to prevent them from being squeezed out when surface area decreases [32].

1.7 CONCLUSION

The primary aim of this chapter is to summarize the important features of the respiratory system by presenting the anatomy and physiology of the respiratory system to provide easy understanding of the various processes of viral infections of the respiratory system. Specialized cellular immune responses and lymphoid tissues are involved in the protection of distinct anatomical microenvironments of the respiratory tract, such as the large airways of the nose and the alveolar airspaces.

The viral pathogenesis represents a major challenge for the respiratory system. It is very important to understand the molecular interactions in between the viruses infecting the respiratory system and the host to understand the cellular machineries exploited by various viruses to enter into the cells and use the same for replication, as well as in the immune evasion process utilized by viruses to escape from the attack of immune responses.

Although there have been significant advances in different fields of medical virology, there are still many questions to answer. The host and viral immunological interactions need further attention to understand the molecular mechanisms of acute and chronic respiratory viral infections. A deeper knowledge and understanding of the cellular interactions with the viruses infecting the human upper and lower respiratory tracts will be helpful in the proper understanding of the respiratory viral pathogenesis and development of tools to combat such viral infections.

REFERENCES

1. Von Hayek H. *The Human Lung*. New York: Hafer; 1960.
2. Nagaishi C. *Functional Anatomy and Histology of the Lung*. Baltimore: University Park Press; 1972.
3. Tortora JG, and Grabowski SR. The respiratory system. *Principles Anat Physiol* 1993; Chapter 23, 7:720–735.
4. Sato K. Functional fine structures of the human vocal fold mucosa. In Rubin, J.S., Sataloff, R.T., and Korovin, G.S. (eds.), *Diagnosis and Treatment of Voice Disorders* (pp. 41–48). Clifton Park, NY: Delmar Learning; 2003.
5. Saunders WH. *The Larynx*. Summit, NJ: Ciba_Geigy Co; 1964.
6. Gail DB, and Lenfant CJM. State of the art—Cells of the lung: Biology and clinical implications. *Am Rev Respir Dis* 1983; 127:366.
7. Godfrey RWA, Severs NJ, and Jeffrey PK. Freeze–fracture morphology and quantification of human bronchial epithelial tight junctions. *Am J Respir Cell Mol Biol* 1992;6:453.
8. Herard AL, Zahm JM, Pierrot D et al. Epithelial barrier integrity during *in vitro* wound repair of the airway epithelium. *Am J Respir Cell Mol Biol* 1996;15:624.
9. Rhodin JAG. The ciliated cell: Ultrastructure and function of the human tracheal mucosa. *Am Rev Respir Dis* 1966;93:1.
10. Ebert RV, and Terracio MJ. The bronchiolar epithelium in cigarette smokers: Observations with the scanning electron microscope. *Am Rev Respir Dis* 1975;111:4.
11. Tamai S. Basal cells of the human bronchiole. *Acta Pathol Jpn* 1983;33:125.
12. Massaro GD, Singh G, Mason R et al. Biology of the Clara cell. *Am J Physiol* 1994;266:L101.
13. Phelps DS, and Floros J. Localization of pulmonary surfactant proteins using immunohistochemistry and tissue *in situ* hybridization. *Exp Lung Res* 1991;17:985.
14. Jorens PG, Sibille Y, Goulding NJ et al. Potential role of Clara cell protein, an endogenous phospholipase A2 inhibitor, in acute lung injury. *Eur Respir J* 1995;8:1647.
15. Evans MJ, Cabral-Anderson LJ, and Freeman G. Role of the Clara cell in renewal of the bronchiolar epithelium. *Lab Invest* 1978;38:648.
16. Becker KL. The coming of age of a bronchial epithelial cell. *Am Rev Respir Dis* 1993;148:1166.

17. Van Haarst JM, Verhoeven GT, de Wit HJ et al. CD1a_ and CD1a_ accessory cells from human bronchoalveolar lavage differ in allostimulatory potential and cytokine production. *Am J Respir Cell Mol Biol* 1996;15:752.
18. Lamb D and Lumsden A. Intraepithelial mast cells in human airway epithelium: Evidence for smoking-induced changes in their frequency. *Thorax* 1982;37:334.
19. Whimster WF, Lord P, and Biles B. Tracheobronchial gland profiles in four segmental airways. *Am Rev Respir Dis* 1984;129:985.
20. Roberts M, Reiss M, and Monger G. *Gaseous Exchange*. In: *Advanced Biology*. Surrey, Nelson. P167; 2007.
21. Ochs M, Nyengaard JR, Jung A, Knudsen L, Voigt M, Wahlers T, Richter J, and Gundersen HJG. The number of alveoli in the human lung. *Am J Respir Crit Care Med* 2004; 169(1): 120–124.
22. Lambrecht BN. Alveolar macrophage in the driver's seat. *Immunity* 2006; 24.4: 366–368.
23. Guyton AC. Physiology of the respiratory system. *Textbook Med Physiol* 2007; Chapter 33, 11:431–433.
24. Stafford JL, Neumann NF, and Belosevic M. Macrophage-mediated innate host defense against protozoan parasites. *Crit Rev Microbiol* 2002; 28.3: 187–248.
25. Holt PG et al. Downregulation of the antigen presenting cell function(s) of pulmonary dendritic cells *in vivo* by resident alveolar macrophages. *J Exp Med* 1993; 177.2: 397–407.
26. Bunn HJ, Hewitt CRA, and Grigg J. Suppression of autologous peripheral blood mononuclear cell proliferation by alveolar macrophages from young infants. *Clin Exp Immunol* 2002; 128.2: 313–317.
27. Lacraz S et al. Suppression of metalloproteinase biosynthesis in human alveolar macrophages by interleukin-4. *J Clin Invest* 1992; 90.2: 382–388.
28. West JB. *Respiratory Physiology—The Essentials*. Baltimore: Williams & Wilkins.
29. Wright JR. Host defense functions of pulmonary surfactant. *Biol Neonate* 2004; 85(4): 326–332. Epub 2004, June 8.
30. Hills BA. An alternative view of the role(s) of surfactant and the alveolar model. *J Appl Physiol* 1999; 87 (5): 1567–1583.
31. Samuel S, Bachofenb H, and Possmayer F. Pulmonary surfactant: Surface properties and function of alveolar and airway surfactant. *Pure Appl Chem* 1992; 64 (11): 1745–1750.
32. Possmayer F, Kaushik N, Rodrigueza K, Qanbarb R, and Schürch S. Surface activity *in situ*, *in vivo*, and in the captive bubble surfactometer. *Comp Biochem Physiol—Part A: Mol Integ Physiol* 2001; 129 (1): 209–220.

2 Lung Defenses
An Overview

Laurent P. Nicod

CONTENTS

2.1 INTRODUCTION

Inspired air is the source of oxygen for the body, but it also introduces numerous particles, toxic gases, and microorganisms in the airways. The upper and lower airways together represent the largest epithelial surface exposed to the outside environment; the alveolar surface being the size of a tennis court. In order to allow gas exchange, foreign substances and microorganisms must be stopped and removed without undue inflammation. The upper and lower airways protect the lung with anatomical barriers. They are associated with the cough reflex and use the mucociliary apparatus with enzymes and secretory immunoglobulin A (IgA), which is the main antibody isotype in mucosal secretions, contributing to the initial defense mechanism.[1] The basal layers of the respiratory mucosa in the nose and the conducting airways contain a tight network of dendritic cells (DCs) that sense and catch any invading organisms and bring them to the draining lymph nodes to generate the adaptive immunity. Particles of size 2 μm reaching the respiratory units beyond the respiratory bronchioles will be caught by alveolar macrophages (AMs) in a milieu that is rich in defense elements, such as IgG, complement, surfactant, and fibronectin. Depending on the load of pathogens and the innate immune processes locally involved, various amounts of inflammatory cells, in particular neutrophils, will be rapidly recruited. Once adaptive immunity is also involved, memory T-cells will be found in the interstitium around the bronchi and vessels, as well as in the alveoli (Table 2.1).

TABLE 2.1
Major Constituents of Lung Defenses

Airways and Their Mucosa
Luminal defense mechanisms
Anatomical barrier
Cough
Mucociliary clearance
Secretory IgA
Lysozymes, lactoferrins, SLPi
Defensins
Epithelial cells
Epithelial barrier
Mucin release
Antimicrobial peptides
Bacterial receptors
Chemotactic factors
Growth factors; cytokines
Blood-derived cells of the mucosa
Dendritic cells (conventional; plasmocytoids, …)
Lymphocytes (T-cells; γδ; NK cells)
B lymphocytes
Eosinophils; mast cells; basophils
Alveolar Spaces
Pneumocyte types I and II
Alveolar macrophages (M1 or M2 phenotypes)
Lymphocytes
Neutrophils
IgG and opsonins
Surfactant

Ig: immunoglobulin; NK: natural killer.

2.2 AIRWAYS AND THEIR MUCOSA

2.2.1 Luminal Defense Mechanisms

The nasopharyngeal anatomy and airway bifurcation represent important anatomical barriers to prevent the penetration of particles or organisms 2–3 μm into the lower airways. Cough generated by forced expiration allows enough turbulence and shearing forces in the major bronchi and trachea to extrude material such as debris or infected mucus.[2] The mucociliary transport allows impacted particles to be removed from the terminal bronchioles to the trachea by the ciliary beats of the epithelial cells in the mucus of bronchi. The airway mucus is composed of the sole phase, a periciliary liquid, 5–10 μm deep, allowing the cilia to beat and a gel phase on the surface of the cilia of 2–20 μm thickness. The flow of the gel is referred to as mucociliary transport. The physical properties of mucus are provided mainly by mucins, which are mucoglycoproteins and proteoglycans secreted from the surface of epithelial cells and from the glands. Phospholipids are also secreted by the epithelial cells and submucosal glands of the airways, weakening the adhesion of the mucus and altering its physical properties. The mucus gel acts as a barrier for bacteria and viruses.[3]

Secretory IgAs are released by the epithelial cells as dimeric molecules, associated with a single J chain of 23,000 daltons. IgAs are particularly important as they neutralize toxins and viruses and block the entry of bacteria across the epithelium by binding to lectin-like bacterial adhesion molecules operating as generic immune barrier. IgAs are poor activators of the classical pathway of complement but can activate the alternate pathway, allowing a better opsonization of bacteria by eosinophils, neutrophils, and monocytes/macrophages.[4]

In human airway, the main classes of antimicrobial peptides are the β-defensins and the cathelicidins. Lysozyme, lactoferrin, or peroxide is also carried within the mucus. These substances participate in the nonspecific first line of defense to invasion by microorganisms. The lysozyme degrades a glycosidic linkage of bacterial membrane peptidoglycans.[5] Epithelial cells, serous cells of submucosal glands, macrophages, and neutrophils can be a source of lysozyme. Lactoferrin is an iron-binding protein that reduces the availability of elemental iron, an obligatory cofactor for bacterial replication. Lactoferrin may also be bactericidal by binding to endotoxin.[6] The secretory protease inhibitor (SLPI), produced by the mucous glands, epithelial cells, and macrophages, has antifungal, antiviral, and antibacterial properties.[7] The peroxides from leukocytes (myeloperoxidases) act on thiocyanate ions or produce oxygen radicals that are bacteriostatic or bactericidal. Active plasma components can also extravasate from the blood vessels to the mucosa during airway inflammations. Igs and complement factors then take part in defense mechanisms, as well as in the inflammatory cascade.[8]

2.2.2 Epithelial Cells

Epithelials provide a mucosal barrier and contribute to the mucociliary clearance function already mentioned. Lining the luminal surface of the airways, they are attached to neighboring cells by several structures: tight junctions, intermediate junctions, gap junctions, and desmosomes.[9] These structures form a barrier between the luminal space and the pulmonary parenchyma. Desmosomes mediate mechanical adhesion of cells to their neighbors and tight junctions completely obliterate the intercellular spaces just below the luminal surface.[10] Transport through gap junctions may be a means for the cells to provide their neighbors with defense molecules, such as antioxidants.[11] This organization of epithelial cells creates an effective mechanical barrier and allows for polarity in function, thus, maintaining an ionic gradient for bidirectional secretion of many substances.

Epithelial cells play a key role in the induction of innate immunity by identifying molecules that are exclusive to microbes: pathogen-associated molecular patterns (PAMPs). Several families of pattern recognition receptors (PRRs) can achieve this recognition and they are expressed on epithelial cells, neutrophils, alveolar macrophages, and DCs. The PRRs include transmembrane Toll-like receptors (TLRs), cytosolic NOD-like receptors (NLRs), and RIG-I-like receptors (RLRs).[12] In addition to PAMPs, PRRs are activated by specific endogenous molecules, released after cell damage: damage-associated molecular patterns (DAMPs). The recognition of PAMPs and DAMPs by PRRs is key in initiating inflammatory response.[13]

Epithelial cells recruit inflammatory cells by releasing arachidonic acid derivates,[14] cytokines and chemokines, in response to a variety of stimuli, such as bacterial products, viral infections, or cigarette smoke.[15–17] Among the chemokines are interleukin (IL)-8, GRO-α; β, monocyte chemotactic protein-1, or lymphocyte chemoattractant factor (IL-16).[18] Epithelial cells upregulate adhesion molecules in response to inflammatory stimuli, allowing the adhesion of neutrophils and mononuclear cells to an inflamed area. Epithelial cells can also express major histocompatibility complex of class I and II, when exposed to cytokines such as interferons (IFNs). Epithelial cells then have a limited capacity for presenting antigens to lymphocytes and potentially to amplify an antigen-driven lymphocyte response.[19] Normal epithelial cells secrete antimicrobial peptides, such as β-defensins and lactoferrins, which directly contribute to host defense.[20]

2.3 BLOOD-DERIVED CELLS OF THE MUCOSA

2.3.1 Dendritic Cells

DCs lie above and below the basement membrane in a resting or immature state and extend their dendrites between the epithelial cells. They form a network optimally situated to sample inhaled antigens.[21,22] There are hundreds of DCs per square millimeter in the rat trachea and they become more numerous in response to inhaled antigens.[23] There is an extraordinary complex network of Langerhans cells, conventional DC, plasmocytoid DC, and monocyte-derived DC subsets contributing either to induction of immune responses or the maintenance of tolerance. The transcription programming of the DC network is much better known[24] and in the lung the influence of local environments might play a key role in their precise phenotypes and functions.[25]

Human lung DCs, like immature DCs derived from blood, are conventional DCs characterized by a high endocytic activity that can be measured with fluorescent isothiocyanate dextran fixation, but show only limited expression of CD40, CD80, and CD86.[26]

Inflammatory stimuli on DCs result in a loss of the antigen capturing machinery and an increase in T-cell stimulatory function, a process referred to as maturation. Once activated, lung DCs migrate to lymphoid structures in the hilar lymph nodes.[27] Using their various pathogen recognition receptors recognizing carbohydrate motifs presented on the surface of several microbial organisms, lung DCs continuously report antigenic information from the airways to pulmonary lymph nodes. DCs can even phagocytose apoptotic bodies derived from viral-infected epithelial cells. Activated by these bodies and their content, they will be able to induce specific cytotoxic T-cells.[28] After antigen uptake, airway DCs migrate to the paracortical T-cell zone of the draining lymph nodes of the lung, where they interact with naive T-cells.[29] Activated CD4 or CD8 memory T-cells will migrate toward other lymphoid structures and nonlymphoid structures of the body, such as the lung.[30] DCs translate their signals from the pulmonary environment into a specific immune response. DCs decrease in number after treatment with glucocorticoids.[31] This might help to decrease immune processes. Cigarette smoke also decreases pulmonary DCs and then impacts on the antiviral immune response.[32]

2.3.2 T-Cells, γδ T-Cells, Natural Killer Cells, and B Lymphocytes

In the absence of inflammation, the epithelium contains few CD4 and CD8 T cells. γδ T-cells and natural killer (NK) cells are part of the innate immunity, independent of DCs. They are likely to play a crucial role in lung immunity, in that they react to pathogens in the absence of preliminary priming. The γδ T-cell clones can also be segregated into T1 or T2, by their cytokine patterns, with a bias toward the production of T1 cytokines.[33] NK cells seem not only involved in viral immunity but also in host defense against *Pseudomonas aeruginosa* in acute infections. CD1d-restricted NK T-cells were shown to be required for good control of such infections and their activation associated with a rapid pulmonary clearance of these pathogens through enhanced phagocytosis by AMs.[34]

In humans, B lymphocytes are scattered in the airways. It is only after recurrent infections or injuries that lymphocytes are found in follicles around the airways. These formations are then called bronchus-associated lymphoid tissues.

2.3.3 Eosinophils, Mast Cells, and Basophils

Eosinophils, mast cells, and basophils are the effector cells of immediate hypersensitivity reactions and allergic diseases. Mature mast cells are found throughout the body, predominantly located near blood vessels, nerves, and beneath epithelia. Although normally not present in tissues, basophils are recruited to some inflammatory sites, usually with eosinophils.[35] Eosinophils are abundant in the infiltrates of late phase reactions and contribute to many of the pathological processes in allergic diseases. Cytokines, produced by Th2 cells, promote their recruitment and activation. Eosinophils release numerous mediators that are toxic to parasitic organisms and may injure normal tissues.

2.4 IMMUNE RESPONSE IN THE ALVEOLAR SPACES

2.4.1 Alveolar Epithelial Cells

The importance of type I epithelial cells and their precursors, the type II pneumocytes, will only be briefly mentioned in this chapter. However, they are crucial in the homeostasis of the alveoli, for instance, in the removal of water and electrolytes. Pneumocytes are also the major source of surfactant proteins (SP). SP A and SP D are members of the collecting family of mammalian lectins that contribute to pulmonary host defenses. SPs enhance the phagocytosis and killing of microbes.[36]

Alteration of epithelial cells in lung reperfusion injury and in acute respiratory distress syndrome is likely to play an important role in the incidence of pneumonia in these conditions.

2.4.2 Alveolar Macrophages

AMs, the resident mononuclear phagocytes of the lung, provide the first line of defense against organisms or particles reaching the lower airways. They must neutralize the invading pathogens or recruit neutrophils and other mononuclear cells. Once the infection or inflammatory process has been controlled, cell debris and exudates must be removed in order to recover the alveolar architecture. The ability of macrophages to interact with pathogens is mediated by surface receptors capable of binding to specific ligands, including toxins, polysaccharides, lipopolysaccharides, complement proteins, and Igs.

TLRs are a family of 11 molecules in human and 13 in mammals that initiate intracellular signaling cascades or specific microbial components.[37] Phagocytic cells, such as macrophages, neutrophils, and DCs, exhibit the broadest repertoire that results in the activation of several intracellular pathways.[38] The modulation/activation of these receptors may be linked to the capacity of mononuclear cells to release IL-12 instead of IL-10,[39] with a marked influence on lung immunity.

AM will initiate lung inflammation by the release of IL-1α and IL-1β or tumor necrosis factor (TNF)-α, leading to inflammatory cascades in the alveolar milieu, such as the appearance of adhesion molecules on endothelial cells or epithelial cells or the release of chemokines and growth factors. IL-1β released stimulates, for instance, Th17 to produce IL-17, which play an important role in defense mechanisms and in profibrotic processes.[40] These events are key in innate immunity, leading to the activation of neighboring cells, and to attract elements from the blood, such as neutrophils.

AM also controls inflammation by the release of inhibitors of IL-1 or TNF-α in the form of IL-1 receptor antagonists or TNF soluble receptors.[41] Macrophages have the capacity to markedly reduce IL-1 or TNF synthesis by their own release of IL-10.[42] The proinflammatory state is often referred to as M1 phenotype, while the M2 phenotype is rather an anti-inflammatory phenotype. M1 and M2 phenotype might not be stably differentiated subsets in the same way as Th1 and Th2 cells, for example. This dynamic transition requires still further investigations despite major steps made.[43]

AM have important bactericidal activities realized by the production of lysozymes or defensins, cationic proteins capable of killing a wide variety of bacteria, including mycobacteria or fungi.[44] Reactive oxygen intermediates (superoxide anion, hydrogen peroxide, hydroxyl radicals and/or reactive nitrogen) are also involved in killing microorganisms. Several components of complement are produced by macrophages, as well as the C1q inhibitor.[45] Complement promotes the clearance of an immune complex, an important means of eliminating antibody-coated bacteria.

AMs can, under circumstances that are currently poorly understood, acquire some characteristics of DCs and may thus be able to activate T-cells.[46] This is in contrast to the fact that they prevent

T-cell activation in normal subjects.[47,48] Thus, macrophages under the influence of innate and adaptive immune mechanisms may change their antigen capacity and/or cytokine production. AMs can indeed produce IL-12 when stimulated by bacterial lipopolysaccharides and IFN-γ, or during the interaction of CD40–CD40 L on T-cells and macrophages.[49]

2.4.3 Lymphocytes

Alveoli contain 10% lymphocytes, of which 50% are CD4, 30% are CD8, 10–15% are killer or NK cells, and 5% B lymphocytes. The CD4/CD8 ratio is 1.5, similar to that of peripheral blood. In the alveolar milieu, lymphocytes have a slightly altered phenotype and function related to those of the interstitium. For instance, NK cells in the alveoli have a reduced cytotoxicity compared with interstitial NK cells.[50] B lymphocytes, CD4, and CD8 T-cells are major components of the adaptive immune response and most T-cells have a memory phenotype. Once they are primed, T lymphocytes may be reactivated by DCs around the airways and vessels.[51] The real importance of epithelial cells, endothelial cells, or fibroblasts for this purpose mostly relay on *in vitro* studies in which endothelial cells appear potentially as the most efficient antigen-presenting cell.[52] CD4 and CD8 cells are not only key elements for the defense against viruses but also appear to play a role in bacterial clearance.[53]

2.4.4 Neutrophils

The recruitment of neutrophils is a major component of the protective host response to bacterial infections and appears to outweigh the contribution of other immune cells, at least in the acute setting.[54] Neutrophils aggregate rapidly at the site of infection with three key actions: phagocytosis, release of the contents of preformed granules, and production of reactive oxygen species (ROS). In the bronchoalveolar (BAL), they normally represent 2% of the cells. However, if AMs in the alveoli are unable to control infectious agents, a massive flux of neutrophils occurs. Thus, depending on the dose of *Staphylococcus aureus* instilled in the airways, they will be neutralized by macrophages only or with the influx of neutrophils, and with higher doses of the pathogens, the mice will die.[55] Chemotactic factors include C5 fragments generated by the activation of the alternative pathways of complement by bacteria. AMs generate products of arachidonic acid, such as leukotriene B_4. Chemokines are also small polypeptides, critically involved in neutrophil recruitment. The C-X-C chemokines include IL8, GRO-α, and GRO-β, found in the BAL of patients with various types of pneumonia.[56]

AMs, endothelial cells, and epithelial cells have the ability to generate chemokines in response to microbial products or cytokines such as TNF-α or IL-1, as part of the innate immune response.

Activated neutrophils eliminate microorganisms by means of a range of mechanisms, which involve phagocytosis, release of oxygen radicals, and production of cytotoxic peptides or proteins. Carbohydrate residues of bacteria are attacked by their enzymes, such as sialidase, x-mannosidase, β-glucuronidase, *N*-acetyl-β-glucosoaminidase, and lysozyme. Cytotoxic protein, such as neutrophil defensins and serine proteinases, damages bacterial membranes.[57] Defects in neutrophil function lead to severe disorders. In Chediak–Higaschi disease, a congenital immunological defect known to be accompanied by severe pyogenic infections, the granules cannot package the protein elastase or the cathepsin-G superfamily.[58]

The respiratory burst results in the release of ROS to facilitate bacterial killing, induced by optimizing conditions via ion flux and pH changes, the enzymes released from granules become more active, facilitating the destruction of pathogens.[59] In chronic granulomatous diseases, affected individuals are susceptible to bacterial infections because their phagocytic cells are unable to generate the products of respiratory burst.[60] This is caused by a defective gene for one of the subunits of nicotinamide adenine dinucleotide phosphate (NADPH) oxidase, resulting in life-threatening bacterial infections and granuloma formation.[61]

Neutrophil migration itself is impaired in leukocyte adhesion deficiencies (LAD); thus, in LAD II, a defect in the expression of sialyl Lewis-x, the counter-receptor for E-selectin and P-selectin has been demonstrated.[62]

2.4.5 Immunoglobulins and Opsonins

Normal bronchoalveolar lavage contains several substances capable of coating bacteria that will enhance phagocytic uptake by AMs, acting as opsonins. Surfactant, fibronectin, and C-reactive protein may all have opsonic activities. IgG, which constitutes 5% of the total protein content of BAL,[63] is the predominant Ig in the alveoli. IgG_1 and IgG_2 are present in greatest concentration (65% and 28%, respectively), whereas IgG_1 and IgG_3 are considered to be the most important, as only these two antibodies fix the complement. IgG_2 is a type-specific antibody against pathogens such as *Streptococcus pneumoniae* or *Haemophilus influenzae*.[64] IgG_4 acts as a reaginic antibody in allergic diseases and increased IgG_4 may lead to hypersensitivity pneumonitis. In the absence of IgG_4, there is however a predisposition to sinopulmonary infections and bronchiectasis.[65]

Many complement components can be produced *in vitro* by monocytes or macrophages. However, most are produced by the liver and carried to the lungs via the blood. Activation of the entire complement pathway in the presence of microbes can result in their lysis and killing. When bacteria activate the alternate pathway, C3b is released, allowing a good opsonization of bacteria for neutrophils or macrophages. Complement and, in particular, the alternative complement pathways are likely to play an important role as the first line of defense against many extracellular microbes as part of the innate immune defenses.[66]

2.5 CHANGES INDUCED IN LUNG DEFENSES

The early childhood environment is linked with changes in immune processes and the role of infection in the evolution of immune defenses and allergies in children is becoming unraveled. It is becoming increasingly clear that allergies are linked with epithelial changes leading to an increased risk of invasive infections.[67] Various particles and active and passive smoking induce many changes in airway mucosa, leading to chronic bronchitis and acute exacerbations.

Viruses have several strategies to evade lung defenses and eventually remain as persistent infections, especially in immunosuppressed patients.[68] Innate and adaptive mechanisms, triggered by viruses and other irritants, may amplify several diseases, including asthma.

Immunosuppressants are commonly used either in allergic phenomena, in autoimmune processes, in relation to chemotherapy, or after various transplantations. Moderate doses of steroids (>30 mg day^{-1}) are sufficient to lead to opportunistic infections after a few weeks in adults.[69] Infections related to a wide array of other immunosuppressions have been the subject of an evidence-based review.[70] Common mechanisms involved in the digestive tract and respiratory tract are currently described. It is becoming clear that the immune processes of these two types of mucosa may even influence each other, either via innate immunity or adaptive immunity. It is, therefore, timely to gather this evidence and hope that modulation of immune processes, either through the respiratory or the digestive tract, may become more understood to decrease infections and perhaps reduce allergies.[71] A recent review[72] discusses the current evidence on how bacterial extracts taken orally can decrease the rate and severity of infections in both children and adults with chronic obstructive pulmonary disease.

2.6 CONCLUSION

Lung defenses are dependent on a complex array of mechanisms in the upper airways, which must to be differentiated from those of the distal airways. However, the first lines of defense in the proximal and distal airways are predominantly based on mechanical barriers and several mechanisms related

45. Hamacher J, Sadallah S, Schifferli JA, Villard J, Nicod LP. Soluble complement receptor type 1 (CD35) in bronchoalveolar lavage of inflammatory lung diseases. *Eur Respir J.* 1998 Jan;11(1):112–9.
46. Nicod LP, Isler P. Alveolar macrophages in sarcoidosis coexpress high levels of CD86 (B7.2), CD40, and CD30 L. *Am J Respir Cell Mol Biol.* 1997 Jul;17(1):91–6.
47. Toews GB, Vial WC, Dunn MM, Guzzetta P, Nunez G, Stastny P et al. The accessory cell function of human alveolar macrophages in specific T cell proliferation. *J Immunol.* 1984 Jan;132(1):181–6.
48. Metzger Z, Hoffeld JT, Oppenheim JJ. Macrophage-mediated suppression. I. Evidence for participation of both hydrogen peroxide and prostaglandins in suppression of murine lymphocyte proliferation. *J Immunol.* 1980 Feb;124(2):983–8.
49. Isler P, de Rochemonteix BG, Songeon F, Boehringer N, Nicod LP. Interleukin-12 production by human alveolar macrophages is controlled by the autocrine production of interleukin-10. *Am J Respir Cell Mol Biol.* 1999 Feb;20(2):270–8.
50. Weissler JC, Nicod LP, Lipscomb MF, Toews GB. Natural killer cell function in human lung is compartmentalized. *Am Rev Respir Dis.* 1987 Apr;135(4):941–9.
51. Lambrecht BN. Dendritic cells and the regulation of the allergic immune response. *Allergy.* 2005 Mar;60(3):271–82.
52. Geppert TD, Lipsky PE. Dissection of defective antigen presentation by interferon-gamma-treated fibroblasts. *J Immunol.* 1987 Jan 15;138(2):385–92.
53. Moser C, Jensen PO, Kobayashi O, Hougen HP, Song Z, Rygaard J et al. Improved outcome of chronic *Pseudomonas aeruginosa* lung infection is associated with induction of a Th1-dominated cytokine response. *Clin Exp Immunol.* 2002 Feb;127(2):206–13.
54. Mizgerd JP. Molecular mechanisms of neutrophil recruitment elicited by bacteria in the lungs. *Semin Immunol.* 2002 Apr;14(2):123–32.
55. Onofrio JM, Toews GB, Lipscomb MF, Pierce AK. Granulocyte-alveolar-macrophage interaction in the pulmonary clearance of *Staphylococcus aureus*. *Am Rev Respir Dis.* 1983 Mar;127(3):335–41.
56. Villard J, Dayer-Pastore F, Hamacher J, Aubert JD, Schlegel-Haueter S, Nicod LP. GRO alpha and interleukin-8 in *Pneumocystis carinii* or bacterial pneumonia and adult respiratory distress syndrome. *Am J Respir Crit Care Med.* 1995 Nov;152(5 Pt 1):1549–54.
57. Whitters D, Stockley R. Immunity and bacterial colonisation in bronchiectasis. *Thorax.* 2012 Nov;67(11):1006–13.
58. Barbosa MD, Barrat FJ, Tchernev VT, Nguyen QA, Mishra VS, Colman SD et al. Identification of mutations in two major mRNA isoforms of the Chediak-Higashi syndrome gene in human and mouse. *Hum Mol Genet.* 1997 Jul;6(7):1091–8.
59. Reeves EP, Lu H, Jacobs HL, Messina CG, Bolsover S, Gabella G et al. Killing activity of neutrophils is mediated through activation of proteases by K+ flux. *Nature.* 2002 Mar 21;416(6878):291–7.
60. Curnutte JT, Whitten DM, Babior BM. Defective superoxide production by granulocytes from patients with chronic granulomatous disease. *N Engl J Med.* 1974 Mar 14;290(11):593–7.
61. Rosenzweig SD. Inflammatory manifestations in chronic granulomatous disease (CGD). *J Clin Immunol.* 2008 May;28 Suppl 1:S67–72.
62. von Andrian UH, Berger EM, Ramezani L, Chambers JD, Ochs HD, Harlan JM et al. *In vivo* behavior of neutrophils from two patients with distinct inherited leukocyte adhesion deficiency syndromes. *J Clin Invest.* 1993 Jun;91(6):2893–7.
63. Reynolds HY, Newball HH. Analysis of proteins and respiratory cells obtained from human lungs by bronchial lavage. *J Lab Clin Med.* 1974 Oct;84(4):559–73.
64. Siber GR, Schur PH, Aisenberg AC, Weitzman SA, Schiffman G. Correlation between serum IgG-2 concentrations and the antibody response to bacterial polysaccharide antigens. *N Engl J Med.* 1980 Jul 24;303(4):178–82.
65. Gross GN, Rehm SR, Pierce AK. The effect of complement depletion on lung clearance of bacteria. *J Clin Invest.* 1978 Aug;62(2):373–8.
66. Robertson J, Caldwell JR, Castle JR, Waldman RH. Evidence for the presence of components of the alternative (properdin) pathway of complement activation in respiratory secretions. *J Immunol.* 1976 Sep;117(3):900–3.
67. Talbot TR, Hartert TV, Mitchel E, Halasa NB, Arbogast PG, Poehling KA et al. Asthma as a risk factor for invasive pneumococcal disease. *N Engl J Med.* 2005 May 19;352(20):2082–90.
68. Hilleman MR. Strategies and mechanisms for host and pathogen survival in acute and persistent viral infections. *Proc Natl Acad Sci U S A.* 2004 Oct 5;101 Suppl 2:14560–6.
69. Lionakis MS, Kontoyiannis DP. Glucocorticoids and invasive fungal infections. *Lancet.* 2003 Nov 29;362(9398):1828–38.

70. Gea-Banacloche JC, Opal SM, Jorgensen J, Carcillo JA, Sepkowitz KA, Cordonnier C. Sepsis associated with immunosuppressive medications: An evidence-based review. *Crit Care Med.* 2004 Nov;32(11 Suppl):S578–90.
71. Marsland BJ. Regulation of inflammatory responses by the commensal microbiota. *Thorax.* 2012 Jan;67(1):93–4.
72. UB S. Prevention of paediatric respiratory tract infections: Emphasis on the role of OM-85. *Eur Respir Rev.* 2005;14(95):74–5.

3 Airway Epithelial and Early Innate Immune Responses to Virus Infections

Alan Chen-Yu Hsu, Su-Ling Loo, Faezeh Fathi Aghdam, Kristy Parsons, Philip M. Hansbro, and Peter A. B. Wark

CONTENTS

3.1 INTRODUCTION

Respiratory viruses are important human pathogens due to their propensity to cause disease and their fast transmission rate among humans via aerosols. They are the most common cause of infection and frequently lead to a large burden of illness and increased mortality, as well as high socioeconomic cost. Rapid mutation and transmission rates of viruses such as influenza can cause annual epidemics. This then leads to increased visits to health care workers, elevated use of prescription medicines, increased absenteeism from school or work, and in the very young, old, immune-compromised, and those with underlying morbidities can result in severe and life-threatening infection.

Many respiratory viruses have been identified that infect humans. Some cause mild diseases while others such as influenza and severe acute respiratory syndrome (SARS) coronavirus can result in marked morbidity and mortality. Some of the clinically important respiratory viruses are listed in Table 3.1.

Respiratory viral infection often leads to symptoms ranging from mild symptoms such as sore throat to severe symptoms, including life-threatening pneumonia. The outcome of these infections is the result of complex interaction between the invading viruses and the host immune system.

The human immune system is a complex defensive response that protects the host from infection. Immune responses to viruses involve both innate and adaptive arms of human immunity (Figure 3.1). Innate responses provide the first line of defense and contain the infection at the site of encounter. They also provide important signals to the adaptive immunity that then initiates final clearance and immunological memory to subsequent infection.

TABLE 3.1
Respiratory Viruses Known to Cause Diseases in Humans

Family	Virus Name
Adenoviridae	Human adenovirus
Bunyaviridae	Hentavirus
Coronaviridae	Human coronavirus (SARS-CoV, HCoV-229E, HCoVOC43, HKU1-CoV, NL63, novel coronavirus)
Herpesviridae	Cytomegalovirus or human herpes virus type 5
	Epstein–Barr virus or human herpes virus type 4
	Varicella-zoster virus or herpes virus type 3
Orthomyxoviridae	Influenza virus A and B
Paramyxoviridae	Human metapneumovirus 1–4
	Human parainfluenza virus 1–4
	Human respiratory syncytial virus (RSV) A and B
Picornaviridae	Human rhinovirus A, B, or C
	Human enterovirus A–D

Since the discovery of pattern-recognition receptors (PRRs), the innate immune system has attracted much attention. This is due to the function of PRRs in specifically recognizing common pathogen products called pathogen-associated molecular patterns (PAMPs), including bacterial (e.g., lipopolysaccharide and peptidoglycan) and viral (RNAs, DNAs) components. The ability of cellular PRRs to recognize viral RNAs in the infected cells enables the host to initiate appropriate innate and subsequently adaptive immune responses to limit the infection. This is particularly important in the airways as unsuccessful containments of infection increase the severity of the disease with enhanced mortality. Advances in immunology have enabled the functional characterization of innate immune signaling proteins involved in innate immunity to viral infection.

Despite the well-developed and structured innate immune response, viruses have adapted mechanisms to evade the host's immunity. Reverse genetic engineering has been used as a valuable tool in identifying novel viral virulence factors and their interaction with the host innate immune signaling proteins. Nevertheless, irrespective of recent discoveries in viral immunology, there are still many immune proteins, signaling, and regulatory mechanisms that have yet to be identified. In this review, we will explore the current understanding of innate immunity to respiratory viral infections in the airways and the mechanisms that viruses utilize to evade host immunity. Furthermore, people with chronic airways diseases such as asthma and chronic obstructive pulmonary disease (COPD) have dysregulated immune responses that are damaging to the airways, but appear to be associated with enhanced susceptible to respiratory viral infections.[1] Upon a viral infection, they suffer acute exacerbation of their preexisting conditions accompanied by severe symptoms with increased mortality. The mechanisms underpinning increased susceptibility to infection and more severe disease are still largely unclear. Therefore, we will also discuss the abnormal innate immunity in those with chronic airways diseases and the host factors that may contribute to the high susceptibility to viral infection.

3.2 BRONCHIAL EPITHELIAL CELLS AND THE INNATE IMMUNE RESPONSE

3.2.1 Airway Epithelium as a Barrier to Infection

The airway epithelium is constantly exposed to noxious agents, potential pathogens, and particles that may damage it and impair its function. An intact epithelial barrier comprises ciliated epithelial cells, mucus-secreting cells, and a functional mucociliary escalator, and is the host's first line of defense to these challenges. The importance of an intact epithelial layer to virus infection was elegantly demonstrated with an *in vitro* model of cultured primary airway epithelial cells (AECs).[2]

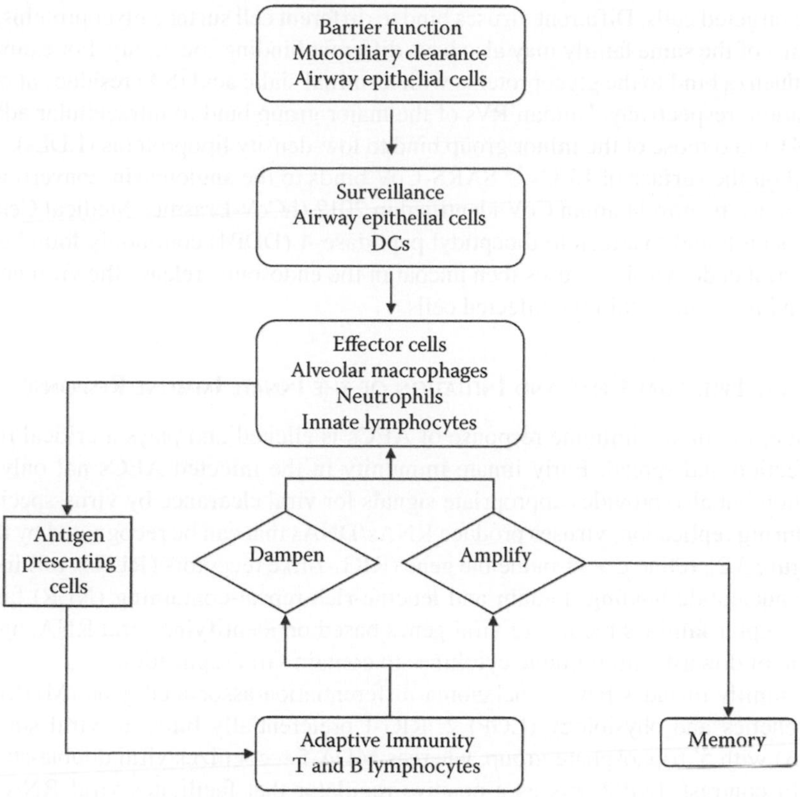

FIGURE 3.1 The immune system. The immune system is broadly divided into functional components known as the innate and adaptive immune responses. The innate immune response is an ancient system that has evolved with the development of multicellular organisms and is remarkably similar in both animals and plants, suggesting that it had evolved prior to the split of these organisms into their separate kingdoms. In contrast, the adaptive immune response is seen only in vertebrates and has evolved only in addition to the innate immune response and is therefore dependent upon it. In the lungs, this encompasses the role of the mucociliary escalator and cough reflex as a barrier, preventing the access of microorganisms, allergens, and noxious agents to the host. The next component involves surveillance against the presence of highly conserved nonanimal molecules. It is at this point that the innate and adaptive response systems begin to interact. The adaptive immune response has developed the ability to react to specific recognition proteins, but in order to do this they must be recruited by an effector cell that has been activated through the innate immune response. These antigen-presenting cells (APCs) travel to regional lymph nodes, internalize and express foreign antigens and then in the presence of costimulatory molecules lead to the clonal expansion and differentiation of T and B lymphocytes. This adaptive immune response is a powerful system that leads to a highly specific reaction, but is reliant upon activation of innate effector cells and is inherently delayed by the need for clonal expansion and differentiation of lymphocytes to occur.

These authors grew primary AECs at the air–liquid interface until they were confluent and differentiated into pseudostratified columnar epithelium that rested upon a layer of basal AEC. They then either left the cultures intact or damaged them, by trauma, proteolysis, or through the removal of the ciliated layer by culturing the cells in the absence of calcium and magnesium. When infected with rhinovirus (RV), the intact differentiated cells were the most resistant, while the damage models that exposed the basal epithelial cells to RV (particularly the scratch model) showed a 50-fold increase in infectivity. These results reinforce the importance of an intact barrier function in reducing viral respiratory infection. Similar results occurred with bacterial infection.

Once the virus has evaded the normal barrier function of the AECs, these cells become the primary site of infection. Viruses initiate infection by first binding to host surface glycoproteins and enter into the targeted cells. Different viruses bind to different cell surface glycoproteins, and different viral strains of the same family may also have different binding specificity. For example, human and avian influenza bind to the glycoproteins with terminal sialic acid (SA) residues at α2,6Gal and α2,3Gal position, respectively. Human RVs of the major group bind to intracellular adhesion molecule (ICAM)-1 and those of the minor group bind to low-density lipoproteins (LDLs), all of which are expressed on the surface of BECs.[3,4] SARS-CoV binds to the angiotensin-converting enzyme 2 (ACE2),[5] whereas the novel human CoV identified in 2012 (hCoV-Erasmus Medical Centre (EMC)) has recently been found to attach to dipeptidyl peptidase-4 (DDP4) commonly found on epithelial cells.[6] After viral endocytosis, viruses then uncoat in the endosome, release the viral genes into the cytoplasm, and replicate within the infected cells.

3.2.2 Airway Epithelial Cells and Initiation of the Innate Immune Response

Upon infection, the innate immune response of AECs is elicited and plays a critical role in limiting viral infection and spread. Early innate immunity in the infected AECs not only suppresses viral replication but also provides appropriate signals for viral clearance by virus-specific adaptive immunity. During replication, viruses produce RNAs/DNAs that can be recognized by three classes of PRRs (Figure 3.2), retinoic acid-inducible gene (RIG)-I-like receptors (RLRs), toll-like receptors (TLRs), and nucleotide-binding domain and leucine-rich-repeat-containing (NLR) family receptors. These receptor families recognize viral genes based on identifying viral RNA, and signal for the expression of downstream immune cytokines to contain viral replication.

The RLR family includes RIG-I, melanoma-differentiation-associated gene (MDA)-5, and laboratory of genetics and physiology (LGP) 2. RIG-I preferentially binds to viral single-stranded RNA (ssRNA) with 5′ triphosphate group, whereas MDA-5 recognizes viral double-stranded RNA (dsRNA).[7,8] In contrast, LGP2 acts as a positive regulator that facilitates viral RNA binding by RIG-I and MDA-5.[8] Once bound to viral genomes, these RLRs are then ubiquitinated by the adaptor

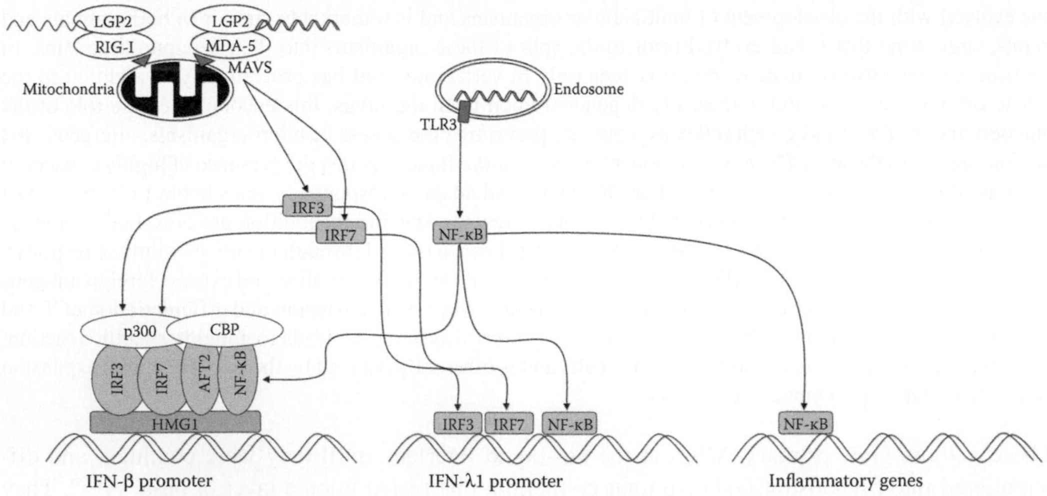

FIGURE 3.2 RLR and TLR viral recognition system and innate immune signaling pathway. During respiratory viral infection, viral RNAs are recognized by the host PRRs, including RIG-I, MDA-5, and TLR3. Upon engagement, RIG-I/MDA-5 with the help of LGP2 binds to MAVS on the mitochondrial membrane, which then facilitates the phosphorylation of IRF3/7. Activated IRF3/7 translocates to the nucleus where it binds with other transcription factor ATF3 and NF-κB, and structural protein HMG1, forming a transcription complex called IFN-β enhanceosome. This complex then drives the transcription of IFN-β gene expression. In contrast, IFN-λ1 gene induction only requires IRF3/7 and NF-κB. TLR3 binding to viral RNAs also activates NF-κB, which is required for the induction of inflammatory genes such as IL-6.

protein tripartite motif protein (TRIM) 25. This results in a conformational change that allows the RLRs to bind to the adaptor protein mitochondrial antiviral signaling (MAVS) on the mitochondrial membrane. Tumor necrosis factor (TNF)-receptor-associated factor (TRAF) 3 then associates with the RIG-I/MDA-5–MAVS complex and activates TRAF family member-associated nuclear factor (NF)-κB activator (TANK)-binding kinase (TBK) 1.[9] These proteins then phosphorylate interferon regulatory factor (IRF) 3 and 7, which then translocate to the nucleus where they act as transcription factors driving the induction of type I (IFN-α/-β) and type III IFNs (IFN-λ1/2/3).[10–12] These IFNs play an important role in subsequent innate and adaptive antiviral responses to infection. Once released, IFNs bind to the same or neighboring cells via type I (IFNAR1/2) and type III IFN (IL-28Rα/IL-10Rβ) receptors, respectively, and induce the expression of over 300 IFN-stimulated genes (ISGs) via activation of signal transducer and activator of transcription (STAT)-1 and STAT-2.[12–16] ISGs, including protein kinase RNA-activated (PKR), 2′,5′-oligoadenylate synthetase (OAS), and MxA protein, suppress viral replication by degrading viral RNAs and initiate apoptosis, a critical antiviral response that causes infected cells to self-destruct, limiting viral replication.[17–22] RIG-I, MDA-5, and IRF7 are also induced following infection, in a positive feedback response to infection to respiratory viral infection.[17,19,23,24]

Ten TLRs have been identified in humans. TLR3 is the predominant viral responsive one and detects viral dsRNAs within the endosomes in BECs. Once engaged, TLR3 activates its direct downstream adaptor protein TIR-domain containing adaptor-inducible IFN-β (TRIF), which then activates NF-κB that translocates to the nucleus where it drives the induction of inflammatory mediators such as CXCL-8 and TNF-α.[25] These mediators then recruit and activate innate immune cells, including neutrophils, resulting in an acute airway inflammation.

NLRs (Figure 3.3) are the third set of PRRs that recognize viral RNAs during infection. NLR protein (NLRP) 3 recognizes viral dsRNA/ssRNAs and then binds to apoptotic speck protein containing caspase activation and recruitment domain (AC), forming a complex known as the NLRP3 inflammasome. This complex then cleaves pro-caspase 1 into a functional caspase 1, which in turn cleaves pro-interleukin (IL)-1 into its active form, IL-1β. The released IL-1β protein then binds to toll/IL-1 receptors on the same or neighboring cells, and induces the expression of inflammatory

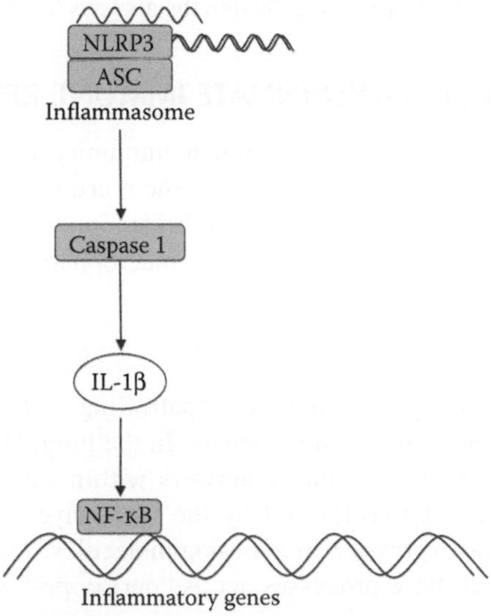

FIGURE 3.3 NLRP3 inflammasome signaling pathway. NLRP3 recognizes viral RNAs during infection and binds to ASC, forming an inflammatory complex called inflammasome. This complex then cleaves and activates caspase 1 protein, which in turn activates IL-1β. The released IL-1β then binds to its receptor IL-1R to activate NF-κB and induces the inflammatory genes expression.

cytokines via NF-κB activation.[26] Another function of IL-1β is to recruit neutrophils and further increase inflammation in the airways.[27–29] Viral infections, including influenza and RV, can also upregulate the protein induction of NLRP3, forming a positive feedback loop that reinforces inflammatory responses.[27,30]

Despite the differential recognition of viral RNAs by the PRRs and their distinct signaling pathways that induce antiviral and inflammatory responses, there also appears to be cross-regulation between the transcription factors in these pathways. Human RV is an ssRNA virus that generates dsRNA during replication that could be recognized by MDA-5, TLR3, and NLRP3.[7,8,30] In contrast, influenza, RSV, and metapneumovirus are ssRNA viruses that have been shown to only generate 5′ppp ssRNA and, therefore, are preferentially recognized by RIG-I.[31–34] However, they have also been shown to activate TLR3, which only binds to dsRNAs, and facilitates NF-κB-mediated inflammatory response in BECs. This is particularly evident in human infection by the highly pathogenic avian influenza H5N1, which induces a lethal inflammatory cytokine storm with 60–70% mortality.[35,36] While it is unknown as to how TLR3 recognizes influenza 5′ppp ssRNA, other PRRs such as NLRP3 have been shown to bind to RNAs from influenza and RV, and induce inflammatory responses via IL-1β. The specific binding mechanism and preference of NLRP3 has not been characterized at the molecular level.

TLR3-mediated NF-κB activation and signaling has also been demonstrated to participate in type I and III IFN induction and signaling. After viral infection transcription factors NF-κB, IRF3, and activating transcription factor (ATF) 3 bind to a structural protein named high mobility group (HMG)-I protein, they form a transcription factor-enhancer complex named the IFN-β enhanceosome. This complex then binds to the transcription coactivator cAMP response element-binding (CREB) binding protein (CBP)/p300, forming another complex called transcription preinitiation complex (PIC). PIC then facilitates the binding of RNA polymerase II to the transcription start site of IFN-β gene, thereby driving the induction of IFN-β.[37,38] NF-κB has also been shown to drive the induction of type III IFN after infection. A cluster of NF-κB binding sites has been found on human IFN-λ1 promoter, and NF-κB and IRF3 have been shown to be critical in the induction of IFN-λ1 during viral infection.[39]

The dynamic recognition of viral RNAs and the induction and regulation of antiviral and inflammatory responses to infection are mounted to contain replicating viruses at the site of infection. These responses concomitantly recruit other immune cells into the airways to enhance the clearance of viruses.

3.3 AIRWAY IMMUNE CELLS AND INNATE IMMUNE RESPONSES

AECs are not alone in their propensity to provide innate immunity to viral pathogens. They are also able to affect other innate immune responses through the recruitment, activation, and maturation of other immune cells, including those that are able to bridge innate and adaptive immune systems. Important airway immune cells include dendritic cells, macrophages, and natural killer cells.

3.3.1 Dendritic Cells

DCs belong to the innate immune system, and these "patrolling sentinels" are unique in their ability to detect viral pathogens and damage in the tissue. In the lung, DCs are the principal resident antigen-presenting cells, forming a surveillance network within and around the airways. DCs are found in the lateral intercellular space formed by the basal layer of epithelial cells, anchoring directly with AECs through the expression of adhesion molecules. Their dentrites form extensions in-between epithelial cells, and these processes act as "periscopes" and are used to sample antigen in the airway lumen providing continuous immune surveillance. DCs are characterized into various subsets, which are thought to perform distinct functions in immunological responses.[40,41] There are two main subsets of DCs, plasmacytoid (pDCs) and myeloid DCs (mDCs) (Figure 3.4).[42]

pDCs play an important role in clearing viral infections and have been extensively studied due to their role as professional type I IFN-producing cells.[43,44] Upon viral infection, pDCs utilize

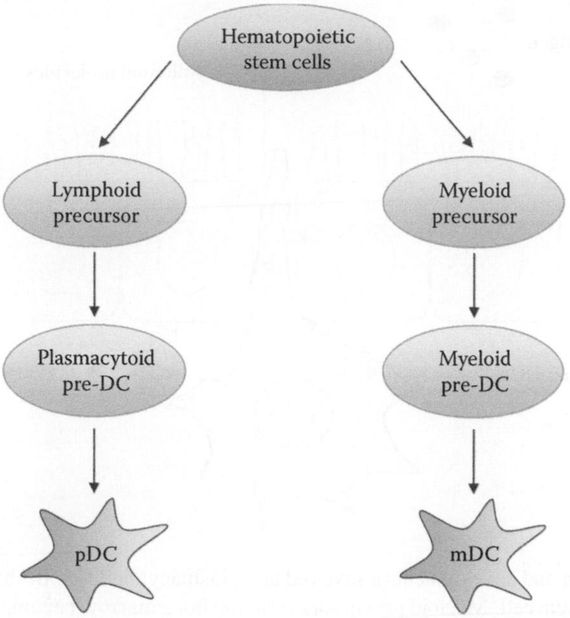

FIGURE 3.4 Airway antigen sampling. Antigens in the airway are sampled by the DC extensions in-between airway epithelial cells. DCs form tight junctions with airway epithelial cells through adhesion interaction. DCs extend long processes between epithelial cells, and these are able to sample antigen directly.

TLR7/8/9 in the endosome, instead of RLRs, to recognize viral RNAs and initiate the same innate immune signaling pathways as found in AECs, leading to the production of antiviral and inflammatory cytokines.[45,46] Many viruses, including influenza, RV, and RSV, have been found to replicate unproductively in pDCs[47–50]; this could be the result of potent type I IFN responses produced by these cells, and may explain the dispensability of RLRs in the clearance of infection. Furthermore, type I IFNs can also promote DC maturation and enhance their ability to educate naïve T cells to become virus-specific cytotoxic T-cells that efficiently clear viruses.[51,52]

mDCs are the predominant population of DCs, and occur directly underneath the mucosal epithelium lining the airways; thus, they are strategically positioned for primary encounters with inhaled particles or pathogens (Figure 3.5). They are named antigen-presenting cells due to their ability to capture and present antigens, including those from viruses, to naïve T cells in lymphoid tissues, which then differentiate into virus-specific cytotoxic T-cells and specifically kill virus-infected cells.[56,57]

DCs can also be activated by a unique subset of T lymphocytes named invariant natural killer T (iNKT) cells. They have been identified to be involved in innate, instead of adaptive, immunity. Influenza-induced IL-1β from AECs and DCs has been shown to activate iNKT cells via NF-κB to produce immune-modulatory cytokines such as the type II IFN, IFN-γ, which further stimulates the induction of inflammatory cytokines from BECs and DCs.[53–55]

3.3.2 Macrophages

Macrophages are the scavenger cells of the innate immune system that detect and phagocytose foreign pathogens and apoptotic cells in the airways. They originate from bone marrow as promonocytes, which then mature into monocytes and differentiate into macrophages as they migrate to the respiratory tract via blood or lymphatic vessels. Macrophages can be recruited into the airways by chemokines such as chemokine (C–C motif) ligand (CCL) 3 (also known as macrophage

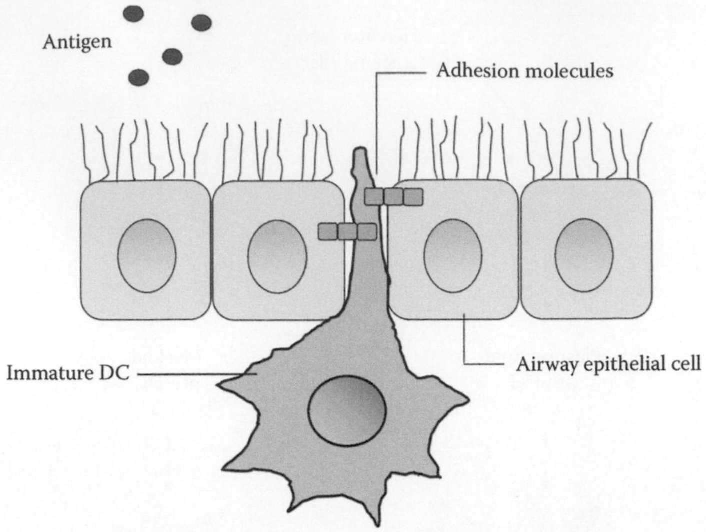

FIGURE 3.5 The origin and development of myeloid and plasmacytoid DCs. Both subsets of DCs originate from the hematopoietic stem cell. Myeloid precursors from the bone marrow become myeloid DCs. Lymphoid precursors develop into plasmacytoid predendritic cells, and form plasmacytoid DCs.

inflammatory protein (MIP)-1α) and CCL5 (also known as regulated and normal T-cell expressed and secreted (RANTES)). These chemokines are produced by virus-infected AECs in an NF-κB-dependent manner. Macrophages recognize features of apoptotic cells, including externalized phospholipids, that is, phosphatidylserine, and initiate phagocytosis.[58–61] These phagocytes also produce surfactant protein (SP)-A that binds to viral surface proteins such as influenza HA protein, and RSV F (fusion) and G (attachment) proteins, which then promotes phagocytosis of invading viruses.[62–64] Once phagocytosed, the virus is then trapped within aphagosome, which then fuses with lysozome, forming a complex called the phagolysosome.[65,66] Hydrolytic enzymes such as nitric oxide (NO) synthase occur in lysozomes and produce NO that directly degrades trapped viruses. Macrophages can also be infected with viruses and elicit similar inflammatory responses via TLR3 and NF-κB, and antiviral responses via RIG-I/MDA-5 induction.[67–70]

3.3.3 Neutrophils

Neutrophils are also the phagocytic cells that ingest invading viruses via similar mechanisms to those that occur in macrophages.[71] Upon infection, neutrophils infiltrate into the airways via neutrophil surface receptors CXC chemokine receptor (CXCR) 1 and 2, and migrate down a chemotactic gradient of CXCL-8 produced by infected cells.[72] Once the infected cells are phagocytosed and incorporated into phagolysosomes, neutrophil elastases, matrix metalloproteases (MMPs), and myeloperoxidase (MPO) are produced to convert reactive oxygen species (ROS) such as hydrogen peroxide into hypochlorous acid that digest viral proteins.[65,66,73,74] This process is called the neutrophil oxidative burst and is now considered as a defensive response against respiratory viruses. Neutrophils can also be infected with viruses and produce inflammatory cytokines such as CXL-8 and TNF-α that then further enhance inflammatory responses in the lung.[75–77] Neutrophils produce SP-D protein that directly binds to influenza HA and adenovirus surface capsid protein, after which human neutrophil peptides (HNP) 1 and 2 then bind to the viral surface protein-SP-D complex that enhances phagocytosis.[78–82]

The multiple levels of innate immune responses induced by airway immune cells provide a critical early defensive system that contains the infection in the local environment and concomitantly signals for efficient viral clearance by adaptive immunity.

3.4 VIRAL INFECTION AND EVASION OF INNATE IMMUNE RESPONSES

In response to the effectiveness of innate immunity in clearing infection, viruses have developed immune evasion mechanisms that enable their persistence. The immune evasion strategies of influenza viruses are one of the most well-characterized among respiratory viruses.

Influenza has a particularly frequent mutation rate that allows it to undergo genetic changes, frequently in the genes encoding for HA and another surface protein neuraminidase (NA). Slight changes in influenza HA and NA can lead to immune evasion from host antibody responses that are generated by vaccination or previous infection. This phenomenon is called antigenic drift, and is the reason for the need for an annual vaccination with new formulations against currently circulating influenza strains.[83] Of even greater concern is that two or more strains of influenza have the potential to recombine in a single host. This has the potential to lead to major genetic changes in the influenza genome, and if the virus is viable, it is a novel influenza strain to which the population has little or no immunity. The resulting strain has unpredictable pathogenicity with the potential to induce a pandemic. This event is called antigenic shift,[84] and has occurred three times in the last 10 years (H5N1 bird flu, H3N2 swine flu, and the most recent H7N9). Antiviral drugs to influenza, including M2 ion channel blocker (adamantine and rimantadine) and NA inhibitor (oseltamivir and zanamavir), are also available as prophylaxis or for treatment.[85–87] However, the rapid mutation rate of influenza and heavy use of these drugs has resulted in the emergence of drug-resistant strains.[88–93] This poses a serious threat as drug resistance could become embedded within the genomes of future epidemic and/or pandemic viruses during mutation and recombination. Vaccination manufacture is also a long process taking several months, further highlighting the urgent need for new drugs in preparation for future pandemics.

Influenza viruses have also developed mechanisms to inhibit host innate antiviral responses, which promote productive infection. The influenza genome encodes a protein called nonstructural (NS) 1 that inhibits RIG-I-induced activation of IRF3, thereby suppressing type I and III IFN responses.[94] NS1 also binds to cellular antiviral ISGs such as PKR to prevent viral RNA degradation and apoptosis.[95–99] As numerous strains of influenza viruses occur, their host's antiviral inhibitory ability also varies. Seasonal human influenza H3N2 has been shown to carry a potent NS1 protein that more effectively inhibits antiviral responses and leads to a more productive viral replication compared to that of low pathogenic avian influenza.[100] In contrast, the NS1 protein of the highly pathogenic avian H5N1 is able to completely suppress antiviral responses in BECs and DCs.[101–106] In addition to the suppression of antiviral responses, the NS1 protein also reduces host protein synthesis by binding to cleavage and polyadenylation specificity factor subunit 30 (CPSF30) and poly A binding protein (PAB) II, thereby controlling the host machinery for viral replication and infection.

Other respiratory viruses also have similar immune evasion strategies. RSV has an NS1/2 protein that binds and degrades STAT2 protein, inhibiting ISGs and antiviral responses in BECs.[107–109] Adenoviruses possess an early region (E) 4 open reading frame (ORF) 3 and 6 that inhibits IFN responses and enables efficient viral replication.[110,111] SARS-CoV has also been shown to produce a highly basic nucleocapsid (N) protein that suppresses type I IFN responses via an unidentified mechanism.[112]

Inhibition of antiviral signaling therefore is an important immune evasion mechanism employed by many viruses to promote their survival, further demonstrating the importance of innate antiviral immunity in respiratory viral infection.

3.5 SUSCEPTIBILITY TO VIRUS INFECTION IN CHRONIC RESPIRATORY DISEASE

The consequence of respiratory viral infections is clearly dependent upon complex interactions between the host and pathogen. The importance of any shift in these interactions is illustrated by the enhanced susceptibility of those with chronic respiratory disease to infection. Viral respiratory tract infections are the most frequent triggers of acute exacerbations of both asthma and COPD; with RV being the most common pathogen.[113,114] In comparison to healthy individuals, asthmatics are more likely to have lower respiratory tract symptoms, which are more severe and last longer.[115] We have previously demonstrated that asthmatic primary bronchial epithelial cells (pBEC) have impaired type I (IFN-β)[116] and type III (IFN λ1/3) IFN responses to RV infection.[117] Although the reasons for these impaired responses have not yet been defined, they are crucial to our understanding of virus-induced acute asthma. Factors contributing to more severe RV infections include host factors, environmental influences, and immunological parameters.[118] These include allergic sensitization, allergen exposure, and virus occurrence, which all increase the odds of being admitted to the hospital with acute asthma.[119] While inhaled steroids reduce the frequency of exacerbations,[120,121] they are also associated with decreases in eosinophilic inflammation.[120] Asthmatics with eosinophilic airway inflammation are considered as being exacerbation-prone[122] and treatments directed at normalizing sputum eosinophil counts reduce asthma exacerbations.[123] It is also noteworthy that some severe exacerbations are associated with an accumulation of neutrophils in the airways.[124] Therefore, there is clearly a complex interplay between the chronic inflammatory process of asthma and susceptibility to virus infection. However, not all studies have demonstrated impaired antiviral immunity in asthma,[125,126] and differences in severity of asthma or inflammatory subtypes may contribute to these conflicting observations.[127] Furthermore, airway cells other than AECs are also involved in the antiviral response, which is highlighted by the observation that only a small fraction of AECs become infected with RV.[128] Interestingly, some asthmatics display reduced IFN-λ,[129] IFN-α (type I IFN),[130] and IFN-γ (type II IFN)[131] levels when their peripheral blood mononuclear cells (PBMCs) were exposed to RV. Neutralization of type I IFN secretion in PBMCs exposed to RV resulted in IL-13 synthesis. This is a Th2 cytokine associated with allergic asthma. Furthermore, depletion of pDCs in these cultures abolished IFN-α release and boosted the production of other Th2 cytokines; IL-5, IL-9, and again IL-13.[132] In contrast, the addition of IFN-β inhibited Th2 cytokine production in the presence of a range of allergen and antigen stimulants *in vitro*.[133] Finally, impaired RV-induced IFN-γ responses, measured as a surrogate for deficient T helper cell (Th) 1 responses, were also associated with increased asthma severity.[134] The effect of modulating antiviral responses in asthmatics for the prevention or treatment of asthma exacerbations has yet to be determined but a proof-of-concept Phase II study using nebulized IFN-β has completed recruitment and results are expected to be released soon.

Despite important differences in the pathogenesis between asthma and COPD, both are disorders characterized by chronic airway inflammation and intriguingly both demonstrate an enhanced susceptibility to the effects of virus infection. In COPD, virus infection is associated with more frequent and severe exacerbations[114] and viral infection may even influence airway inflammation acutely in COPD.[135] Enhanced susceptibility to RV infection in COPD was best demonstrated when Mallia et al.,[136] used an experimental RV model to show that subjects with COPD would exacerbate following RV infection. This was associated with features of worsened airway inflammation and reduced lung function, and they also demonstrated impaired IFN-α/λ responses to RV in bronchial lavage specimens. Even less is known about why this susceptibility may occur in COPD compared to asthma but such studies illustrate that there is an important link between conditions characterized by chronic airway inflammation and impaired antiviral responses.

3.6 CONCLUSIONS

Viral respiratory tract infections remain an important medical and social problem, ranging from trivial infections to life-threatening episodes. As knowledge in regard to the innate immune response in the airways has increased, it is becoming increasingly recognized that this early response is crucial in determining the outcome of virus infection. From the host's perspective, this innate immune response needs to rapidly identify viral pathogens as nonself, and then limit the virus's ability to infect and replicate. As the epithelium is the initial site of this interaction, most studies have focused on these initial steps. Viruses have evolved to adhere and gain access to the epithelium, while early responses that prevent virus replication and the infection of neighboring epithelial cells, centered around the type I IFN responses remain the first line of the host's defense. Such responses are fast and limit infection and damage to the host by minimizing inflammation. To counteract this robust system, successful, respiratory viruses have developed the means to subvert to some extent this innate response, allowing them to become successful pathogens. New insights gained into other cellular components of the innate immune response are now starting to illustrate how the initial triggering events of infection lead to the development of a more specific adaptive immune response. A greater understanding of these processes will ultimately enable us to consider novel strategies to combat the effects of these infections, especially in those most vulnerable to them.

REFERENCES

1. Hansbro NG, Horvat JC, Wark PA, Hansbro PM. Understanding the mechanisms of viral induced asthma: New therapeutic directions. *Pharmacol Ther* 2008; 117(3): 313–53.
2. Jakiela B, Brockman-Schneider R, Amineva S, Lee WM, Gern JE. Basal cells of differentiated bronchial epithelium are more susceptible to rhinovirus infection. *Am J Respir Cell Mol Biol* 2008; 38(5): 517–23.
3. Suzuki T, Yamaya M, Kamanaka M et al. Type 2 rhinovirus infection of cultured human tracheal epithelial cells: Role of LDL receptor. *Am J Physiol Lung Cell Mol Physiol* 2001; 280(3): L409–20.
4. Papi A, Johnston SL. Rhinovirus infection induces expression of its own receptor intercellular adhesion molecule 1 (ICAM-1) via increased NF-kappaB-mediated transcription. *J Biol Chem* 1999; 274(14): 9707–20.
5. Li W, Moore MJ, Vasilieva N et al. Angiotensin-converting enzyme 2 is a functional receptor for the SARS coronavirus. *Nature* 2003; 426(6965): 450–4.
6. Raj VS, Mou H, Smits SL et al. Dipeptidyl peptidase 4 is a functional receptor for the emerging human coronavirus-EMC. *Nature* 2013; 495(7440): 251–4.
7. Kato H, Takeuchi O, Sato S et al. Differential roles of MDA5 and RIG-I helicases in the recognition of RNA viruses. *Nature* 2006; 441(7089): 101–5.
8. Satoh T, Kato H, Kumagai Y et al. LGP2 is a positive regulator of RIG-I- and MDA5-mediated antiviral responses. *Proc Natl Acad Sci U S A* 2010; 107(4): 1512–7.
9. Oganesyan G, Saha SK, Guo B et al. Critical role of TRAF3 in the Toll-like receptor-dependent and -independent antiviral response. *Nature* 2006; 439(7073): 208–11.
10. Fitzgerald KA, McWhirter SM, Faia KL et al. IKKepsilon and TBK1 are essential components of the IRF3 signaling pathway. *Nat Immunol* 2003; 4(5): 491–6.
11. Doyle SE, Schreckhise H, Khuu-Duong K et al. Interleukin-29 uses a type 1 interferon-like program to promote antiviral responses in human hepatocytes. *Hepatology* 2006; 44(4): 896–906.
12. Kotenko SV, Gallagher G, Baurin VV et al. IFN-lambdas mediate antiviral protection through a distinct class II cytokine receptor complex. *Nat Immunol* 2003; 4(1): 69–77.
13. Levy DE, Garcia-Sastre A. The virus battles: IFN induction of the antiviral state and mechanisms of viral evasion. *Cytokine Growth Factor Rev* 2001; 12(2–3): 143–56.
14. Stark GR, Kerr IM, Williams BR, Silverman RH, Schreiber RD. How cells respond to interferons. *Annu Rev Biochem* 1998; 67: 227–64.
15. Pestka S, Langer JA, Zoon KC, Samuel CE. Interferons and their actions. *Annu Rev Biochem* 1987; 56: 727–77.
16. Sheppard P, Kindsvogel W, Xu W et al. IL-28, IL-29 and their class II cytokine receptor IL-28R. *Nat Immunol* 2003; 4(1): 63–8.
17. Kujime K, Hashimoto S, Gon Y, Shimizu K, Horie T. p38 mitogen-activated protein kinase and c-jun-NH2-terminal kinase regulate RANTES production by influenza virus-infected human bronchial epithelial cells. *J Immunol* 2000; 164(6): 3222–8.
18. Kumar A, Haque J, Lacoste J, Hiscott J, Williams BR. Double-stranded RNA-dependent protein kinase activates transcription factor NF-kappa B by phosphorylating I kappa B. *Proc Natl Acad Sci U S A* 1994; 91(14): 6288–92.
19. Garcia MA, Gil J, Ventoso I et al. Impact of protein kinase PKR in cell biology: From antiviral to antiproliferative action. *Microbiol Mol Biol Rev* 2006; 70(4): 1032–60.
20. Gil J, Esteban M. Induction of apoptosis by the dsRNA-dependent protein kinase (PKR): Mechanism of action. *Apoptosis* 2000; 5(2): 107–14.
21. Zhang P, Samuel CE. Protein kinase PKR plays a stimulus- and virus-dependent role in apoptotic death and virus multiplication in human cells. *J Virol* 2007; 81(15): 8192–200.

22. Chen Z, Li Y, Krug RM. Influenza A virus NS1 protein targets poly(A)-binding protein II of the cellular 3'-end processing machinery. *EMBO J* 1999; 18(8): 2273–83.
23. Pavlovic J, Haller O, Staeheli P. Human and mouse Mx proteins inhibit different steps of the influenza virus multiplication cycle. *J Virol* 1992; 66(4): 2564–9.
24. Slater L, Bartlett NW, Haas JJ et al. Co-ordinated role of TLR3, RIG-I and MDA5 in the innate response to rhinovirus in bronchial epithelium. *PLoS Pathog* 2010; 6(11): e1001178.
25. Chaouat A, Savale L, Chouaid C et al. Role for interleukin-6 in COPD-related pulmonary hypertension. *Chest* 2009; 136(3): 678–87.
26. Takeda K, Kaisho T, Akira S. Toll-like receptors. *Annu Rev Immunol* 2003; 21: 335–76.
27. Allen IC, Scull MA, Moore CB et al. The NLRP3 inflammasome mediates *in vivo* innate immunity to influenza A virus through recognition of viral RNA. *Immunity* 2009; 30(4): 556–65.
28. Akira S, Uematsu S, Takeuchi O. Pathogen recognition and innate immunity. *Cell* 2006; 124(4): 783–801.
29. Ting JP, Lovering RC, Alnemri ES et al. The NLR gene family: A standard nomenclature. *Immunity* 2008; 28(3): 285–7.
30. Schneider D, Ganesan S, Comstock AT et al. Increased cytokine response of rhinovirus-infected airway epithelial cells in chronic obstructive pulmonary disease. *Am J Respir Crit Care Med* 2010; 182(3): 332–40.
31. Pichlmair A, Schulz O, Tan CP et al. RIG-I-mediated antiviral responses to single-stranded RNA bearing 5'-phosphates. *Science (New York, NY)* 2006; 314(5801): 997–1001.
32. Loo YM, Fornek J, Crochet N et al. Distinct RIG-I and MDA5 signaling by RNA viruses in innate immunity. *J Virol* 2008; 82(1): 335–45.
33. Le Goffic R, Pothlichet J, Vitour D et al. Cutting edge: Influenza A virus activates TLR3-dependent inflammatory and RIG-I-dependent antiviral responses in human lung epithelial cells. *J Immunol* 2007; 178(6): 3368–72.
34. Saito T, Gale M, Jr. Differential recognition of double-stranded RNA by RIG-I-like receptors in antiviral immunity. *J Exp Med* 2008; 205(7): 1523–7.
35. Chotpitayasunondh T, Ungchusak K, Hanshaoworakul W et al. Human disease from influenza A (H5N1), Thailand, 2004. *Emerg Infect Dis* 2005; 11(2): 201–9.
36. Tran TH, Nguyen TL, Nguyen TD et al. Avian influenza A (H5N1) in 10 patients in Vietnam. *New England J Med* 2004; 350(12): 1179–88.
37. Yie J, Senger K, Thanos D. Mechanism by which the IFN-beta enhanceosome activates transcription. *Proc Natl Acad Sci U S A* 1999; 96(23): 13108–13.
38. Kim TK, Maniatis T. The mechanism of transcriptional synergy of an *in vitro* assembled interferon-beta enhanceosome. *Mol Cell* 1997; 1(1): 119–29.
39. Thomson SJ, Goh FG, Banks H et al. The role of transposable elements in the regulation of IFN-lambda1 gene expression. *Proc Natl Acad Sci U S A* 2009; 106(28): 11564–9.
40. Nelson EL, Strobl S, Subleski J, Prieto D, Kopp WC, Nelson PJ. Cycling of human dendritic cell effector phenotypes in response to TNF-{alpha}: Modification of the current 'maturation' paradigm and implications for *in vivo* immunoregulation. *FASEB J* 1999; 13(14): 2021–30.
41. Hart DNJ. Dendritic cells: Unique leukocyte populations which control the primary immune response. *Blood* 1997; 90(9): 3245–87.
42. Vermaelen K, Pauwels R. Pulmonary dendritic cells. *Am J Respir Crit Care Med* 2005; 172(5): 530–51.
43. Birmachu W, Gleason, RM, Bulbulian, BJ, Riter, CL, Vasilakos, JP, Lipson, KE and Nikolsky, Y. Transcriptional networks in plasmacytoid dendritic cells stimulated with synthetic TLR7 agonists. *BMC Immunol* 2007; 12(8): 26.
44. Haeryfar SMM. The importance of being a pDC in antiviral immunity: The IFN mission versus Ag presentation? *Trends Immunol* 2005; 26(6): 311–7.
45. Takeda K, Akira S. Toll-like receptors in innate immunity. *Int Immunol* 2005; 17(1): 1–14.
46. Honda K, Taniguchi T. IRFs: Master regulators of signalling by Toll-like receptors and cytosolic pattern-recognition receptors. *Nat Rev Immunol* 2006; 6(9): 644–58.
47. Fonteneau JF, Gilliet M, Larsson M et al. Activation of influenza virus-specific CD4+ and CD8+ T cells: A new role for plasmacytoid dendritic cells in adaptive immunity. *Blood* 2003; 101(9): 3520–6.
48. Smed-Sorensen A, Chalouni C, Chatterjee B et al. Influenza A virus infection of human primary dendritic cells impairs their ability to cross-present antigen to CD8 T cells. *PLoS Pathogens* 2012; 8(3): e1002572.
49. Boogaard I, van Oosten M, van Rijt LS et al. Respiratory syncytial virus differentially activates murine myeloid and plasmacytoid dendritic cells. *Immunology* 2007; 122(1): 65–72.

50. Schrauf C, Kirchberger S, Majdic O et al. The ssRNA genome of human rhinovirus induces a type I IFN response but fails to induce maturation in human monocyte-derived dendritic cells. *J Immunol* 2009; 183(7): 4440–8.
51. Luft T, Pang KC, Thomas E et al. Type I IFNs enhance the terminal differentiation of dendritic cells. *J Immunol* 1998; 161(4): 1947–53.
52. Spadaro F, Lapenta C, Donati S et al. IFN-alpha enhances cross-presentation in human dendritic cells by modulating antigen survival, endocytic routing, and processing. *Blood* 2012; 119(6): 1407–17.
53. Ho LP, Denney L, Luhn K, Teoh D, Clelland C, McMichael AJ. Activation of invariant NKT cells enhances the innate immune response and improves the disease course in influenza A virus infection. *Eur J Immunol* 2008; 38(7): 1913–22.
54. Paget C, Ivanov S, Fontaine J et al. Interleukin-22 is produced by invariant natural killer T lymphocytes during influenza A virus infection: Potential role in protection against lung epithelial damage. *J Biol Chem* 2012.
55. Boehm U, Klamp T, Groot M, Howard JC. Cellular responses to interferon-gamma. *Annu Rev Immunol* 1997; 15: 749–95.
56. Heil F, Hemmi H, Hochrein H et al. Species-specific recognition of single-stranded RNA via Toll-like receptor 7 and 8. *Science* 2004; 303(5663): 1526–9.
57. Coccia EM. IFN regulation and functions in myeloid dendritic cells. *Cytokine Growth Factor Rev* 2008; 19(1): 21–32.
58. Piccolo MT, Wang Y, Sannomiya P et al. Chemotactic mediator requirements in lung injury following skin burns in rats. *Exp Mol Pathol* 1999; 66(3): 220–6.
59. Shukaliak JA, Dorovini-Zis K. Expression of the beta-chemokines RANTES and MIP-1 beta by human brain microvessel endothelial cells in primary culture. *J Neuropathol Exp Neurol* 2000; 59(5): 339–52.
60. Shiratsuchi A, Kaido M, Takizawa T, Nakanishi Y. Phosphatidylserine-mediated phagocytosis of influenza A virus-infected cells by mouse peritoneal macrophages. *J Virol* 2000; 74(19): 9240–4.
61. Hashimoto Y, Moki T, Takizawa T, Shiratsuchi A, Nakanishi Y. Evidence for phagocytosis of influenza virus-infected, apoptotic cells by neutrophils and macrophages in mice. *J Immunol* 2007; 178(4): 2448–57.
62. Malhotra R, Haurum JS, Thiel S, Sim RB. Binding of human collectins (SP-A and MBP) to influenza virus. *Biochem J* 1994; 304 (Pt 2): 455–61.
63. Barr FE, Pedigo H, Johnson TR, Shepherd VL. Surfactant protein-A enhances uptake of respiratory syncytial virus by monocytes and U937 macrophages. *Am J Respir Cell Mol Biol* 2000; 23(5): 586–92.
64. Ghildyal R, Hartley C, Varrasso A et al. Surfactant protein A binds to the fusion glycoprotein of respiratory syncytial virus and neutralizes virion infectivity. *J Infect Dis* 1999; 180(6): 2009–13.
65. Tate MD, Ioannidis LJ, Croker B, Brown LE, Brooks AG, Reading PC. The role of neutrophils during mild and severe influenza virus infections of mice. *PLoS ONE* 2011; 6(3): e17618.
66. Tate MD, Brooks AG, Reading PC. The role of neutrophils in the upper and lower respiratory tract during influenza virus infection of mice. *Respir Res* 2008; 9: 57.
67. Cheung CY, Poon LL, Lau AS et al. Induction of proinflammatory cytokines in human macrophages by influenza A (H5N1) viruses: A mechanism for the unusual severity of human disease? *Lancet* 2002; 360(9348): 1831–7.
68. Laza-Stanca V, Stanciu LA, Message SD, Edwards MR, Gern JE, Johnston SL. Rhinovirus replication in human macrophages induces NF-kappaB-dependent tumor necrosis factor alpha production. *J Virol* 2006; 80(16): 8248–58.
69. Senft AP, Taylor RH, Lei W et al. Respiratory syncytial virus impairs macrophage IFN-alpha/beta- and IFN-gamma-stimulated transcription by distinct mechanisms. *Am J Respir Cell Mol Biol* 2010; 42(4): 404–14.
70. Wang J, Nikrad MP, Travanty EA et al. Innate immune response of human alveolar macrophages during influenza A infection. *PLoS ONE* 2012; 7(3): e29879.
71. Cowburn AS, Condliffe AM, Farahi N, Summers C, Chilvers ER. Advances in neutrophil biology: Clinical implications. *Chest* 2008; 134(3): 606–12.
72. Woolhouse IS, Bayley DL, Stockley RA. Sputum chemotactic activity in chronic obstructive pulmonary disease: effect of alpha(1)-antitrypsin deficiency and the role of leukotriene B(4) and interleukin 8. *Thorax* 2002; 57(8): 709–14.
73. Yamamoto K, Miyoshi-Koshio T, Utsuki Y, Mizuno S, Suzuki K. Virucidal activity and viral protein modification by myeloperoxidase: A candidate for defense factor of human polymorphonuclear leukocytes against influenza virus infection. *J Infect Dis* 1991; 164(1): 8–14.
74. Lambeth JD. NOX enzymes and the biology of reactive oxygen. *Nat Rev Immunol* 2004; 4(3): 181–9.

cells to the infected tissue and provide the adequate substrate for an immune response. In some cases vascular injury may occur altering the basic function of the lung and leading to respiratory failure. This is mainly due to fluid accumulation in the air spaces and parenchyma of the lung, a state described as pulmonary edema. This complication is caused by increased vascular permeability and constitutes the main characteristic of acute respiratory distress syndrome (ARDS). In this chapter we will present the basic functions of the pulmonary endothelial cell (EC) and how this is affected by viral infections.

4.2 DEVELOPMENT AND HETEROGENEITY

The mesoderm consists the developmental origin of ECs. A pluripotent stem cell will eventually form an EC via differentiation of hemangioblasts and/or angioblasts, responding to endoderm signaling. After proliferation, the ECs migrate through the extracellular matrix (ECM) forming cell-to-cell junctions.[1] This procedure will develop the intimal lining of all blood vessels, occupying in the human lung a surface of approximately 130 square meters.[2] This continuous monolayer formed by squamous ECs was considered for many years to be nothing more than a semi-permeable homogenous cellular layer that separated blood from the surrounding tissues and in the case of the lung, blood from air. However, years of research initiated in the 1970s established that ECs are highly specialized, metabolically active cells that exhibit heterogeneity in structure and function depending on organ and vascular bed location.[2] For example, lung blood vessels present remarkable distinctions among the arterial–capillary–venous axis. The arterial ECs reside on a thick basement membrane that separates the intima from underlying smooth muscle layers, while capillary ECs are based on a thin basement membrane. Additionally, arterial ECs present an alignment following the blood flow, a phenotype not seen in the capillary ECs.[3]

4.3 BASIC FUNCTIONS

Despite anatomic distinctions, there are major physiological properties shared among all ECs (Table 4.1). These include among others: (i) the promotion of antiaggregation and hemofluidity, (ii) an enforced barrier function, (iii) synthesis, metabolism, or uptake of vasoactive compounds that modulate the systemic, as well as the pulmonary vascular tone, and (iv) participation in immune reactions. The major properties of pulmonary endothelium in health are shown in Figure 4.1.

TABLE 4.1
Major Pulmonary Endothelial Functions

- Semi-permeable cellular barrier function
- Metabolic activity. Expression of enzymes such as angiotensin-converting enzyme, endothelin converting enzyme, and nitric oxide (NO) synthase
- Regulation of pulmonary and systemic vascular resistance
- Control of smooth muscle cell via production of prostanoids and endothelins. Regulation of vascular tone
- Innate and adaptive immunity. Interactions with leukocytes and binding of immune complexes
- Preservation of hemofluidity via regulation of coagulation and thrombolysis
- Leukocyte trafficking and regulation of hemostasis
- Production of membrane receptors and junction molecules
- Production of growth factors
- Production of cytokines and chemokines
- Regulation of redox activity

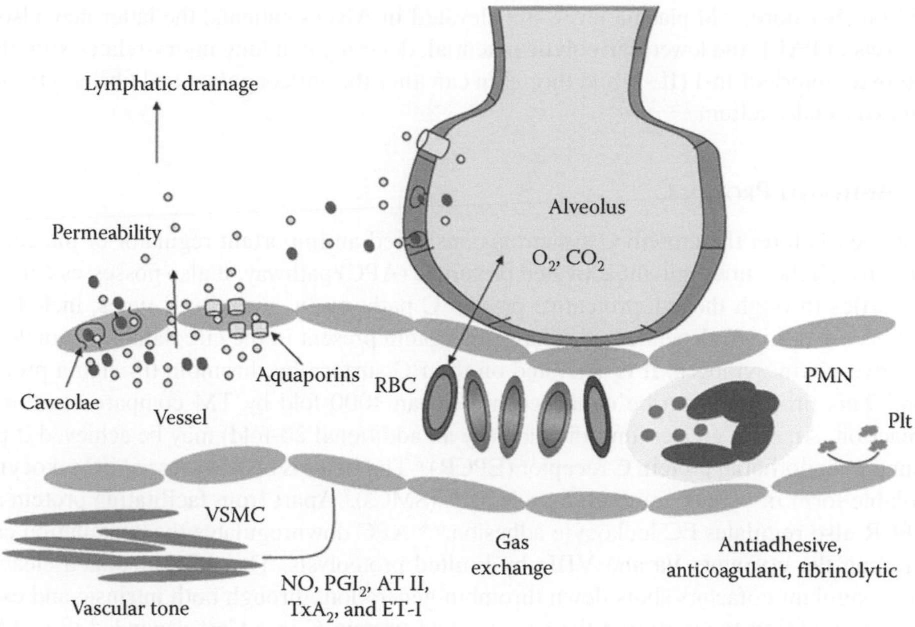

FIGURE 4.1 **(See color insert.)** Schematic illustration of the basic endothelial functions in health. The structure of pulmonary microvessels and ECs is adapted in such a way as to enable efficient gas exchange of the entire cardiac output at baseline and under exertion. Synthesis and release of several vasoactive compounds such as angiotensin II (AT II), prostacyclin (PGI_2), thromboxane A_2 (TxA_2), nitric oxide (NO), and endothelin-1 (ET-1) regulate, permeability and vascular tone so perfusion is matched to ventilation. Additionally, ECs maintain hemofluidity and regulate coagulation via expression of several agents. Furthermore, lung ECs express enzymes (such as angiotensin converting enzyme, endothelin converting enzyme, nucleotidases, NO synthase and lipoprotein lipase), receptors, and signal transduction molecules, and synthesizing anticoagulant and hemostatic factors. Other important functions of lung EC include, participation in immune reactions, binding of immune complexes, internalization blood components such as leukocytes and platelets. RBC: red blood cells, PMN: polymorphonuclear granulocytes; VSMC: vascular smooth muscle cells, Plt: platelets, dark blue circles: albumin; light blue circles: water. (Reproduced from Maniatis NA et al. *Vasc Pharmacol* 2008; **49**(4–6): 119–33. With permission.)

4.4 PULMONARY ENDOTHELIUM AND HEMOFLUIDITY

The hemostatic system serves the following features: (a) platelet aggregation, (b) blood coagulation, and (c) fibrinolysis.[2] ECs can modulate all three functions through a variety of interacting factors. Platelet function is mediated through synthesis of nitric oxide (NO), prostacyclin (PGI_2) and von Willebrand factor (vWF), removal of serotonin from the pulmonary circulation, as well as conversion of adenosine diphosphate (which can induce platelet aggregation) to adenosine monophosphate, mediated by the endothelial ectoenzyme adenosine diphosphatase. The anticoagulant properties of ECs are driven mainly through antithrombin III (AT III), which is an inhibitor of thrombin and blood coagulation.[2] The reaction is facilitated by glycosaminoglucans and sulfated proteoglycans on the surface of ECs, such as thrombomodulin (TM). Thrombin reacts with TM, producing an increase of the thrombin-catalyzed activation of protein C (PC), which in turn deactivates the coagulation factors VA and VIIIA. The procoagulant properties of ECs are normally covered by the predominant anticoagulant activity. Studies have shown that lung injury-related stimuli can induce the normally low activity of the EC-associated procoagulant factor, thromboplastin.[2] The fibrinolytic properties of ECs are driven through expression of tissue-type (t-PA) and urokinase-type (u-PA) plasminogen activators, as well as plasminogen activator inhibitors (PAI). All the above metabolic functions can be altered in cases of injury, such as ARDS.[2] In patients with ARDS the pulmonary extraction of serotonin is lowered, while vWF plasma levels are elevated consisting a marker of EC activation or injury.[2,4] Furthermore, TM plasma levels are elevated in ARDS patients; the latter may also carry higher levels of PAI 1 and lower fibrinolytic potential, denoting that lung injury-related stimuli, such as, endotoxin, interleukin-1 (IL-1) and thrombin can alter the anticoagulant and fibrinolytic activity of pulmonary endothelium.[2,5]

4.4.1 Activated Protein C

As mentioned before, the protein C system is considered an important regulator of the coagulant cascade through the anticoagulant activated protein C (APC) pathway. It also possesses cytoprotective properties through the cytoprotective protein C pathway in several cell types, including EC. Protein C is a vitamin K-dependent plasma glycoprotein present in the circulation as a biologically inactive, two-chain zymogen. It is activated on the EC surface by thrombin through a proteolytic reaction.[6] This procedure can be enhanced more than 1000-fold by TM compared to thrombin-alone reaction. An even greater amplification (by an additional 20-fold) may be achieved if protein C is bound to endothelial protein C receptor (EPCR).[6] The latter is also expressed in leukocytes and in its soluble form in vascular smooth muscle cells (SMCs).[7] Apart from facilitating protein activation, EPCR also regulates EC leukocyte adhesion.[6–8] APC downregulates the coagulation cascade by degrading the cofactors Va and VIIIa by limited proteolysis. The APC-mediated cleavage of these procoagulant cofactors shuts down thrombin generation, through both intrinsic and extrinsic pathways. In addition to promoting the activation of protein C in a Ca^{2+} depended way, TM also inhibits the activity of thrombin toward the procoagulant substrates fibrinogen, PAR-1, and cofactors V and VIII. TM can bind to a basic exosite on thrombin (exosite-1), thereby enabling the protease to recognize and rapidly activate protein C. The high-affinity interaction of TM with exosite-1 competitively inhibits the binding of procoagulant substrates to this site and, hence, the cofactor essentially converts thrombin from a procoagulant to a potent anticoagulant protease upon binding.[6]

The cytoprotective effects of APC can be related to: (a) gene-expression alteration, (b) anti-inflammatory activities, (c) antiapoptotic activity, and (d) stabilization of the EC barrier. Most of these effects require the activation of protease-activated receptor-1 (PAR-1), while EPCR serves as a co-receptor. PAR-1 is a G-protein, which is activated via a proteolytic reaction. The anti-inflammatory properties of APC act through reduced expression of NF-κB, while cytokine signaling is inhibited by preventing the expression of cell surface adhesion molecules. Additionally, APC facilitates the production of prostacyclins via upregulation of inducible cyclo-oxygenase (COX) and appears to inhibit inducible NO synthase (iNOS) through decreased tumor necrosis factor (TNF)-α production.[9–11] Furthermore, APC attenuates IL-1β- and thrombin-induced barrier disruption[12] while in a more recent study induced barrier protection via cytoskeletal regulation mediated by sphingosine 1 phosphate receptor transactivation, combined with EPCR ligation.[13] Regarding the above, a paradox arises referring to the beneficial effects of APC via PAR-1, while the same receptor is used by thrombin to exert its pro-inflammatory action. This leads to a hypothesis that PAR-1 can regulate either pro- or anti-inflammatory signals depending on the cell type and protease concentration.

4.5 BARRIER FUNCTION

The continuous nature of the pulmonary endothelium facilitates one of its most important functions, the maintenance of a semi-permeable barrier. Due to the strategic location of the lungs and the enormous surface area of the capillary endothelium, the latter is allowed to filter the entire volume of circulating blood. The endothelial barrier function (Figure 4.1) is crucial for establishing the transendothelial protein gradient required for tissue fluid homeostasis. There are several ways through which the endothelium manages to accomplish this function, but they can be separated in two basic categories, the paracellular and the transcellular way.[1]

The paracellular way refers to a route "around" the cell. The molecules that use this way are small, such as urea and glucose, and their transportation is size-selected, depending on their molecular radii

(M_r), which cannot exceed 3 nm.[1] The "continuous layer" of the endothelial structure is achieved through a complex set of junctional proteins forming tight junctions (TJs) and adherens junctions (AJs), giving shape to a zipper-like frame. Adherens junctions are formed mainly by vascular-endothelial (VE)-cadherin, a member of the cadherin family. These are single-span transmembrane glycoproteins. They mediate cell-to-cell adhesion in a calcium-dependent way.[1] A potent disruptor of vascular permeability is vascular endothelial growth factor (VEGF). VE-cadherin maintains vascular permeability by binding to tyrosine kinase VEGF receptor 2 (VEGF-R2). In the presence of VEGF, the degradation of VE-cadherin is initiated and the AJs are disrupted.[14,15] Tight junctions are formed by claudins, occluding and junctional adhesion molecules (JAMs). These three protein complexes bind zona occludens (ZO) to cytoplasmic signaling molecules and the actin cytoskeleton. AJs and TJs, composing the interendothelial junctions (IEJs) maintain vascular integrity via actin remodeling.[1] Another type of connection between ECs is gap junctions (GJs). These are formed by hydrophilic transmembrane proteins called connexons (Cx), such as Cx37, Cx40, and Cx43.[1] Moreover, the paracellular pathway is affected by the interaction of ECs with ECM. Integrins are expressed by ECs and are bound to the ECM serving as protein receptors. The specific integrin binding sites of the ECM are named "focal contacts" or "focal adhesions." Signaling pathways regulate paracellular permeability through a complex interaction between adhesive and counteradhesive forces, which adjust the opening and closing of the IEJs. The GJs signaling pathways also regulate the interactions between ECs and the ECM.[1]

The transcellular pathway is used by water and molecules with a M_r greater than 3 nm. The former uses channels across the lipid bilayer formed by proteins named aquaporins (Figure 4.1).[16] Under normal conditions, the plasma proteins can also be transported through the endothelium via a fluid phase or using a receptor-mediated manner. Additionally, transcellular channels are often formed transiently in order to facilitate protein transportation, such as albumin by caveolae.[17] The latter are vesicular carriers established as clusters in the membrane. The major component of caveolae is the protein caveolin-1. It plays an important role in caveolae formation, as well as molecule capture and transcytosis.[1,17,18]

ECs respond to a variety of insults, such as hyperoxia, drugs, mechanic stress, and viruses by converting from a low to a high permeability barrier (Figure 4.2). The disruption of the endothelial barrier is a *sine qua non* of lung injury and ARDS leading to increased vascular permeability, which is the hallmark of disease pathogenesis, and, inevitably, to pulmonary edema formation. The endothelial actin cytoskeleton is a complex network of actin molecules polymerized into filaments creating multiple connections to junctional proteins, glycocalyx (negatively charged, luminal structure of the EC) and focal adhesions. Stimuli, such as shear stress, activate signaling pathways, leading to upregulation of transcription factors and subsequent gene expression of various vasoactive substances, growth factors, and adhesion molecules. Active cytoskeletal rearrangement begins rapidly and continues to occur over several hours as ECs orient themselves to reduce both peak shear stresses and shear stress gradients.[19] Additionally, lung injury-related cytokines can affect cytoskeletal modulation leading to barrier disruption. In this respect, ARDS patients, especially nonsurvivors, appear to have elevated levels of plasma VEGF.[20]

4.6 ENDOTHELIAL AND LEUKOCYTE INTERACTIONS

ECs provide an adequate substrate for leukocyte adhesion and facilitate their transportation through the barrier. The cell-to-cell interactions developed between ECs and leukocytes play a key role for the latters' migration from capillaries to lung parenchyma in order for the immune response to unfold. The main cell type that participates in lung injury and the ARDS pathogenesis are neutrophils, while macrophages and eosinophils are also involved.[21,22] The adhesion of leukocytes is a multistep procedure. The initial phase is referred to as cell capture and rolling. The main protein family implicated in this procedure is the selectin family. Selectins constitute a family of cell adhesion receptors that mediate the initial tethering and rolling of leukocytes on inflamed endothelium

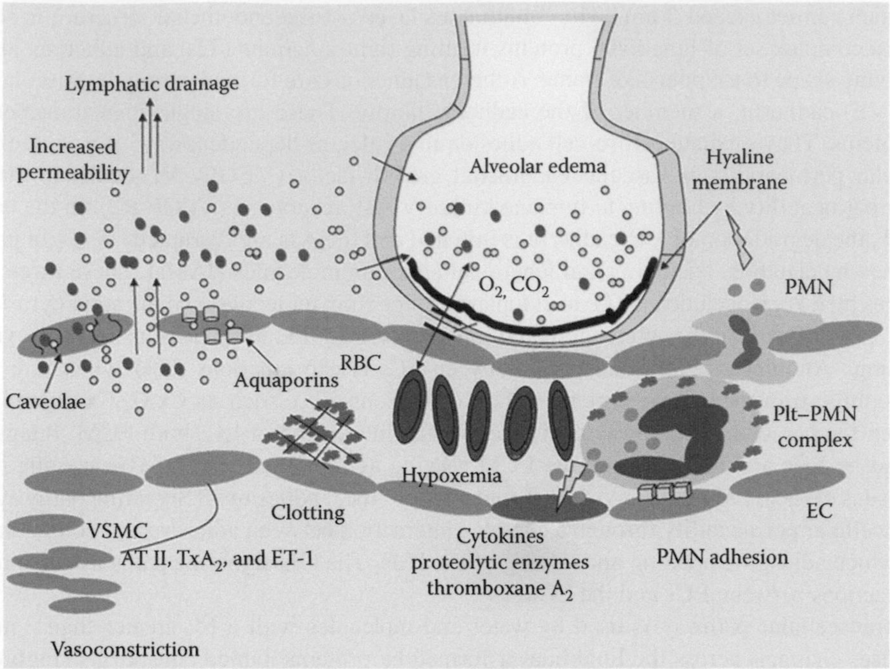

FIGURE 4.2 **(See color insert.)** Schematic illustration of EC response in lung injury. EC respond to a variety of insults by converting from an antiadhesive, low permeability barrier to an adhesive, high permeability cell layer, as described in detail in the text. Common endothelial insults include microbes (e.g., bacteria, viruses, protozoa), hyperoxia, radiation, immune complexes, drugs, ischemia/reperfusion, toxins, mechanical stretch and microemboli. Adhesion molecules on the surface of EC orchestrate transmigration of circulating immune cells, which secrete microbicidal and cytotoxic substances such as oxygen free radicals and proteolytic enzymes. Increased endothelial permeability and vascular tone is mediated by vasoactive substances, including thrombin, angiotensin II (AT II), endothelin-1 (ET-1), thromboxane A_2 (TxA_2), tumor necrosis factor-α and interleukin-8, which are secreted by a number of cell types (EC, platelets, neutrophils, airway epithelia, macrophages). The rationale for these responses seems to be the clearance of infectious agents and damaged host cells; however, life-threatening pulmonary dysfunction and respiratory failure can occur as a consequence of lung flooding and hemodynamic compromise. These alterations trigger a set of anti-inflammatory and repair processes, which, in many cases, successfully restore vascular integrity. RBC: red blood cells, PMN: polymorphonuclear granulocytes; VSMC: vascular smooth muscle cells, Plt: platelets, dark blue circles: albumin; light blue circles: water. (Reproduced from Maniatis NA et al. *Vasc Pharmacol* 2008; **49**(4–6): 119–33. With permission.)

as a prelude to their firm attachment and extravasation into tissues.[23] There are three members of the selectin family; E-selectin is expressed only in the ECs, P-selectin is found in platelets, as well as the EC, and L-selectin is constitutively expressed in neutrophils. The latter is expressed within minutes on the EC surface following its activation by stimuli, such as histamine, thrombin, bradykinin, leukotriene C4, or free radicals. P-selectin interacts with neutrophil counter-receptors, such as the P-selectin glycoprotein-1. E-selectin is rapidly synthesized by the ECs after its activation by cytokines, such as TNF-α and IL-1, or endotoxin.[24]

Firm adhesion is the second phase of endothelial–leukocyte interaction. In this procedure, the β_2 (CD18) integrin family and more specifically the CD11/CD18 integrins are involved. These are expressed in neutrophils and interact with the intercellular adhesion molecule-1 (ICAM-1), a member of the immunoglobulin family that is expressed in EC.[2]

The third phase of the adhesion cascade refers to the migration of leukocytes through the endothelium. It requires the platelet-EC adhesion molecule 1 (PECAM-1), which is expressed in the EC junctions.[24] Leukocyte migration also requires a chemeotactic gradient, while a firm adherence is not always needed.[24] Cytokines that induce neutrophil activation and, thus enhance EC leukocyte interaction include, among others, TNF-α and IL-1, which play an essential role in the early stages of ARDS.[2] Other factors include endotoxin/lipopolysaccharide (LPS) and oxidative stress.

More specifically, neutrophil adhesion as a response to cytokine stimuli can cause the establishment of an oxidant-rich environment, due to production of reactive oxidant species (ROS) and proteases as a massive burst, enhancing cell death at the place of injury.[25] With regard to the above, EC–neutrophil interaction could provide valuable therapeutic solutions. Many research studies have shown that neutralization of several molecules, such as CD18,[26] as well as ICAM-1,[27] or members of the selectin family[28,29] can attenuate lung injury in multiple animal models, through the inactivation of neutrophils.[30,31] To this end, human studies tried to provide endothelial markers that could predict ARDS development or outcome.[2] Nonsurviving ARDS patients presented elevated soluble plasma P-selectin levels.[32] Septic patients in risk to develop ARDS had elevated levels of plasma vWF antigen, soluble ICAM-1, and soluble E-selectin. Trauma patients did not present the same phenotype.[33] Plasma-soluble (s) L-selectin levels measured in at-risk for ARDS patients were significantly lower in those who subsequently progressed to ARDS than in those who did not or in normal controls.[34] Significant correlations were found between the above low (s) L-selectin levels and the requirement for ventilation, the degree of respiratory failure, and patient mortality.[32–34] As a therapeutic approach, a selective in cell and inflammation manner β_2 CD11/CD18 antagonist managed to prevent neutrophil adhesion in LPS-activated pulmonary arterial ECs, and lung injury development in a bacterial-induced animal model. Conditional blocking of β_2 integrin function appears to provide a potential treatment procedure.[2]

4.7 ENDOTHELIAL CELL ACTIVATION

ECs exert active control over the vascular tone and regulate thrombolysis and coagulation. They also determine the extent to which the vasculature is permeable to cells and molecules, through the synthesis and release of a wide variety of substances. Under inflammatory conditions, EC activation occurs. The normal phenotype is reversed from anti- to pro-thrombotic, followed by loss of vascular integrity, increased expression of leukocyte adhesion molecules, cytokine production and upregulation of human leukocyte antigen (HLA) molecules.[35,36] The activation occurs in two steps. The first is EC stimulation or Type I activation, which does not require *de novo* protein synthesis or genotypic upregulation. ECs retract from each other, express P-selectin leading to increased neutrophil adhesion and release von Willebrand factor, which regulates platelet adherence to the sub-endothelium. The second step is type II activation that requires upregulation of mRNA expression and *de novo* protein synthesis, particularly of cytokines and especially of TNF-α and IL-1, adhesion molecules, such as vascular cell adhesion molecule-1 (VCAM-1), ICAM-1 and ICAM-2 molecules, and E-selectin. Transcription factors are major components of EC activation. One of the most crucial is nuclear factor-κB (NF- κB).[37,38] This is the final receptor of a signaling pathway from the cell surface to the nucleus. Among the factors that trigger enhanced gene expression by NF-κB are TNF-α and IL-1, ROS, and viral and bacterial derivatives, such as LPS. Endotoxin stimulates NF-κB through Toll-like receptors (TLRs). Upon stimulation, NF-κB alters the normal production of NO, endothelins (ETs) and COX products, thus changing the normal phenotype of low vascular resistance and appropriate ventilation–perfusion matching (Figure 4.3).

4.8 ENDOTHELIUM AND VASOACTIVE COMPOUNDS

Pulmonary endothelium under nonpathologic status regulates smooth muscle tone through the secretion of vasodilators, which also possess antiproliferative and anti-inflammatory effects (e.g., NO, PGI_2) in favor of vasoconstrictors, which also induce cell proliferation, hypertrophy, and inflammation (ET-1, TxA_2, AT II).[38] This phenomenon is reversed under injury.

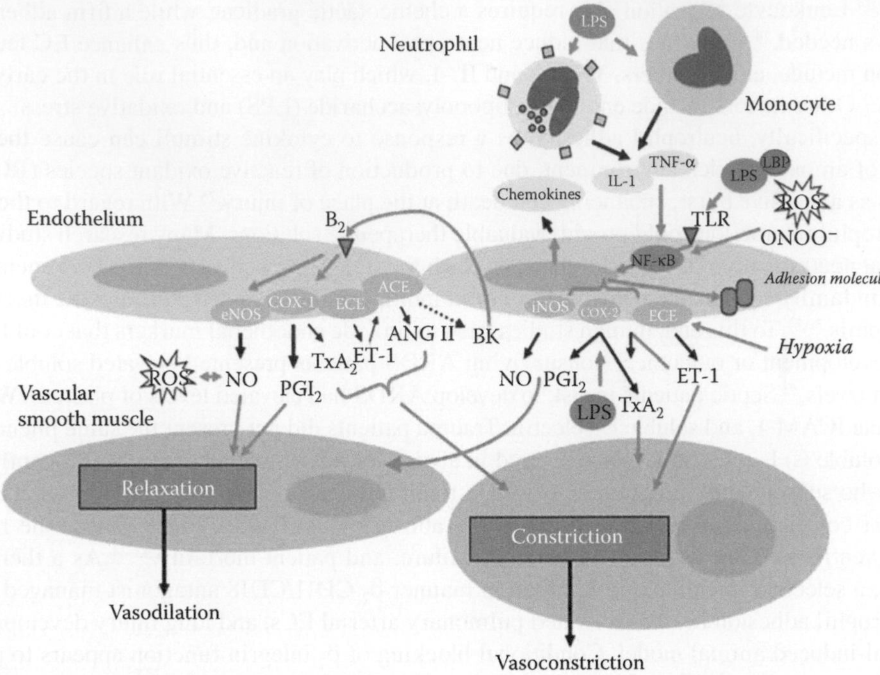

FIGURE 4.3 **(See color insert.)** Schematic illustration of physiologic endothelial–smooth muscle interactions and EC response to inflammatory stimuli. Inflammatory stimuli induce the activation of nuclear factor-κB (NF-κB) or other transcription factors. NF-κB promotes the synthesis of vasoactive agents regulating vascular tone. TNF-α: tumor necrosis factor-α; IL-1: interleukin-1; NO: nitric oxide; ONOO−: peroxynitrite; ET-1: endothelin-1; PGI_2: prostacyclin; TxA_2: thromboxane A_2; ANG II: angiotensin II; BK: bradykinin; ROS: reactive oxygen species; eNOS: endothelial NO synthase; iNOS: inducible NO synthase; COX-1: constitutive cyclooxygenase; COX-2: inducible cyclooxygenase; ACE: angiotensin-converting enzyme; ECE: endothelin-converting enzyme; B_2: B_2 kinin receptor. Red arrows action; black arrows synthesis (and uptake for ET-1); dotted arrow breakdown. (Reproduced from Orfanos SE et al. *Intensive Care Med* 2004; **30**(9): 1702–14. With permission.)

Nitric oxide is a free radical belonging to the family of reactive nitrogen species (RNS) with a very short half-life and is very unstable in biological systems. Other members of the family include nitrogen dioxide (NO_2), and peroxynitrite ($ONOO^-$). Together with the ROS family, that includes superoxide anion (O_2^-), hydrogen peroxide (H_2O_2) and the hydroxyl radical (OH^-) they represent the main oxidant molecules and participate in important biological signaling procedures.[39] However, at high concentrations they can have toxic effects and contribute to tissue damage. Especially NO is a potent vasodilator and inhibitor of hypoxic pulmonary vasoconstriction, as well as platelet aggregation. NO synthase (NOS) forms NO from l-arginine. Deficiency of l-arginine or the NOS cofactor tetrahydrobiopterin may result in production of O_2^- instead of or along with NO, promoting the formation of highly reactive RNS, such as $ONOO^-$.[39] There are three known NOS isoenzymes: (1) neuronal (n) NOS, also expressed in pulmonary arterial smooth muscle cells (SMC), (2) inducible (i) NOS, induced by several pro-inflammatory mediators, which upon expression produces NO at very high rates with profound effects on cardiovascular homeostasis, and (3) endothelial (e) NOS, a constitutive isoenzyme expressed principally in EC[2]. The latter is the main isoenzyme involved in vascular tone regulation. NO activates soluble granulate cyclase, thus producing 3,5-cyclic guanosine monophosphate (cGMP) and eliciting cGMP-mediated SMC relaxation and other cell-specific functions.[39] Following the exposure to various inflammatory stimuli, pulmonary endothelial, epithelial, and alveolar macrophages are among the cell types of the lung that contribute to increased generation of ROS and RNS, which including the deficiency of antioxidant defenses, cause molecular/cellular damage in ARDS patients. Among other features, this oxidant stress alters endothelial barrier function and increases endothelial permeability through activation of protein kinase C (PKC), myosin light-chain kinase (MLCK), and other signaling pathways.[1] In the lung, hypoxia reduces the production of NO facilitating the development of hypoxic pulmonary vasoconstriction (HPV),[40] a unique physiological feature of the pulmonary circulation that maintains proper ventilation/perfusion match and optimizes oxygenation; this feature is lost in ARDS.[40] As a therapeutic agent, inhaled NO improved oxygenation in animal models of lung injury, as well as in ARDS patients.[41] In contrast, a meta-analysis of studies on ARDS patients revealed that inhaled NO failed to make a difference in the clinical outcome of ARDS, despite the initial oxygenation improvement, while it increased the risk of renal dysfunction.[42] Thus, NO may have beneficial or deleterious effects, depending on the type and the amount of oxygen radicals present.[41]

The prostanoids are part of a family of biologically active lipids derived from the action of COX. They can be further subdivided into three main groups; (a) prostacyclins, (b) prostaglandins, and (c) thromboxanes.[2] PGI_2 is considered to be a potent vasodilator and platelet aggregation inhibitor produced downstream of cyclooxygenase by prostacyclin synthase. Another COX product is prostaglandin E_1 (PGE_1), which has similar properties to PGI_2. COX products contribute to HPV, but in contrast with NO, their action seems to be dependent on the size of the artery and the species involved.[2] Another difference between PGI_2 and NO is that the latter predominantly activates cGMP, while the former acts through cyclic adenosine monophosphate (cAMP).

A third prostanoid that participates in the regulation of the vascular tone is thromboxane A_2 (TxA_2). Apart from EC, thromboxane A2 is secreted by platelets, as well. TxA_2 is a potent vasoconstrictor in contrast with PGI_2 and PGE_1; it enhances platelet aggregation and capillary permeability through barrier disruption.[38] A particular role for eicosanoids in several lung injury models is their contribution to the regulation of perfusion redistribution that diverts blood flow to healthier lung regions.[2] In a similar respect, selective inhibition of the inducible COX isoform protects against endotoxin-related loss of perfusion redistribution in an oleic acid-induced canine lung injury model, an effect mediated by PGI_2.[43–45]

Endothelins have matching vasoactive properties with TxA_2. The ET family represents one of the most potent naturally occurring vasoconstrictors. Three isoforms have been identified; ET-1, ET-2, and ET-3.[2] These three isoforms have similar structures. ET-1 is a 21-residue peptide produced from preproendothelin, and is encoded by three different genes found in the genomic DNA library of several species, including humans and rodents. Preproendothelins generate 38-residue biologically inactive intermediates, termed big ETs that are processed in mature ETs. Big ET-1 is cleaved to ET-1 by the endothelin-converting enzyme-1 (ECE-1), which is a membrane-bound metalloprotease.[35] ET-1 has numerous and diverse actions, including vasoconstriction, bronchoconstriction, and growth promotion. The effects of the ETs are mediated by two principal specific receptors; ET-A, which has a substantially greater affinity for ET-1 than for ET-2 and ET- 3, and ET-B, with a similar affinity for ET-1, ET-2, and ET-3.[35] Endothelin-1 is produced mainly by EC, and its production is induced by several factors, including hypoxia, endotoxin, TNF-α, interferon, and epinephrine.[35] The main area of ET-1 release is located in the abluminal direction where the EC interacts with SMC. The main ET receptor that is expressed on SMC is ET-A, also expressed in EC, facilitating vasoconstriction.[39] The second ET-1 receptor, ET-B, is expressed primarily in EC, causing transient vasodilation through NO and prostaglandin signaling pathways.[39] Upon EC activation, as ET-1 increases, eNOS is reduced, revealing a coordination between the two vasoactive molecules.[39] The human lung is an important site for ET-1 clearance, a function achieved through the ET-B receptors. Approximately 50% of circulating ET-1 is cleared in a single transpulmonary passage with simultaneous equal production.[46] Human studies have shown that this balance between pulmonary ET-1 clearance and release was decreased in early stages of acute lung injury and it was reversed in patients who subsequently recovered.[47] Additionally, plasma ET-1 values are increased in septic patients with and without ARDS, possibly contributing to lung injury-associated pulmonary hypertension.[46–48]

4.8.1 Renin–Angiotensin–Aldosterone System

The renin–angiotensin–aldosterone system (RAAS) is a potent biological system that plays a key role in pulmonary and systemic vascular homeostasis. The main participant in this system is the angiotensin converting enzyme (ACE) that is highly expressed and uniformly distributed on the luminal surface of EC. The main functions of pulmonary endothelium-bound (PE) ACE are the hydrolysis of angiotensin-I to angiotensin-II and the breakdown of bradykinin.[38] Angiotensin-II is an inducer of SMC constriction, growth, and proliferation, while it also possesses pro-inflammatory properties.[38] On the contrary, bradykinin that escapes inactivation by ACE, acts as a vasodilator, as well as an anti-inflammatory and antithrombotic factor, through the endothelial B_2 receptors (Figure 4.3).[2] The latter pathway acts through the release of PGI_2 and NO, produced by COX-1 and eNOS, respectively[2] The pro-inflammatory functions of angiotensin-II act through angiotensin receptor 1 (AT_1). This receptor stimulates the expression of cytokines, such as IL-1, IL-6, IL-8, adhesion molecules such as ICAM-1 and VCAM-1, and enhances the production of the transcription factor NF-κB.[38] In contrast, activation of the second angiotensin receptor (AT_2) leads to an anti-inflammatory response suppressing IL-1 and NF-κB and upregulating the expression of IL-10.[49] A third function of PE-ACE appears to be as a signal transduction molecule in EC outside-in signaling, involving c-Jun N-terminal kinase (JNK).[50]

The catalytic site of PE-ACE is exposed on the luminal side of the blood vessels. Since the enzyme is in direct contact with blood-borne substrates, its activity can be measured by indicator-dilution type techniques. In the surface of the capillaries are located high numbers of the enzyme, thus monitoring PE-ACE activity equals to monitoring pulmonary capillary endothelium-bound (PCEB)-ACE activity. This method offers quantifiable indices that may distinguish between abnormalities secondary to endothelial dysfunction per se and decreased pulmonary vascular surface area.[50,51] A second index of pulmonary endothelial dysfunction, is plasma-soluble ACE (sACE), which has a surrogate role compared to PCEB-ACE activity. Both PCEB-ACE and sACE are decreased in several lung injury animal models, as well as in human ARDS patients[49,50,52,53] PCEB-ACE activity was estimated in mechanically ventilated patients belonging to high-risk groups for ARDS development or to patients already suffering from ARDS of diverse severity.[49] Enzyme activity was expressed as transpulmonary substrate hydrolysis (reflecting enzyme activity per capillary) and as functional capillary surface area (FCSA; originally termed A_{max}/K_m and reflecting enzyme activity per vascular bed), relating to both enzyme quantity and functional integrity.[53] Both indices decreased early during the ARDS continuum and were inversely related to lung injury score, suggesting that the clinical severity of the syndrome is related to the degree of PCEB-ACE activity depression (i.e., the underlying pulmonary endothelial dysfunction).[49]

An ACE homologue called ACE-2 appears to have anti-inflammatory properties, thus counterbalancing the known pro-inflammatory role of angiotensin II.[38] ACE-2 presents the function of a carboxypeptidase, producing angiotensins (1–9) from angiotensin I and angiotensins (1–7) from angiotensin II, by cleaving one residue from each molecule. Treatment with recombinant ACE-2 seems to improve lung injury in animal models, since it controls vascular permeability thus preventing edema formation.[38] Additional interest in ACE-2 provides the fact that it serves as a receptor for the SARS-corona virus (see below). This fact may trigger SARS-mediated ARDS through ACE-2 dysfunction.[54–56]

4.9 PULMONARY ENDOTHELIUM AND GROWTH FACTORS

The development of the vascular system is a complicated procedure that involves several agents and pathways. Two major growth factor families play a key role in the coordination of the process: (i) the angiopoietins (Angs) and (ii) the vascular endothelial growth factors (VEGFs).

Four members have been identified in the angiopoietin family. Three of these members, angiopoietin-1 (Ang-1), angiopoietin-2 (Ang-2), and angiopoietin-4 (Ang-4) are expressed in humans. Ang-1 is an oligomeric-secreted glycoprotein that exerts its effects through the receptor TIE2, an endothelial-specific tyrosine kinase. The basic functions of Ang-1 are induction of EC migration, formation of capillary-like structures, inhibition of EC apoptosis, reduction of vascular permeability, and inflammation and maintenance of vascular integrity.[38] The expression of Ang-1 and TIE2 is present during development of blood vessels. Ang-1 is expressed and secreted by vascular SMCs, while TIE2 is a transmembrane receptor expressed in ECs. In the adult lung vasculature, Ang-1 expression is reduced significantly, showing minimal presence,[57] while the expression of TIE2 remains unaltered.[57,58] The second member of the angiopoietin family, Ang-2, is a TIE2 receptor agonist or, mainly, antagonist. Both Ang-1 and Ang-2 appear to have the same affinity for TIE2. Ang-2, however, has a context-specific effect depending on the cell type and condition. In the presence of Ang-1 (i.e., a TIE2 agonist), Ang-2 will mostly act as an antagonist and block TIE2 signaling, preventing cytoprotection. Activation of Ang-2/TIE2 signaling promotes vascular destabilization and VEGF-induced angiogenesis.[58,59]

Since Angs participate in angiogenesis and maintenance of vascular integrity, they play an important role in pathological conditions, such as tumor metastasis, pulmonary hypertension, sepsis, and ARDS. Genetically modified mice that lack Ang-1 or its receptor TIE2, are found to have disrupted angiogenesis in mouse embryos.[60] In more recent studies, the Angl/Tie2 signals have been shown to contribute to tumor progression by increasing vascular entry and exit of tumor cells to facilitate tumor dissemination and establishment of metastases; inhibition of Ang-2 prevents tumor metastasis in adult mice by enhancing the endothelial cell-to-cell junctions.[61,62]

Pulmonary hypertension in humans has been characterized by overexpression of Ang-1 and enhanced activation of TIE2 via phosphorylation, regulating pathological SMC hyperplasia.[63,64] Viral-mediated overexpression of Ang-1 may lead to pulmonary arterial hypertension, while molecular inhibition of the Ang-1/TIE2 pathway blocks the development of the disease in animals.[65,66] On the other hand, studies in a monocrotaline-induced and a hypoxia-induced animal model of pulmonary hypertension supported a protective role for Ang-1, enhancing the controversy in the field.[66] Ang-1 has been shown to inhibit endothelin-1 in ECs, restricting its pro-inflammatory and vasoconstrictive effects.[67] Moreover, treatment with mesenchymal stem cell-based Ang-1 attenuated LPS-induced lung injury.[68] Additionally, Ang-1 prevented endotoxin-induced vascular leakage in a p190 RhoGAP-dependent way, activating Racl and inhibiting RhoA. These findings suggest that Ang-1 prevents vascular permeability by regulating the endothelial cytoskeleton.[69]

Ang-2 has been related with endothelial barrier disruption and vascular leak in lung injury.[70,71] NOS is implicated in hyperoxia induced-lung injury protecting against the Ang-2-induced injury.[72] In contrast, a protective role for Ang-2 by blocking the vascular leak through an autocrine effect on stressed ECs has been suggested.[73] In humans, serum Ang-2 levels are increased during severe sepsis. They are related with serum TNF-α levels and the disease severity.[74] The ratio of Ang-2 to Ang-1 may be a prognostic biomarker of endothelial activation in ARDS patients and, along with pulmonary dead-space fraction, may be useful for risk stratification of such patients.[75]

VEGF (also known as VEGF-A) is a member of the VEGF family that includes several other members of growth factors, such as VEGF-B, -C, -D, and the placental growth factor. It is a multipotent growth factor expressed in high levels in the lung and is required in several physiological EC functions. It is also involved in the development and maintenance of the structure in the adult lung.[1,2] VEGF exerts its functions through several receptors. VEGFR-2 is the main receptor through which VEGF can regulate angiogenesis, vascular permeability, cell proliferation, prostacyclin, and NO production. The latter can also be mediated through VEGFR-1.[76] Additional properties of VEGF include inhibition of apoptosis and, survival and differentiation of ECs. There are several mechanisms through which VEGF mediates its properties. Binding to VEGFR-2 will cause receptor autophosphorylation, leading to activation of pathways, such as c-Src and Akt.[77] Both of these pathways lead to release of NO. The c-Src pathway also promotes prostacyclin release, as well as cell proliferation via activation of protein kinase C (PKC) and the Raf–MEK–ERK pathway. The Akt pathway, apart from NO release, enhances cell survival by inhibiting the proteins caspase-9, Bad, and p38MAPK and regulates cell cycle proteins, such as cyclin D and E2F.[77] In addition,

N-terminal fragment of the protein ligand Slit (SlitN2) in mice affected with H5N1.[95] Slit family includes proteins sending neurovascular guidance messages, aiming at the inhibition of vascular hyperpermeability, caused by VEGF.[98] Slit2N interacts with the endothelial-specific receptor Robo-4, reducing the vascular permeability caused by the cytokine storm.[99] The subsequent integrity of endothelial barrier was produced by the stabilization of cell surface VE-cadherin, the major constituent of adherens intercellular endothelial junctions.[100] Inflammatory mediators cause endocytosis of VE-cadherin, leading to vascular hyperpermeability.[89,101]

The influenza virus infection has also been associated with activation of the coagulation cascade, in terms of disseminated intravascular coagulation and atherothrombosis.[102] This issue has been attributed to the invasion of ECs by enveloped and nonenveloped respiratory viruses, including influenza and adenoviruses, respectively. Visseren et al. have studied *in vitro* the accentuated procoagulant endothelial activity following respiratory viral infections.[102] The infection of umbilical vein ECs (HUVEC) by various viruses including influenza H1N1 and H3N2 and influenza B, resulted in accentuated activity of tissue factor (TF) and subsequent activation of prothrombinase complex and thrombin generation.

To conclude, influenza-mediated endothelial injury might play a significant role in the pathogenesis of pulmonary vascular leak. Novel therapeutics approaches could aim on strengthening the endothelial barrier.

4.10.2 Herpes Viruses

4.10.2.1 Herpes Simplex Virus

Herpes simplex virus (HSV) is occasionally found in oropharyngeal swab or specimen drawn from the lower respiratory tract of critically ill patients.[103,104] Aspiration of the virus might lead to life-threatening HSV pneumonia and subsequent evolution to ARDS.[103,105] The exact pathologic mechanism of HSV-related lung injury is not clarified, since biopsies are rarely performed in those patients, because of the risk of complications. However, there are clinical and experimental data showing that HSV might interact with ECs, playing a crucial role in the activation of coagulation cascade and in the development of human atherosclerosis.[106,102] Histological studies of HSV mucosal lesions are consistent with leukocytoclastic vasculitis and intravascular fibrin deposits.[107] Key et al.[106] reported that HUVEC contaminated with HSV-1 showed accentuated TF expression on their cell surface and significant reduction on the activation of protein C, attributed to TM reduced activity. The expression of tissue factor of ECs leads to the activation of extrinsic coagulation cascade, whereas the inhibition of activation of protein C promotes the procoagulant activity. Moreover, enhanced thrombin production by HSV in HUVEC, stimulated PAR1, leading to further propagation of HSV.[108] Whether a similar mechanism might occur in vivo, leading to increase procoagulant activity of lung endothelium in the case of HSV pneumonia is not yet clarified.

4.10.2.2 Human Cytomegalovirus

Human cytomegalovirus (HCMV) is a betaherpes enveloped virus, causing a life-threatening pneumonia especially in immunocompromised patients. HCMV pneumonia is a frequent complication occurring after organ transplants, resulting in increased morbidity and mortality.[109] Additionally, chronic HCMV infection, might affect transplant recipients, leading to subclinical pulmonary dysfunction, characterized by reduced lung diffusing capacity.[110] Chronic vascular infection caused by HCMV has been associated with atherosclerosis and sclerosis of transplant vessels.[111,112] The diagnosis of HCMV-viremia is established by measuring the number of pp65 polymorphonuclear cells per 50,000 leukocytes.[113]

HCMV infects human cells including monocytes–macrophages, neutrophils, epithelial cells, SMCs, and ECs.[114] Indeed, high levels of pp65 antigenemia have been associated to the revealing of cytomegalic endothelial cells (CEC) in blood.[115] A possible explanation for the HCMV-related lung dysfunction and reduced diffusing capacity might be the dissemination of active replicative virus by circulating CEC and mononuclear cells to the pulmonary endothelium.[116,117] The subsequent activation of pulmonary endothelium stimulates proinflammatory signaling leading to the expression of mediators as IL-1, IL-6, RANTES (chemokine regulated on activation, normal T cell expressed and secreted), and TNF-α.[118] This local inflammatory procedure, pneumonitis, leads to the loss of vascular integrity of the pulmonary capillary bed, resulting in pulmonary edema and reduced diffusing capacity.

Moreover, HCMV-related endothelial damage promotes the activation of prothrombinase complex, enhancing thrombin generation.[102,111] The latter may result in recruitment of inflammatory cells, thus contributing to tissue injury. This prothrombotic process may be accentuated by anchoring leukocytes and leukocyte-derived microparticles.[119,120]

HCMV infection has been associated with thrombosis in deep veins and in pulmonary arteries.[121] Interestingly, it has been reported that HCMV infection has been associated with pulmonary embolism and the presence of antiphospholipid antibodies.[122]

In conclusion, the amplification of the inflammation process and coagulation cascade might be a possible explanation for the HCMV-related acute and chronic pulmonary injury, and the accompanying vascular pathology.

4.10.2.3 Human Herpesvirus-8

Human herpesvirus-8 (HHV-8) or Kaposi's sarcoma-associated herpesvirus belongs to the family of Rhadinovirus. HHV-8 is causatively associated to Kaposi's sarcoma, Castleman's disease, and primary effusion lymphoma.[123] The virus insults various cells, including B lymphocytes and monocytes, in which HHV-8 stays in latent state.[124] Recently, it has been reported that HHV-8 infects human ECs and modifies cellular gene expressions.[125] The clinical consequence of this latent infection is not well established. Since there are several cases of coincidence of Castleman's disease and pulmonary hypertension, Cool et al.[126] reported the possible etiologic association of HHV-8 infection with PAH. They found an increased expression of HHV-8 latency-associated nuclear antigen 1 in plexiform lesions of PAH patients. However, this possible relationship was not confirmed and the issue remains under investigation.[127] Recently it has been reported that HHV-8 downregulates VE-cadherin, a prominent element of the endothelial barrier, thus influencing vascular permeability.[128,129] Therefore, it seems that HHV-8 insults endothelium by a variety of means.

4.10.3 Parvovirus B19

Parvovirus B19 (B19) is a nonenveloped DNA virus etiologically associated with the childhood exanthem fifth disease.[130] Recently, B19 infection has been associated with vasculitic syndromes. Wegener's granulomatosis, Henoch–Schonlein purpura, Kawasaki disease, dermatomyositis, and scleroderma.[131–133] Moreover, B12 has been documented as an endotheliotropic agent implicated in pathogenesis of idiopathic pulmonary fibrosis.[134] In a recent report, 12 patients with interstitial lung disease and chronic parvovirus B19 infection were studied.[135] The performed direct and indirect immunofluorescence revealed the presence of antiendothelial cell antibodies, antiphospholipid antibodies, and deposition of complement, IgG, IgA, and IgM in pulmonary vascular bed. Factor VIII, an important index of microvascular damage was elevated in some patients.[136]

The autoimmune endothelial damage caused by B19 is attributed to the stimulation of TNF-α pathway and propagation of apoptosis. Therefore, B19 can insult pulmonary endothelium by an autoimmune mechanism, leading to the development of a capillary injury syndrome potentially associated with pulmonary fibrosis.

4.10.4 Hantaviruses

Hantaviruses, RNA viruses belonging to the family *Bunyaviridae,* are causatively related to a hemorrhagic fever associated with renal syndrome (HFRS) and hantavirus pulmonary syndrome (HPS).[137]

HPS in North and South America is caused by Sin Nombre virus and Andes virus, included in the New World hantaviruses.[138] HPS begins with “flu like illness” and progressively evolves to pulmonary edema and shock. Pulmonary edema is mainly noncardiogenic, in terms of ARDS. However, in fatal cases a cardiopulmonary syndrome might develop, characterized by cardiogenic shock.[139] Microvascular endothelium is the prominent target of the hantavirus, and microvascular leakage is the cornerstone of pathology of the relevant syndrome.[139]

The etiology of lung microvascular leakage in HPS is multifactorial. Indirect host immunologic reactions to the virus, in combination with direct endothelial damage caused by viral replication, contributes to the development of pulmonary edema.[140] The innate and subsequent immune host response to hantavirus aims to virus elimination: PAMPs of the virus are recognized by extracellular domains of TLR’s of endothelial host cells, leading to the production of proinflammatory cytokines and chemokines, such as IFN-γ, IL-1a, IL-6, and TNF-α.[141] The “cytokine storm,” in parallel with its contribution to the host defense against hantavirus, might affect endothelial integrity and lead to disturbed vascular permeability.[142]

However, there is increasing evidence that HPS is not only an immune-modulated disease. Hantavirus might directly insult pulmonary endothelium and regulate vascular permeability by interacting with the endothelial cellular receptor β3 integrin.[143,144] Additionally it has been found that hantavirus infection of human primary lung ECs lead to the increase of secreted levels of VEGF and downregulation of VE-cadherin.[138] Moreover, virus replication per se might affect the integrity of endothelial barrier. VEGF normally increases vascular permeability and binds to tyrosine kinase receptor VEGF-R2 expressed on ECs. VEGF-R2 interrelates to VE-cadherin contributing to the integrity of adherens junctions between ECs.[145] VEGF binding to VEGF-R2 leads to the degradation of VE-cadherin and loss of the integrity of adherens junctions.[101] Therefore, the concomitant increase in VEGF levels during hantavirus infection, might lead to EC leakage. Experimental data are highlighting the role of hantavirus on influencing the VEGF–VEGFR2–VE–cadherin cascade. Hantavirus-infected cells exposed to high levels of exogenous VEGF showed a decrease in VE-cadherin levels.[146] Moreover, in patients with HFRS-attenuated Ang-1 expression has been found, possibly contributing to increased vascular permeability.[147]

In conclusion, hantaviruses are causative agents of HPS, interacting with pulmonary endothelium and leading to increased vascular permeability by a variety of direct and indirect mechanisms.

4.10.5 Ebola Virus

Ebola virus (EBOV) is the cause of Ebola hemorrhagic fever, characterized by shock, generalized edema, and disseminated intravascular coagulation (DIC). DIC is characterized by activation of coagulation cascade, widespread consuming of clotting factors, inhibition of fibrinolysis, and deposition of fibrin to the vessels of several organs, leading to multiorgan dysfunction syndrome (MODS) with increased morbidity and mortality.[148] The pathophysiologic mechanism of EBOV-related MODS is not well understood. Postmortem studies have shown the EBOV infection of ECs.[149] It has been reported that EBOV glycoprotein might directly insult ECs leading to bleeding disorders and DIC.[150] Additionally, the “cytokine storm” induced by activated ECs, monocytes, and leukocytes might influence vascular tone and activate a coagulation cascade.[151]

However, animal studies showed that the EBOV infection of ECs did not induce degeneration of the vascular endothelial structure.[148] Interestingly, human lung-derived ECs seem to be infected by EBOV only in late states of the disease. Additionally, virus replication triggers neither endothelial damage nor increased apoptosis of ECs. Therefore, the pathogenesis of EBOV-induced DIC and MODS appears related to the effects of cytokines, and other agents secreted by activated cells, on vascular integrity.[152] Direct EBOV-related damage of EC is rather of minimal importance, in terms of deregulation of coagulation mechanism and subsequent organ dysfunction.

4.10.6 Dengue Virus

Dengue virus (DV) is a member of *Flaviviruses.* The clinical spectrum of disease caused by Dengue virus varies from mild disease, to hemorrhagic fever and dengue shock syndrome (DHF/DSS). The main characteristic of this most severe DV-related clinical entity is increased capillary permeability, while capillary endothelium remains morphologically intact.[153] The subsequent plasma leakage affects cavities of the body (pleura, pericardium, abdomen), and almost all of the organs (lung alveolar compartment, brain, gut, kidney, reproductive tract) and may become fatal because of the concomitant shock syndrome. The pathophysiologic mechanism of DV-derived morbidity is not well understood. However, the role of vascular endothelium as a main target of the virus is well established.[155] According to histopathological studies performed on tissues of patients with DHF/DSS, viral antigens have been found in macrophages and lung vascular endothelium.[154] Nevertheless, ECs did not reveal morphological injury, whereas high levels of adhesion molecules (ICAM-a and VCAM-1) in blood, witnessed activation of endothelium. Further production of cytokines plays an important role to the pathogenesis of DHF/DSS, by affecting vascular permeability. The severity of the disease is related to high levels of IL-8 and low levels of IL-12.[155,156] Moreover, plasma levels of VEGFR2 correlate inversely to the severity of leakage, while the degree of reduction of VEGFR2 levels, is associated with the viral load.[157]

In vitro studies in HUVEC confirmed the latent mechanisms of DV-related endothelial activation and damage, focusing on the role of "cytokine storm."[158] Furthermore, according to Zhang et al.,[160] increased TM expression has been described in HUVEC leading to extreme coagulation. B3 integrin, the cellular receptor of DV, is upregulated after DV infection, playing pivotal role in regulation of capillary permeability.[159]

Conclusively, DV infection is characterized by plasma leakage and edema formation. Host immune response combined with other host factor cascades contribute to the pathology of the disease, while ECs remain morphologically intact.

4.10.7 Human Immunodeficiency Virus

Human immunodeficiency virus (HIV) is a virus impairing the host's immune system. Several lung diseases have been associated with HIV infection, such as bacterial pneumonia, *Pneumocystis pneumonia* and tuberculosis. However, given the longer survival of HIV patients, noninfectious complications of HIV infection have become apparent and might significantly affect morbidity and mortality.[160] Among these pulmonary complications are PAH and atherosclerosis.[161] The incidence of HIV-related PAH is reported to be 0.5% of HIV-infected patients.[162] Histology of vascular lesions is similar to the lesions found in other patients with PAH: An angioproliferative disease with laminar intimal fibrosis, medial hypotrophy, and plexiform lesions.[163]

It appears that vascular endothelium is a possible target of HIV, albeit the exact pathogenic mechanism is not clarified. HIV does not directly insult pulmonary endothelium.[164] However, HIV proteins might be noxious to the endothelium. The most important HIV proteins involved in cardiopulmonary complications are envelope glycoprotein-120 (gp-120), trans-activator of transcription (Tat protein) and the negative factor (Nef). Gp-120 has been found to induce the production of proinflammatory cytokines, accentuate endothelin secretion and increase apoptosis of ECs.[165] Tat protein activates lung ECs and might play a role in angiogenesis.[166] Nef protein probably exhibits the most important role in the pathogenesis of HIV-related PAH. Nef is associated to the maintenance of high viral loads, and influences the clinical evolution to AIDS.[167] Interestingly, specific chemokine receptors allow the entrance of extracellular Nef in lung ECs, even in the absence of HIV infection.[168]

An experimental study performed in HIV-Nef-treated porcine pulmonary arterial rings and human pulmonary arterial ECs, showed that Nef significantly reduced endothelium-dependent vasorelaxation.[169] The same protein was found to significantly reduce NO levels, by decreasing vessel NOS expression. NO plays a key role in supporting vascular integrity, as it determines the production of growth factors regulating angiogenesis and smooth muscle proliferation, and modulates cell adhesion and platelet aggregation.[170] The Nef-induced decreased NO production, may lead to endothelial damage and consequent pulmonary hypertension.

To conclude, HIV infection is an established risk factor for the development of PAH, carrying poor prognosis and high mortality. The implicating pathophysiological mechanism might be related to the deleterious effect of viral proteins on lung ECs.

4.10.8 Severe Acute Respiratory Syndrome Coronavirus

Severe acute respiratory syndrome (SARS) is an infectious disease with significant mortality (10%), etiologically related to a coronavirus (SARS-CoV). SARS-CoV infection contributes to systemic vasculitis affecting small vessels of lung and other organs of the body.[171] The prominent clinical characteristic of the syndrome is respiratory distress due to pulmonary edema, whereas the accompanying histological finding is diffuse alveolar damage.[172] It has been recently discovered that the functional receptor for SARS-CoV is ACE-2.[173] ACE-2 is a metallopeptidase expressed on lung alveolar epithelial cells, in arterial and venous ECs and arterial smooth muscle cells.[174] As previously analyzed, it plays a significant role in vascular permeability and the regulation of inflammatory mediators: In mutant mice, loss of ACE-2 expression led to increased vascular permeability and neutrophil accumulation, while ACE-2 improved acute lung injury in ACE-2 knockout mice.[175]

According to recent research, ACE-2 is highly expressed in pneumocytes type I and type II and in ECs of many human organs, in cases of proven SARS.[174] The increased expression of ACE-2 enhances viral replication and contributes to the disruption of alveolar wall, resulting in diffuse alveolar damage and pulmonary edema.

4.11 CONCLUSION

Pulmonary endothelium is a major metabolic organ, the functional integrity of which is of paramount importance for the maintenance of pulmonary and systemic vascular homeostasis. Among others, pulmonary endothelium in health promotes barrier integrity and hemofluidity, additionally acting as an anti-inflammatory, antiproliferative, and vasodilation promoter mainly through its paracrine and endocrine properties. Exposure of the pulmonary EC to noxious stimuli and pathogens like viruses will derange or even reverse the above-mentioned protective features transforming the friend to a foe and promoting lung vascular injury. Understanding further the virus-induced pathogenesis of pulmonary endothelial functional and structural injury should allow the addition of new weapons in our armamentarium in an effort to prevent and treat lung-related pathologies.

REFERENCES

1. Mehta D, Malik AB. Signaling mechanisms regulating endothelial permeability. *Physiol Rev* 2006; **86**(1): 279–367.
2. Orfanos SE, Mavrommati I, Korovesi I, Roussos C. Pulmonary endothelium in acute lung injury: From basic science to the critically ill. *Intensive Care Med* 2004; **30**(9): 1702–14.
3. Stevens T, Phan S, Frid MG, Alvarez D, Herzog E, Stenmark KR. Lung vascular cell heterogeneity: Endothelium, smooth muscle, and fibroblasts. *Proc Am Thorac Soc* 2008; **5**(7): 783–91.
4. Morel DR, Dargent F, Bachmann M, Suter PM, Junod AF. Pulmonary extraction of serotonin and propranolol in patients with adult respiratory distress syndrome. *Am Rev Respir Dis* 1985; **132**(3): 479–84.
5. Block ER. Pulmonary endothelial cell pathobiology: Implications for acute lung injury. *Am J Med Sci* 1992; **304**(2): 136–44.
6. Esmon CT. Protein C anticoagulant system—Anti-inflammatory effects. *Semin Immunopathol* 2012; **34**(1): 127–32.
7. Bretschneider E, Uzonyi B, Weber AA et al. Human vascular smooth muscle cells express functionally active endothelial cell protein C receptor. *Circ Res* 2007; **100**(2): 255–62.
8. Mosnier LO, Zlokovic BV, Griffin JH. The cytoprotective protein C pathway. *Blood* 2007; **109**(8): 3161–72.

9. Brueckmann M, Horn S, Lang S et al. Recombinant human activated protein C upregulates cyclooxygenase-2 expression in endothelial cells via binding to endothelial cell protein C receptor and activation of protease-activated receptor-1. *Thromb Haemost* 2005; **93**(4): 743–50.
10. Isobe H, Okajima K, Uchiba M et al. Activated protein C prevents endotoxin-induced hypotension in rats by inhibiting excessive production of nitric oxide. *Circulation* 2001; **104**(10): 1171–5.
11. Rezaie AR. Regulation of the protein C anticoagulant and anti-inflammatory pathways. *Curr Med Chem* 2010; **17**(19): 2059–69.
12. Zeng W, Matter WF, Yan SB, Um SL, Vlahos CJ, Liu L. Effect of drotrecogin alfa (activated) on human endothelial cell permeability and Rho kinase signaling. *Crit Care Med* 2004; **32**(5 Suppl): S302–8.
13. Finigan JH, Dudek SM, Singleton PA et al. Activated protein C mediates novel lung endothelial barrier enhancement: Role of sphingosine 1-phosphate receptor transactivation. *J Biol Chem* 2005; **280**(17): 17286–93.
14. Lampugnani MG, Orsenigo F, Gagliani MC, Tacchetti C, Dejana E. Vascular endothelial cadherin controls VEGFR-2 internalization and signaling from intracellular compartments. *J Cell Biol* 2006; **174**(4): 593–604.
15. Quadri SK. Cross talk between focal adhesion kinase and cadherins: Role in regulating endothelial barrier function. *Microvasc Res* 2012; **83**(1): 3–11.
16. Schnitzer JE, Oh P. Aquaporin-1 in plasma membrane and caveolae provides mercury-sensitive water channels across lung endothelium. *Am J Physiol* 1996; **270**(1 Pt 2): H416–22.
17. Sowa G. Caveolae, caveolins, cavins, and endothelial cell function: New insights. *Front Physiol* 2012; **2**: 120.
18. Maniatis NA, Chernaya O, Shinin V, Minshall RD. Caveolins and lung function. *Adv Exp Med Biol* 2012; **729**: 157–79.
19. Dudek SM, Garcia JG. Cytoskeletal regulation of pulmonary vascular permeability. *J Appl Physiol* 2001; **91**(4): 1487–500.
20. Thickett DR, Armstrong L, Christie SJ, Millar AB. Vascular endothelial growth factor may contribute to increased vascular permeability in acute respiratory distress syndrome. *Am J Respir Crit Care Med* 2001; **164**(9): 1601–5.
21. Hallgren R, Samuelsson T, Venge P, Modig J. Eosinophil activation in the lung is related to lung damage in adult respiratory distress syndrome. *Am Rev Respir Dis* 1987; **135**(3): 639–42.
22. Rowen JL, Hyde DM, McDonald RJ. Eosinophils cause acute edematous injury in isolated perfused rat lungs. *Am Rev Respir Dis* 1990; **142**(1): 215–20.
23. Somers WS, Tang J, Shaw GD, Camphausen RT. Insights into the molecular basis of leukocyte tethering and rolling revealed by structures of P- and E-selectin bound to SLe(X) and PSGL-1. *Cell* 2000; **103**(3): 467–79.
24. Albelda SM, Smith CW, Ward PA. Adhesion molecules and inflammatory injury. *FASEB J* 1994; **8**(8): 504–12.
25. Lum H, Roebuck KA. Oxidant stress and endothelial cell dysfunction. *Am J Physiol Cell Physiol* 2001; **280**(4): C719–41.
26. Folkesson HG, Matthay MA. Inhibition of CD18 or CD11b attenuates acute lung injury after acid instillation in rabbits. *J Appl Physiol* 1997; **82**(6): 1743–50.
27. Sato N, Suzuki Y, Nishio K et al. Roles of ICAM-1 for abnormal leukocyte recruitment in the microcirculation of bleomycin-induced fibrotic lung injury. *Am J Respir Crit Care Med* 2000; **161**(5): 1681–8.
28. Azuma A, Takahashi S, Nose M et al. Role of E-selectin in bleomycin induced lung fibrosis in mice. *Thorax* 2000; **55**(2): 147–52.
29. Folch E, Salas A, Panes J et al. Role of P-selectin and ICAM-1 in pancreatitis-induced lung inflammation in rats: Significance of oxidative stress. *Ann Surg* 1999; **230**(6): 792–8; discussion 8–9.
30. Moriuchi H, Zaha M, Fukumoto T, Yuizono T. Activation of polymorphonuclear leukocytes in oleic acid-induced lung injury. *Intensive Care Med* 1998; **24**(7): 709–15.
31. Sheridan BC, McIntyre RC, Jr., Moore EE, Meldrum DR, Agrafojo J, Fullerton DA. Neutrophils mediate pulmonary vasomotor dysfunction in endotoxin-induced acute lung injury. *J Trauma* 1997; **42**(3): 391–6; discussion 6–7.
32. Sakamaki F, Ishizaka A, Handa M et al. Soluble form of P-selectin in plasma is elevated in acute lung injury. *Am J Respir Crit Care Med* 1995; **151**(6): 1821–6.
33. Moss M, Gillespie MK, Ackerson L, Moore FA, Moore EE, Parsons PE. Endothelial cell activity varies in patients at risk for the adult respiratory distress syndrome. *Crit Care Med* 1996; **24**(11): 1782–6.
34. Donnelly SC, Haslett C, Dransfield I et al. Role of selectins in development of adult respiratory distress syndrome. *Lancet* 1994; **344**(8917): 215–9.

35. Wort SJ, Evans TW. The role of the endothelium in modulating vascular control in sepsis and related conditions. *Br Med Bull* 1999; **55**(1): 30–48.
36. Aird WC. Phenotypic heterogeneity of the endothelium: II. Representative vascular beds. *Circ Res* 2007; **100**(2): 174–90.
37. Blackwell TS, Christman JW. The role of nuclear factor-kappa B in cytokine gene regulation. *Am J Respir Cell Mol Biol* 1997; **17**(1): 3–9.
38. Maniatis NA, Kotanidou A, Catravas JD, Orfanos SE. Endothelial pathomechanisms in acute lung injury. *Vasc Pharmacol* 2008; **49**(4–6): 119–33.
39. Mawji IA, Marsden PA. Perturbations in paracrine control of the circulation: Role of the endothelial-derived vasomediators, endothelin-1 and nitric oxide. *Microsc Res Tech* 2003; **60**(1): 46–58.
40. Liu SF, Crawley DE, Barnes PJ, Evans TW. Endothelium-derived relaxing factor inhibits hypoxic pulmonary vasoconstriction in rats. *Am Rev Respir Dis* 1991; **143**(1): 32–7.
41. Hart CM. Nitric oxide in adult lung disease. *Chest* 1999; **115**(5): 1407–17.
42. Adhikari NK, Burns KE, Friedrich JO, Granton JT, Cook DJ, Meade MO. Effect of nitric oxide on oxygenation and mortality in acute lung injury: systematic review and meta-analysis. *BMJ* 2007; **334**(7597): 779.
43. Chen X, Orfanos SE, Catravas JD. Effects of indomethacin on PMA-induced pulmonary endothelial enzyme dysfunction in vivo. *Am J Physiol* 1992; **262**(2 Pt 1): L153–62.
44. Gust R, Kozlowski JK, Stephenson AH, Schuster DP. Role of cyclooxygenase-2 in oleic acid-induced acute lung injury. *Am J Respir Crit Care Med* 1999; **160**(4): 1165–70.
45. Moloney ED, Evans TW. Pathophysiology and pharmacological treatment of pulmonary hypertension in acute respiratory distress syndrome. *Eur Respir J* 2003; **21**(4): 720–7.
46. Dupuis J, Stewart DJ, Cernacek P, Gosselin G. Human pulmonary circulation is an important site for both clearance and production of endothelin-1. *Circulation* 1996; **94**(7): 1578–84.
47. Langleben D, DeMarchie M, Laporta D, Spanier AH, Schlesinger RD, Stewart DJ. Endothelin-1 in acute lung injury and the adult respiratory distress syndrome. *Am Rev Respir Dis* 1993; **148**(6 Pt 1): 1646–50.
48. Sanai L, Haynes WG, MacKenzie A, Grant IS, Webb DJ. Endothelin production in sepsis and the adult respiratory distress syndrome. *Intensive Care Med* 1996; **22**(1): 52–6.
49. Orfanos SE, Armaganidis A, Glynos C et al. Pulmonary capillary endothelium-bound angiotensin-converting enzyme activity in acute lung injury. *Circulation* 2000; **102**(16): 2011–8.
50. Kohlstedt K, Brandes RP, Muller-Esterl W, Busse R, Fleming I. Angiotensin-converting enzyme is involved in outside-in signaling in endothelial cells. *Circ Res* 2004; **94**(1): 60–7.
51. Linz W, Wohlfart P, Scholkens BA, Malinski T, Wiemer G. Interactions among ACE, kinins and NO. *Cardiovasc Res* 1999; **43**(3): 549–61.
52. Casey L, Krieger B, Kohler J, Rice C, Oparil S, Szidon P. Decreased serum angiotensin converting enzyme in adult respiratory distress syndrome associated with sepsis: A preliminary report. *Crit Care Med* 1981; **9**(9): 651–4.
53. Orfanos SE, Langleben D, Khoury J et al. Pulmonary capillary endothelium-bound angiotensin-converting enzyme activity in humans. *Circulation* 1999; **99**(12): 1593–9.
54. Donoghue M, Hsieh F, Baronas E et al. A novel angiotensin-converting enzyme-related carboxypeptidase (ACE2) converts angiotensin I to angiotensin 1–9. *Circ Res* 2000; **87**(5): E1–9.
55. Kaparianos A, Argyropoulou E. Local renin-angiotensin II systems, angiotensin-converting enzyme and its homologue ACE2: Their potential role in the pathogenesis of chronic obstructive pulmonary diseases, pulmonary hypertension and acute respiratory distress syndrome. *Curr Med Chem* 2011; **18**(23): 3506–15.
56. Turner AJ, Hiscox JA, Hooper NM. ACE2: From vasopeptidase to SARS virus receptor. *Trends Pharmacol Sci* 2004; **25**(6): 291–4.
57. Morrell NW, Adnot S, Archer SL et al. Cellular and molecular basis of pulmonary arterial hypertension. *J Am Coll Cardiol* 2009; **54**(1 Suppl): S20–31.
58. Kim KT, Choi HH, Steinmetz MO et al. Oligomerization and multimerization are critical for angiopoietin-1 to bind and phosphorylate Tie2. *J Biol Chem* 2005; **280**(20): 20126–31.
59. Albini A, Noonan DM. Angiopoietin2 and tie2: Tied to lymphangiogenesis and lung metastasis. New perspectives in antimetastatic antiangiogenic therapy. *J Natl Cancer Inst* 2012; **104**(6): 429–31.
60. Carlson TR, Feng Y, Maisonpierre PC, Mrksich M, Morla AO. Direct cell adhesion to the angiopoietins mediated by integrins. *J Biol Chem* 2001; **276**(28): 26516–25.
61. Holopainen T, Huang H, Chen C et al. Angiopoietin-1 overexpression modulates vascular endothelium to facilitate tumor cell dissemination and metastasis establishment. *Cancer Res* 2009; **69**(11): 4656–64.
62. Holopainen T, Saharinen P, D'Amico G et al. Effects of angiopoietin-2-blocking antibody on endothelial cell–cell junctions and lung metastasis. *J Natl Cancer Inst* 2012; **104**(6): 461–75.

63. Dewachter L, Adnot S, Fadel E et al. Angiopoietin/Tie2 pathway influences smooth muscle hyperplasia in idiopathic pulmonary hypertension. *Am J Respir Crit Care Med* 2006; **174**(9): 1025–33.
64. Sullivan CC, Du L, Chu D et al. Induction of pulmonary hypertension by an angiopoietin 1/TIE2/serotonin pathway. *Proc Natl Acad Sci USA* 2003; **100**(21): 12331–6.
65. Chu D, Sullivan CC, Du L et al. A new animal model for pulmonary hypertension based on the overexpression of a single gene, angiopoietin-1. *Ann Thorac Surg* 2004; **77**(2): 449–56; discussion 56–7.
66. Kido M, Du L, Sullivan CC, Deutsch R, Jamieson SW, Thistlethwaite PA. Gene transfer of a TIE2 receptor antagonist prevents pulmonary hypertension in rodents. *J Thorac Cardiovasc Surg* 2005; **129**(2): 268–76.
67. McCarter SD, Mei SH, Lai PF et al. Cell-based angiopoietin-1 gene therapy for acute lung injury. *Am J Respir Crit Care Med* 2007; **175**(10): 1014–26.
68. Xu J, Qu J, Cao L et al. Mesenchymal stem cell-based angiopoietin-1 gene therapy for acute lung injury induced by lipopolysaccharide in mice. *J Pathol* 2008; **214**(4): 472–81.
69. Mammoto T, Parikh SM, Mammoto A et al. Angiopoietin-1 requires p190 RhoGAP to protect against vascular leakage in vivo. *J Biol Chem* 2007; **282**(33): 23910–8.
70. Parikh SM, Mammoto T, Schultz A et al. Excess circulating angiopoietin-2 may contribute to pulmonary vascular leak in sepsis in humans. *PLoS Med* 2006; **3**(3): e46.
71. Bhandari V, Choo-Wing R, Lee CG et al. Hyperoxia causes angiopoietin 2-mediated acute lung injury and necrotic cell death. *Nat Med* 2006; **12**(11): 1286–93.
72. Bhandari V, Choo-Wing R, Harijith A et al. Increased hyperoxia-induced lung injury in nitric oxide synthase 2 null mice is mediated via angiopoietin 2. *Am J Respir Cell Mol Biol* 2012; **46**(5): 668–76.
73. Daly C, Pasnikowski E, Burova E et al. Angiopoietin-2 functions as an autocrine protective factor in stressed endothelial cells. *Proc Natl Acad Sci USA* 2006; **103**(42): 15491–6.
74. Orfanos SE, Kotanidou A, Glynos C et al. Angiopoietin-2 is increased in severe sepsis: Correlation with inflammatory mediators. *Crit Care Med* 2007; **35**(1): 199–206.
75. Ong T, McClintock DE, Kallet RH, Ware LB, Matthay MA, Liu KD. Ratio of angiopoietin-2 to angiopoietin-1 as a predictor of mortality in acute lung injury patients. *Crit Care Med* 2010; **38**(9): 1845–51.
76. Ahmad S, Hewett PW, Wang P et al. Direct evidence for endothelial vascular endothelial growth factor receptor-1 function in nitric oxide-mediated angiogenesis. *Circ Res* 2006; **99**(7): 715–22.
77. Lahm T, Crisostomo PR, Markel TA, Wang M, Lillemoe KD, Meldrum DR. The critical role of vascular endothelial growth factor in pulmonary vascular remodeling after lung injury. *Shock* 2007; **28**(1): 4–14.
78. Akeson AL, Greenberg JM, Cameron JE et al. Temporal and spatial regulation of VEGF-A controls vascular patterning in the embryonic lung. *Dev Biol* 2003; **264**(2): 443–55.
79. Gerber HP, Hillan KJ, Ryan AM et al. VEGF is required for growth and survival in neonatal mice. *Development* 1999; **126**(6): 1149–59.
80. Le Cras TD, Markham NE, Tuder RM, Voelkel NF, Abman SH. Treatment of newborn rats with a VEGF receptor inhibitor causes pulmonary hypertension and abnormal lung structure. *Am J Physiol Lung Cell Mol Physiol* 2002; **283**(3): L555–62.
81. Waltenberger J, Claesson-Welsh L, Siegbahn A, Shibuya M, Heldin CH. Different signal transduction properties of KDR and Flt1, two receptors for vascular endothelial growth factor. *J Biol Chem* 1994; **269**(43): 26988–95.
82. Abadie Y, Bregeon F, Papazian L et al. Decreased VEGF concentration in lung tissue and vascular injury during ARDS. *Eur Respir J* 2005; **25**(1): 139–46.
83. Medford AR, Millar AB. Vascular endothelial growth factor (VEGF) in acute lung injury (ALI) and acute respiratory distress syndrome (ARDS): Paradox or paradigm? *Thorax* 2006; **61**(7): 621–6.
84. Nicolls MR, Mizuno S, Taraseviciene-Stewart L et al. New models of pulmonary hypertension based on VEGF receptor blockade-induced endothelial cell apoptosis. *Pulm Circ* 2012; **2**(4): 434–42.
85. Armstrong SM, Wang C, Tigdi J et al. Influenza infects lung microvascular endothelium leading to microvascular leak: Role of apoptosis and claudin-5. *PLoS One* 2012; **7**(10): e47323.
86. Dominguez-Cherit G, Lapinsky SE, Macias AE et al. Critically Ill patients with 2009 influenza A(H1N1) in Mexico. *JAMA* 2009; **302**(17): 1880–7.
87. Teijaro JR, Walsh KB, Cahalan S et al. Endothelial cells are central orchestrators of cytokine amplification during influenza virus infection. *Cell* 2011; **146**(6): 980–91.
88. Kobasa D, Jones SM, Shinya K et al. Aberrant innate immune response in lethal infection of macaques with the 1918 influenza virus. *Nature* 2007; **445**(7125): 319–23.
89. de Jong MD, Simmons CP, Thanh TT et al. Fatal outcome of human influenza A (H5N1) is associated with high viral load and hypercytokinemia. *Nat Med* 2006; **12**(10): 1203–7.

140. Macneil A, Nichol ST, Spiropoulou CF. Hantavirus pulmonary syndrome. *Virus Res* 2011; **162**(1–2): 138–47.
141. Markotic A, Hensley L, Daddario K, Spik K, Anderson K, Schmaljohn C. Pathogenic hantaviruses elicit different immunoreactions in THP-1 cells and primary monocytes and induce differentiation of human monocytes to dendritic-like cells. *Coll Antropol* 2007; **31**(4): 1159–67.
142. Marsac D, Garcia S, Fournet A et al. Infection of human monocyte-derived dendritic cells by ANDES Hantavirus enhances pro-inflammatory state, the secretion of active MMP-9 and indirectly enhances endothelial permeability. *Virol J* 2011; **8**: 223.
143. Geimonen E, Neff S, Raymond T, Kocer SS, Gavrilovskaya IN, Mackow ER. Pathogenic and nonpathogenic hantaviruses differentially regulate endothelial cell responses. *Proc Natl Acad Sci USA* 2002; **99**(21): 13837–42.
144. Gavrilovskaya IN, Gorbunova EE, Mackow ER. Pathogenic hantaviruses direct the adherence of quiescent platelets to infected endothelial cells. *J Virol* 2010; **84**(9): 4832–9.
145. Shay-Salit A, Shushy M, Wolfovitz E et al. VEGF receptor 2 and the adherens junction as a mechanical transducer in vascular endothelial cells. *Proc Natl Acad Sci USA* 2002; **99**(14): 9462–7.
146. Gorbunova E, Gavrilovskaya IN, Mackow ER. Pathogenic hantaviruses Andes virus and Hantaan virus induce adherens junction disassembly by directing vascular endothelial cadherin internalization in human endothelial cells. *J Virol* 2010; **84**(14): 7405–11.
147. Hwang JY, Park JW, Hong SY, Park HS. Reduced expression of angiopoietin-1 in Hantaan virus-infected human umbilical vein endothelial cell increases their permeability. *Acta Virol* 2009; **53**(1): 7–13.
148. Geisbert TW, Young HA, Jahrling PB et al. Pathogenesis of Ebola hemorrhagic fever in primate models: Evidence that hemorrhage is not a direct effect of virus-induced cytolysis of endothelial cells. *Am J Pathol* 2003; **163**(6): 2371–82.
149. Zaki SR, Goldsmith CS. Pathologic features of filovirus infections in humans. *Curr Top Microbiol Immunol* 1999; **235**: 97–116.
150. Yang ZY, Duckers HJ, Sullivan NJ, Sanchez A, Nabel EG, Nabel GJ. Identification of the Ebola virus glycoprotein as the main viral determinant of vascular cell cytotoxicity and injury. *Nat Med* 2000; **6**(8): 886–9.
151. Mantovani A, Bussolino F, Dejana E. Cytokine regulation of endothelial cell function. *FASEB J: Off Publ Fed Am Soc Exp Biol* 1992; **6**(8): 2591–9.
152. Peters CJ, Zaki SR. Role of the endothelium in viral hemorrhagic fevers. *Crit Care Med* 2002; **30**(5 Suppl): S268–73.
153. Basu A, Chaturvedi UC. Vascular endothelium: The battlefield of dengue viruses. *FEMS Immunol Med Microbiol* 2008; **53**(3): 287–99.
154. Jessie K, Fong MY, Devi S, Lam SK, Wong KT. Localization of dengue virus in naturally infected human tissues, by immunohistochemistry and *in situ* hybridization. *J Infect Dis* 2004; **189**(8): 1411–8.
155. Pacsa AS, Agarwal R, Elbishbishi EA, Chaturvedi UC, Nagar R, Mustafa AS. Role of interleukin-12 in patients with dengue hemorrhagic fever. *FEMS Immunol Med Microbiol* 2000; **28**(2): 151–5.
156. Raghupathy R, Chaturvedi UC, Al-Sayer H et al. Elevated levels of IL-8 in dengue hemorrhagic fever. *J Med Virol* 1998; **56**(3): 280–5.
157. Srikiatkhachorn A, Ajariyakhajorn C, Endy TP et al. Virus-induced decline in soluble vascular endothelial growth receptor 2 is associated with plasma leakage in dengue hemorrhagic fever. *J Virol* 2007; **81**(4): 1592–600.
158. Carr JM, Hocking H, Bunting K et al. Supernatants from dengue virus type-2 infected macrophages induce permeability changes in endothelial cell monolayers. *J Med Virol* 2003; **69**(4): 521–8.
159. Zhang JL, Wang JL, Gao N, Chen ZT, Tian YP, An J. Up-regulated expression of beta3 integrin induced by dengue virus serotype 2 infection associated with virus entry into human dermal microvascular endothelial cells. *Biochem Biophys Res Commun* 2007; **356**(3): 763–8.
160. Braithwaite RS, Justice AC, Chang CC et al. Estimating the proportion of patients infected with HIV who will die of comorbid diseases. *Am J Med* 2005; **118**(8): 890–8.
161. Crum NF, Riffenburgh RH, Wegner S et al. Comparisons of causes of death and mortality rates among HIV-infected persons: Analysis of the pre-, early, and late HAART (highly active antiretroviral therapy) eras. *J Acquir Immune Defic Syndr* 2006; **41**(2): 194–200.
162. Almodovar S, Hsue PY, Morelli J, Huang L, Flores SC. Pathogenesis of HIV-associated pulmonary hypertension: potential role of HIV-1 Nef. *Proc Am Thoracic Soc* 2011; **8**(3): 308–12.
163. Petitpretz P, Brenot F, Azarian R et al. Pulmonary hypertension in patients with human immunodeficiency virus infection. Comparison with primary pulmonary hypertension. *Circulation* 1994; **89**(6): 2722–7.

164. Marecki JC, Cool CD, Parr JE et al. HIV-1 Nef is associated with complex pulmonary vascular lesions in SHIV-nef-infected macaques. *Am J Resp Crit Care Med* 2006; **174**(4): 437–45.
165. Kanmogne GD, Primeaux C, Grammas P. Induction of apoptosis and endothelin-1 secretion in primary human lung endothelial cells by HIV-1 gp120 proteins. *Biochem Biophys Res Commun* 2005; **333**(4): 1107–15.
166. Albini A, Barillari G, Benelli R, Gallo RC, Ensoli B. Angiogenic properties of human immunodeficiency virus type 1 Tat protein. *Proc Natl Acad Sci USA* 1995; **92**(11): 4838–42.
167. Lindwasser OW, Chaudhuri R, Bonifacino JS. Mechanisms of CD4 downregulation by the Nef and Vpu proteins of primate immunodeficiency viruses. *Curr Mol Med* 2007; **7**(2): 171–84.
168. Roeth JF, Collins KL. Human immunodeficiency virus type 1 Nef: Adapting to intracellular trafficking pathways. *Microbiol Mol Biol Rev* 2006; **70**(2): 548–63.
169. Duffy P, Wang X, Lin PH, Yao Q, Chen C. HIV Nef protein causes endothelial dysfunction in porcine pulmonary arteries and human pulmonary artery endothelial cells. *J Surg Res* 2009; **156**(2): 257–64.
170. Ganz P, Vita JA. Testing endothelial vasomotor function: Nitric oxide, a multipotent molecule. *Circulation* 2003; **108**(17): 2049–53.
171. Kuiken T, Fouchier RA, Schutten M et al. Newly discovered coronavirus as the primary cause of severe acute respiratory syndrome. *Lancet* 2003; **362**(9380): 263–70.
172. Ding Y, Wang H, Shen H et al. The clinical pathology of severe acute respiratory syndrome (SARS): A report from China. *J Pathol* 2003; **200**(3): 282–9.
173. Imai Y, Kuba K, Penninger JM. Angiotensin-converting enzyme 2 in acute respiratory distress syndrome. *Cell Mol Life Sci* 2007; **64**(15): 2006–12.
174. Hamming I, Timens W, Bulthuis ML, Lely AT, Navis G, van Goor H. Tissue distribution of ACE2 protein, the functional receptor for SARS coronavirus. A first step in understanding SARS pathogenesis. *J Pathol* 2004; **203**(2): 631–7.
175. Kuba K, Imai Y, Penninger JM. Angiotensin-converting enzyme 2 in lung diseases. *Curr Opin Pharmacol* 2006; **6**(3): 271–6.

5 Cough Formation in Viral Infections in Children

Kerry-Ann F. O'Grady, Ian M. Mackay, and Anne B. Chang

CONTENTS

5.1 INTRODUCTION

Cough is a defensive and clearing mechanism that functions to remove mechanical and chemical irritants and debris from the airways.[1] In lay terms, cough is usually defined as a forceful release of air from the lungs accompanied by a sudden sharp sound. In medical terms, the definition of cough becomes more complex. It is commonly referred to as a three-phase event: an initial inspiration (the inspiratory phase), followed by closure of the glottis and a forced expiratory effort (the compressive phase), followed by opening of the glottis and vigorous expiration (the expulsive phase).[2] Cough may occur as a single event or as a cough "epoch" (or "bout" or "attack") that includes several or many expiratory efforts in a single episode.[2]

The importance of cough ranges from it being a transient cause of discomfort and nuisance,[3] to being a sentinel symptom of many chronic airway diseases.[3] Infectious and noninfectious, acute and chronic, upper and lower respiratory illnesses and injuries that have cough as a symptom remain leading causes of morbidity and mortality worldwide,[4–6] contributing to substantial disability-adjusted life years lost, poor quality of life, and reduced life expectancy.[4–6]

Here, we discuss the epidemiology and burden of cough, the physiology of cough as it relates to viral infection and the viruses commonly associated with cough in children. Finally, we discuss the gaps in clinical and public health knowledge that need to be addressed by high-quality studies.

5.2 COUGH

The etiologies that underpin the formation of cough are not a homogenous entity. The classification and differentiation of cough into specific phenotypes (acute/chronic, wet/dry, day/night, male/female, trigger-related) is becoming an increasingly important area of research in both adults and children.[7] Historically, this has been driven by a focus on the early identification of asthma in children and chronic obstructive pulmonary disease (COPD) in adults.[7–11] In children, the pivotal Tuscon Children's Respiratory Study[12,13] made a substantial contribution to the understanding of respiratory illnesses, their symptoms and etiologies, risk factors, and outcomes, and to understanding of the development of childhood asthma in particular. In adults, the "British hypothesis,"[9] that is, that recurrent bronchial infections in smokers were associated with progressive lung function decline, led to decades of research into the role of infections, chronic cough, and sputum production in airway and alveolar damage and disease progression.[9]

More recently, increases in asthma prevalence[14] and the importance of chronic lung diseases as leading causes of morbidity and mortality has driven the development of standardized tools and surveys to characterize and measure respiratory symptoms, including cough,[15–19] and cough burden.[20–22] To date, however, there remains a high degree of variability in the reporting of cough prevalence, type, intensity, and severity reflecting different study designs, study populations, selection and recall biases, cough definitions, objective versus subjective cough reporting, and perceptions of cough.[7,23] Furthermore, there remains scarce data on the nature and burden of acute cough in children given the predominant focus on asthma and, to some degree, chronic cough.

5.2.1 Basic Physiology of Cough

To appreciate the physiology of cough related to viral infections, one needs a basic understanding of the physiology of the three phases of cough.[24] The inspiratory phase consists of inhaling a variable amount of air, which serves to lengthen the expiratory muscles, optimizing the length–tension relationship. The compressive phase consists of a very brief (200 ms) closure of the glottis to maintain lung volume as intrathoracic pressure builds (up to 300 mm Hg in adults) due to isometric contraction of the expiratory muscles against a closed glottis. The expiratory phase starts with opening of the glottis, releasing a brief (30–50 ms) supramaximal expiratory flow[25] (up to 12 L/s in adults, also termed the "cough spike") followed by lower (3–4 L/s) expiratory flows lasting a further 200–500 ms.[24] Dynamic compression of the airways occurs during the expiratory phase and the high-velocity expulsion of gas (air) sweeps airway debris along. Airway debris and secretions are also swept proximally by ciliary activity, which cough enhances in both healthy individuals as well as those with lung disease.[26]

Cough can be voluntarily initiated or suppressed except when it is part of the laryngeal expiratory reflex when the larynx is mechanically stimulated by foreign materials. Physiologists describe two basic types of cough; laryngeal cough (a true reflex, also known as "expiratory reflex") and tracheo-bronchial cough. Laryngeal cough thus protects the airways from aspiration. Tracheo-bronchial cough is initiated distal to the larynx and can be volitional. It is primarily stimulated by chemoreceptors in the lower airways and can also be mechanically stimulated.[27] The primary function of tracheo-bronchial cough is airway clearance and maintenance of the mucociliary apparatus. Physiologists have argued that differentiating tracheo-bronchial cough from a expiration reflex and what constitutes a cough (e.g., the different phases and/or the sound) is important.[28] However, clinicians remain certain about what a cough is in the clinical setting.

The knowledge of cough neurophysiology has significantly advanced in recent years, although much of the work is based on animal models and may have limited applicability to humans as significant interspecies differences exist.[29] Readers are referred to recent reviews[29–32] for in-depth aspects of cough-related neurophysiology. As a gross over-simplification, the cough pathway can be compartmentalized to the afferent arm (from cough stimulus to the respiratory center) and efferent arms (from respiratory center to respiratory muscles, larynx, and pelvic muscles) of the cough pathway. These are likely to be influenced by a bidirectional feedback loop, but this has not yet been clearly established. Receptors involved in cough are terminations of vagal afferents in airway mucosa and submucosa.[29,33,34] These afferent receptors have different sensitivity to different stimuli and are unequally distributed in the airways; generally, the larynx and proximal large airways are more mechanosensitive and less chemosensitive than peripheral large airways. The existence of distinct cough receptors, widely assumed to be present and first proposed by Widdicombe,[35] is now proven.[30,33] Generation of action potentials (depolarization of the terminal membrane) from these receptors are subclassified into ionotropic receptors (cause generator potentials by acting on ligand-gated ion channels) and metabotropic receptors (act indirectly on ligand-gated ion channels via G-protein-coupled receptors).[29,36] These include the transient receptor-potential cation channel subfamily V member 1 (TRPV1), transient receptor-potential cation channel subfamily A member 1 (TRPA1), and G-protein-coupled opioid-like receptor-1 (NOP1) receptors.[37]

These cough and airway receptors mediate through the vagus nerve, jugular, and nodose ganglions and extend to the nucleus tractus solitaris (NTS), which is the first central nervous system (CNS) synaptic contact for these afferent fibers.[38] Second-order neurons from the NTS have polysynaptic connections with the central cough generator, which is also the respiratory pattern generator.[32,38] NTS is postulated to be the site of greatest modulatory influence and plasticity. The mechanisms underpinning chronic cough have been likened to that of chronic pain[27] and increased neurogenic markers have been described in children with increased cough receptor sensitivity.[39] The intrathoracic pressure and effects of it generated by cough may also perpetuate the chronic cough cycle as suggested by a recent animal study that showed pressure effects enhance cough sensitivity.[40]

5.2.1.1 Physiology of Cough in Relation to Viruses

As described in the section on the epidemiology of cough and viral infections, viral-induced cough is likely the most common cause of acute cough. However, viruses are also a likely trigger of chronic cough in people with established lung diseases. In the clinical context, cough related to viral infections is acute bronchitis. The precise mechanisms underpinning acute bronchitis will vary depending on the insulting agent (properties of the infectious agent) and the host characteristics (e.g., preexisting conditions) and response (such as the host's innate and adaptive immunity, genetic predispositions to intensity of inflammation). This is briefly discussed below.

The pathophysiology by which cough occurs in the context of a viral infection is manyfold, but proving cause and effect is difficult in human studies. These mechanisms include trigger points of the cough reflex as exemplified below.

5.2.1.1.1 Airway Inflammation

The cellular responses to protect the host in response to a viral infection include an inflammation cascade and cytokine release. Inflammation of the lower respiratory tract (LRT) has been described in children with clinically trivial colds, and can persist for up to 1 week after complete resolution of coryzal symptoms.[41] Various inflammation components can directly enhance or stimulate the cough reflex such as bradykinin,[42] substance P,[31] prostaglandins, lipid mediators,[37] and calcitonin gene-related peptide (CGRP).

5.2.1.1.2 Airway Narrowing

Viruses can trigger airway hyperresponsiveness.[42] The resultant airway narrowing can trigger cough due to mechanical deformation, which stimulates cough receptors in the airways. In the laboratory, bronchoconstriction and cough pathways can be separately inhibited. Medications (lignocaine, oral codeine) can inhibit cough and have no effect on bronchoconstriction. Conversely, medications (cromoglygate, atropine) can inhibit the pharmacologically induced bronchoconstriction, but have no effect on the cough response of adults.[27]

Alterations of the central cough pathway: Viral infections also likely alter the central mechanisms of cough.[43]

5.2.1.1.3 Mucus Hypersecretion

In large conducting airways, cough receptors and the submucosal gland ducts are colocalized.[44] Viral infections stimulate mucosal glands and the mucin produced then causes cough. One mechanism involves stimulation of the epidermal growth factor receptor cascade.[44]

Cough receptors and sensory nerve hypersensitivity: The mechanism is not understood but cough receptor sensitivity occurs in almost all conditions associated with cough. This has also been described in people with an upper respiratory tract (URT) infection.[45] In many, this is temporary and when the cough abates, the hypersensitivity resolves.[46,47] However, in some, akin to the pathological pain,[27] this persists and is associated with chronic cough.

5.2.1.1.4 Epithelial Cell Necrosis

Viruses such as influenza virus (IFV) can cause epithelial cell necrosis and apoptosis, which then induces an inflammatory process[48,49] and hence cough.

5.2.1.1.5 Virus–Bacteria Coinfection

Respiratory infections, ostensibly viral in nature, can prepare the way for bacterial superinfections and increased morbidity.[50,51] A brief discussion of viruses and bacteria in the upper airways is described in a later section of this chapter. Bacteria infection following a viral infection is most obvious in the polymicrobial diseases sinusitis,[52] otitis media,[53] cystic fibrosis,[54] and pneumonia.[55] While virus-alone or bacteria-alone infections are associated with disease,[56] there is also a risk of disease when both viruses and bacteria or different bacteria, co-occur or when viral infection upsets a balance between host and colonized bacteria.[57,58] Animal studies show that virus–bacteria interactions have a role in disease development[53] and that immune modulation by IFV can induce microenvironmental change.[59] Viruses are also associated with increased adherence of bacteria in human epithelial cell cultures.[60] Carriage of bacteria is at its most widespread in early childhood,[61] a time when repeated cytopathic viral infections are thought to create the acute inflammatory setting upon which chronic inflammatory disease develops. Preventing excessive acute inflammation from virulent virus infections may prevent a bacterial passenger from becoming a bacterial pathogen.

These relationships are receiving greater attention via recent pneumococcal vaccine trials. A small 2×2 factorial trial of antenatal influenza vaccination of mothers and 7-valent pneumococcal conjugate vaccination of their infants in Bangladesh found an efficacy of this vaccine strategy during an influenza season of 72.4% (95%CI 30.2–89.1%) against febrile respiratory illness and 66.4% against medically attended acute respiratory illness (ARI) in the first six months of infancy.[62] These findings support previous observations of the interaction between influenza virus and *Streptococcus pneumoniae*.[63–65]

Protracted bacterial bronchitis (PBB), a type of chronic airway inflammation in children, is a recent diagnostic clinical entity.[66] PBB is associated with persistent bacterial infection in the airways[66] and it is widely accepted that persistent bacterial infection is harmful to the airways.[67] The organisms most commonly identified in the airways (sputum or bronchoalveolar lavage, BAL) of children with PBB are common respiratory bacteria, that is, nontypeable *Haemophilus influenzae, S. pneumoniae*, and *Moraxella catarrhalis*.[66] However, transient viral ARIs in early childhood commonly precede PBB as the most common initiating event; more recent studies have found virus–bacteria coinfections in the BAL of children with PBB and wet cough.[68] Disease mechanisms involved in PBB include neutrophilic inflammation, innate immunity upregulation in the airways,[69] and altered expression of both the toll-like receptor (TLR)-4 and the preprotachykinin gene, TAC1, that encodes substance P.[70]

5.2.1.2 Physiology in Otherwise Well People

Bronchitis occurs in almost all (if not all) airway diseases, at least intermittently during exacerbation phases. In the literal translation of the word, bronchitis refers to inflammation of the bronchus or bronchi. Cough usually occurs when bronchitis is present, other than when bronchitis is very mild.

Any pathogen that infects the respiratory tract can cause bronchitis and these include viruses, bacteria, fungi, and helminths. However, only viruses, bacteria, mycoplasma, and chlamydia are considered in the clinical phenotype of acute bronchitis. Respiratory viruses are the most common etiology.[71,72] Importantly, many infections involve both viruses (single or multiple) and bacteria.[73,74] In developed countries, both viral and bacterial infections are likely to be self-limited. Common respiratory viruses in children are rhinoviruses (HRVs), coronaviruses (hCoVs), respiratory syncytial virus (RSV) (A and B), parainfluenza viruses (1–3), influenza viruses human bocavirus (hBoV), adenoviruses (hAdVs), and human metapneumovirus (hMPV).[72] In the first year of life of a birth cohort (668 samples from 305 infants),[71] the most common respiratory pathogens were HRVs (73% of the samples), RSV (11%), and coronaviruses (8%). Another birth cohort (Switzerland)[75] described that all infants with ARI had a cough and one or more respiratory viruses were found in 88 of the 112 infants (79%); HRVs (23% of all viruses) and hCoVs (18%) were also the most common. In the Swiss cohort,[75] HRV, coronaviruses hBoV, and hMPV accounted for 60% of viruses identified, but symptom scores were similar for the various viral infections other than those for RSV cases who had more severe symptoms. Increasingly, previously unknown respiratory viruses are identified and recent additions to respiratory viruses include a third species of HRV, additional human enteroviruses (EVs), and parechoviruses (HPeVs).[76]

Although some viruses are more commonly associated with certain syndromes (e.g., RSV causing bronchiolitis and parainfluenza and hCoV-NL63 causing croup, both of which are associated with a coughing illness), any of these respiratory pathogens can cause acute bronchitis. With modern molecular techniques, coinfections are also found[76] in both symptomatic and asymptomatic children.[72,75] In the lower airways (broncho-alveolar lavage), viruses can be detected in 16.9% of cough-free children despite having no acute viral LRT infection symptoms.[68]

5.2.1.3 Physiology in People with an Underlying Disease

In people with an underlying lung disease such as asthma, COPD, and bronchiectasis, differentiating viral or bacterial infections as the initiator and/or cause of cough is very difficult. However, in many of these conditions, viral infections often trigger an exacerbation where cough is a dominant symptom.[77,78] The underlying cellular mechanisms associated with cough are likely similar to that discussed above but in a more exaggerated manner. For example, in people with bronchiectasis, the mucous glands are already in a stimulated state and, thus, an additional trigger from virus infection would likely exaggerate the response. Further, the response to viral infection in well people has been shown to be different to that from people with an underlying disease such as COPD.[79]

In a study on children with asthma and not hospitalized, viral infections were found in >50% and viral codetections occurred in 25.6% of children.[77] Coinfections were associated ($p = 0.04$) with lower asthma quality of life scores upon presentation than were single viral detections but the recovery phase (including symptoms of acute bronchitis) was not influenced by the undifferentiated presence or absence of virus.[76] In another study, multiple pathogens were significantly more common (17%) in the symptomatic episodes than asymptomatic episodes (3%).[72] However, there is no consensus in the literature about the relationship between clinical severity and presence of codetections. Persistent symptoms may relate to a bacterial infection, as either a consequence of altered immunity from initial viral insult[80] or a primary infection.[81]

Recent experimental studies have clearly demonstrated that HRV infections precipitate secondary bacterial infections in people with COPD.[79,82] The mechanism involved in this includes release

Prior hospitalization with ALRI is becoming recognized as a risk factor for the development of chronic cough, particularly wet cough.[118–122] The role of hospitalization because of acute viral ALRI in the development of chronic cough has not been well defined and follow-up studies are limited by selection biases, in particular loss to follow-up. Although somewhat limited by these biases, a small prospective study of 94 New Zealand children assessed by a respiratory physician 12 months after a hospital admission for pneumonia or severe bronchiolitis[122] found 30% of children had a history of chronic wet cough and 32% had a wet cough and/or crackles on examination in clinic. Follow-up of native Alaskan children enrolled in a case-control study of RSV hospitalizations before 2 years of age reported hospitalization for RSV infection in early childhood was associated with increased respiratory symptoms and increased chronic productive cough at 5–8 years of age.[123] In this study, however, less than half of the original study population was enrolled and other specific infections in the intervening period were not accounted for.

Data on the risk factors associated with the development of chronic cough after an acute ARI are scarce, including a paucity of differentiation between viral and bacterial risks and coinfection. Importantly, there are no data on whether the persistence of pathogens in the airways over the course of a cough illness is a factor in chronic cough development. Preliminary multivariate analyses of data from an Australian cohort study did not identify the presence of virus and/or bacteria at the time of acute illness to be independent predictors of chronic cough development.[117] In that study, a gestational age of less than 37 weeks, being indigenous, family history of chronic lung disease, and antibiotic use in the emergency department at the time of acute presentation were all associated with cough persistence.[117] In a case-control study of children with respiratory sequelae following severe RSV infection, the only factor suggestive of an association with chronic cough was the presence of a dog in the house (OR: 2.35; 95% CI: 0.89–6.11),[123] a finding also reported with respect to the development of asthma post RSV infection bronchiolitis.[124] These studies, however, have not examined the acquisition and persistence of other pathogens in the intervening period. In a UK study of the outcomes of hospitalization for community acquired pneumonia (median period since admission 5.6 years (range 4.4–7.4)) that did not differentiate between viral and bacterial etiology, only paternal eczema and preexisting asthma at the time of pneumonia were associated with chronic moist cough at follow-up.[119] Recurrent episodes of ALRI in infancy are associated with the development of bronchiectasis in Central Australian Aboriginal children together with other factors such as gestational age, birth weight, and nutritional status.[120]

5.6 THE BURDEN OF COUGH IN CHILDREN

Studies that have addressed the burden of cough as a symptom, particularly cough that is not associated with asthma and COPD, are limited. Even in studies of asthma and COPD burden, cough is usually one part of an overall tool designed to provide a composite rather than component score.[7] This is of particular relevance in attempts to describe the burden of cough due to infectious etiologies, and even more problematic when differentiating between viral and bacterial causes.

In one study in the United Kingdom, designed to test the repeatability of a parent-completed respiratory questionnaire, cough in the absence of other common cold symptoms was reported by a third of parents of young children (median age 17.7 months) and cough at night was reported by one in five parents.[125] The reported prevalence of pediatric nocturnal cough in the absence of a cold, associated with sleeplessness in both parents and the child, varies geographically (27% of children in the United States, up to 42% in Mozambique, and 13% in Japan). In the United Kingdom, 30% of hospital pediatric medical encounters (including emergency departments) are due to respiratory illnesses, with cough as a symptom accounting for over 8% of all presentations.[84] In the United States, cough as a symptom is the fourth leading reason for emergency department attendance, accounting for 3% of all visits (all ages).[83] Cough and cold medicines remain one of the most commonly purchased over-the-counter medicines by parents of young children[126]; in a given week, approximately 1 in 10 children in the United States are given these preparations.[127]

The burden of acute cough in children has been inadequately described and there are currently no validated pediatric acute cough-specific quality of life tools to evaluate this burden. An Italian study of 433 children (mean age 6.1 years) presenting with an URTI to 1 of 4 family care pediatric services over a 3 month period, 81% reported cough intensity as moderate to severe and 71% reported cough occurrence as frequent to continuous.[128] Disturbed sleep was reported in 88% of children and adversely affected school and sporting activities were reported in 76% and 61% of children, respectively.[128] In a study of 104 children (median age 2.6 years; interquartile range (IQR) 1.32–4.79) designed to assess the burden to parents of acute cough in their children, more than half had sought medical attention more than once for their child's cough and stress was the predominant factor of parental burden.[129]

Chronic cough is an under-recognized but important cause of decreased quality of life in children.[66] It accounts for substantial direct and indirect costs for health service providers, patients, and their families.[130] Parents of children with chronic cough may seek ≥5 medical consultations for their child prior to referral to respiratory specialists for investigation.[130] In one study, the greatest contributors to parental burden were feeling frustrated, helpless, upset, and sorry for the child and being awoken at night or having sleepless nights.[130] Reasons of worry or concern were the cause of cough, outcomes of serious illness, the cough causing damage, and the child having poor sleep.[130] Total burden was shown to be significantly negatively correlated with doctor visits in the preceding 12 months.[130]

5.7 VIRUSES INVOLVED IN COUGH

There are a large number of endemic and zoonotic viruses capable of infecting and replicating in the URT or LRT, respectively, of children and adults, worldwide. These include a number of viral families comprising over 200 distinct viruses, many of which circulate in seasonal patterns, generate distinct host-specific immunity, and have been associated with or detected in children and adults with cough. Viruses are linked with cough among the healthy, in children or the elderly,[131,132] or those with underlying conditions such as immunosuppression,[133] asthma, and COPD.[134] It is important to remember that the reliability of data presented by studies seeking or claiming to link virus and cough rely entirely upon the detection methods used. Prior to the 1980s, these methods were culture- and serology-based. Typical culture could not grow around 70 respiratory viruses and was a subjective, lengthy, and insensitive method for those it could grow. After the 1980s, PCR began to be used more often and today the most reliable studies employ PCR-based methods in panels capable of detecting 17 viruses or viral families.

5.7.1 Family *Picornaviridae*

The picornaviruses are the largest family of viruses infecting humans. The HRVs are the most frequent infections of humans with over 70 types circulating at a single site in a given time period.[135] Children in the community can be infected by at least six distinct HRVs in a 12-month period. HRVs have a bimodal peak that brackets winter. All three species, including the HRV-Cs have been found in patients with cough, and some, like HRV-C3, in patients with persistent or hacking cough clinically similar to whooping cough.[136] Similarly, the respiratory route is a major transmission path for the EV, and they are also associated with cough.[137] EV-specific studies confirm the association, for example, infection by EV-68[138] and EV-109[139] are detected from coughing patients.

5.7.2 Family *Orthomyxoviridae*

The human influenza viruses spread by small or large droplets and contaminated surfaces[140] are associated with cough among the community and in healthcare workers exposed to virus in aerosols in the emergency room.[140,141] Influenza virus traditionally exhibits a winter epidemic peak, although this can change with origin; influenza A(H1N1) 2009 (the "swine flu") peaked during spring and summer in the United States and the European Union. The newest influenza A virus, H7N9, is strongly associated with cough.[142,143]

5.7.3 Family *Adenoviridae*

HAdVs feature strongly in patients, particularly among children, with acute URT illnesses presenting to hospital[144] as well as in influenza-like illnesses.[137] The hAdVs also associate strongly with cough and dyspnea in more severe LRT diseases in children of all ages, including a small proportion of radiologically confirmed pneumonia.[145]

5.7.4 Family *Herpesviridae*

Epstein–Barr virus (EBV), which infects via an oropharyngeal route, infection frequently produces cough in the infants of HIV-positive mothers.[146] Among the seronegative, there is a risk of pneumonia developing following adult chickenpox, a consequence of infection with Varicella Zoster virus, and cough manifests in this group in nearly a quarter of cases.[147] Although not of use for differential diagnosis, cough is also found in human herpesvirus-6 infections[148] and herpes simplex virus 2 has been implicated in a case of persistent coughing and pneumonia in an HIV-positive adult.[149]

5.7.5 Family *Paramyxoviridae*

RSV is a frequent cause of acute bronchiolitis, a disease of children under 1 year of age, in which a dry cough is a well-known symptom.[150] It has a winter epidemic peak. Similarly, human metapneumovirus (hMPV) was associated with cough in nearly two-thirds of 273 predominantly children, more often than any other clinical feature during a four year-long study.[151]

The human parainfluenzaviruses (PIV 1–3) are frequently associated with initial clinical presentation of cough, usually with accompanying fever,[152] and have a particularly strong association with croup during the cooler months in children and the elderly.[153,154] Both mumps virus (MuV) and measles virus (MV) infections occur most often during childhood. MV infection is characterized by dry cough during the prodromal phase of infection[155,156] and is part of a more sensitive case definition for measles when combined with fever and rash.[157] Cough is not a clinical feature of MuV infection.[158]

5.7.6 Family *Coronaviridae*

The alphacoronavirus HCoV-229E and the betacoronavirus HCoV-OC43 are well-established causes of URT infections with HCoV-OC43 much more prevalent than the former virus.[159] HCoV-OC43 is detected more frequently, most often in children, is associated with cough in over two-thirds of detections, and is found with another virus in a third of HCoV-OC43 positive patients.[160] HCoV-HKU1 is also more frequently detected than HCoV-229E overall, and over half those patients a cough is present.[161] Among children in whom HCoV-NL63 was detected, over 80% coughed[162] and cough is also strongly associated with HcoV-NL63-infected cases with immunocompromise.[163] This virus has since been shown to be strongly associated with tracheobronchitis (croup).[164] Cough was found most often in HCoV-HKU1 cases during a rare year when we found all four human HCoVs cocirculating.[165] The HCoVs display a seasonal epidemic peak that favors winter.[165] Case definitions of potential human infection by the newly emerged Middle East respiratory syndrome (MERS) CoV also include cough as part of the acute respiratory illness.[166]

5.7.7 Family *Parvoviridae*

Parvovirus B19, agent of slapped cheek or fifth disease, can be transmitted through an aerosol route and has been described, albeit infrequently, in patients with an acute onset dry cough.[167] Human bocavirus-1 (HBoV1), only identified in 2005, has been detected in 1.5–19% of hospitalized, with cough as a major clinical feature[168] and a role in asthma exacerbation also proposed.[169] HBoV1 is also frequently detected with other viruses, making its causal role in disease difficult to discern.

5.8 IMMUNE RESPONSE TO VIRUSES AND VIRUS–VIRUS INTERACTIONS

Virus-induced inflammation begins at "first contact," outpacing the ability of humoral immunity (antibody) to confer a sterilizing defense. Thus, the early (within hours after infection) innate response is a most promising target for primary and broadly active intervention and moderation of viral disease progression. Frequent and repeated exposures to multiple cytopathic viruses may lead to long-term inflammation and microenvironmental changes that underpin asthma and other chronic respiratory disease. However, there is great diversity in the degree of inflammation ascribed to each respiratory virus; very similar viruses can exhibit very different inflammatory profiles and can modulate the innate immune response against them, to differing degrees. Interaction between viruses (virus interference) is an evident but infrequently mentioned feature of respiratory virus infections and may extend to an influence on the length and strength of their epidemic seasons.[135,170–173] For example, in 2009, a newly emerged influenza virus reached pandemic levels. In Europe, unusually high HRV activity co-occurred. We previously noted that detection of an HRV significantly reduced the likelihood of detecting another respiratory pathogens.[174] It appears that Influenza A(H1N1)pdm09 had a significantly reduced impact in the locations with high HRV activity. For some period, infection by HRVs render a population less affected by other viruses.

These complex interactions appear to occur among all the viruses capable of triggering cough, the extent of which is likely governed by the nature of their triggering of innate immunity and interferon.[175] We have noted virus–virus interactions in both hospital and community populations.[135,170] Virus interference (from which the name interferon was derived) constricts the epidemic or pandemic periods of other viruses by reducing the number of fully susceptible hosts, for a brief, perhaps 2-week, period. At the cellular level, virus interference exploits the blockade of superinfection by a preceding viral infection.[176]

5.9 VIRUSES AND BACTERIA IN THE UPPER AIRWAYS

While viruses are the most frequent and repeated cause of human infection, acute illness, and exacerbation of underlying respiratory disease, they are not alone at the site of infection. The nasopharynx is often colonized by pathogenic bacteria, including *S. pneumoniae*, *H. influenzae*, and *Neisseria meningitidis* and is a major site for carriage of bacteria in the population.[177,178] The use of antibacterial drugs and of pneumococcal vaccines has played a role in changing the bacterial ecology of the airways. Killed or vaccine-targeted bacteria are replaced by nontarget serotypes, eventually filling the vacancy.

Next-generation or high-throughput sequencing has been used to examine the diversity of bacteria in the URT.[179,180] This diversity is usually quantified in terms of the 16S rDNA sequence. The healthy adult nasopharynx is notable for the presence of skin lineages, including Staphylococcaceae, Propionibacteriaceae, and Corynebacteriaceae, and those found in the oral cavity such as Streptococcaceae, Veillonellaceae, and Prevotellaceae, but that each adult's URT and LRT microbial communities are more similar to within individuals than between individuals.[180]

It is well established that PCR-based methods afford high specificity and sensitivity and are the methods of choice for detecting viruses and bacteria in the airways.[181,182] These are strengths that are especially important for laboratory confirmation of an agent of cough since the anatomical cause of cough may lag behind the peak levels of pathogen, requiring a robust diagnostic method.

It should be noted that a proportion of every virus might be detected by PCR in hosts that do not present overt clinical illness (signs) and may only have mild feelings of illness (symptomatic), or none at all (asymptomatic). This is not unexpected, rather it is a feature of the impressive array of human innate and adaptive responses designed to block, contain, or at least moderate disease due to being constantly challenged by viruses. Nonetheless, the immune response itself, in the form of inflammation, underpins much of the disease resulting from viral infection.

5.10 NEED TO ADDRESS GAPS IN KNOWLEDGE

There remain substantial gaps in knowledge around cough relating to ARIs. To address this, there is a need for high-quality, prospective nonexperimental and experimental studies that can be replicated and are generalizable across different populations.[88,183–186] This research needs to be driven by clearly defined and standardized cough case definitions and ascertainment methods, cough classification (e.g., acute/chronic, wet/dry) and objective measures of disease burden and outcomes.[183,184,186] Validated tools for making cough-specific quality of life measurements are now, or will be shortly, available for outcome-focused research in children in urban settings in industrialized countries.[129,187] These tools need to be evaluated in a broader range of settings and similar tools need to be developed for alternate populations, particularly in cross-cultural settings with a high incidence and burden of disease.

Cough management guidelines are available in some countries[188–191]; however, to date only one study has evaluated a cough management algorithm in a randomized controlled trial and that study focused on chronic cough.[192] There is limited high-quality evidence to assist clinicians in primary care settings with management choices for children presenting with acute cough, including the evidence for factors that predict prognosis.[115,186] Alternatives are needed to current over-the-counter cough therapies as these are no longer recommended for young children given the lack of evidence for their efficacy and some safety concerns.[193] Such alternatives need to be investigated in high-quality randomized controlled trials that account for the known problems with the use of placebos in cough studies.[185,194]

The development of highly sensitive laboratory techniques that can detect a broad spectrum of respiratory pathogens, both viruses and bacteria, has opened up new possibilities in defining etiology, further elucidating the natural history and outcomes of cough, identifying the most effective time at which to intervene and which interventions to use. Rather than pathogen-specific studies that do not account for other potential etiologies, nonexperimental and experimental studies need to incorporate this broad spectrum and, in particular, include evaluating the role of virus–virus and virus–bacteria interactions in etiology, clinical course, and outcomes.

5.11 CONCLUSION

Specific and nonspecific cough are major contributors to poor quality of life, morbidity, and mortality in children worldwide. Viruses play a major role in cough formation, cough severity, recurrence, and duration and can be associated with long-term, adverse, lung health outcomes. Over recent decades, our knowledge of viruses (known and newly identified) and the role they play in respiratory pathology has become increasingly sophisticated. This knowledge should pave the way for the development of effective and safe prophylactic and therapeutic approaches to acute and chronic cough in children, incorporating measures that reduce the burden of cough.

REFERENCES

1. Widdicombe J, Chung KF. Cough. *Pulm Pharmacol Ther* 2007; 20(4): 305–306.
2. Fontana GA, Widdicombe J. What is cough and what should be measured? *Pulm Pharmacol Ther* 2007; 20(4): 307–312.
3. Chung KF, Widdicombe J. Acute and chronic cough. *Pulm Pharmacol Ther* 2004; 17(6): 471–473.
4. Lozano R, Naghavi M, Foreman K et al. Global and regional mortality from 235 causes of death for 20 age groups in 1990 and 2010: A systematic analysis for the Global Burden of Disease Study 2010. *Lancet* 2012; 380(9859): 2095–2128.

5. Murray CJ, Vos T, Lozano R et al. Disability-adjusted life years (DALYs) for 291 diseases and injuries in 21 regions, 1990–2010: A systematic analysis for the Global Burden of Disease Study 2010. *Lancet* 2012; 380(9859): 2197–2223.
6. Vos T, Flaxman AD, Naghavi M et al. Years lived with disability (YLDs) for 1160 sequelae of 289 diseases and injuries 1990–2010: A systematic analysis for the Global Burden of Disease Study 2010. *Lancet* 2012; 380(9859): 2163–2196.
7. Kauffmann F, Varraso R. The epidemiology of cough. *Pulm Pharmacol Ther* 2011; 24(3): 289–294.
8. Ranciere F, Clarisse B, Nikasinovic L, Just J, Momas I. Cough and dyspnoea may discriminate allergic and infectious respiratory phenotypes in infancy. *Pediatr Allergy Immunol* 2012; 23(4): 367–375.
9. Anthonisen NR. The British hypothesis revisited. *Eur Respir J* 2004; 23(5): 657–658.
10. Fletcher C, Peto R. The natural history of chronic airflow obstruction. *BMJ* 1977; 1(6077): 1645–1648.
11. Vestbo J, Prescott E, Lange P. Association of chronic mucus hypersecretion with FEV1 decline and chronic obstructive pulmonary disease morbidity. Copenhagen City Heart Study Group. *Am J Resp Crit Care Med* 1996; 153(5): 1530–1535.
12. Wright AL, Taussig LM, Ray CG, Harrison HR, Holberg CJ. The Tucson Children's Respiratory Study. II. Lower respiratory tract illness in the first year of life. *Am J Epidemiol* 1989; 129(6): 1232–1246.
13. Taussig LM, Wright AL, Morgan WJ, Harrison HR, Ray CG. The Tucson Children's Respiratory Study. I. Design and implementation of a prospective study of acute and chronic respiratory illness in children. *Am J Epidemiol* 1989; 129(6): 1219–1231.
14. Anandan C, Nurmatov U, van Schayck OC, Sheikh A. Is the prevalence of asthma declining? Systematic review of epidemiological studies. *Allergy* 2010; 65(2): 152–167.
15. Samet JM. A historical and epidemiologic perspective on respiratory symptoms questionnaires. *Am J Epidemiol* 1978; 108(6): 435–446.
16. Jones PW, Quirk FH, Baveystock CM, Littlejohns P. A self-complete measure of health status for chronic airflow limitation. The St. George's Respiratory Questionnaire. *Am Rev Respir Dis* 1992; 145(6): 1321–1327.
17. Voll-Aanerud M, Eagan TM, Plana E et al. Respiratory symptoms in adults are related to impaired quality of life, regardless of asthma and COPD: Results from the European community respiratory health survey. *Health Quality Life Outcomes* 2010; 8: 107.
18. ISAAC Committee. The International Study of Asthma and Allergies in Childhood. http://isaac.auckland.ac.nz/index.html (accessed 12 April 2013).
19. Chang AB, Newman RG, Carlin JB, Phelan PD, Robertson CF. Subjective scoring of cough in children: Parent-completed vs child-completed diary cards vs an objective method. *Eur Respir J* 1998; 11(2): 462–466.
20. Birring SS, Prudon B, Carr AJ, Singh SJ, Morgan MD, Pavord ID. Development of a symptom specific health status measure for patients with chronic cough: Leicester Cough Questionnaire (LCQ). *Thorax* 2003; 58(4): 339–343.
21. Newcombe PA, Sheffield JK, Chang AB. Parent cough-specific quality of life: Development and validation of a short form. *J Allergy Clin Immunology* 2013; 131(4): 1069–1074.
22. Newcombe PA, Sheffield JK, Juniper EF et al. Development of a parent-proxy quality-of-life chronic cough-specific questionnaire: Clinical impact vs psychometric evaluations. *Chest* 2008; 133(2): 386–395.
23. Burgel PR, Wedzicha JA. Chronic cough in chronic obstructive pulmonary disease: Time for listening? *Am J Resp Crit Care Med* 2013; 187(9): 902–904.
24. McCool FD. Global physiology and pathophysiology of cough: ACCP evidence-based clinical practice guidelines. *Chest* 2006; 129(1 Suppl): 48S–53S.
25. Bennett WD, Zeman KL. Effect of enhanced supramaximal flows on cough clearance. *J Appl Physiol* 1994; 77(4): 1577–1583.
26. Oldenburg FA, Jr., Dolovich MB, Montgomery JM, Newhouse MT. Effects of postural drainage, exercise, and cough on mucus clearance in chronic bronchitis. *Am Rev Respir Dis* 1979; 120(4): 739–745.
27. Chang AB. Cough, cough receptors, and asthma in children. *Pediatr Pulmonol* 1999; 28(1): 59–70.
28. Widdicombe J, Fontana G. Cough: What's in a name? *Eur Respir J* 2006; 28(1): 10–15.
29. Canning BJ. Anatomy and neurophysiology of the cough reflex: ACCP evidence-based clinical practice guidelines. *Chest* 2006; 129(1 Suppl): 33S–47S.
30. Canning BJ, Mazzone SB, Meeker SN, Mori N, Reynolds SM, Undem BJ. Identification of the tracheal and laryngeal afferent neurones mediating cough in anaesthetized guinea-pigs. *J Physiol* 2004; 557(Pt 2): 543–558.
31. Haji A, Kimura S, Ohi Y. A model of the central regulatory system for cough reflex. *Biol Pharm Bull* 2013; 36(4): 501–508.

32. Shannon R, Baekey DM, Morris KF, Nuding SC, Segers LS, Lindsey BG. Production of reflex cough by brainstem respiratory networks. *Pulm Pharmacol Ther* 2004; 17(6): 369–376.
33. Mazzone SB. Sensory regulation of the cough reflex. *Pulm Pharmacol Ther* 2004; 17(6): 361–368.
34. Undem BJ, Carr MJ, Kollarik M. Physiology and plasticity of putative cough fibres in the Guinea pig. *Pulm Pharmacol Ther* 2002; 15(3): 193–198.
35. Widdicombe J. The race to explore the pathway to cough: Who won the silver medal? *Am J Resp Crit Care Med* 2001; 164(5): 729–730.
36. Lee MG, Kollarik M, Chuaychoo B, Undem BJ. Ionotropic and metabotropic receptor mediated airway sensory nerve activation. *Pulm Pharmacol Ther* 2004; 17(6): 355–360.
37. Spina D, Page CP. Regulating cough through modulation of sensory nerve function in the airways. *Pulm Pharmacol Ther* 2013; 26(5): 486–490.
38. Bonham AC, Sekizawa SI, Joad JP. Plasticity of central mechanisms for cough. *Pulm Pharmacol Ther* 2004; 17(6): 453–457; discussion 69–70.
39. Chang AB, Gibson PG, Ardill J, McGarvey LP. Calcitonin gene-related peptide relates to cough sensitivity in children with chronic cough. *Eur Respir J* 2007; 30(1): 66–72.
40. Hara J, Fujimura M, Ueda A et al. Effect of pressure stress applied to the airway on cough-reflex sensitivity in Guinea pigs. *Am J Resp Crit Care Med* 2008; 177(6): 585–592.
41. Grigg J, Riedler J, Robertson CF. Bronchoalveolar lavage fluid cellularity and soluble intercellular adhesion molecule-1 in children with colds. *Pediatr Pulmonol* 1999; 28(2): 109–116.
42. Folkerts G, Busse WW, Nijkamp FP, Sorkness R, Gern JE. Virus-induced airway hyperresponsiveness and asthma. *Am J Resp Crit Care Med* 1998; 157(6 Pt 1): 1708–1720.
43. Mazzone SB, McGovern AE, Yang SK et al. Sensorimotor circuitry involved in the higher brain control of coughing. *Cough* 2013; 9(1): 7.
44. Nadel JA. Mucous hypersecretion and relationship to cough. *Pulm Pharmacol Ther* 2013; 26(5): 510–513.
45. O'Connell F, Thomas VE, Studham JM, Pride NB, Fuller RW. Capsaicin cough sensitivity increases during upper respiratory infection. *Respir Med* 1996; 90(5): 279–286.
46. Chang AB, Phelan PD, Robertson CF. Cough receptor sensitivity in children with acute and non-acute asthma. *Thorax* 1997; 52(9): 770–774.
47. O'Connell F, Thomas VE, Pride NB, Fuller RW. Capsaicin cough sensitivity decreases with successful treatment of chronic cough. *Am J Resp Crit Care Med* 1994; 150(2): 374–380.
48. Brydon EW, Smith H, Sweet C. Influenza A virus-induced apoptosis in bronchiolar epithelial (NCI-H292) cells limits pro-inflammatory cytokine release. *J Gen Virol* 2003; 84(Pt 9): 2389–2400.
49. Takizawa T, Tatematsu C, Ohashi K, Nakanishi Y. Recruitment of apoptotic cysteine proteases (caspases) in influenza virus-induced cell death. *Microbiol Immunol* 1999; 43(3): 245–252.
50. Hament JM, Kimpen JL, Fleer A, Wolfs TF. Respiratory viral infection predisposing for bacterial disease: A concise review. *FEMS Immunol Med Microbiol* 1999; 26(3–4): 189–195.
51. Peltola VT, McCullers JA. Respiratory viruses predisposing to bacterial infections: Role of neuraminidase. *Pediatr Infect Dis J* 2004; 23(1 Suppl): S87–S97.
52. Pitkaranta A, Arruda E, Malmberg H, Hayden FG. Detection of rhinovirus in sinus brushings of patients with acute community-acquired sinusitis by reverse transcription-PCR. *J Clin Microbiol* 1997; 35(7): 1791–1793.
53. Chonmaitree T, Heikkinen T. Role of viruses in middle-ear disease. *Ann N. Y. Acad Sci* 1997; 830: 143–157.
54. Wark PA, Tooze M, Cheese L et al. Viral infections trigger exacerbations of cystic fibrosis in adults and children. *Eur Respir J* 2012; 40(2): 510–512.
55. Ruuskanen O, Mertsola J. Childhood community-acquired pneumonia. *Seminars Respiratory Infections* 1999; 14(2): 163–172.
56. Casey JR, Adlowitz DG, Pichichero ME. New patterns in the otopathogens causing acute otitis media six to eight years after introduction of pneumococcal conjugate vaccine. *Pediatr Infect Dis J* 2010; 29(4): 304–309.
57. Nokso-Koivisto J, Pyles RB, Miller AL, Patel JA, Loeffelholz M, Chonmaitree T. Viral load and acute otitis media development after human metapneumovirus upper respiratory tract infection. *Pediatr Infect Dis J* 2012; 31(7): 763–766.
58. Ruohola A, Pettigrew MM, Lindholm L et al. Bacterial and viral interactions within the nasopharynx contribute to the risk of acute otitis media. *J Infect* 2013; 66(3): 247–5466.
59. Hussell T, Cavanagh MM. The innate immune rheostat: Influence on lung inflammatory disease and secondary bacterial pneumonia. *Biochem Soc Trans* 2009; 37(Pt 4): 811–813.
60. George RC, Broadbent DA, Drasar BS. The effect of influenza virus on the adherence of *Haemophilus influenzae* to human cells in tissue culture. *Brit J Exp Pathol* 1983; 64(6): 655–659.

61. Leach AJ, Boswell JB, Asche V, Nienhuys TG, Mathews JD. Bacterial colonization of the nasopharynx predicts very early onset and persistence of otitis media in Australian aboriginal infants. *Pediatr Infect Dis J* 1994; 13(11): 983–989.
62. Omer SB, Zaman K, Roy E et al. Combined effects of antenatal receipt of influenza vaccine by mothers and pneumococcal conjugate vaccine receipt by infants: Results from a randomized, blinded, controlled trial. *J Infect Dis* 2013; 207(7): 1144–1147.
63. McCullers JA. Insights into the interaction between influenza virus and pneumococcus. *Clin Microbiol Rev* 2006; 19(3): 571–582.
64. McCullers JA, Rehg JE. Lethal synergism between influenza virus and *Streptococcus pneumoniae*: Characterization of a mouse model and the role of platelet-activating factor receptor. *J Infect Dis* 2002; 186(3): 341–350.
65. Madhi SA, Klugman KP. A role for *Streptococcus pneumoniae* in virus-associated pneumonia. *Nat Med* 2004; 10(8): 811–813.
66. Marchant JM, Masters IB, Taylor SM, Cox NC, Seymour GJ, Chang AB. Evaluation and outcome of young children with chronic cough. *Chest* 2006; 129(5): 1132–1141.
67. Stockley RA. Lung infections. 1. Role of bacteria in the pathogenesis and progression of acute and chronic lung infection. *Thorax* 1998; 53(1): 58–62.
68. Wurzel D, Marchant J, Clark JE et al. Wet cough in children: Infective and inflammatory characteristics in broncho-alveolar fluid. *Pediatr Pulmonol* 2013; Jun 20. doi: 10.1002/ppul.22792.
69. Chang AB, Yerkovich ST, Gibson PG et al. Pulmonary innate immunity in children with protracted bacterial bronchitis. *J Pediatrics* 2012; 161(4): 621–625 e1.
70. Grissell TV, Chang AB, Gibson PG. Reduced toll-like receptor 4 and substance P gene expression is associated with airway bacterial colonization in children. *Pediatr Pulmonol* 2007; 42(4): 380–385.
71. van der Zalm MM, Uiterwaal CS, Wilbrink B et al. Respiratory pathogens in respiratory tract illnesses during the first year of life: A birth cohort study. *Pediatr Infect Dis J* 2009; 28(6): 472–476.
72. van der Zalm MM, van Ewijk BE, Wilbrink B, Uiterwaal CS, Wolfs TF, van der Ent CK. Respiratory pathogens in children with and without respiratory symptoms. *J Pediatrics* 2009; 154(3): 396–400, e1.
73. Bonzel L, Tenenbaum T, Schroten H, Schildgen O, Schweitzer-Krantz S, Adams O. Frequent detection of viral coinfection in children hospitalized with acute respiratory tract infection using a real-time polymerase chain reaction. *Pediatr Infect Dis J* 2008; 27(7): 589–594.
74. Cheuk DK, Tang IW, Chan KH, Woo PC, Peiris MJ, Chiu SS. Rhinovirus infection in hospitalized children in Hong Kong: A prospective study. *Pediatr Infect Dis J* 2007; 26(11): 995–1000.
75. Regamey N, Kaiser L, Roiha HL et al. Viral etiology of acute respiratory infections with cough in infancy: A community-based birth cohort study. *Pediatr Infect Dis J* 2008; 27(2): 100–105.
76. Arden KE, Chang AB, Lambert SB, Nissen MD, Sloots TP, Mackay IM. Newly identified respiratory viruses in children with asthma exacerbation not requiring admission to hospital. *J Med Virol* 2010; 82(8): 1458–1461.
77. Chang AB, Clark R, Acworth JP, Petsky HL, Sloots TP. The impact of viral respiratory infection on the severity and recovery from an asthma exacerbation. *Pediatr Infect Dis J* 2009; 28(4): 290–294.
78. Kapur N, Masters IB, Morris PS, Galligan J, Ware R, Chang AB. Defining pulmonary exacerbation in children with non-cystic fibrosis bronchiectasis. *Pediatr Pulm* 2012; 47(1): 68–75.
79. Mallia P, Message SD, Gielen V et al. Experimental rhinovirus infection as a human model of chronic obstructive pulmonary disease exacerbation. *Am J Resp Crit Care Med* 2011; 183(6): 734–742.
80. Didierlaurent A, Goulding J, Patel S et al. Sustained desensitization to bacterial Toll-like receptor ligands after resolution of respiratory influenza infection. *J Exp Med* 2008; 205(2): 323–329.
81. Pettigrew MM, Gent JF, Revai K, Patel JA, Chonmaitree T. Microbial interactions during upper respiratory tract infections. *Emerg Infect Dis* 2008; 14(10): 1584–1591.
82. Mallia P, Footitt J, Sotero R et al. Rhinovirus infection induces degradation of antimicrobial peptides and secondary bacterial infection in chronic obstructive pulmonary disease. *Am J Resp Crit Care Med* 2012; 186(11): 1117–1124.
83. Nawar EW, Niska RW, Xu J. National hospital ambulatory medical care survey: 2005 emergency department summary. *Adv Data* 2007; (386): 1–32.
84. Whitburn S, Costelloe C, Montgomery AA et al. The frequency distribution of presenting symptoms in children aged six months to six years to primary care. *Prim Health Care Res Dev* 2011; 12(2): 123–134.
85. Bruijnzeels MA, Foets M, van der Wouden JC, van den Heuvel WJ, Prins A. Everyday symptoms in childhood: Occurrence and general practitioner consultation rates. *Br J Gen Pract* 1998; 48(426): 880–884.

86. Hay AD, Heron J, Ness A, team As. The prevalence of symptoms and consultations in pre-school children in the Avon Longitudinal Study of Parents and Children (ALSPAC): A prospective cohort study. *Fam Pract* 2005; 22(4): 367–374.
87. Zar HJ, Mulholland K. Global burden of pediatric respiratory illness and the implications for management and prevention. *Pediatr Pulmonol* 2003; 36(6): 457–461.
88. Everard ML. 'Recurrent lower respiratory tract infections' going around in circles, respiratory medicine style. *Paediatr Respir Rev* 2012; 13(3): 139–143.
89. Glezen WP, Loda FA, Clyde WA, Jr. et al. Epidemiologic patterns of acute lower respiratory disease of children in a pediatric group practice. *J Pediatrics* 1971; 78(3): 397–406.
90. Monto AS, Cavallaro JJ. The Tecumseh study of respiratory illness. II. Patterns of occurrence of infection with respiratory pathogens, 1965–1969. *Am J Epidemiol* 1971; 94(3): 280–289.
91. Lambert SB, Allen KM, Druce JD et al. Community epidemiology of human metapneumovirus, human coronavirus NL63, and other respiratory viruses in healthy preschool-aged children using parent-collected specimens. *Pediatrics* 2007; 120(4): e929–e937.
92. von Linstow ML, Holst KK, Larsen K, Koch A, Andersen PK, Hogh B. Acute respiratory symptoms and general illness during the first year of life: A population-based birth cohort study. *Pediatr Pulmonol* 2008; 43(6): 584–593.
93. Latzin P, Frey U, Roiha HL et al. Prospectively assessed incidence, severity, and determinants of respiratory symptoms in the first year of life. *Pediatr Pulmonol* 2007; 42(1): 41–50.
94. Houben ML, Bont L, Wilbrink B et al. Clinical prediction rule for RSV bronchiolitis in healthy newborns: Prognostic birth cohort study. *Pediatrics* 2011; 127(1): 35–41.
95. Gove S. Integrated management of childhood illness by outpatient health workers: Technical basis and overview. The WHO Working Group on Guidelines for Integrated Management of the Sick Child. *Bull World Health Organization* 1997; 75 Suppl 1: 7–24.
96. Ostergaard MS, Nantanda R, Tumwine JK, Aabenhus R. Childhood asthma in low income countries: An invisible killer? *Prim Care Respir J* 2012; 21(2): 214–219.
97. Feikin DR, Olack B, Bigogo GM et al. The burden of common infectious disease syndromes at the clinic and household level from population-based surveillance in rural and urban Kenya. *PLoS One* 2011; 6(1): e16085.
98. Lee G, Cama V, Gilman RH et al. Comparison of two types of epidemiological surveys aimed at collecting daily clinical symptoms in community-based longitudinal studies. *Ann Epidemiol* 2010; 20(2): 151–158.
99. Homaira N, Luby SP, Petri WA et al. Incidence of respiratory virus-associated pneumonia in urban poor young children of Dhaka, Bangladesh, 2009–2011. *PLoS One* 2012; 7(2): e32056.
100. Ekalaksananan T, Pientong C, Kongyingyoes B, Pairojkul S, Teeratakulpisarn J, Heng S. Etiology of acute lower respiratory tract infection in children at Srinagarind Hospital, Khon Kaen, Thailand. *Southeast Asian J Trop Med Public Health* 2001; 32(3): 513–519.
101. Forgie IM, Campbell H, Lloyd-Evans N et al. Etiology of acute lower respiratory infections in children in a rural community in the Gambia. *Pediatr Infect Dis J* 1992; 11: 466–473.
102. Berkley JA, Munywoki P, Ngama M et al. Viral etiology of severe pneumonia among Kenyan infants and children. *JAMA* 2010; 303(20): 2051–2057.
103. Aujard Y, Fauroux B. Risk factors for severe respiratory syncytial virus infection in infants. *Respir Med* 2002; 96 Suppl B: S9–S14.
104. Madhi SA, Kuwanda L, Cutland C, Klugman KP. Five-year cohort study of hospitalization for respiratory syncytial virus associated lower respiratory tract infection in African children. *J Clin Virol* 2006; 36(3): 215–221.
105. Cardoso MR, Cousens SN, de Goes Siqueira LF, Alves FM, D'Angelo LA. Crowding: Risk factor or protective factor for lower respiratory disease in young children? *BMC Public Health* 2004; 4: 19.
106. Duffy DL, Mitchell CA. Lower respiratory tract symptoms in Queensland schoolchildren: Risk factors for wheeze, cough and diminished ventilatory function. *Thorax* 1993; 48(10): 1021–1024.
107. Glezen WP, Paredes A, Allison JE, Taber LH, Frank AL. Risk of respiratory syncytial virus infection for infants from low-income families in relationship to age, sex, ethnic group, and maternal antibody level. *J Pediatrics* 1981; 98(5): 708–715.
108. Glezen WP, Taber LH, Frank AL, Kasel JA. Risk of primary infection and reinfection with respiratory syncytial virus. *Am J Dis Children (1960)* 1986; 140(6): 543–546.
109. Holberg CJ, Wright AL, Martinez FD, Ray CG, Taussig LM, Lebowitz MD. Risk factors for respiratory syncytial virus-associated lower respiratory illnesses in the first year of life. *Am J Epidemiol* 1991; 133(11): 1135–11351.

110. Koch A, Molbak K, Homoe P et al. Risk factors for acute respiratory tract infections in young Greenlandic children. *Am J Epidemiol* 2003; 158(4): 374–384.
111. Ramakrishnan K, Harish PS. Hemoglobin level as a risk factor for lower respiratory tract infections. *Indian J Pediatrics* 2006; 73(10): 881–883.
112. Savitha MR, Nandeeshwara SB, Pradeep Kumar MJ, ul-Haque F, Raju CK. Modifiable risk factors for acute lower respiratory tract infections. *Indian J Pediatrics* 2007; 74(5): 477–482.
113. Sigauque B, Roca A, Bassat Q et al. Severe pneumonia in Mozambican young children: Clinical and radiological characteristics and risk factors. *J Trop Pediatrics* 2009; 55(6): 379–387.
114. Hay AD, Wilson A, Fahey T, Peters TJ. The duration of acute cough in pre-school children presenting to primary care: A prospective cohort study. *Fam Pract* 2003; 20(6): 696–705.
115. Hay AD, Wilson AD. The natural history of acute cough in children aged 0 to 4 years in primary care: A systematic review. *Br J Gen Pract* 2002; 52(478): 401–409.
116. Drescher BJ, Chang AB, Phillips N et al. Chronic cough following acute respiratory illness in children. Thoracic Society of Australia and New Zealand Annual Scientific Meeting. Darwin; 2013.
117. Drescher BJ, Chang AB, Phillips N et al. Chronic cough following acute respiratory illness in children. In: ESPID, editor. 31st Annual Meeting of the European Society for Paediatric Infectious Diseases. Milan, Italy; 2013.
118. Chang AB, Masel JP, Boyce NC, Torzillo PJ. Respiratory morbidity in central Australian Aboriginal children with alveolar lobar abnormalities. *Med J Aust* 2003; 178(10): 490–494.
119. Eastham KM, Hammal DM, Parker L, Spencer DA. A follow-up study of children hospitalised with community-acquired pneumonia. *Arch Dis Child* 2008; 93(9): 755–759.
120. Valery PC, Torzillo PJ, Mulholland K, Boyce NC, Purdie DM, Chang AB. Hospital-based case-control study of bronchiectasis in indigenous children in Central Australia. *Pediatr Infect Dis J* 2004; 23(10): 902–908.
121. Puchalski Ritchie LM, Howie SR, Arenovich T et al. Long-term morbidity from severe pneumonia in early childhood in The Gambia, West Africa: A follow-up study. *Int J Tuberc Lung Dis* 2009; 13(4): 527–532.
122. Trenholme AA, Byrnes CA, McBride C et al. Respiratory health outcomes 1 year after admission with severe lower respiratory tract infection. *Pediatr Pulmonol* 2012; 48(8): 772–779.
123. Singleton RJ, Redding GJ, Lewis TC et al. Sequelae of severe respiratory syncytial virus infection in infancy and early childhood among Alaska Native children. *Pediatrics* 2003; 112(2): 285–290.
124. Sigurs N, Bjarnason R, Sigurbergsson F, Kjellman B. Respiratory syncytial virus bronchiolitis in infancy is an important risk factor for asthma and allergy at age 7. *Am J Resp Crit Care Med* 2000; 161(5): 1501–1507.
125. Strippoli MP, Silverman M, Michel G, Kuehni CE. A parent-completed respiratory questionnaire for 1-year-old children: Repeatability. *Arch Dis Child* 2007; 92(10): 861–865.
126. Trajanovska M, Manias E, Cranswick N, Johnston L. Use of over-the-counter medicines for young children in Australia. *J Paediatr Child Health* 2010; 46(1–2): 5–9.
127. Vernacchio L, Kelly JP, Kaufman DW, Mitchell AA. Cough and cold medication use by US children, 1999–2006: Results from the slone survey. *Pediatrics* 2008; 122(2): e323–e329.
128. De Blasio F, Dicpinigaitis PV, Rubin BK, De Danieli G, Lanata L, Zanasi A. An observational study on cough in children: Epidemiology, impact on quality of sleep and treatment outcome. *Cough* 2012; 8(1): 1.
129. Anderson-James S, Newcombe P, Marchant JM et al. Defining the parental burden of acute cough in children. Thoracic Society of Australia and New Zealand Annual Scientific Meeting; 2013 March; Darwin, Australia; 2013.
130. Marchant JM, Newcombe PA, Juniper EF, Sheffield JK, Stathis SL, Chang AB. What is the burden of chronic cough for families? *Chest* 2008; 134(2): 303–309.
131. Falsey AR, McCann RM, Hall WJ et al. The "common cold" in frail older persons: Impact of rhinovirus and coronavirus in a senior daycare center. *J Am Geriatr Soc* 1997; 45(6): 706–711.
132. Jartti T, Jartti L, Ruuskanen O, Soderlund-Venermo M. New respiratory viral infections. *Curr Opin Pulm Med* 2012; 18(3): 271–278.
133. Milano F, Campbell AP, Guthrie KA et al. Human rhinovirus and coronavirus detection among allogeneic hematopoietic stem cell transplantation recipients. *Blood* 2010; 115(10): 2088–2094.
134. Althani A, Bushra S, Shaath N, Sattar HA. Characterisation of winter respiratory viral infections in patients with asthma and COPD in Qatar. *Arch Virol* 2013; 158(5): 1079–1083.
135. Mackay IM, Lambert SB, Faux CE et al. Community-Wide, contemporaneous circulation of a broad spectrum of human rhinoviruses in healthy Australian preschool-aged children during a 12-month period. *J Infect Dis* 2012; 207(9): 1433–1441.

136. McErlean P, Shackelton LA, Lambert SB, Nissen MD, Sloots TP, Mackay IM. Characterisation of a newly identified human rhinovirus, HRV-QPM, discovered in infants with bronchiolitis. *J Clin Virol* 2007; 39(2): 67–75.
137. Bellei N, Carraro E, Perosa A, Watanabe A, Arruda E, Granato C. Acute respiratory infection and influenza-like illness viral etiologies in Brazilian adults. *J Med Virol* 2008; 80(10): 1824–1827.
138. Linsuwanon P, Puenpa J, Suwannakarn K et al. Molecular epidemiology and evolution of human enterovirus serotype 68 in Thailand, 2006–2011. *PLoS One* 2012; 7(5): e35190.
139. Debiaggi M, Ceresola ER, Sampaolo M et al. Epidemiological, molecular and clinical features of enterovirus 109 infection in children and in adult stem cell transplant recipients. *Virol J* 2012; 9: 183.
140. Hall CB. Influenza virus: Here, there, especially air? *J Infect Dis* 2013; 207: 1027–1029.
141. Cunha BA. Swine Influenza (H1N1) pneumonia: Clinical considerations. *Infect Dis Clin Nth America* 2010; 24(1): 203–228.
142. Chen Y, Liang W, Yang S et al. Human infections with the emerging avian influenza A H7N9 virus from wet market poultry: Clinical analysis and characterisation of viral genome. *Lancet* 2013; 381(9881): 1916–1925.
143. Gao R, Cao B, Hu YY, Feng Z, Wang D, Hu W. Human infection with a novel avian-origin influenza A (H7N9) virus. *N Engl J Med* 2013; 368(20): 1888–1897.
144. Kwon HJ, Rhie YJ, Seo WH et al. Clinical manifestations of respiratory adenoviral infection among hospitalized children in Korea. *Pediatr Int* 2013; 55(4): 450–454.
145. Chen SP, Huang YC, Chiu CH et al. Clinical features of radiologically confirmed pneumonia due to adenovirus in children. *J Clin Virol* 2013; 56(1): 7–12.
146. Slyker JA, Casper C, Tapia K et al. Clinical and virologic manifestations of primary Epstein-Barr Virus (EBV) infection in kenyan infants born to HIV-infected women. *J Infect Dis* 2013; 207(12): 1798–1806.
147. Pugh RN, Omar RI, Hossain MM. Varicella infection and pneumonia among adults. *Int J Infect Dis* 1998; 2(4): 205–210.
148. Chua KB, Lam SK, AbuBakar S, Koh MT, Lee WS. The incidence of human herpesvirus 6 infection in children with febrile convulsion admitted to the University Hospital, Kuala Lumpur. *Med J Malaysia* 1997; 52(4): 335–341.
149. Calore EE. Herpes simplex type 2 pneumonia. *Braz J Infect Dis* 2002; 6(6): 305–308.
150. Shields MD, Thavagnanam S. The difficult coughing child: Prolonged acute cough in children. *Cough* 2013; 9(1): 11.
151. Sloots TP, Mackay IM, Bialasiewicz S et al. Human metapneumovirus, Australia, 2001–2004. *Emerg Infect Dis* 2006; 12(8): 1263–1266.
152. Chambers R, Takimoto T. Parainfluenza viruses. 2011. http://dx.doi.org/10.1002/9780470015902.a0001078.pub3.
153. Falsey AR, Walsh EE. Viral pneumonia in older adults. *Clin Infect Dis* 2006; 42(4): 518–524.
154. Zoorob R, Sidani M, Murray J. Croup: An overview. *Am Fam Phys* 2011; 83(9): 1067–1073.
155. Rima BK, Duprex WP. Measles virus. 2011. http://dx.doi.org/10/1002/9780470015902.a0000418.pub3.
156. Gold E. Almost extinct diseases: Measles, mumps, rubella, and pertussis. *Pediatrics in Review/American Academy of Pediatrics* 1996; 17(4): 120–127.
157. Choe YJ, Hu JK, Song KM et al. Evaluation of an expanded case definition for vaccine-modified measles in a school outbreak in South Korea in 2010. *Japanese J Infect Dis* 2012; 65(5): 371–375.
158. Duprex WP, Rima BK. Mumps virus. 2011. http://dx.doi.org/10.1002/9780470015902.a0000419.pub3.
159. McIntosh K, Kapikian AZ, Turner HC, Hartley JW, Parrott RH, Chanock RM. Seroepidemiologic studies of coronavirus infection in adults and children. *Am J Epidemiol* 1970; 91(6): 585–592.
160. Jean A, Quach C, Yung A, Semret M. Severity and outcome associated with human coronavirus OC43 infections among children. *Pediatr Infect Dis J* 2013; 32(4): 325–329.
161. Lee WJ, Chung YS, Yoon HS, Kang C, Kim K. Prevalence and molecular epidemiology of human coronavirus HKU1 in patients with acute respiratory illness. *J Med Virol* 2013; 85(2): 309–314.
162. Arden KE, Nissen MD, Sloots TP, Mackay IM. New human coronavirus, HCoV-NL63, associated with severe lower respiratory tract disease in Australia. *J Med Virol* 2005; 75(3): 455–462.
163. Abdul-Rasool S, Fielding BC. Understanding uman Coronavirus HCoV-NL63. *Open Virol J* 2010; 4: 76–84.
164. van der Hoek L, Sure K, Ihorst G et al. Croup is associated with the novel coronavirus NL63. *PLoS Med* 2005; 2(8): e240.
165. Mackay IM, Arden KE, Speicher DJ et al. Co-circulation of four human coronaviruses (HCoVs) in Queensland children with acute respiratory tract illnesses in 2004. *Viruses* 2012; 4(4): 637–653.
166. Organization WH. Interim surveillance recommendations for human infection with novel coronavirus. 2013. http://www.who.int/csr/disease/coronavirus_infections/InterimRevisedSurveillanceRecommendations_nCoVinfection_18Mar13.pdf (accessed 18 March 2013).

167. Lipsker D, Boeckler P. Acute urticaria and dry cough with interstitial pneumonia: A clue for the diagnosis of primary parvovirus B19 infection. *Clin Exp Dermatol* 2006; 31(3): 473–474.
168. Schildgen O, Muller A, Allander T et al. Human bocavirus: Passenger or pathogen in acute respiratory tract infections? *Clin Microbiol Rev* 2008; 21(2): 291–304, table of contents.
169. Allander T, Jartti T, Gupta S et al. Human bocavirus and acute wheezing in children. *Clin Infect Dis* 2007; 44(7): 904–910.
170. Greer RM, McErlean P, Arden KE et al. Do rhinoviruses reduce the probability of viral co-detection during acute respiratory tract infections? *J Clin Virol* 2009; 45(1): 10–15.
171. Hamano-Hasegawa K, Morozumi M, Nakayama E et al. Comprehensive detection of causative pathogens using real-time PCR to diagnose pediatric community-acquired pneumonia. *J Infect Chemother* 2008; 14(6): 424–432.
172. Rhedin S, Hamrin J, Naucler P et al. Respiratory viruses in hospitalized children with influenza-like illness during the H1n1 2009 pandemic in Sweden. *PLoS One* 2012; 7(12): e51491.
173. Yang Y, Wang Z, Ren L et al. Influenza A/H1N1 2009 pandemic and respiratory virus infections, Beijing, 2009–2010. *PLoS One* 2012; 7(9): e45807.
174. Arden KE, McErlean P, Nissen MD, Sloots TP, Mackay IM. Frequent detection of human rhinoviruses, paramyxoviruses, coronaviruses, and bocavirus during acute respiratory tract infections. *J Med Virol* 2006; 78(9): 1232–1240.
175. Smorodintsev AA, Beare AS, Bynoe ML, Head B, Tyrrell DA. The formation of interferon during acute respiratory virus infection of volunteers. *Archiv Fur Die Gesamte Virusforschung* 1971; 33(1): 9–16.
176. Hitchcock G, Tyrrell DA. Some virus isolations from common colds. II. Virus interference in tissue cultures. *Lancet* 1960; 1(7118): 237–239.
177. Bogaert D, Keijser B, Huse S et al. Variability and diversity of nasopharyngeal microbiota in children: A metagenomic analysis. *PLoS One* 2011; 6(2): e17035.
178. Dunne EM, Smith-Vaughan HC, Robins-Browne RM, Mulholland EK, Satzke C. Nasopharyngeal microbial interactions in the era of pneumococcal conjugate vaccination. *Vaccine* 2013; 31(19): 2333–2342.
179. Biesbroek G, Sanders EA, Roeselers G et al. Deep sequencing analyses of low density microbial communities: Working at the boundary of accurate microbiota detection. *PLoS One* 2012; 7(3): e32942.
180. Charlson ES, Bittinger K, Haas AR et al. Topographical continuity of bacterial populations in the healthy human respiratory tract. *Am J Resp Crit Care Med* 2011; 184(8): 957–963.
181. Mackay IM. Real-time PCR in the microbiology laboratory. *Clin Microbiol Infect* 2004; 10(3): 190–212.
182. Mackay IM, Arden KE, Nissen M, Sloots T. *Challenges Facing Real Time PCR Characterization of Acute Respiratory Tract Infections. Real-Time PCR in Microbiology: From Diagnosis to Characterization.* Norfolk: Caister Academic Press; 2007.
183. Chang AB, Landau LI, van Asperen PP, Masters IB, Mellis CM. The plea for rigorous studies on cough in children. *Chest* 2010; 137(3): 741; author reply -2.
184. Dicpinigaitis PV. Cough: An unmet clinical need. *Br J Pharmacol* 2011; 163(1): 116–124.
185. Eccles R. Importance of placebo effect in cough clinical trials. *Lung* 2010; 188 Suppl 1: S53–S61.
186. Hayward G, Thompson M, Hay AD. What factors influence prognosis in children with acute cough and respiratory tract infection in primary care? *BMJ* 2012; 345: e6212.
187. Newcombe PA, Sheffield JK, Juniper EF, Petsky HL, Willis C, Chang AB. Validation of a parent-proxy quality of life questionnaire for paediatric chronic cough (PC-QOL). *Thorax* 2010; 65(9): 819–823.
188. Chang AB, Glomb WB. Guidelines for evaluating chronic cough in pediatrics: ACCP evidence-based clinical practice guidelines. *Chest* 2006; 129(1 Suppl): 260S–83S.
189. Gibson PG, Chang AB, Glasgow NJ et al. CICADA: Cough in children and adults: Diagnosis and assessment. Australian cough guidelines summary statement. *Med J Aust* 2010; 192(5): 265–271.
190. Irwin RS, Gutterman DD. American college of chest physicians' cough guidelines. *Lancet* 2006; 367(9515): 981.
191. Keeley D. Cough in children: New guidelines from the British Thoracic Society. *Postgrad Med J* 2008; 84(995): 449.
192. Chang AB, Robertson CFPP, van Asperen PP et al. A cough algorithm on chronic cough in children: A multicentre randomized controlled study. *Pediatrics* 2012; 131: e1576–e1583.
193. Vassilev ZP, Kabadi S, Villa R. Safety and efficacy of over-the-counter cough and cold medicines for use in children. *Expert Opin Drug Safety* 2010; 9(2): 233–242.
194. Smith SM, Schroeder K, Fahey T. Over-the-counter (OTC) medications for acute cough in children and adults in ambulatory settings. *Cochrane Database Syst Rev* 2012; 8: CD001831.

6 Aerosol Spread and Communicability of Respiratory Viruses

Samira Mubareka, Thomas G. Voss, Daniel Verreault, and Chad J. Roy

CONTENTS

6.1 INTRODUCTION

Aerosol spread and transmissibility of pathogenic viruses by that route had plagued the human race since time immemorial. It is only within the last hundred years that the concept of airborne transmissibility has been endorsed as a plausible mode of transfer of viral agent from an infected to naïve host. As early as the 1940s, nearly 75 years ago, William Furth Wells, who was preeminent in developing the initial concepts of airborne infection in those early years, summarized these important properties in a treatise published by the Commonwealth Fund.[1] The concepts laid out so eloquently in his book still seem valid today. Although most of the focus on airborne transmission in his early text was centered on studies that dealt almost exclusively with bacterial diseases, viral disease transmission shares many of the conclusions reached from these studies. Only within the last few decades has there been a genuine uptick in the interest in airborne transmission of infectious diseases, triggered primarily by increased global travel that has given rise to emerging pathogenic agents with a penchant for causing outbreaks in locales that rarely fit the ecological niche of the particular virus. Sensational epidemics caused by novel viruses, such as severe acute respiratory syndrome-coronavirus (SARS-CoV), have brought the question of aerosol transmissibility to the forefront of scientific discussion, and have cast many of the long archived aerosol transmission studies described in the 1940–1960s in a completely new light. Many of the most comprehensive studies of viral transmission and our understanding of airborne infection came from military-funded laboratories including the U.S. Army Chemical Corps Biological Laboratories located at Fort Detrick, Maryland (presently the U.S. Army Medical Research Institute for Infectious Disease) and the Microbiological Research Establishment (presently the Defense Science and Technology Laboratories) at Porton, England.

Present day approaches to investigation of viral aerosols and transmission studies, in contrast to descriptive early studies, rely heavily upon inference and epidemiology as surrogate measures for establishing patterns and exposure-effect relationships for a variety of airborne viral pathogens. The key, however, to establishing the cause (the virus) and the effect (an infected host) in aerosol transmission studies lies in an empiric approach to studies that may or may not involve animal models. Focused studies demonstrate the airborne spread of infectious disease from an environmental or natural generator source to naïve host and initial infection via the respiratory system. The study of both aerosol and other forms of spread of infectious disease will distinguish which viral agents readily spread by the airborne modality. This chapter attempts to capture the important aspects of viral aerosols and aerosol transmission and the unique characteristics of viruses that influence the ability to cause disease by this route.

6.2 PARTICLE SIZE AND EXPOSURE

Aerosolized particles are measured according to their aerodynamic diameter rather than their actual physical size. This measurement is used to predict and understand the behavior of airborne particles by attributing to the particle the diameter it would have if it had the same aerodynamic behavior but was perfectly spherical and had the density of a pure water droplet (1000 kg/m^3).[2] The size of aerosolized particles is thus normalized for shape and density. Furthermore, the size of viral-laden particles is governed by the content of the initial droplet suspended in the air. The size of the virus itself will most likely be negligible in the granulometric distribution of the aerosol.[3]

Aerosol particles are required to be quite small in order to be respirable, generally 10 μm or less, allowing the particles to remain suspended in the air for an appreciable amount of time. To place into perspective, terminal-settling velocity dictates that a 100 μm aerosol particle will fall the height of a room (about 8 feet) in less than a minute, and in about 20 min for the same distance for a 10 μm particle. In contrast, a 1–2 μm particle of the approximate same density can remain suspended for days. Aerosols generated by natural sources both directly (e.g., coughing, sneezing) and indirectly (e.g., fomite formation) are known to be very heterogeneous in size distribution. Sizes from particles from these sources may range from >50 to <1 μm and the measurement of aerosols generated from normal human activities[4,5] and expiratory maneuvers have shown particle size distributions to be heterogeneous across individuals.[6] Determination of the particle size distribution in natural aerosol infection is too diffuse a variable to draw conclusions about the particular area of the respiratory system that is targeted, and thus can be problematic in predicting disease outcome from such exposures.

Basic deposition patterns within the human respiratory system based upon particle size are known,[7] as well as the main physical mechanisms of particle deposition that govern the process. Aerosols from natural sources that contain a biologic load, such as viruses, share commonalities such as hygroscopicity, which allow some conclusions about respiratory deposition. In addition, physiologic interaction with the host, including the flow and depth of respiration, will affect rates and anatomic location of particle deposition. The percent of deposition of particular fractions of aerosol particles during normal breathing is perhaps the most important parameter when considering aerosol transmission of viruses. Respiratory deposition for particles <3.5 μm have been estimated to range from between 20% and 70% when measured during normal breathing, indicating a highly variable process from person to person.[8] The health status and use of tobacco products (smokers vs. nonsmokers) with impaired lung function will also affect the location of particle deposition; the velocity of inhalation is dramatically reduced in the diseased lung, thereby causing highly respirable particles to deposit in the tracheobronchial region of the respiratory system rather than the pulmonary (alveolar) spaces. Mucociliary clearance, resident pulmonary macrophages, and other components of the host defense system introduce additional variables that are dependent on host health and genetics. Deposition location and inoculum within the lung may ultimately affect the type and severity of viral disease that ensues in the susceptible population.

The composition of the materials at the aerosol source generation can impact the disease initiation and relative dose and disease initiation. Generally, fluids serving as a source for viral particle formation (e.g., mucus on mucosal linings) may have vastly different pathogen titers compared to source materials from indirect sources (e.g., fomites from bed sheets of an infectious individual). Thus, the biologic loading in individual aerosol particles within a particular distribution may be dramatically divergent. Similarly, particles of discrete sizes (1 vs. 10 μm) may not contain a uniformly distribution of viral particles within the aerosol particles comprising the distribution.[9] The relative contribution of high titer, respirable particles (<3.5 μm) may contrast sharply with minimally respirable (>5 μm) particles with a lower viral titer. Nonetheless, direct generation of viral aerosols from activities such as sneezing and coughing continue to be a predominant source of aerosol transmission of disease.

6.3 ENVIRONMENTAL SUSCEPTIBILITY OF VIRUSES IN NATURALLY GENERATED AEROSOLS

Viral aerosols may persist in the environment, given the appropriate size, based upon prevailing meteorological conditions, thus increasing the probability of aerosol transmission. Location largely affects transmission occurrence; outdoor venues promote rapid dispersion of aerosols whereas poorly ventilated indoor environments may increase airborne particle concentrations and subsequent exposure probability. The relative humidity from seasonal changes has also been shown to affect the survival of viral aerosols; humidity has been shown to have deleterious effects upon viruses with particular characteristics and morphologies. Viral species containing lipid envelopes, for example, will survive in aerosol at a much higher rate in lower humidity environments.[6,10] This includes a variety of pathogenic viruses from a constellation of viral families including *Paramyxoviridae* (measles, mumps), *Orthomyxoviridae* (influenza), *Herpesviridae* (varicella), and *Togaviridae* (rubella).[4] Incidence of these viral infections tends to increase in the winter months, when humidity is generally lower.

Other viruses, in contrast, thrive in high-humidity environments. These include viruses primarily from the *Picornaviridae* family (coxsackie virus, echovirus, and foot and mouth disease virus) and are nonenveloped.[4] The correlation of the timing and seasonal patterns of increased incidence of particular viral infection and structural similarities suggest that transmission by aerosol is partially dictated by prevailing environmental conditions. Thus, virus morphology, in part, has some control over inactivation in this exposure pathway, as is the case of viral inactivation on contaminated surfaces. Lipid-containing viruses and the protein coat are highly susceptible to water interaction found in high humidity environments, whereas nonenveloped viruses may be rendered inactive when in dry environments. Of course humidity is only one of many different variables in the environment that impacts the replicative potential of an aerosolized virus and there are no absolute guidelines to predict the susceptibility of a virus to its environment based on its structural properties. Other factors include the native fluid suspension, mechanical shear, dramatic changes in humidity and temperature, and radiological (solar) exposure.

6.4 DROPLET NUCLEI AND CONTACT TRANSMISSION

Transmission of an infectious virus by large particles (droplet nuclei) which impact directly upon surfaces via high-velocity expulsion (cough) is an alternative and potentially important exposure pathway that contrasts with small particle (<5 μm) disease transmission. The mouth and nose are the primary sites for viral entry in the case of large particle transmission. This involves direct impaction of large droplet nuclei entering the mouth or nose immediately upon expulsion from the infected host. Alternatively infectious large particle droplets contaminate surfaces that effectively transmit virus via hand-to-mouth activities.[4] This latter pathway has been shown to readily transmit rhinovirus among individuals. Similar studies of the efficiency of large particle droplets to transmit rhinovirus via direct oral inoculation (via impaction) resulted in no infection. Studies of clinical infection models using influenza and respiratory syncytial virus (RSV) have yielded similar results.[4,6] Past human experimental work and epidemiological studies suggest that fomites and droplet aerosols are routes for transmission of RSV, though there are conflicting data regarding the contribution of fomites to transmission. The results of focused clinical infection studies and understanding how viruses interact with the host through direct mucosal inoculation suggest that direct physical contact with an infected host remains an important means of virus transmission. Other viruses causing disease via transmission by small particle aerosols bypass the upper respiratory mucosa and infect the alveolar region of the lung, the main deposition site.

6.5 RESPIRATORY VIRUS INFECTIONS: THE PATHOGENS AND THEIR PATHOGENESIS

Viral respiratory diseases of humans are associated with infection by a wide array of agents shown in Table 6.1. Other viruses are also associated with respiratory pathology, but are not considered communicable by the respiratory route. Infection by respiratory viruses through direct contact with infectious aerosols from infected individuals is associated with influenza viruses, paramyxoviruses, coronaviruses, and picornaviruses. Transmission of hantavirus pulmonary syndrome-associated viruses (bunyaviruses) is typically by inhalation of infectious aerosolized rodent excreta with one exception where human to human, aerosol transmission with Andes virus was reported.[11] Contact with fomites is a common route of infection with adenoviruses, and there is evidence of gastrointestinal infection with adenoviruses, coronaviruses, and even influenza viruses which can lead to respiratory pathology, but often is manifested clinically as gastroenteritis.

The pathogenesis of acute respiratory virus infections is typically a combination of direct viral effects on infected respiratory epithelial cells, and immune-mediated pathology. Immune responses to virus replication are most often cited as the cause of acute lung damage in influenza virus, RSV, and SARS-CoV infections. Significant morbidity and mortality in patients with influenza virus and other respiratory pathogens is associated with secondary bacterial infection often due to virus or immune-mediated damage to the epithelium allowing colonization by bacterial pathogens including *Streptococcus* and *Staphylococcus* species.[12–17] In addition to direct damage resulting in bacterial secondary infection, alteration of key toll-like receptor (TLR)-triggered mediators of bacterial clearance by bacterial/viral coinfection has been proposed to play a key role in morbidity and mortality in respiratory virus infection. It was shown that coinfection by influenza virus and *Staphylococcus aureus* in mice resulted in increased type I and type II interferon production compared to virus alone, and that this is associated with reduction in IL-17, IL-22, and IL-23 production after infection and reduced bacterial clearance.[17,18] Hantavirus pulmonary syndrome-associated virus infections are responsible for development of acute respiratory distress syndrome (ARDS) characterized by pulmonary edema which has been shown to be the result of loss of endothelial cell barrier integrity in the lung resulting from proinflammatory cytokine and other mediators expressed

TABLE 6.1
Major Viral Pathogens Associated with Human Respiratory Disease

Virus Family	Viral Pathogens
Orthomyxoviridae	Influenza A, B, C
Paramyxoviridae	RSV, PIV, measles virus, mumps virus, nipah virus, hendra virus, hMPV
Coronaviridae	Human coronaviruses (229E, OC43, NL63), SARS-CoV, MERS-CoV
Picornaviridae	Rhinovirus
Adenoviridae	Adenovirus
Bunyaviridae	Hantaviruses associated with hantavirus pulmonary syndrome

in response to infection of the endothelium of the lung.[17–19] A similar role for the endothelium in the pathogenesis of influenza virus has recently been reported with sphingosine-1-phosphate ($S1P_1$) signaling, a key modulator of immune cell trafficking and immune responses, to be important in initiation of proinflammatory cytokine amplification or "cytokine storm."[14,15] These studies showed efficacy of selective inhibitors of $S1P_1$ receptor inhibits early proinflammatory cytokine expression and innate cell accumulation in the lungs of influenza virus-infected mice.

These studies are focused on the pathogens, the induction of respiratory tract pathology and the role of immune response in acute respiratory tract damage resulting from infection. Understanding the underlying mechanisms of virus–host interactions, and the development of acute respiratory pathology may have broader implications with regard to transmission by aerosol due to the physiologic responses to infection in humans, and in valid animal models. It clearly implicates a critical role for the host in transmission of respiratory viruses, and is an active area of research in a number of laboratories.

6.6 ANIMAL MODELS

Animal models have been used extensively to study the transmission of respiratory viruses, specifically influenza virus. Unfortunately, mice do not demonstrate sustained animal-to-animal transmission by aerosol route. Thus, the ferret model is currently the most widely accepted *in vivo* system for influenza virus transmission work.[20,21] The ferret model has the following advantages: (1) ferrets are susceptible to human influenza viruses and viral adaptation is not required, (2) the transmission phenotype reflects what is observed in humans, whereby human influenza viruses transmit among human hosts but avian influenza viruses do not, (3) the clinical phenotype reflects what is observed in humans whereby ferrets develop fever, expulsion events (sneezing), and lethargy. Young ferrets have more severe diseases, and ferrets infected with highly pathogenic avian influenza viruses demonstrate mortality, as observed among humans. The principle disadvantages of this model include ferrets' difficult temperament, high cost, housing needs, and importantly, the absence of readily available reagents (e.g., species-specific cytokine ELISAs).

In order to circumvent some of these challenges, a guinea pig model has been developed.[22] Guinea pigs are easier to work with, less expensive, and demonstrate similar transmission phenotypes to ferrets and humans. The principal limitation of this model is the absence of a clinical (and histopathological) phenotype. Also, much like the ferret model, it suffers from a lack of available reagents for further analysis. This model has been used for larger scale experiments examining the impact of environmental factors such as temperature and relative humidity on transmission efficiency, the effect of neuraminidase-inhibitor resistance on transmission phenotype, and the abrogation of transmission through vaccination.

The majority of transmission studies have focused heavily on transmission phenotypes and the effects of various interventions. A substantial proportion of studies have investigated viral determinants for transmission and have been invaluable with respect to understanding why avian influenza viruses do not transmit efficiently among mammals, and the minimal viral requirements for efficient transmission. Although several studies have used aerosol challenge, inoculation is generally done by large droplets (intranasal deposition by pipet). Few studies have used these models to interrogate the aerosols generated by infected animals. NIOSH cyclone samplers have been used to compare viral recovery from the air exhaled by guinea pigs infected with different strains of influenza virus.[23] In addition, a ferret aerosol exposure and analytical system has been used at the CDC to inoculate ferrets and subsequently interrogate exhaled bioaerosols.[24] Using these system investigators noted that a viable virus was recovered during quiet breathing as well as sneezing, and that the infectious dose was lower for aerosol-inoculation (compared to droplet). In addition, ferrets infected with seasonal human (vs. avian) influenza viruses produce a higher volume of particles in their exhaled breaths and importantly, a significant proportion of these particles are in the respirable range. The major challenge in animal studies remains the investigation of the viable viral content of the aerosol. While particle counting and recovery of viral RNA is readily done, recovery of infectious (and potentially transmissible) viruses from the air remains a substantial challenge. Although this can be done using a cyclone sampler or a cascade impactor, viral titers are low and variable, making it difficult to obtain statistical significance and gain an accurate understanding of the aerosol dynamics and kinetics. This challenge is principally attributed to technical issues, since viruses may be sheared during sampling, and thus inactivated. In addition, the concentration of infectious virus in an exhaled bioaerosol may be too low to detect accurately using live culture methods.

6.6.1 Simulation Models and Human Studies

Although animal models and clinical sampling data have been quite informative, these approaches are not amenable to testing certain interventions, such as mask types. Several groups have used a mannequin head to simulate an infected person, and a simulated patient examination room has been established at NIOSH.[25] This system was used to demonstrate that a properly fitted respirator blocked 99.8% of virus compared to a poorly fitted respirator or a surgical mask which blocked only approximately 65% of virus.

A safe human model would be the ideal system to fill knowledge gaps regarding the dynamics and determinants for respiratory virus transmission, and to evaluate means to abrogate spread. This type of work was done in the past[26] and after decades of minimal activity in this area, human studies using influenza virus have resumed.[27] Others have made use of human challenge studies to extrapolate dose response, revealing that not unlike ferrets, the infectious dose is lower when inoculated by the aerosol (vs. the intranasal) route.[28]

Another approach is to assess bioaerosols produced by naturally infected humans. Although less controlled with respect to viral strain and inocula, these bioaerosols are more reflective of real exposures. Different systems have been used for aerosol capture and analysis, including cough boxes and modified masks. These studies have revealed that surgical masks reduced large droplet recovery from the air exhaled by naturally infected participants with influenza virus, but finer particles escape, albeit with lower viral RNA copies, and viral RNA recovery declines with time from symptom onset.[29,30] Recovery of viral RNA from fine (respirable) exhaled particles in this setting represents a significant advance in our understanding of the mode of transmission for influenza virus, and implies that the possibility of airborne spread cannot be completely discarded.

6.7 HUMAN ENVIRONMENTS

Sampling natural (e.g., nonexperimental) human environments has been a valuable and informative approach. Initial studies were performed among military recruits during periods of high adenovirus activity.[31] Since then, sampling of high-risk environments has been performed in emergency department and clinic waiting rooms, as well as at the bedside. In this context, sampling may be done using static samplers left in place in specific areas, and/or worn as personal samplers, generally by healthcare workers. In the latter case, the sampler is worn in the healthcare worker's breathing zone to more accurately reflect exposure risk. Approximately 40% of influenza virus-infected patients emit measurable amounts of virus into the air and viral RNA may be detectable at 6 feet in some cases, especially if the infected individual is symptomatic and is shedding a high amount of virus from the nose. Approximately one in five people may shed high titers of virus. It is unknown whether this can be attributed to intrinsic host determinants, viral determinants, or is simply dependent on the natural course of disease. The specter of the "super shedder" arose during the SARS outbreak in the early 2000s, and the existence of such a host has yet to be confirmed and defined. Viral recovery from fine particles has also been demonstrated, and over half of viral particles recovered are in the respirable range (<5 μm). A poorly understood issue which was highlighted during SARS was that of aerosol-generating procedures. The highest risk procedures appear to be tracheal intubation, manual ventilation ("bagging"), tracheotomy, and noninvasive ventilation; procedures such as suctioning, chest compressions, bronchoscopy, and nebulization were not strongly associated with SARS transmission events. Needless to say, this is a very challenging area of study that is not amenable to animal models or clinical trials, and underscores the need for more field study to garner sufficient data for robust risk assessments.

6.7.1 Epidemiology

Infections due to respiratory viruses account for substantial morbidity, mortality, lost productivity, and financial losses globally. Of the common respiratory viruses, only influenza virus is vaccine preventable. Noninfluenza respiratory viruses account for the majority of virus-associated respiratory illness, which most frequently manifests as the common cold. Estimates reveal that approximately 500 million colds occur annually and that associated direct and indirect costs are in the order of 40 billion dollars.[32] Some simple observations such as the reduction of influenza virus transmission in the presence of upper room UV radiation devices or the lower infective doses for aerosol infection versus large droplet infection suggest that aerosol transmission is the natural route of transmission of influenza virus.[33] A mathematical modeling study on the transmission of influenza suggested that aerosols account for half of the transmission events in a household,[34] thus suggesting that aerosol transmission has a much more important role than previously believed. Although experimental data is essential for understanding the aerosol spread of viral diseases, the complexity of air sampling and sample analysis for studies on the aerosol transmission over long distances has rendered epidemiology a very practical alternative. This approach has been used to study the transmission of the foot and mouth disease (FMD) virus between swine herds. Computer modeling based on environmental factors affecting aerosol transport strongly suggests that infective viruses can travel from contaminated herds to susceptible hosts over distances of 20,[35] 60,[36] and 70 km.[37] A "worst case scenario" model predicted that infection could even occur over distances as far as 300 km.[38]

A seasonal pattern has been well described for influenza virus in temperate regions. Similarly, other respiratory viruses also have a predilection to certain times of the year, with the sharpest peaks in temperate regions; sporadic disease tends to occur around the equator and some viruses are associated with rainy seasons in tropical climates. RSV tends to circulate in January with human metapneumovirus (hMPV) generally following two months after; coronaviruses tend to peak in February. Rhinoviruses account for the majority of viral upper respiratory tract infections (URTIs) and circulate predominantly in September and May[39] though sporadic activity is often observed. Though human hosts mount immune responses to respiratory viruses, antibodies may wane or are not cross-protective between viral strains. Thus, recurrent infection with rhinovirus, coronavirus, or influenza virus is not uncommon; North American children experience five to seven episodes of the common cold per year; adults experience two to three annually.[40]

The incubation period for the majority of respiratory viruses is approximately 2–6 days, but can be as short as 24 h in the case of enterovirus (coxsackie/echovirus)-associated hemorrhagic conjunctivitis. Incubation time for adenovirus can be as long as 14 days past initial exposure. Generally speaking, humans are the principal reservoirs for respiratory viruses and asymptomatic young children in particular may be responsible for a proportion of viral dispersion[41] and up to 12–32% of children with rhinovirus infections may be asymptomatic.[42] In addition, up to 47% of children with respiratory illnesses may harbor more than one virus, and viral shedding may be prolonged,[43,44] thus enhancing their role in the spread of respiratory viral pathogens.

In addition to asymptomatic infections described above, viral infection of the respiratory tract often results in symptomatic disease. The clinical presentation is frequently reflected in the site of viral replication and host response. The respiratory epithelium is present throughout the upper and lower respiratory tracts and includes the conjunctiva, nasal cavity, paranasal sinuses, nasopharynx, oropharynx, hypopharynx (including the larynx), middle ear, trachea, bronchioles, and alveoli.

The majority of respiratory viruses replicate in the upper respiratory tract (above the trachea) where the temperature is lower (approximately 33°C).

The conjunctiva may be the primary site of infection for adenovirus replication resulting in conjunctivitis or "pink eye," which is highly contagious. Viruses such as coxsackie A24 and enterovirus 70 may cause hemorrhagic conjunctivitis leading to corneal scarring; this presentation is uncommon in North America but has been well described in resource-limited settings. The influenza virus receptor (α2,6-linked sialic acid) is present on the conjunctiva and has been shown to be a site of viral infection for seasonal as well as avian strains of influenza virus.[45,46]

URTIs such as the common cold are associated with sore throat, rhinorrhea, sneezing, congestion, and cough, frequently in that order of onset. Fever and malaise may also be reported. Purulent nasal discharge is not necessarily an indicator of bacterial infection and likely represents host immune cell activation. Rhinovirus accounts for approximately half of viral URTIs, with coronaviruses being the second most common group of agents. RSV, hMPV, parainfluenza viruses (PIVs), and influenza virus are also frequently implicated. Duration of illness is host and virus-dependent, and varies from 3 to 25 days. It is not uncommon for coughing to persist for several weeks. Complications of the cold may include bacterial sinusitis, otitis media (especially in children), and exacerbations of underlying airway diseases such as asthma and chronic obstructive pulmonary disease. Also, URTI-triggered wheezing among young children has been well described in the absence of asthma.

Lower respiratory tract infection is a serious complication of respiratory virus infections. Croup and laryngotracheobronchitis is well described among children and associated with PIV, particularly PIV-1. A barking cough and in severe cases, stridor denote this condition. Bronchiolitis is not uncommon in cases of RSV, hMPV, and some strains of PIV. Influenza virus may also cause viral pneumonia. In addition, postinfluenza bacterial pneumonia due to *Streptococcus pneumoniae*, *Haemophilus influenzae*, and *S. aureus* (including methicillin-resistant *S. aureus*) is observed during seasonal epidemics and was implicated as a major cause of death during the 1918 pandemic. It remains an important contributor to the severity of influenza on an annual basis.

Common risk factors for complicated URTI include individuals at the extremes of age, immunocompromised states, underlying lung disease, and exposure to cigarette smoke. During the most recent influenza pandemic in 2009, populations at risk included pregnant women, obese individuals, and First Nations people. Multiple immunogenetic factors including HLA type, changes in the NLRP3 gene (a component of the inflammasome) CCR5 (a chemokine receptor) have been implicated in severity of influenza illness, but studies have been limited in power and scope.[47,48] RSV-induced wheezing has been associated with single nucleotide polymorphisms (SNPs) in genes encoding IL-8, mannose-binding lectins and interferon-γ, among several others.[49] These genes are involved in important immune responses against viral infection.[50]

The mainstay of management for viral respiratory tract infections is generally supportive. Antiviral such as neuraminidase inhibitors (oseltamivir and zanamivir) are administered in cases of severe influenza and to individuals at risk for complications. Similarly, the use of ribavirin for RSV is restricted to certain populations, particularly severe cases and profoundly immunocompromised individuals. The timing of antivirals is an important aspect of management, with optimal efficacy when administered early in disease (within 48 h of symptom onset). For severe influenza, late antiviral administration is superior to no effective antivirals at all. There are no antivirals available for other respiratory viruses. As mentioned above, primary vaccination is available only for influenza virus. Immunoglobulins are available to high-risk individuals for passive immunization for RSV, but a vaccine has yet to be developed. Community-based control of the spread of respiratory viruses therefore relies on proper cough etiquette, hand washing, and self-isolation. In hospitals, droplet precautions (isolation, gowning, gloving, surgical masks, etc.) are used to prevent person-to-person transmission of respiratory viruses. Use of airborne precautions (negative pressure isolation and use of N95 respirators) is currently recommended in cases of suspected or confirmed Middle East respiratory syndrome-coronavirus (MERS-CoV) and avian influenza virus infections.

6.8 CONCLUSION

There are a number of hallmarks of airborne virus transmission previously established that can be used collectively to better explain this exposure pathway. Naturally generated viral aerosols are produced from expiratory maneuvers such as coughing and sneezing and indirectly from normal human activities (e.g., contaminated bed sheets). Although the particles generated from these sources are heterodisperse in size, a proportion of the distribution is composed of small (<5 μm), highly respirable aerosols. Aerosol sampling in proximity of infected individuals have shown that the virus can be recovered from this aerosol fraction. Clinical infection studies performed with both susceptible laboratory animals and humans have demonstrated that airborne infection with aerosolized virus is possible under tightly controlled experimental conditions.

Large particle spread of infectious virus, however, remains a significant means for transmission of disease and in some cases, predominates transport and exposure of viruses via small particle aerosol. There are some families of viruses wherein the morphology of the viral structure and rapid transmission through a population suggest that small particle aerosol is the primary exposure route. *Orthomyxoviridae,* including influenza virus, is a prime example of a family of viruses that prefers transmission via small particle aerosols, and many studies have substantiated the case for this exposure pathway.[28] Other viruses such as rhinovirus, in contrast, will readily transmit by casual contact or hand-to-mouth activity. Strategies for intervention to further reduce viral transmission could be better designed if more information was available on the mechanisms of airborne transmission. Influenza is a good example of a disease whose incidence could be dramatically impacted; it remains to this day a major cause of morbidity and mortality in the industrialized and developing world. Incidence and prevalence in the population is seasonal and episodic. Controlled studies could better correlate the epidemiological phenomena with empirically derived transmission data.

REFERENCES

1. Wells W. *Airborne Contagion and Air Hygiene: An Ecological Study of Droplet Infections.* 1955, The Commonwealth Fund, Harvard University Press, Cambridge.
2. Hinds WC. *Aerosol Technology*, 2009, 2nd edition. Wiley-Interscience, New York.
3. Hogan CJ Jr., Kettleson EM, Lee MH, Ramaswami B, Angenent LT, Biswas P. Sampling methodologies and dosage assessment techniques for submicrometre and ultrafine virus aerosol particles. *J Appl Microbiol* 2005; 99: 1422–1434.
4. Knight V. Viruses as agents of airborne contagion. *New York Academy of Sciences* 1980; 80: 147–155.
5. Roy CJ, Milton DK. Airborne transmission of communicable infection-the elusive pathway. *N Engl J Med* 2004; 350: 1710–1712.
6. Couch RB, Douglas RG, Lindgren KM, Gerone PJ, Knight. Airborne transmission of respiratory infection with coxsackievirus A type 21. *Am J Epi* 1970; 91(1): 78–86.
7. Hatch TF, Gross P. *Pulmonary Deposition and Retention of Inhaled Aerosols.* 1964, American Industrial Hygiene Association, Cincinnati.
8. Brown JH, Cook KM, Ney FG, Hatch TF. Influence of particle size upon the retention of particulate matter in the human lung. *Am J Public Health* 1950; 40: 45–480.
9. Martinelli CA, Harley NH, Lippmann M, Cohen BS. Monitoring real-time aerosol distribution in the breathing zone. *Am Ind Hyg Assoc J* 1983;44(4): 280–285.
10. Verreault D, Moineau S, Duchaine C. Methods for sampling of airborne viruses. *Microbiol Mol Biol Rev* 2008; 72(3): 413–444.
11. Martinez VP, C. Bellomo et al. Person-to-person transmission of Andes virus. *Emerg Infect Dis* 2005; 11(12): 1848–1853.
12. Matheu MP, JR Teijaro et al. Three phases of CD8 T cell response in the lung following H1N1 influenza infection and sphingosine 1 phosphate agonist therapy. *PLoS One* 2013; 8(3): e58033.
13. Syha R, R Beck et al. Human metapneumovirus (HMPV) associated pulmonary infections in immunocompromised adults—initial CT findings, disease course and comparison to respiratory-syncytial-virus (RSV) induced pulmonary infections. *Eur J Radiol* 2013; 81(12): 4173–4178.
14. Teijaro J R., KB. Walsh et al. Endothelial cells are central orchestrators of cytokine amplification during influenza virus infection. *Cell* 2011; 146(6): 980–991.

15. Walsh KB, JR Teijaro et al. Quelling the storm: Utilization of sphingosine-1-phosphate receptor signaling to ameliorate influenza virus-induced cytokine storm. *Immunol Res* 2011; 51(1): 15–25.
16. Walsh KB, JR Teijaro et al. Suppression of cytokine storm with a sphingosine analog provides protection against pathogenic influenza virus. *Proc Natl Acad Sci USA* 2011; 108(29): 12018–12023.
17. Ahmed R, MB Oldstone et al. Protective immunity and susceptibility to infectious diseases: Lessons from the 1918 influenza pandemic. *Nat Immunol* 2007; 8(11): 1188–1193.
18. Borges AA, GM Campos et al. Hantavirus cardiopulmonary syndrome: Immune response and pathogenesis. *Microbes Infect* 2006; 8(8): 2324–2330.
19. Casali P, GP Rice et al. Viruses disrupt functions of human lymphocytes. Effects of measles virus and influenza virus on lymphocyte-mediated killing and antibody production. *J Exp Med* 1984; 159(5): 1322–1337.
20. Hutchinson KL, PE Rollin et al. Pathogenesis of a North American hantavirus, Black Creek Canal virus, in experimentally infected *Sigmodon hispidus*. *Am J Trop Med Hyg* 1998; 59(1): 58–65.
21. Stark GV, Long JP, Ortiz DI, Gainey M, Carper BA, Feng J. Clinical profiles associated with influenza disease in the ferret model. *PLoS One*. 2013; 8(3): e58337.
22. Lowen AC, Mubareka S, Tumpey TM, Garcia-Sastre A, Palese P. The guinea pig as a transmission model for human influenza viruses. *Proc Natl Acad Sci USA* 2006; 17; 103(26): 9988–9992.
23. Mubareka S, Lowen AC, Steel J, Coates AL, Garcia-Sastre A, Palese P. Transmission of influenza virus via aerosols and fomites in the guinea pig model. *J Infect Dis* 2009; 15: 199(6): 858–865.
24. Gustin KM, Belser JA, Wadford DA, Pearce MB, Katz JM, Tumpey TM et al. Influenza virus aerosol exposure and analytical system for ferrets. *Proc Natl Acad Sci USA* 2011; 108(20): 8432–8437.
25. Noti JD, Lindsley WG, Blachere FM, Cao G, Kashon ML, Thewlis RE et al. Detection of infectious influenza virus in cough aerosols generated in a simulated patient examination room. *Clin Infect Dis* 2012; 54(11): 1569–1577.
26. Alford RH, Kasel JA, Gerone PJ, Knight V. Human influenza resulting from aerosol inhalation. *Proc Soc Exp Biol Med* 1966; 122(3): 800–804.
27. Killingley B, Enstone JE, Greatorex J, Gilbert AS, Lambkin-Williams R, Cauchemez S et al. Use of a human influenza challenge model to assess person-to-person transmission: Proof-of-concept study. *J Infect Dis* 2012; 205(1): 35–43.
28. Teunis PF, Brienen N, Kretzschmar ME. High infectivity and pathogenicity of influenza A virus via aerosol and droplet transmission. *Epidemics* 2010; 2(4): 215–222.
29. Milton DK, Fabian MP, Cowling BJ, Grantham ML, McDevitt JJ. Influenza virus aerosols in human exhaled breath: Particle size, culturability, and effect of surgical masks. *PLoS Pathog*. 2013; 9(3): e1003205.
30. Fabian P, McDevitt JJ, DeHaan WH, Fung RO, Cowling BJ, Chan KH et al. Influenza virus in human exhaled breath: An observational study. *PLoS One* 2008;3(7): e2691.
31. Artenstein MS, Miller WS, Rust JH, Jr., Lamson TH. Large-volume air sampling of human respiratory disease pathogens. *Am J Epidemiol* 1967; 85(3): 479–485.
32. Fendrick AM, Monto AS, Nightengale B, Sarnes M. The economic burden of non-influenza-related viral respiratory tract infection in the United States. *Arch Intern Med* 2003; 24; 163(4): 487–494.
33. Tellier, R. Aerosol transmission of influenza A virus: A review of new studies. *J R Soc Interface* 2009; 6;6 Suppl 6: S783–S790.
34. Cowling BJ, Fang VJ, Suntarattiwong S, Olsen S, Levy J, Uyeki TM et al. Aerosol transmission is an important mode of influenza A virus spread. *Nat Commun* 2013; 4: 1935.
35. Daggupaty SM, Sellers RF. Airborne spread of foot-and-mouth disease in Saskatchewan, Canada, 1951–1952. *Can J Vet Res* 1990; 54: 465–468.
36. Gloster J, Freshwater A, Sellers RF, Alexandersen S. Reassessing the likelihood of airborne spread of foot-and-mouth disease at the start of the 1967–1968 UK foot-and-mouth disease epidemic. *Epidemiol Infect* 2005; 133: 767–783.
37. Christensen LS, Normann P, Thykier-Nielsen S, Sorensen JH, de Stricker K, Rosenorn S. Analysis of the epidemiological dynamics during the 1982–1983 epidemic of foot-and-mouth disease in Denmark based on molecular high-resolution strain identification. *J Gen Virol* 2005; 86: 2577–2584.
38. Donaldson AI, Alexandersen S. Predicting the spread of foot and mouth disease by airborne virus. *Rev Sci Tech* 2002; 21: 569–575.
39. Marks PJ, Vipond IB, Carlisle D, Deakin D, Fey RE, and Caul EO. Evidence for airborne transmission of Norwalk-like virus (NLV) in a hotel restaurant. *Epidemiol Infect* 2000; 124: 481–487.
40. Marks PJ, Vipond IB, Regan IF, Wedgwood K, Fey RE, Caul EO. A school outbreak of Norwalk-like virus: Evidence for airborne transmission. *Epidemiol Infect* 2005; 131: 727–736.

41. Litwin CM, Bosley JG. Seasonality and prevalence of respiratory pathogens detected by multiplex PCR at a tertiary care medical center. *Arch Virol* 2013; Jul 24.
42. Monto AS. Studies of the community and family: Acute respiratory illness and infection. *Epidemiol Rev* 1994; 16(2): 351–373.
43. Milstone AM, Perl TM, Valsamakis A. Epidemiology of respiratory viruses in children admitted to an infant/toddler unit. *Am J Infect Control* 2012; 40(5): 462–464.
44. Jacobs SE, Lamson DM, St George K, Walsh TJ. Human rhinoviruses. *Clin Microbiol Rev* 2013; 26(1): 135–162.
45. Martin ET, Fairchok MP, Stednick ZJ, Kuypers J, Englund JA. Epidemiology of multiple respiratory viruses in childcare attendees. *J Infect Dis* 2013; 15;207(6): 982–989.
46. Nguyen-Van-Tam JS, Nair P, Acheson P, Baker A, Barker M, Bracebridge S et al. Outbreak of low pathogenicity H7N3 avian influenza in UK, including associated case of human conjunctivitis. *Euro Surveill* 2006; 11(5): E060504 2.
47. Belser JA, Davis CT, Balish A, Edwards LE, Zeng H, Maines TR et al. Pathogenesis, transmissibility, and ocular tropism of a highly pathogenic avian influenza A (H7N3) virus associated with human conjunctivitis. *J Virol* 2013; 87(10): 5746–5754.
48. Juno J, Fowke KR, Keynan Y. Immunogenetic factors associated with severe respiratory illness caused by zoonotic H1N1 and H5N1 influenza viruses. *Clin Dev Immunol* 2012; 797180.
49. Horby P, Nguyen NY, Dunstan SJ, Baillie JK. The role of host genetics in susceptibility to influenza: A systematic review. *PLoS One* 2012; 7(3): e33180.
50. Drysdale SB, Milner AD, Greenough A. Respiratory syncytial virus infection and chronic respiratory morbidity—is there a functional or genetic predisposition? *Acta Paediatr* 2012; 101(11): 1114–1120.

7 Environmental Variables in the Transmission of Respiratory Viruses

Nicole M. Bouvier

CONTENTS

7.1 INTRODUCTION

Although human respiratory diseases of viral origin can be virtually indistinguishable clinically, the causative viruses are quite heterogeneous, not only in their virion structure and genome composition but also in the routes by which they transmit among humans (Table 7.1). The modes by which these viruses spread from person to person are critical in understanding how the environment impacts their transmission. For instance, transmission of respiratory syncytial virus (RSV) appears to be mediated mainly by direct and indirect contact, while SARS coronavirus (SARS-CoV) spread via airborne routes, including droplet spray and aerosol, seemed to play the prominent role in its

TABLE 7.1
Modes of Transmission of Several Human Respiratory Tract Viruses

Respiratory Virus	Family	Genome Composition	Primary Mode(s) of Respiratory Transmission Among Humans
Human adenoviruses (HAdV)	Adenoviridae	Double-stranded linear DNA	Contact, possibly droplet spray and/or aerosol (limited evidence)[1–5]
Influenza viruses	Orthomyxoviridae	Single-stranded negative-sense segmented RNA	Contact, droplet spray and/or aerosol (unresolved)[6–10]
Human parainfluenza viruses (HPIV)	Paramyxoviridae	Single-stranded negative-sense RNA	Unclear (limited evidence); perhaps similar to RSV[11–14]
Human meta-pneumovirus (HMPV)	Paramyxoviridae	Single-stranded negative-sense RNA	Unclear (limited evidence)[4]
Respiratory syncytial virus (RSV)	Paramyxoviridae	Single-stranded negative-sense RNA	Direct and indirect contact,[8,15–18] possibly droplet spray[15]
Rhinoviruses	Picornaviridae	Single-stranded positive-sense RNA	Contact, droplet spray and/or aerosol (unresolved)[8,19–21]
SARS Coronavirus (SARS-CoV)	Coronaviridae	Single-stranded positive-sense RNA	Droplet spray and aerosol,[1,4,22] possibly contact[23]

Source: Adapted from Pica N, Bouvier NM. *Curr Opin Virol.* 2012;2(1):90–95.

dissemination in the 2003 outbreak. With other viruses, evidence is either sparse or contradictory, and mode(s) of transmission are yet to be fully elucidated.

In the United States, the Centers for Disease Control and Prevention (CDC) has established a consensus definition for the modes of transmission of influenza virus; their classification scheme is broadly applicable to other respiratory viruses that spread from person to person without an intermediate vector (Box 7.1). For consistency, CDC terminology will be employed throughout this discussion of environment and virus transmission. Thus, "contact transmission" encompasses both direct and indirect transmission, while "airborne transmission," comprising both droplet spray and aerosol modes, describes the inoculation of virus particles from the air directly into the respiratory tract without an intermediate, such as a contaminated door handle or hand.

Though the impact of environmental variables on the transmission of human respiratory viruses has been much more thoroughly studied for some viruses than others, the goal of this discussion is to summarize the existing body of evidence in the biomedical literature and, where possible, to identify knowledge gaps that require further study.

7.2 THE SEASONAL EPIDEMIOLOGY OF RESPIRATORY VIRUS TRANSMISSION

7.2.1 Early Observations

Many theories have been proposed to explain the specific effect of environmental variables on the pronounced seasonality of influenza and, to a lesser extent, disease caused by RSV and "common cold" viruses.[24–28] Many of these hypotheses have been based upon epidemiological observations made in temperate climates at different times of the year, such as a study conducted in the Netherlands in the winter of 1925–1926. Nearly 7000 persons were followed weekly for the development of upper respiratory tract infections (URIs), which were then further classified as "nose cold, sore throat (angina), hoarseness (laryngitis), cold with cough (bronchitis) or slight influenza."[29] This study found that similar URI syndromes tended to be reported simultaneously from different areas

BOX 7.1 MODES OF PERSON-TO-PERSON TRANSMISSION OF RESPIRATORY VIRUSES

Contact transmission: In both modes of contract transmission, contaminated hands play an important role in carrying virus to the mucous membranes of the respiratory tract.

Direct transmission: Virus is transferred from an infected person directly to a susceptible person's hand without a contaminated intermediate object (fomite).

Indirect transmission: Virus is transferred by hand contact with a contaminated intermediate object (fomite) that has been touched by an infected person.

Airborne transmission: In both modes of airborne transmission, virus particles in the air are inoculated directly into the respiratory tract; intermediates such as contaminated hands or fomites are not involved.

Droplet spray transmission: Virus transmits through the air in a plume of large, water-laden droplets (such as those produced by coughing or sneezing); a key feature is deposition of droplets by impaction on exposed mucous membranes.

Aerosol (droplet nuclei) transmission: Virus transmits through the air by desiccated aerosols (droplet nuclei) in the inspirable size range; aerosol particles are small enough to remain suspended in the air for hours and to be inhaled into the oronasopharynx and distally into the trachea and lung.

Source: Adapted from Pica N, Bouvier NM. Environmental factors affecting the transmission of respiratory viruses. *Curr Opin Virol.* 2012;2(1):90–95.

of the country, despite many intervening miles. Most interestingly, when the data were compared to outdoor temperature, a correlation between falling outdoor temperatures and rising incidence of illness was appreciated (Figure 7.1).[29]

For much of the twentieth century, the association between cold weather and respiratory illness in temperate climates was attributed not to the cold itself but rather to other variables associated with inclement weather, such as changes in host behavior (e.g., more time spent indoors, in closed environments, during cold or rainy weather),[30] changes in host defense mechanisms (e.g., impaired mucociliary clearance with inhalation of cold, dry air),[31,32] and changes in airborne or surface-contaminating virus viability (e.g., enhanced virus stability and infectivity under different temperature and humidity conditions).[33–41] It has been commonly proposed that, unlike in the summertime, cold, rainy, or otherwise inhospitable weather drives people inside, where they spend more time in poorly ventilated spaces in close contact with other, potentially infectious people. Though somewhat intuitive and thus regularly proffered, the "crowding" hypothesis actually has very little experimental evidence to support it.[30] In 1965, Sir Christopher Andrewes, one of the discoverers of influenza A virus in 1933,[42] noted, "Many people regard [crowding indoors] as the likeliest 'winter factor' to explain the facts [of respiratory virus seasonality]. I have always had doubts about this.... There may be rather better ventilation in summer, but that is the only likely difference. If close contact were all, one would think that London Transport would ensure an all-the-year round epidemic."[43]

In 1958, a British general practitioner, Dr. R.E. Hope Simpson, offered the hypothesis that it was not low temperatures or behaviors associated with it, but rather relative humidity (RH), that influenced the seasonality of respiratory viruses such as influenza, RSV, and other common cold viruses. Similar to the Netherlands study,[29] he found a near-perfect inverse correlation between common cold incidence among his own patients and decreasing temperature—so perfect, in fact, that he estimated that for every 1°F (0.56°C) decrease in outdoor temperature, morbidity due to URI increased by 1% in his patient cohort. However, because most of his patients spent far

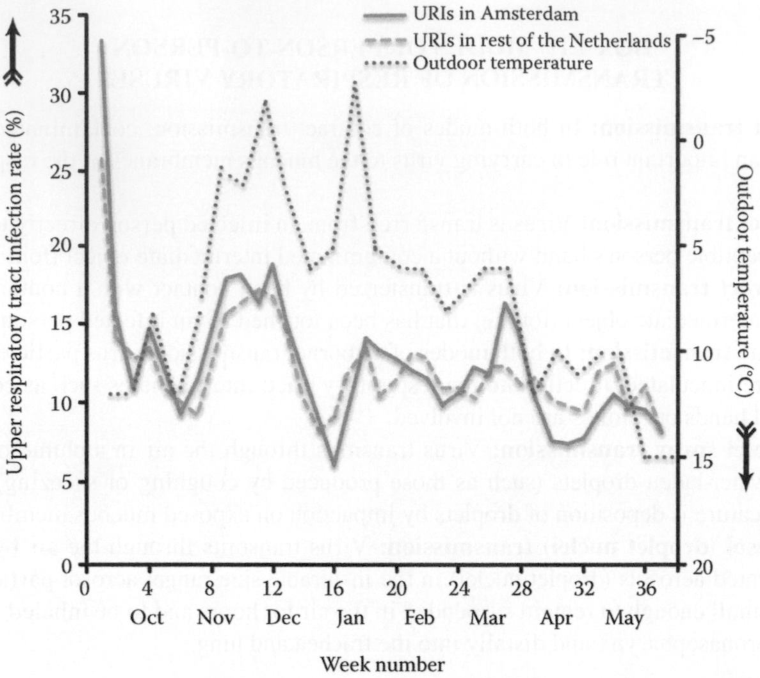

FIGURE 7.1 Incident URI and ambient temperature are inversely correlated. The percentages of cohort subjects reporting URI symptoms during the winter of 1925–1926 in Amsterdam ($n = 1159$) and in the rest of the Netherlands ($n = 5774$), as compared with the average air temperatures in the same period, reveal a strong epidemiological association between cooling weather and the onset of respiratory infections. (Redrawn from van Loghem JJ. An epidemiological contribution to the knowledge of the respiratory diseases. *J Hyg (Lond).* 1928;28(1):33–54.)

more time indoors than outside during the winter, he proposed that the relationship between cold weather and URI was indirect. Rather, he implicated indoor RH as the causative variable, specifically the "drying and warming of the air by the artificial heating in our houses."[44] He specifically hypothesized that drying of the respiratory mucosa at low RH, such as is found in heated buildings during the temperate winter, impeded mucociliary clearance, which in turn led to "irritation and damage to the underlying cells" that "would impair the cleansing mechanism of the respiratory tract."[44] Though experiments performed three decades later confirmed that nasal mucociliary clearance is indeed slowed in subjects breathing dry air,[31] Hope–Simpson's hypothesis still provides an incomplete picture, failing to account for respiratory virus transmission that is observed in the hot, humid tropics.

7.2.2 Geography, Season, and Climate

7.2.2.1 Influenza

Since epidemiological observations such as those discussed above were made, numerous studies have been performed to investigate the incidence, timing, magnitude, and peak of influenza and other respiratory virus epidemics in various climates around the world. Although few of these studies are adequately powered individually to shed definitive light on the question of environmental variables that play a role in respiratory virus seasonality, several recent systematic reviews have analyzed these data in aggregate, revealing interesting patterns of respiratory virus behavior with regards to geography and climate.

To describe the timing of influenza activity globally, Azziz Baumgartner et al.[45] performed a descriptive analysis of laboratory-confirmed seasonal influenza data, culled either from the published medical literature or from publicly available databases, such as the World Health Organization (WHO) FluNet or those maintained by national public health agencies. The final analysis, comprising data from 85 countries, concluded that annual influenza epidemics occur in consistent temporal patterns depending on climate. In the countries with available data, influenza viruses typically caused 1 or 2 predictable annual epidemics, lasting an average of 4 months, worldwide. In this analysis, local weather perhaps influenced the timing of peak influenza activity in temperate climates, where it was associated with the coldest month or the following one in significantly more temperate countries than tropical or subtropical ones. Multiple influenza epidemics per year were more common in tropical countries than in temperate countries, and year-round activity (defined as laboratory-confirmed influenza virus identified in every week of the year in which ≥10 specimens were submitted for testing) was most often observed in tropical countries and least often in temperate countries. In aggregate, influenza activity tended to peak in Southeast Asia and Oceania in June and July; in Australia in August; in the Middle East, North Africa, and Mexico in December; in Europe and North America in February and March; and in South America and South Africa in May and June. However, the authors noted that their analysis was limited by a relative paucity of data from the Middle East and Africa.[45]

A more recent and larger analysis, by Bloom-Feshbach et al.,[46] reviewed similar source data (i.e., published studies and electronic databases) to assess quantitatively the seasonal patterns of laboratory-confirmed influenza and RSV epidemics in 137 locations on 5 continents. This systematic review examined climate and influenza activity data from individual cities or regions and was thus more spatially resolved than that of Azziz-Baumgartner et al., which utilized data compiled on a national level.[45] Bloom-Feshbach et al. found that the seasonal patterns of epidemic influenza and RSV are generally similar, with both viruses exhibiting sharp peaks of activity during winter months in temperate climates and longer-lasting, less temporally concentrated epidemic activity in the tropics. In contrast to the prevailing view that respiratory viruses circulate essentially year-round in the tropics,[47] in this analysis, the authors failed to identify any location with consistent viral activity throughout the year; an epidemic peak could always be defined. The aggregation of data from multiple sites revealed that 80% of tropical regions have RSV seasons lasting a maximum of 6 months and 50% have similarly distinct influenza seasons, though with lower-amplitude, broader peaks than those at higher latitudes.[46]

Influenza epidemics in temperate regions tended to have defined peaks, with modes in February and July in Northern and Southern Hemispheres, respectively, and generally later onset with increasing latitude away from the equator. However, in some temperate zones, particularly in Asia, influenza activity occurred in two discrete semi-annual peaks, in January–February and then again in June–August of the same year. Tropical climates experienced more variability in influenza epidemic timing and duration than did temperate climates, although, as the authors noted, the data were limited by undersampling in some areas, such as tropical regions of Africa and parts of the Southern Hemisphere.[46]

A separate analysis of similar source data by Tamerius et al.[48] likewise found that the relationship between seasonal climate and influenza peaks was not completely consistent worldwide. At higher latitudes, in temperate climates, influenza epidemics were correlated with low temperatures and low specific humidity (SH), which is a ratio between the mass of water vapor in air to the total mass of the air and water vapor together. However, in tropical areas at lower latitudes, peak influenza activity correlated with high levels of precipitation and, accordingly, high humidity. Interestingly, the association between peak influenza activity and temperature or SH was most significant when the influenza epidemic occurred with a one-month lag behind these environmental predictors.[48]

Tamerius et al. found a significant relationship between influenza epidemics and climatic variables according to extremes of latitude. Between latitudes 25°N/S and the poles, peak influenza

7.4.1.1 Influenza

Early investigations into the survival of airborne influenza virus under differing humidity conditions revealed somewhat different results. In 1943, Loosli and colleagues examined the effect of humidity on aerosolized influenza virus and found a monotonic increase in influenza virus viability with decrease in RH.[26] Shortly thereafter, in 1950, Shechmeister reassessed the airborne infectivity, in mice, of influenza virus, aerosolized by means of a Wells atomizer. Unlike Loosli et al., Shechmeister observed a bimodal relationship between virus viability and RH, such that airborne virus was more infectious to mice at humidity extremes—32% and 68%RH—than at a mid-range RH of 60%.[41]

In the early 1960s, Hemmes et al.,[33] Harper et al.,[34] and Hood et al.[38] independently derived experimental data that, like the measurements of Loosli et al., suggested a monotonic inverse relationship between airborne influenza virus survival and RH, in which virus viability increased with decreasing RH. In addition to enhanced virus survival at low RH (Figure 7.3), Harper et al. also found that virus stability was maximized at low temperatures.[34] Reviewing previous data, Hemmes et al. suggested that, given the rather narrow range of indoor temperatures in modern heated buildings, the effect of temperature on influenza virus viability should be relatively small, compared to that of RH. Assessing the infectiousness of airborne influenza virus aerosolized at room temperature at various RH levels, they found that loss of viability was high at 50–90%RH and low at 15–40%RH. Between 40% and 50%RH, a sharp transition occurred, with the virus death rate *K* increasing exponentially with increasing RH. Hemmes et al. concluded that the loss of viability with increasing RH was a monotonic relationship, and their data reveal three RH-dependent, kinetically distinct phases of decay: <40%RH; 40–70%RH; and >70%RH (Figure 7.3), although there appears to be more significant scatter in the data points in mid-range RH levels.[33]

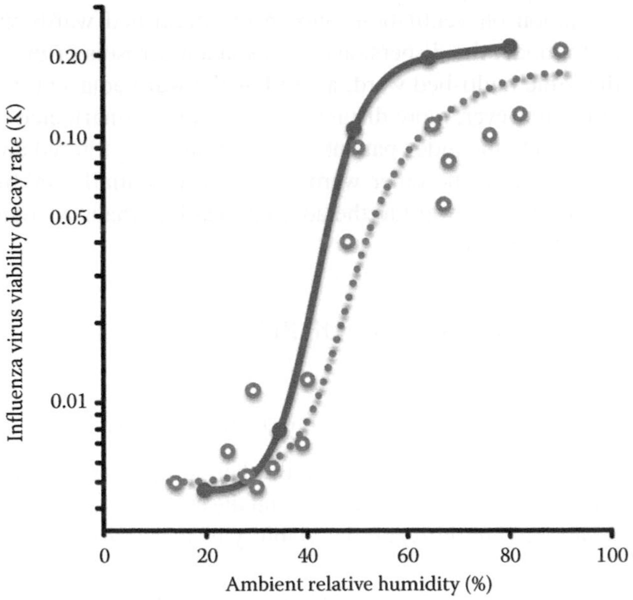

FIGURE 7.3 Aerosolized influenza viruses remain infectious longer in drier air. The data of Hemmes et al.[19] (dotted line and open symbols) present the influenza virus "death rate" or its rate of viability decay (*K*), graphed as a function of RH at room temperature. The data of Harper et al.[21] (solid line and closed symbols) were used to calculate, in arbitrary units, the decay rate *K* for a different influenza virus aerosolized at ambient RH between 20% and 80%. Graphed logarithmically as a function of RH, Hemmes' and Harper's data reveal a similar pattern of RH-dependent, monotonic decrease in airborne influenza virus viability with increasing RH.

In 1976, Schaffer et al., like Shechmeister in 1950, observed a nonmonotonic, U-shaped curve describing the correspondence between influenza virus viability and RH, with maximal stability at low RH (20–40%), minimal stability at mid-range RH (40–60%), and moderate stability at high RH (60–80%).[40] Though these laboratory data overall are conflicting, it is important to recall that the experimental methods, including the buffer solutions in which the influenza viruses were suspended and the techniques for aerosolizing virus into airborne droplets, were not standardized, and thus the resulting droplet size and composition were different in each case.

Influenza virus stability is generally enhanced on nonporous surfaces, compared to being suspended in the air or deposited onto porous surfaces.[108] On stainless steel, aqueous suspensions of influenza A virus have been found to lose infectivity more rapidly at higher temperatures (60°C and 65°C, relative to 55°C) and at higher RH levels (50%, and 75%, relative to 25%RH). These relationships could be simplified by replacing temperature and RH with AH; virus inactivation increased linearly with increasing AH with a high degree of correlation. These results suggest that thermal inactivation in the presence of moisture may be an effective way of sanitizing heat-resistant surfaces.[109]

7.4.1.2 Other Respiratory Viruses

Though fewer experimental data exist to describe the airborne stability of respiratory viruses other than influenza virus, some general trends have been observed. In aerosol viability experiments, the paramyxoviruses, parainfluenza virus and RSV, like the orthomyxovirus influenza virus, have generally demonstrated maximal stability at lower RH levels and temperatures. Experiments with aerosolized HPIV-3 revealed minimal infectivity decay at 20%RH, compared to 50% and 80%RH.[39] Other investigators found that, at 6°C, the stability of airborne bovine PIV-3 was roughly equivalent at 30% and 90%RH; however, at 32°C, infectiousness declined more rapidly at 90%RH than at 30%RH.[36] At room temperature, Rechsteiner et al. discovered that aerosolized RSV was maximally unstable between 70% and 90%RH and moderately unstable at 30%RH, with maximal stability at 20% and 40–60%RH. Due to the bimodal nature of the observed virus decay curves, the authors suggested that at these two RH levels, different processes of virus inactivation were likely at work; however, these processes are not fully understood.[110]

In contrast to the para- and orthomyxoviruses, adenovirus[35,39] and rhinovirus[111] appear to be more stable at high RH, though there is some evidence to suggest that they are still vulnerable to more rapid decay at high temperatures. Aerosolized HAdV-4 and -7 have demonstrated maximal stability at 80%RH, compared to 20% or 50%RH.[39] Airborne bovine AdV-3 was observed to maintain infectiousness longer at 90%RH than at 30%RH and at 6°C than at 32°C. In the latter experiments, after 2 h storage time, aerosolized BAdV-3 held at 6°C and 90%RH remained almost 3000 times more infectious than a similar aerosol kept at 32°C and 30%RH.[35] At room temperature, airborne rhinovirus-14 infectivity decayed rapidly at low (30 ± 5%) and medium (50 ± 5%) RH; however, at high (80 ± 5%) RH, this rhinovirus demonstrated a half-life of almost 14 h.[111]

Coronavirus stability, including that of SARS-CoV, has mainly been assessed on surfaces, not in aerosols. The animal coronaviruses transmissible gastroenteritis virus (TGEV, a swine virus) and mouse hepatitis virus (MHV) maintained infectiousness on stainless steel for up to 28 days at 4°C, with maximal stability at 20%RH. Infectivity decay rates increased with higher temperatures (20 and 40°C). With these viruses, the relationship between RH and decay rates was nonmonotonic, such that decay was more rapid at 50%RH than at 20% or 80%RH.[24]

In separate experiments, SARS-CoV dried on plastic lost only 10% viability after 5 days at 22–25°C and 40–50%RH. High humidity (>95%RH) at comparatively low temperature (28 and 33°C), or high temperature (38°C) at comparatively low humidity (80–90%RH), had only modest effects on virus infectivity, but the combination of high humidity and high temperature (>95%RH and 38°C) resulted in maximal decay of virus infectivity.[112]

The temperature and humidity dependence of airborne virus survival may be linked to virion structure. The para- and orthomyxoviruses (HPIV, RSV, and influenza virus) are all enveloped, meaning that the virus particle is surrounded by a lipid envelope, which is derived from the host cell membrane.

humidity and temperature, and meteorological events, like precipitation and wind, are involved in modulating human respiratory virus transmission, and which variables are causative and which are merely correlated or confounding, remains an open question.[26] Most likely, some or all of these variables, and perhaps others still to be elucidated, play partial roles in respiratory virus seasonality, and this complex web of interactions has yet to be fully unraveled.

Thus, what Andrewes noted in 1965 remains, to some extent, true today: "All this is fascinating but very speculative. So, as to why we get more colds in the winter, we must at present admit that we just do not know."[43]

REFERENCES

1. Forgie S, Marrie TJ. Healthcare-associated atypical pneumonia. *Semin Respir Crit Care Med.* 2009;30(1):67–85.
2. Lynch JP, 3rd, Fishbein M, Echavarria M. Adenovirus. *Semin Respir Crit Care Med.* 2011;32(4):494–511.
3. Musher DM. How contagious are common respiratory tract infections? *N Engl J Med.* 2003;348(13):1256–1266.
4. Sandrock C, Stollenwerk N. Acute febrile respiratory illness in the ICU: Reducing disease transmission. *Chest.* 2008;133(5):1221–1231.
5. Tebruegge M, Curtis N. Adenovirus: An overview for pediatric infectious diseases specialists. *Pediatr Infect Dis J.* 2012;31(6):626–627.
6. Belser JA, Maines TR, Tumpey TM, Katz JM. Influenza A virus transmission: Contributing factors and clinical implications. *Expert Rev Mol Med.* 2010;12:e39.
7. Brankston G, Gitterman L, Hirji Z, Lemieux C, Gardam M. Transmission of influenza A in human beings. *Lancet Infect Dis.* 2007;7(4):257–265.
8. Goldmann DA. Transmission of viral respiratory infections in the home. *Pediatr Infect Dis J.* 2000;19(10 Suppl):S97–S102.
9. Tellier R. Review of aerosol transmission of influenza A virus. *Emerg Infect Dis.* 2006;12(11):1657–1662.
10. Tellier R. Aerosol transmission of influenza A virus: a review of new studies. *J R Soc Interface.* 2009;6 Suppl 6:S783–S790.
11. Ansari SA, Springthorpe VS, Sattar SA, Rivard S, Rahman M. Potential role of hands in the spread of respiratory viral infections: Studies with human parainfluenza virus 3 and rhinovirus 14. *J Clin Microbiol.* 1991;29(10):2115–2119.
12. Brady MT, Evans J, Cuartas J. Survival and disinfection of parainfluenza viruses on environmental surfaces. *Am J Infect Control.* 1990;18(1):18–23.
13. Henrickson KJ. Parainfluenza viruses. *Clin Microbiol Rev.* 2003;16(2):242–264.
14. Meissner HC, Murray SA, Kiernan MA, Snydman DR, McIntosh K. A simultaneous outbreak of respiratory syncytial virus and parainfluenza virus type 3 in a newborn nursery. *J Pediatr.* 1984;104(5):680–684.
15. Hall CB, Douglas RG, Jr. Modes of transmission of respiratory syncytial virus. *J Pediatr.* 1981;99(1):100–103.
16. Hall CB, Douglas RG, Jr., Geiman JM. Possible transmission by fomites of respiratory syncytial virus. *J Infect Dis.* 1980;141(1):98–102.
17. Hall CB, Douglas RG, Jr., Schnabel KC, Geiman JM. Infectivity of respiratory syncytial virus by various routes of inoculation. *Infect Immun.* 1981;33(3):779–783.
18. Wright M, Piedimonte G. Respiratory syncytial virus prevention and therapy: Past, present, and future. *Pediatr Pulmonol.* 2011;46(4):324–347.
19. Dick EC, Jennings LC, Mink KA, Wartgow CD, Inhorn SL. Aerosol transmission of rhinovirus colds. *J Infect Dis.* 1987;156(3):442–448.
20. Pica N, Bouvier NM. Environmental factors affecting the transmission of respiratory viruses. *Curr Opin Virol.* 2012;2(1):90–95.
20. Gwaltney JM, Jr., Moskalski PB, Hendley JO. Hand-to-hand transmission of rhinovirus colds. *Ann Intern Med.* 1978;88(4):463–467.
21. Winther B. Rhinovirus infections in the upper airway. *Proc Am Thorac Soc.* 2011;8(1):79–89.
22. Hui DS, Chan PK. Severe acute respiratory syndrome and coronavirus. *Infect Dis Clin North Am.* 2010;24(3):619–638.
23. Peiris JS, Yuen KY, Osterhaus AD, Stohr K. The severe acute respiratory syndrome. *N Engl J Med.* 2003;349(25):2431–2441.

24. Casanova LM, Jeon S, Rutala WA, Weber DJ, Sobsey MD. Effects of air temperature and relative humidity on coronavirus survival on surfaces. *Appl Environ Microbiol*. 2010;76(9):2712–2717.
25. Sloan C, Moore ML, Hartert T. Impact of pollution, climate, and sociodemographic factors on spatiotemporal dynamics of seasonal respiratory viruses. *Clin Transl Sci*. 2011;4(1):48–54.
26. Tamerius J, Nelson MI, Zhou SZ, Viboud C, Miller MA, Alonso WJ. Global influenza seasonality: Reconciling patterns across temperate and tropical regions. *Environ Health Perspect*. 2011;119(4):439–445.
27. Welliver RC, Sr. Temperature, humidity, and ultraviolet B radiation predict community respiratory syncytial virus activity. *Pediatr Infect Dis J*. 2007;26(11 Suppl):S29–S35.
28. Yusuf S, Piedimonte G, Auais A, Demmler G, Krishnan S, Van Caeseele P et al. The relationship of meteorological conditions to the epidemic activity of respiratory syncytial virus. *Epidemiol Infect*. 2007;135(7):1077–1090.
29. van Loghem JJ. An epidemiological contribution to the knowledge of the respiratory diseases. *J Hyg (Lond)*. 1928;28(1):33–54.
30. Lofgren E, Fefferman NH, Naumov YN, Gorski J, Naumova EN. Influenza seasonality: Underlying causes and modeling theories. *J Virol*. 2007;81(11):5429–5436.
31. Salah B, Dinh Xuan AT, Fouilladieu JL, Lockhart A, Regnard J. Nasal mucociliary transport in healthy subjects is slower when breathing dry air. *Eur Respir J*. 1988;1(9):852–855.
32. Diesel DA, Lebel JL, Tucker A. Pulmonary particle deposition and airway mucociliary clearance in cold-exposed calves. *Am J Vet Res*. 1991;52(10):1665–1671.
33. Hemmes JH, Winkler KC, Kool SM. Virus survival as a seasonal factor in influenza and polimyelitis. *Nature*. 1960;188:430–431.
34. Harper GJ. Airborne micro-organisms: Survival tests with four viruses. *J Hyg (Lond)*. 1961;59:479–486.
35. Elazhary MA, Derbyshire JB. Aerosol stability of bovine adenovirus type 3. *Can J Comp Med*. 1979;43(3):305–312.
36. Elazhary MA, Derbyshire JB. Aerosol stability of bovine parainfluenza type 3 virus. *Can J Comp Med*. 1979;43(3):295–304.
37. Hall CB. The spread of influenza and other respiratory viruses: Complexities and conjectures. *Clin Infect Dis*. 2007;45(3):353–359.
38. Hood AM. Infectivity of influenza virus aerosols. *J Hyg (Lond)*. 1963;61:331–335.
39. Miller WS, Artenstein MS. Aerosol stability of three acute respiratory disease viruses. *Proc Soc Exp Biol Med*. 1967;125(1):222–227.
40. Schaffer FL, Soergel ME, Straube DC. Survival of airborne influenza virus: Effects of propagating host, relative humidity, and composition of spray fluids. *Arch Virol*. 1976;51(4):263–273.
41. Shechmeister IL. Studies on the experimental epidemiology of respiratory infections. III. Certain aspects of the behavior of type A influenza virus as an air-borne cloud. *J Infect Dis*. 1950;87(2):128–132.
42. Smith W, Andrewes CH, Laidlaw PP. A virus obtained from influenza patients. *The Lancet*. 1933;222(5732):66–68.
43. Andrewes C. *Season, Weather, and Climate. The Common Cold*. London: Weidenfeld and Nicolson; 1965. p. 133–145.
44. Hope Simpson RE. Discussion on the common cold. *Proc R Soc Med*. 1958;51(4):267–271.
45. Azziz Baumgartner E, Dao CN, Nasreen S, Bhuiyan MU, Mah EMS, Al Mamun A et al. Seasonality, timing, and climate drivers of influenza activity worldwide. *J Infect Dis*. 2012;206(6):838–846.
46. Bloom-Feshbach K, Alonso WJ, Charu V, Tamerius J, Simonsen L, Miller MA et al. Latitudinal variations in seasonal activity of influenza and respiratory syncytial virus (RSV): A global comparative review. *PLoS One*. 2013;8(2):e54445.
47. Viboud C, Alonso WJ, Simonsen L. Influenza in tropical regions. *PLoS Med*. 2006;3(4):e89.
48. Tamerius JD, Shaman J, Alonso WJ, Bloom-Feshbach K, Uejio CK, Comrie A et al. Environmental predictors of seasonal influenza epidemics across temperate and tropical climates. *PLoS Pathogens*. 2013;9(3):e1003194.
49. Chowell G, Towers S, Viboud C, Fuentes R, Sotomayor V, Simonsen L et al. The influence of climatic conditions on the transmission dynamics of the 2009 A/H1N1 influenza pandemic in Chile. *BMC Infect Dis*. 2012;12:298.
50. Rambaut A, Pybus OG, Nelson MI, Viboud C, Taubenberger JK, Holmes EC. The genomic and epidemiological dynamics of human influenza A virus. *Nature*. 2008;453(7195):615–619.
51. Nelson MI, Simonsen L, Viboud C, Miller MA, Holmes EC. Phylogenetic analysis reveals the global migration of seasonal influenza A viruses. *PLoS Pathog*. 2007;3(9):1220–1228.

52. Chan J, Holmes A, Rabadan R. Network analysis of global influenza spread. *PLoS Comput Biol.* 2010;6(11):e1001005.
53. Moorthy M, Castronovo D, Abraham A, Bhattacharyya S, Gradus S, Gorski J et al. Deviations in influenza seasonality: Odd coincidence or obscure consequence? *Clin Microbiol Infect.* 2012;18(10):955–962.
54. Weber MW, Mulholland EK, Greenwood BM. Respiratory syncytial virus infection in tropical and developing countries. *Trop Med Int Health.* 1998;3(4):268–280.
55. Monto AS. Occurrence of respiratory virus: Time, place and person. *Pediatr Infect Dis J.* 2004;23 (1 Suppl):S58–S64.
56. Leecaster M, Gesteland P, Greene T, Walton N, Gundlapalli A, Rolfs R et al. Modeling the variations in pediatric respiratory syncytial virus seasonal epidemics. *BMC Infect Dis.* 2011;11:105.
57. Wilcox MH, Williams O, Camp SJ, Spencer RC, Barker I. Characteristics of successive epidemics of respiratory syncytial virus infection. *Lancet.* 1991;338(8772):943–944.
58. Eriksson M, Bennet R, Rotzen-Ostlund M, von Sydow M, Wirgart BZ. Population-based rates of severe respiratory syncytial virus infection in children with and without risk factors, and outcome in a tertiary care setting. *Acta Paediatr.* 2002;91(5):593–598.
59. Waris M. Pattern of respiratory syncytial virus epidemics in Finland: Two-year cycles with alternating prevalence of groups A and B. *J Infect Dis.* 1991;163(3):464–469.
60. Hagglund S, Hjort M, Graham DA, Ohagen P, Tornquist M, Alenius S. A six-year study on respiratory viral infections in a bull testing facility. *Vet J.* 2007;173(3):585–593.
61. Ampuero JS, Ocana V, Gomez J, Gamero ME, Garcia J, Halsey ES et al. Adenovirus respiratory tract infections in Peru. *PLoS One.* 2012;7(10):e46898.
62. Ji W, Chen ZR, Guo HB, Wang MJ, Yan YD, Zhang XL et al. Characteristics and the prevalence of respiratory viruses and the correlation with climatic factors of hospitalized children in Suzhou children's hospital. *Zhonghua Yu Fang Yi Xue Za Zhi.* 2011;45(3):205–210.
63. Nascimento-Carvalho CM, Cardoso MR, Barral A, Araujo-Neto CA, Oliveira JR, Sobral LS et al. Seasonal patterns of viral and bacterial infections among children hospitalized with community-acquired pneumonia in a tropical region. *Scand J Infect Dis.* 2010;42(11–12):839–844.
64. Shult PA, Polyak F, Dick EC, Warshauer DM, King LA, Mandel AD. Adenovirus 21 infection in an isolated Antarctic station: Transmission of the virus and susceptibility of the population. *Am J Epidemiol.* 1991;133(6):599–607.
65. Monto AS. Medical reviews. Coronaviruses. *Yale J Biol Med.* 1974;47(4):234–251.
66. van der Hoek L, Pyrc K, Jebbink MF, Vermeulen-Oost W, Berkhout RJ, Wolthers KC et al. Identification of a new human coronavirus. *Nat Med.* 2004;10(4):368–373.
67. Lau SK, Woo PC, Yip CC, Tse H, Tsoi HW, Cheng VC et al. Coronavirus HKU1 and other coronavirus infections in Hong Kong. *J Clin Microbiol.* 2006;44(6):2063–2071.
68. Chiu SS, Chan KH, Chu KW, Kwan SW, Guan Y, Poon LL et al. Human coronavirus NL63 infection and other coronavirus infections in children hospitalized with acute respiratory disease in Hong Kong, China. *Clin Infect Dis: Off Publ Infect Dis Soc Am.* 2005;40(12):1721–1729.
69. Cleri DJ, Ricketti AJ, Vernaleo JR. Severe acute respiratory syndrome (SARS). *Infect Dis Clin North Am.* 2010;24(1):175–202.
70. Monto AS. The seasonality of rhinovirus infections and its implications for clinical recognition. *Clin Ther.* 2002;24(12):1987–1997.
71. Wright PF. Parainfluenza viruses. In: Mandell GL, Bennett JE, Dolin R, eds. *Mandell, Douglas, and Bennett's Principles and Practice of Infectious Diseases.* 7th ed. Philadelphia: Churchill Livingstone Elsevier; 2009. p. 2195–2199.
72. Nicholls N. El nino-southern oscillation and vector-borne disease. *Lancet.* 1993;342(8882):1284–1285.
73. McPhaden MJ, Zebiak SE, Glantz MH. ENSO as an integrating concept in earth science. *Science.* 2006;314(5806):1740–1745.
74. Maelzer D, Hales S, Weinstein P, Zalucki M, Woodward A. El Nino and arboviral disease prediction. *Environ Health Perspect.* 1999;107(10):817–818.
75. Shaman J, Lipsitch M. The El Nino-Southern Oscillation (ENSO)-pandemic influenza connection: Coincident or causal? *Proc Natl Acad Sci USA.* 2013;110 Suppl 1:3689–3691.
76. Ebi KL, Exuzides KA, Lau E, Kelsh M, Barnston A. Association of normal weather periods and El Nino events with hospitalization for viral pneumonia in females: California, 1983–1998. *Am J Public Health.* 2001;91(8):1200–1208.
77. Viboud C, Pakdaman K, Boelle PY, Wilson ML, Myers MF, Valleron AJ et al. Association of influenza epidemics with global climate variability. *Eur J Epidemiol.* 2004;19(11):1055–1059.

78. Choi KM, Christakos G, Wilson ML. El Nino effects on influenza mortality risks in the state of California. *Public Health*. 2006;120(6):505–516.
79. Zaraket H, Saito R, Tanabe N, Taniguchi K, Suzuki H. Association of early annual peak influenza activity with El Nino southern oscillation in Japan. *Influenza Other Respi Viruses*. 2008;2(4):127–130.
80. Dawood FS, Jain S, Finelli L, Shaw MW, Lindstrom S, Garten RJ et al. Emergence of a novel swine-origin influenza A (H1N1) virus in humans. *N Engl J Med*. 2009;360(25):2605–2615.
81. Neumann G, Noda T, Kawaoka Y. Emergence and pandemic potential of swine-origin H1N1 influenza virus. *Nature*. 2009;459(7249):931–939.
82. Hammond GW, Raddatz RL, Gelskey DE. Impact of atmospheric dispersion and transport of viral aerosols on the epidemiology of influenza. *Rev Infect Dis*. 1989;11(3):494–497.
83. Rohani P, Breban R, Stallknecht DE, Drake JM. Environmental transmission of low pathogenicity avian influenza viruses and its implications for pathogen invasion. *Proc Natl Acad Sci USA*. 2009;106(25):10365–10369.
84. Spekreijse D, Bouma A, Koch G, Stegeman JA. Airborne transmission of a highly pathogenic avian influenza virus strain H5N1 between groups of chickens quantified in an experimental setting. *Vet Microbiol*. 2011;152(1–2):88–95.
85. Ssematimba A, Hagenaars TJ, de Jong MC. Modelling the wind-borne spread of highly pathogenic avian influenza virus between farms. *PLoS One*. 2012;7(2):e31114.
86. Ypma RJ, Jonges M, Bataille A, Stegeman A, Koch G, van Boven M et al. Genetic data provide evidence for wind-mediated transmission of highly pathogenic avian influenza. *J Infect Dis*. 2013;207(5):730–735.
87. Firestone SM, Cogger N, Ward MP, Toribio JA, Moloney BJ, Dhand NK. The influence of meteorology on the spread of influenza: Survival analysis of an equine influenza (A/H3N8) outbreak. *PLoS One*. 2012;7(4):e35284.
88. Spokes PJ, Marich AJ, Musto JA, Ward KA, Craig AT, McAnulty JM. Investigation of equine influenza transmission in NSW: walk, wind or wing? *N S W Public Health Bull*. 2009;20(9–10):152–156.
89. Davis J, Garner MG, East IJ. Analysis of local spread of equine influenza in the Park Ridge region of Queensland. *Transbound Emerg Dis*. 2009;56(1–2):31–38.
90. Yuan J, Yun H, Lan W, Wang W, Sullivan SG, Jia S et al. A climatologic investigation of the SARS-CoV outbreak in Beijing, China. *Am J Infect Control*. 2006;34(4):234–236.
91. McKinney KR, Gong YY, Lewis TG. Environmental transmission of SARS at Amoy Gardens. *J Environ Health*. 2006;68(9):26–30; quiz 51–52.
92. Yu IT, Li Y, Wong TW, Tam W, Chan AT, Lee JH et al. Evidence of airborne transmission of the severe acute respiratory syndrome virus. *N Engl J Med*. 2004;350(17):1731–1739.
93. Li Y, Leung GM, Tang JW, Yang X, Chao CY, Lin JZ et al. Role of ventilation in airborne transmission of infectious agents in the built environment—A multidisciplinary systematic review. *Indoor Air*. 2007;17(1):2–18.
94. Rudnick SN, Milton DK. Risk of indoor airborne infection transmission estimated from carbon dioxide concentration. *Indoor Air*. 2003;13(3):237–245.
95. Moser MR, Bender TR, Margolis HS, Noble GR, Kendal AP, Ritter DG. An outbreak of influenza aboard a commercial airliner. *Am J Epidemiol*. 1979;110(1):1–6.
96. Myatt TA, Johnston SL, Zuo Z, Wand M, Kebadze T, Rudnick S et al. Detection of airborne rhinovirus and its relation to outdoor air supply in office environments. *Am J Respir Crit Care Med*. 2004;169(11):1187–1190.
97. Goyal SM, Anantharaman S, Ramakrishnan MA, Sajja S, Kim SW, Stanley NJ et al. Detection of viruses in used ventilation filters from two large public buildings. *Am J Infect Control*. 2011;39(7):e30–e38.
98. Korves TM, Johnson D, Jones BW, Watson J, Wolk DM, Hwang GM. Detection of respiratory viruses on air filters from aircraft. *Lett Appl Microbiol*. 2011;53(3):306–312.
99. Blachere FM, Lindsley WG, Pearce TA, Anderson SE, Fisher M, Khakoo R et al. Measurement of airborne influenza virus in a hospital emergency department. *Clin Infect Dis*. 2009;48(4):438–440.
100. Blachere FM, Lindsley WG, Slaven JE, Green BJ, Anderson SE, Chen BT et al. Bioaerosol sampling for the detection of aerosolized influenza virus. *Influenza Other Respi Viruses*. 2007;1(3):113–120.
101. Lindsley WG, Blachere FM, Davis KA, Pearce TA, Fisher MA, Khakoo R et al. Distribution of airborne influenza virus and respiratory syncytial virus in an urgent care medical clinic. *Clin Infect Dis*. 2010;50(5):693–698.
102. Li Y, Huang X, Yu IT, Wong TW, Qian H. Role of air distribution in SARS transmission during the largest nosocomial outbreak in Hong Kong. *Indoor Air*. 2005;15(2):83–95.
103. Wong TW, Lee CK, Tam W, Lau JT, Yu TS, Lui SF et al. Cluster of SARS among medical students exposed to single patient, Hong Kong. *Emerg Infect Dis*. 2004;10(2):269–276.

104. Yu IT, Wong TW, Chiu YL, Lee N, Li Y. Temporal-spatial analysis of severe acute respiratory syndrome among hospital inpatients. *Clin Infect Dis*. 2005;40(9):1237–1243.
105. Chen C, Zhao B, Yang X, Li Y. Role of two-way airflow owing to temperature difference in severe acute respiratory syndrome transmission: revisiting the largest nosocomial severe acute respiratory syndrome outbreak in Hong Kong. *J R Soc Interface*. 2011;8(58):699–710.
106. Wong BC, Lee N, Li Y, Chan PK, Qiu H, Luo Z et al. Possible role of aerosol transmission in a hospital outbreak of influenza. *Clin Infect Dis*. 2010;51(10):1176–1183.
107. Shaman J, Kohn M. Absolute humidity modulates influenza survival, transmission, and seasonality. *Proc Natl Acad Sci USA*. 2009;106(9):3243–3248.
108. Bean B, Moore BM, Sterner B, Peterson LR, Gerding DN, Balfour HH, Jr. Survival of influenza viruses on environmental surfaces. *J Infect Dis*. 1982;146(1):47–51.
109. McDevitt J, Rudnick S, First M, Spengler J. Role of absolute humidity in the inactivation of influenza viruses on stainless steel surfaces at elevated temperatures. *Appl Environ Microbiol*. 2010;76(12):3943–3947.
110. Rechsteiner J, Winkler KC. Inactivation of respiratory syncytial virus in aerosol. *J Gen Virol*. 1969;5:405–410.
111. Karim YG, Ijaz MK, Sattar SA, Johnson-Lussenburg CM. Effect of relative humidity on the airborne survival of rhinovirus-14. *Can J Microbiol*. 1985;31(11):1058–1061.
112. Chan KH, Peiris JS, Lam SY, Poon LL, Yuen KY, Seto WH. The effects of temperature and relative humidity on the viability of the SARS coronavirus. *Adv Virol*. 2011;2011:734690.
113. Minhaz Ud-Dean SM. Structural explanation for the effect of humidity on persistence of airborne virus: Seasonality of influenza. *J Theor Biol*. 2010;264(3):822–829.
114. Polozov IV, Bezrukov L, Gawrisch K, Zimmerberg J. Progressive ordering with decreasing temperature of the phospholipids of influenza virus. *Nat Chem Biol*. 2008;4(4):248–255.
115. Bouvier NM, Lowen AC. Animal models for influenza virus pathogenesis and transmission. *Viruses*. 2010;2(8):1530–1563.
116. Schulman JL. Experimental transmission of influenza virus infection in mice. IV. Relationship of transmissibility of different strains of virus and recovery of airborne virus in the environment of infector mice. *J Exp Med*. 1967;125(3):479–488.
117. Schulman JL, Kilbourne ED. Airborne transmission of influenza virus infection in mice. *Nature*. 1962;195:1129–1130.
118. Schulman JL, Kilbourne ED. Experimental transmission of influenza virus infection in mice. Ii. Some factors affecting the incidence of transmitted infection. *J Exp Med*. 1963;118:267–275.
119. Lowen AC, Mubareka S, Steel J, Palese P. Influenza virus transmission is dependent on relative humidity and temperature. *PLoS Pathog*. 2007;3(10):1470–1476.
120. Lowen AC, Steel J, Mubareka S, Palese P. High temperature (30 degrees C) blocks aerosol but not contact transmission of influenza virus. *J Virol*. 2008;82(11):5650–5652.
121. Halloran SK, Wexler AS, Ristenpart WD. A comprehensive breath plume model for disease transmission via expiratory aerosols. *PLoS One*. 2012;7(5):e37088.
122. Yang W, Marr LC. Dynamics of airborne influenza a viruses indoors and dependence on humidity. *PLoS One*. 2011;6(6):e21481.
123. Shaman J, Pitzer VE, Viboud C, Grenfell BT, Lipsitch M. Absolute humidity and the seasonal onset of influenza in the continental United States. *PLoS Biol*. 2010;8(2):e1000316.
124. Shoji M, Katayama K, Sano K. Absolute humidity as a deterministic factor affecting seasonal influenza epidemics in Japan. *Tohoku J Exp Med*. 2011;224(4):251–256.
125. Yang W, Elankumaran S, Marr LC. Relationship between humidity and influenza A viability in droplets and implications for influenza's seasonality. *PLoS One*. 2012;7(10):e46789.
126. Lowen AC, Mubareka S, Tumpey TM, Garcia-Sastre A, Palese P. The guinea pig as a transmission model for human influenza viruses. *Proc Natl Acad Sci USA*. 2006;103(26):9988–9992.
127. Steel J, Palese P, Lowen AC. Transmission of a 2009 pandemic influenza virus shows a sensitivity to temperature and humidity similar to that of an H3N2 seasonal strain. *J Virol*. 2011;85(3):1400–1402.
128. Ciencewicki J, Jaspers I. Air pollution and respiratory viral infection. *Inhal Toxicol*. 2007;19(14):1135–1146.
129. Hope-Simpson RE. The role of season in the epidemiology of influenza. *J Hygiene*. 1981;86(1):35–47.

8 Animal Models of Human Respiratory Viral Infections

Kayla A. Weiss, Cory J. Knudson, Allison F. Christiaansen, and Steven M. Varga

CONTENTS

8.1 INTRODUCTION

Viral respiratory infections are a leading cause of morbidity and mortality worldwide, especially in young children and the elderly, due primarily to the physiological effects associated with virus-induced pulmonary injury. Animal models that recapitulate the infection and disease of these human pathogens serve as a critical tool to develop therapeutic treatments and vaccines. This chapter will outline the anatomical and general considerations for the use of various animal species used most frequently to model human respiratory disease. In addition, this chapter will discuss the most widely used animal models for a number of medically important human respiratory viruses. When appropriate, the use of other animal viruses that are used to model the disease induced by the human pathogen will also be discussed. The content provided in this chapter will convey the general considerations and current information for the most commonly studied animal models of human respiratory viral infections and disease.

8.2 PULMONARY MECHANICS AND ANATOMY OF COMMON ANIMAL MODELS FOR RESPIRATORY VIRAL INFECTIONS

8.2.1 Mice

Mice and rats comprise approximately 95% of all animals used in laboratory research.[1] Murine biological processes and genetic makeup share many similarities to humans.[2] Approximately 80% of murine genes have an identifiable orthologue in the human genome, and less than 1% of the murine genome does not have a corresponding human homologue.[3–5] Mice are commonly used as models to study respiratory viral infections because they share major features of pulmonary physiology and anatomy with humans.

8.2.1.1 Anatomy

The general composition of the respiratory tract of mice is similar to humans. Both mice and humans have comparable tissues and organs in the lower and upper respiratory tracts that perform similar functions. However, the murine upper respiratory tract contains several unique structural features.

The primary role of the nasal cavity of both mice and humans is air uptake. However, the murine nose is also specialized for olfaction. Mice have a more complex turbinate structure as compared to humans.[6] Turbinates are long scroll-shaped spongy bones that protrude into the lumen of the nasal cavity forming groove-like structures to direct airflow. Turbinates are rich in blood vessels and lined with mucosal epithelium to help humidify, heat and filter inhaled air to aid in respiration. While a larger fraction of nasal epithelium in mice is olfactory epithelium, roughly 50% as compared to only 3% in humans, the relative surface area of the murine turbinate structure is also five times greater than in humans. The complex murine turbinate structure may allow for better protection of the lower respiratory tract due to increased filtration within the nasal cavity.[7] However, this may lead to a higher incidence of lesion formation in the upper respiratory tract as noted in toxicology studies.[8] There are also a few minor differences in the shape and tissue composition of the pharynx and larynx of mice as compared to humans.[6] However, these minor structural differences likely have a negligible overall impact on pulmonary mechanics and immune responses to viral infections as compared to humans.

The lower respiratory tract of mice also contains a number of similarities and distinctions to humans. The size and proportion of the murine trachea is similar in comparison to humans.[10] In contrast, the murine bronchial tree consists of relatively wider airways as compared to large animals and is comprised of a monopodial branching pattern distinct from the dichotomous branching pattern observed in humans.[11] Therefore, main bronchi in mice extend further throughout the lung prior to branching into smaller bronchi. Due to the monopodial branching pattern, particle deposition in the murine lower airways is believed to be more uniform.[12] While mice and humans have similar epithelial cell types in the respiratory tract, the presence of submucosal glands in the murine intrapulmonary airways is very rare.[13–15] Furthermore, the tracheobronchial region of the murine respiratory tract is lined with a greater fraction of Clara cells and a reduced number of goblet cells.[14,16,17] There is currently no data to suggest that the altered composition of mucin-secreting cells has a significant impact on pulmonary function during infection or respiratory illness. However, the low frequency of goblet cells together with relatively wider airways may reduce overall susceptibility to lower respiratory tract dysfunction and illness.

8.2.1.2 Physiology and Mechanics

Differences in the anatomy of the respiratory tract of mice as compared to humans have a significant impact on particular aspects of pulmonary physiology and baseline mechanics. The complex turbinate structure of mice significantly increases the turbulence of airflow within the nasal cavity. Because mice are obligate nose breathers, particle deposition in the nasal cavity is significantly increased as compared to humans.[7] This may provide the lower airways of mice more protection from inhalation of harmful chemicals or pathogens. Mice also exhibit differences in lymphoid tissue organization in the upper respiratory tract. Distinct organized tertiary lymphoid tissues, specifically nasal-associated lymphoid tissues (NALT), form above the nasopharyngeal region of mice following immune responses in the upper airways.[18,19] Though the pattern is more diffuse and disorganized, NALT formation has been observed post-mortem in the nasal cavities of children who died from either sudden infant syndrome or other undefined causes.[20] The more distinct and highly organized NALT structures observed in mice is likely due to the lack of tonsils in the pharyngeal region.[6] These NALT structures serve as the critical induction site for the generation of mucosal IgA antibody.[18,21]

The organization of the murine bronchial tree has a profound impact on airway resistance. Mice exhibit a monopodial branching pattern for the bronchial tree in comparison to humans that have a dichotomous branching pattern.[11] The dichotomous branching pattern in humans leads to more turbulent airflow that may contribute to greater airway resistance.[22] However, the relatively larger airways and laminar airflow in the murine lower respiratory tract likely contributes to a greater ventilatory dead space that is compensated for by a higher frequency of breathing.

Despite these differences mice exhibit altered airway mechanics similar to humans during respiratory distress or illness. The challenge of mice with bronchoconstrictor agonists, a common method to assess airway function during asthma, results in increased airway resistance and reduced lung compliance.[23–25] Increased airway resistance has also been observed during common respiratory viral infections, such as human respiratory syncytial virus (HRSV) or influenza A virus (IAV) in both humans and mice.[26–29] Thus, although mice exhibit altered baseline airway mechanics, the changes in these parameters during respiratory infection are similar to humans.

8.2.1.3 Additional Considerations

Mice are the most commonly used animal models in biomedical research due to their accessibility, availability of tools, and cost effectiveness. Mice have large litter sizes with short gestation periods in comparison to larger mammals so it is easy to generate sizable colonies in a short period of time. Their small size also makes them easier to handle as well as inexpensive to house and feed. The relatively short life span of mice makes them ideal for aging studies. Furthermore, there are a number of commercial facilities devoted to breeding and maintenance of common murine strains making them readily available. Genetic variation is minimized through breeding of siblings paired with genotypic screening. Genetic modification is also common in the murine model allowing for an evaluation of the role of individual genes *in vivo*. Owing to their prominent use, mice also have the most extensive catalog of tools and reagents available. This is especially important when considering the evaluation of lung function, as there are a number of machines tailored to measure pulmonary mechanics in mice, such as whole body plethysmography and mechanical ventilators. These benefits allow for analysis of a large sample size with little genetic variability at a fraction of the cost it would require for larger animal or human studies.[30]

8.2.2 Cotton Rats

In contrast to other small mammals, cotton rats are highly permissive to infection and replication by a wide number of respiratory viruses. This makes cotton rats an ideal model to evaluate new vaccine strategies prior to testing in humans.

8.2.2.1 Anatomy

There are no comparative studies of lung morphology between cotton rats and humans. Gross anatomy is likely comparable to other small rodents with a more complex turbinate structure in the nasal cavity. It is unclear if cotton rats have altered cellular composition in the tracheobronchial region or a monopodial bronchial tree similar to mice. Further investigation is necessary to more fully compare cotton rat lung morphology to humans.

8.2.2.2 Physiology and Mechanics

Cotton rats are permissive to infection by a number of human respiratory viruses such as IAV, HRSV, parainfluenza, and human metapneumovirus (HMPV).[31–34] However, there has been virtually no evaluation of pulmonary mechanics following respiratory viral infection. While immune responses are detectable in the cotton rats following infection with these respiratory viruses, is unclear if pulmonary function and airway resistance are significantly altered.

8.2.2.3 Additional Considerations

The cotton rat is commercially available as an inbred strain making them reasonably accessible with limited genetic variability. The gestation period of the cotton rat is approximately 27 days with an average litter size of 5. While cotton rats are more expensive to house and feed as compared to mice, they are relatively inexpensive as compared to the high costs associated with either nonhuman primate or human studies. The relatively short life span of a laboratory cotton rat ranges from 12 to 18 months and allows for the evaluation of aged cotton rats in a reasonably brief period of time. A limitation to using cotton rats as a model is the lack of currently available reagents. However, a number of antibodies and polymerase chain reaction primers and probes specific to cytokines and chemokines for other species can be utilized due to their cross-reactivity and sequence homology, respectively.[35] Cotton rats are also more difficult to handle due to their larger size and increased aggressiveness as compared to mice.

8.2.3 Hamsters

Hamsters are the fifth most commonly used laboratory animal in research.[36] Approximately 90% of hamsters used in research are Syrian hamsters, and therefore the majority of investigations on respiratory illness in hamsters are performed with this species.[37] Hamsters can be infected with a number of common respiratory viruses and serve as a good model to study particular aspects of respiratory disease.

8.2.3.1 Anatomy

The gross anatomy of the respiratory tract of hamsters is similar to other small rodents such as mice. Few comparative studies of the upper respiratory tract between hamsters and humans have been conducted. While overall tissue organization of the upper respiratory tract is similar to humans, hamsters have a more complex nasal passage and turbinate structure though not as intricate as previously documented with mice.[38,39] These differences likely impact airflow by increasing turbulence and particle deposition in the upper respiratory tract, however this has not been thoroughly investigated.

A number of similarities and differences in the lower respiratory tract have been observed in comparative studies between hamsters and humans. The length and diameter of the trachea is directly proportional to the body size in hamsters and humans.[10] The branching pattern of the bronchial tree has been described as unequal or irregular dichotomous.[40] Unlike humans, there is a lack of symmetry in the airway branching and the pattern can be occasionally trichotomous, diverging from the main into three bronchi.

Furthermore, the angle of branching is greater in the hamster as compared to humans, making bronchi more lateral in relation to the primary bronchi.[41] It is unclear if this has a significant impact on airflow though it may alter particle deposition patterns in the lung due to the lack of symmetry.

The composition of respiratory epithelium in hamsters is similar to humans; however, there is a significant decrease in the number of mucus secreting cells as observed in mice.[38,40] While there is a high density of submucosal glands present in the upper region of the trachea near the larynx of hamsters, there is an absence of these glands in the tracheobronchial region similar to mice.[42] Goblet cells are present in both the trachea and bronchial tree of hamsters similar to humans.[40] While both humans and hamsters have Clara cells present in the bronchioles of the lower airways, hamsters have a greater number of these cells in the bronchi.[43] It is important to note that the concentration of secretory granules are diminished in Clara cells and secretory granules do not coalesce in goblet cells as observed in humans, which may contribute to the reduced detection of mucin-secreting cells in the lower airways.[40,44] It is unclear if these distinctions in mucus secreting cells in hamsters alter disease and pulmonary mechanics during respiratory viral infection.

8.2.3.2 Physiology and Mechanics

Although the respiratory tract of hamsters contains a number of unique features as compared to humans, it is unclear if there are significant differences in pulmonary mechanics and physiology. In addition to the reduced number of submucosal glands in the respiratory tract of hamsters, there is also a scarce distribution of lymphoid tissue in the tracheobronchial region.[40] This is likely due to the more complex nasal passage of hamsters as compared to humans that improves filtration of air. However, similar to mice, distinct arrangements of NALT are present at the end of the nasal cavity leading to the pharynx.[45]

The increased complexity of the nasal passage and altered branching pattern of the bronchial tree likely contribute to increased baseline airway resistance. However, there are an inadequate number of studies that have investigated the pulmonary mechanics of hamsters. Treatment of hamsters with the bronchoconstrictor reagent methacholine induces airway obstruction and gas trapping.[46] Hamsters also exhibit a significant increase in total lung capacity and functional residual capacity following elastase administration, making them an excellent model for pulmonary emphysema.[47] Hamsters are susceptible to infection by a number of common respiratory viruses including IAV, severe acute respiratory syndrome coronavirus (SARS-CoV), and HMPV allowing for the evaluation of new vaccines or pharmacological agents.[48,49] However, due to the lack of disease signs in hamsters following respiratory viral infections, there are virtually no published studies examining pulmonary mechanics during respiratory disease.

8.2.3.3 Additional Considerations

Hamsters are one of the more commonly used animal models due to their accessibility and cost effectiveness. Commercial vendors sell hamsters making them readily available and there are a number of inbred strains. The gestation period for hamsters is relatively short at approximately 16–24 days with a litter size of 5–10. This allows for the accumulation of a large number of animals in a short time frame. Hamsters can also live up to 2–3 years permitting long-term experimentation and aging studies. Furthermore, hamsters are generally tame, easy to handle, and cheaper to house and feed as compared to larger mammals.

The major drawback to using hamsters in research studies is the lack of available reagents, particularly antibodies. This makes it difficult to assess specific aspects of the immune response in hamsters following respiratory viral infection. Furthermore, the most commonly used hamster strain, *Mesocricetus auratus* or Syrian hamsters, are outbred and will have greater genetic variability.

8.2.4 Guinea Pigs

Guinea pigs remain one of the most commonly used animal models in biomedical research since the seventeenth century though their use has been gradually replaced by other rodents such as mice and rats.[36] Guinea pigs can be infected with many common respiratory viruses and serve as an excellent model for pulmonary disease.

8.2.4.1 Anatomy

The morphology of the respiratory tract in guinea pigs is similar to humans and other small rodents. The nasopharynx in guinea pigs consists of a central structure with a number of air pockets that is similar to humans.[7] The larynx and laryngopharynx region are similar in morphology between guinea pigs and humans.

Guinea pigs lack a significant number of goblet cells and submucosal glands in the tracheobronchial region as well as ciliated cells lining the tracheal wall.[50,51] The composition of respiratory epithelium is otherwise relatively similar in guinea pigs as compared to humans. However, there are a greater number of Clara cells specifically in the terminal bronchioles of guinea pigs.[52] The branching pattern of the bronchial tree in guinea pigs is similar to hamsters in that it is irregularly dichotomous.[39,53] Furthermore, while there are several generations of bronchioles similar to humans, guinea pigs have far fewer respiratory bronchioles that eventually branch into alveoli.[53–55]

8.2.4.2 Physiology and Mechanics

The unique structural features of the respiratory tract of guinea pigs likely contributes to altered baseline mechanics, it is unclear to what extent these morphological differences individually contribute to pulmonary mechanics. Guinea pigs exhibit increased baseline airway resistance as compared to mice.[56] This is likely due to the irregular dichotomous branching pattern of the bronchial tree and smaller bronchi relative to mice.

Guinea pigs are an established animal model to study asthma and exhibit decreased lung function and increased airway resistance in response to common bronchoconstrictor agents.[57–59] Interestingly, guinea pigs exhibit constitutive expression of the chemokine eotaxin in the lower airways, which may make their lung environment more prone to Th2-biased immune responses following allergen challenge.[60] However, evaluation of the lower airway pulmonary mechanics following respiratory viral infection has not been thoroughly investigated in guinea pigs. Similar to hamsters, guinea pigs do not display signs of disease to respiratory viral infections, with the exception of histamine-treated animals following human parainfluenza (HPIV) type 3 infection, as discussed in detail later.[61] This may make guinea pigs a poor model for the evaluation of pulmonary mechanics following respiratory virus infection though further investigation is necessary. In contrast to the majority of animal models, guinea pigs exhibit a cough and sneeze reflex and can transmit IAV to uninfected guinea pigs in separate nearby cages.[8] Thus guinea pigs are a useful model to study viral transmission.

8.2.4.3 Additional Considerations

Inbred strains of guinea pigs are commercially available for purchase making them accessible and reducing genetic variability. Furthermore, guinea pigs have a relatively short gestation period of approximately 59–72 days with a litter size of 1–6. The above, in combination with a reduced cost to house and feed as compared to nonhuman primates, makes guinea pigs as an alternative model to study respiratory viral infections. However, a major limitation is that there are very few reagents specific for guinea pigs. Genetic manipulation of guinea pigs is also very limited making evaluation of immune responses and physiological processes difficult.

8.2.5 Ferrets

Ferrets are a common animal model to investigate multiple aspects of human respiratory virus-induced disease. Due to their similarities in lung structure to humans, ferrets are commonly used to assess pathogenesis, transmission, and pulmonary function following respiratory viral infections.

8.2.5.1 Anatomy

While few studies have directly compared the morphological features of ferrets to humans in detail, the gross anatomy of both is similar.[64–66] One notable difference is that ferrets have a relatively long trachea that contributes to increased baseline pulmonary resistance. In addition, histological studies have revealed similar lung cell composition in the tracheobronchial region with a large number of mucus-secreting cells.[67,68] The relative proportion of submucosal glands is far greater in number than other small animal models making ferrets more similar to humans.[69] This makes ferrets a suitable model for the study of mucus hypersecretion during respiratory disease. Ferrets also have a greater number of terminal bronchioles as compared to other small animals, although it is still fewer than the number found in humans.[64] Lastly, the ferret lung and lower airways are disproportionately large for its body size.[64] Together these factors make the ferret an appealing model to assess lung disease and pulmonary mechanics.

8.2.5.2 Physiology and Mechanics

The total lung capacity of the ferret is approximately three times larger than expected according to its body size.[70] The relatively large airways of ferrets also contributes to decreased airway resistance, which is more similar to humans.[71] This is ideal, as the longer trachea in ferrets increases baseline pulmonary resistance. Ferrets also exhibit increased airway resistance and reduced lung compliance in response to common bronchoconstrictor agonists.[64,72] This would suggest that the

8.4.2 Disease

Adenovirus types 1, 2, 3, 5, 6, and 7 can induce respiratory tract disease in infants. Infections are associated with mild upper respiratory illness, pharyngitis, bronchitis, and pneumonia.[48–51] Fatalities in children with adenovirus infection reveal that lung consolidation, airway occlusion, lesions, fibrin deposits, and alveolar thickening occurs.[52] In addition, adenovirus types 4 and 7 induce acute respiratory disease (ARD) in military training camps.[53] In affected trainee units, up to 80% of individuals were hospitalized for ARD due to acute symptoms of fever, myalgia, headache, dizziness, pharyngitis, and dry cough following adenovirus infection.[54–56] In addition, approximately 90% of pneumonia cases in military training camps are associated with adenovirus infection.[57–59]

Ad5 infection of cotton rats induces pneumonia. Following Ad5 infection in cotton rats, similarities with human disease are observed—including bronchiolar epithelial cell damage, mononuclear infiltration, and intranuclear inclusions.[41,52,60,61] However, infection with a high dose of Ad5 results in 100% mortality within seven days p.i.[41] Therefore, inoculum dose should be carefully considered when attempting to recapitulate human disease in the cotton rat model. Inoculation of various inbred strains of mice with a high dose of Ad5 intranasally resulted in the development of pneumonia with a hierarchy of disease severity as follows: C57BL/6 > CBA/ > C3H/ > C57BL/10.[42] Similar to cotton rats, pneumonia developed and is described as two phases—thickening of alveolar walls in the first phase and immune cellular infiltration in both phases.[42] Ad3 or Ad7 induce similar disease following intratracheal infection of C57BL/6 mice.[43] Increased perivascular infiltration and cytopathology of the bronchial epithelium are observed in mice as compared to cotton rats.[42] Thus, mice are able to model the pneumonia aspect of adenovirus-induced ARD in humans. However, since mice do not support viral replication, this model is limited in assessing the role of viral replication in human disease.

8.4.3 Immune Response

Macrophages and neutrophils are present in the airways of children with fatal adenovirus infection, while the lamina propria is infiltrated with lymphocytes, plasma cells, and macrophages.[52] Alveolar infiltration and peribronchiolar and perivascular lymphocytic infiltration is observed following intranasal Ad5 infection in cotton rats.[41] Development of pneumonia occurs in two phases following infection of C57BL/6 mice with a high dose of Ad5 intranasally.[42] In the first phase intraalveolar monocyte, macrophage, and lymphocyte infiltration is observed, followed by perivascular and peribronchial infiltration by lymphocytes in the second phase.[42] Similar cellular infiltration and inflammation was observed following infection of C57BL/6 mice with Ad3 or Ad7.[43] However, at early time points post-Ad3 or Ad7 infection (days 1–2), the majority of cellular infiltration was neutrophils accounting for 70–80% of the total cellularity.[43]

8.4.4 Vaccines and Genetic Vectors

A live oral vaccine against types 4 and 7 was developed and administered to new military recruits, yielding a significant decrease in the frequency of reported ARD outbreaks in military camps.[62] The use of Ad4 and Ad7 vaccines resulted in a 50–60% decrease in total disease induced by respiratory infections and decreased adenovirus-induced disease by 95–99%.[63–65] Given the immunogenicity of adenoviruses and their success as immunizations in the military, the use of adenoviruses as either vaccines or genetic vectors has been of interest. However this strategy has complications since over 90% of the population have antibodies reactive to at least one type of human adenovirus limiting their potential use as vaccines and genetic vectors.[66,67] In addition, their robust natural immunogenicity limits their use as long-term genetic vectors in immunocompetent individuals. Therefore, the use of alternative approaches to overcome the preexisting immunity and their immunogenicity in the human population is required to further develop the use of adenoviruses as vaccines and vectors.[68]

8.5 CORONAVIRIDAE: CORONAVIRUS

8.5.1 Infection

Alpha and beta human coronaviruses (HCoV) induce disease in the human population. From alphacoronaviruses, humans are infected by HCoV-229E and HCoV-NL63, and HCoV-OC43, HCoV-HKU1, and SARS-CoV from betacoronaviruses. In the summer of 2012 there was the emergence of another betacoronavirus, HCoV-EMC, which induced respiratory disease in humans.[69] With the exception of SARS-CoV, productive infection of HCoVs is limited to humans. A transgenic immunocompromised mouse strain expressing the human aminopeptidase N (hAPN) protein, the putative receptor for HCoV-229E, was developed to permit the replication of an adapted HCoV-229E in an animal model.[70] HCoV-NL63 and -HKU1 viruses are recently identified human pathogens[71,72] and no animal models have been described to date for these viruses.

In humans SARS-CoV initially replicates in the lung, but the virus is also detectable in the stool, urine, and sweat of infected patients, indicating virus dissemination and development of systemic infection.[73,74] SARS-CoV also exhibits efficient cross-species transmission. This is due to the unique receptor for SARS-CoV, ACE2, and the SARS-CoV spike protein associating with multiple species' ACE2 permitting virus entry. The relative virulence of various SARS-CoV strains is attributed to the ability of the spike protein to interact with various species' ACE2 protein.[75–78]

SARS-CoV is capable of replicating in the respiratory tracts of cynomolgus and rhesus macaques, African green monkeys, and marmosets. Cynomolgus macaques shed the virus from the nasal passageway between days 2 and 6 p.i.[79,80] In rhesus macaques viral RNA is detected up to 16 days p.i.[81] Viral RNA is detectable in the lungs of marmosets on day 4 and 7 p.i. at the time of necropsy.[82] Thus, SARS-CoV is able to efficiently replicate in multiple nonhuman primate species.

In BALB/c and C57BL/6 mice, SARS-CoV replicates in the upper and lower respiratory tracts.[83,84] Peak viral replication was observed at day 2 and 3 p.i. and clearance in the lungs occurs by day 7 and 9 p.i. in BALB/c and C57BL/6 mice, respectively.[83,84] However, mouse adapted SARS-CoV have been developed and are used to model CoV-SARS infection in humans.[85] SARS-CoV replicates in the respiratory tract of ferrets following intranasal infection with viral shedding occurring between days 2 and 14 p.i.[86] In golden Syrian hamsters, virus replication occurs with antigen primarily localized to the respiratory epithelium in the airways and trachea and virus is no longer detectable in the lungs by day 7 p.i.[87]

8.5.2 Disease

The respiratory disease in humans is dependent upon the infecting coronavirus strain. HCoV-OC43 and -229E both generally induce mild disease following infection with the development of common cold symptoms, including coughing, nasal discharge, pharyngitis, and sneezing. In contrast, infection with HCoV-HKU1 and -NL63 result in more severe disease, with pneumonia in the elderly, and bronchiolitis, croup, and pneumonia in young children observed, respectively.[71,72,88,89]

Intranasal HCoV-OC43 infection of mice results in the development of encephalitis and is used as a model for diseases in humans, such as multiple sclerosis.[90] Therefore, HCoV-OC43 infection of mice is not used as a model for respiratory disease in humans. However, HCoV-229E infection of transgenic immunocompromised mice, expressing the human receptor for HCoV-229E, induces mild disease as measured by slight weight loss, mild fever, and hemorrhagic areas in the lung as determined by histological analysis.[70] Although transgenic immunocompromised mice are required to establish infection and disease, this model is the most appealing current model for respiratory tract disease induced by common coronaviruses due to reagent availability for the species and because the model recapitulates critical aspects of the human disease.

A recent pandemic of a newly emerged HCoV, SARS-CoV, induced significant morbidity and mortality in the human population. Human infection with SARS-CoV generally results in clinical symptoms of fever, dyspnea, and lower respiratory tract disease (LRTD).[91,92] In addition the development of enteric disease occurs in approximately 30–40% of patients.[93] In fatal cases of SARS-CoV infection of humans, histopathology reveals the presence of edema, alveolar damage, giant cells, and epithelium hyperplasia in the lower respiratory tract.[94,95]

SARS-CoV infection of cynomolgus macaques results in clinical disease. On day 3 p.i., lethargy is observed followed by the development of an acute skin rash by day 4 p.i.[79] Pneumonia assessed by histological analysis on day 6 p.i. was present with tissue lesions, alveolar damage, cellular necrosis, edema, and cellular infiltration observed.[79] These histological observations in cynomolgus macaques are similar to reports from the autopsies of SARS patients.[94,95] However, a separate study found that SARS-CoV infection in both cynomolgus and rhesus macaques results in very acute mild disease constrained to the upper respiratory tract, unlike human disease.[96] The histological analysis on days 12–14 p.i. revealed patches of edema and inflammation without the presence of syncytia and damage to the lung airways unlike the observations made for humans.[96] An additional study reported SARS-CoV replication in rhesus macaques, as well as African green monkeys and cynomolgus macaques, without the development of clinical illness.[97] In addition, the effect of SARS-CoV infection in rhesus macaques for a longer duration was assessed, with interstitial pneumonia present at 60 days p.i.[81] Overall, no nonhuman primate is able to model the severe disease observed in humans following SARS-CoV infection.

SARS-CoV infection of either BALB/c or C57BL/6 mice does not result in the development of clinical disease.[83,84] In BALB/c mice, peribronchiolar mononuclear infiltration was observed, although it was mild and focal in the lung tissue.[84] However, infection of aged BALB/c mice with SARS-CoV resulted in the development of clinical disease.[98] Ferrets infected with SARS-CoV fail to exhibit clinical respiratory disease symptoms, however lethargy and pulmonary lesions were observed.[86] Similarly, no clinical disease was observed following SARS-CoV infection of golden Syrian hamsters.[87] However, on day 3 p.i., inflammation was observed in the lung tissue along with mononuclear and polymorphonuclear infiltrates, which resolved by day 5 p.i.[87] Thus, no small animal model is able to fully model the disease observed in humans following SARS-CoV infection.

8.5.3 Immune Response

T-cell lymphopenia was observed following SARS-CoV infection in humans with severe disease.[99–101] However, animal models recapitulating T-cell lymphopenia following infection have not been described. It will be of interest to develop an animal model to recapitulate this aspect of the disease if surviving SARS-CoV individuals with lymphopenia exhibit adverse long-term outcomes.

Development of a SARS-CoV neutralizing antibody response occurs in humans following infection.[102,103] SARS-CoV infection in African green monkeys induces a neutralizing antibody response able to prevent secondary infections two months later with no detectable virus replication or clinical disease.[97] In addition, neutralizing antibodies are detectable by day 15 p.i. and are at the highest level on day 60 p.i. in rhesus macaques following SARS-CoV infection.[81]

Neutralizing antibodies have been shown to mediate protection from SARS-CoV infection in BALB/c mice.[84] Neutralizing antibodies develop following SARS-CoV infection in golden Syrian hamsters and are detectable starting day 7 p.i.[87] This response is able to provide complete protection from lower respiratory tract infection following a secondary challenge.[87] Infected ferrets also develop a SARS-CoV specific-antibody response by four weeks p.i.[86] These data demonstrate the protective role neutralizing antibodies play in preventing subsequent infections with SARS-CoV.

8.5.4 Animal Viruses to Model Human Disease

There are multiple porcine coronaviruses that cause enteric and respiratory disease resulting in large economic losses due to the high mortality following infection of neonates in the agricultural industry.[104] Transmissible gastroenteritis coronavirus (TGEV) infection primarily results in gastroenteritis, but is capable of infecting the respiratory tract as well.[105] Although TGEV can cause significant disease in neonates, disease is very mild in adult pigs. Porcine respiratory virus (PRCoV) is a variant of TGEV with their genomes being 96% homologous.[105] PRCoV replicates in lung epithelium and alveolar macrophages, and results in the development of interstitial pneumonia.[105] Porcine epidemic diarrhea coronavirus (PEDV) is another porcine coronavirus that is genetically similar to the human coronavirus 229E.[105]

The avian coronavirus IBV replicates in the upper respiratory tract and in young animals severe disease from lower respiratory tract infections are observed.[93] IBV is a highly virulent virus primarily infecting chickens and is a large concern for the poultry industry. Some strains can induce systemic disease following infection of the respiratory tract, which is believed to be due to insufficient antibodies to prevent the dissemination of the virus from the lung.[106] Maternal antibodies can protect a neonate from IBV infection, as well as adoptive transfer of CD8 T cells.[106] Owing to the economic importance of porcine and avian coronaviruses, several vaccine strategies have been developed. Live-attenuated vaccines provided no or short-lived immunity in pigs and chickens, whereas inactivated vaccines were beneficial in boosting preexisting immunity in animals.[105–107] However, the lack of cross reactivity between serotypes and/or viruses is a challenge in providing broadly protective immunity. Although the strategies for vaccine development against porcine and avian coronaviruses have been unsuccessful to date, the attempts may be relevant to human vaccines against coronavirus infections.

Two biotypes comprise feline coronaviruses—feline enteric coronavirus (FeCoV) and feline infectious peritonitis virus (FIPV). FeCoV induces asymptomatic disease, whereas FIPV infection causes severe disease with significant mortality. FIPV is able to replicate in macrophages leading to systemic spread of the virus.[108]

Bovine coronavirus (BCoV) infects the respiratory and gastrointestinal tract in cattle. BCoV is a ubiquitous global pathogen resulting in calf diarrhea and adult winter dysentery from enteric disease and shipping fever from respiratory disease.[105,106] The majority of morbidity is more severe and observed in young animals and thus may be a good model to investigate for severe disease following HCoV-NL63 and HCoV-HKU1 in young children.

There are multiple strains of mouse hepatitis virus (MHV) with tropisms for the liver and brain, making these murine coronaviruses a commonly used animal model for investigating hepatitis and encephalitis in humans. In addition, intranasal infection of A/J mice with MHV-1 has been described as a model for SARS-CoV-induced disease and pathology in humans.[109] MHV-1 primarily replicates in the lungs of A/J mice; although it does disseminate from the lungs with virus detected in the brain, liver, and spleen.[109] Cellular infiltration, pulmonary edema, alveolar thickening, fibrin deposits, and multinucleated giant cells are observed early following MHV-1 infection similar to fatal SARS-CoV infection in humans.[94,109] In addition, lung consolidation was observed by day 10 p.i. following virus-induced mortality of A/J mice.[109] Work in this model demonstrates that T cells contribute to the morbidity and mortality observed in A/J mice following MHV-1 infection.[110] These data support the use of MHV-1 infection in A/J mice as a model for the clinical disease and pulmonary pathology of SARS-CoV in humans.

8.6 PARAMYXOVIRIDAE: PARAINFLUENZA

8.6.1 Infection

Humans are infected by four parainfluenza viruses—HPIV1 to HPIV4. Viral shedding from the upper respiratory tract in humans is variable depending on age, medical condition, and reinfection.[111] In nonhuman primate models, HPIV1 replicates most efficiently in African green monkeys, with prolonged virus shedding for at least 10 days p.i. in both the upper and lower respiratory tracts.[112] HPIV1 replication in chimpanzees was similar to African green monkeys in the upper respiratory tract, but did not reach the same magnitude in the lower respiratory tract.[112] The respiratory tracts yields clinical disease from upper respiratory tract infection including rhinorrhea, sneezing, and coughing.[126] However, no disease symptoms from LRTD are observed.[126] HRSV infection of owl monkeys results in development of mild nasal discharge, but no signs of LRTD.[127] Rhesus macaques, and squirrel and cebus monkeys do not exhibit any signs of disease following HRSV infection.[126]

HRSV infection of cotton rats results in histological changes in the lung tissue including bronchiolitis, pneumonia, sloughing of epithelial cells, edema, and localized atelectasis.[129] However, clinical symptoms of URTD and LRTD are not observed in cotton rats following HRSV infection.[129] One of the most permissive mouse strains to HRSV infection is BALB/c mice,[132] which are commonly used as a laboratory model for HRSV disease in humans. Following infection with a high inoculum of 10^5–10^7 PFU per mouse, BALB/c mice develop clinical disease as measured by airway hyperreactivity and weight loss.[135,136]

Neonatal lambs exhibit upper and lower respiratory tract disease following HRSV infection. URTD is evident by day 6 p.i. with clinical signs of coughing in some of the lambs.[133] LRTD has been characterized in neonatal lambs by the presence of bronchiolitis, epithelial cell sloughing, alveolar consolidation, and interstitial pneumonia assessed by histology.[133]

8.7.3 Immune Response

HRSV-induced disease in experimentally infected adults positively correlates with the cytokines and chemokines, IL-6, IL-8, TNF-α, RANTES, and MIP-1α.[137] In mice, the increased expression of these cytokines and chemokines (with the murine analog of IL-8 being KC) in the lung throughout the course of infection has been observed.[136,138–141] Therefore, mice are a good model to investigate viral interactions with host cells following HRSV infection resulting in this cytokine and chemokine profile.

HRSV protection from disease in humans strongly correlates with the presence of neutralizing maternal or acquired antibodies.[135] Children with certain immunodeficiencies and immunocompromised adults, especially hematopoietic stem cell transplant patients fail to clear virus, shedding virus for many months.[135] Likely CD8 T cells are required for humans to clear RSV from the infected epithelium.

Chimpanzees, and cebus and squirrel monkeys develop an anti-HRSV antibody response by four weeks p.i., with chimpanzees developing the highest serum antibody response correlating with the highest load of shedding virus.[126] Passive administration of antibodies on day 5 p.i. in owl monkeys infected with HRSV yields increased kinetics of virus clearance with an approximate 30-fold reduction in viral load.[127] Currently, chimpanzees are predominantly used as model for HRSV vaccines.[142–147]

Cotton rats infected with HRSV develop a strong neutralizing antibody response that is detected by day 5 p.i.[129] Passive immunity to HRSV infection is attained in the lower respiratory tract of cotton rats administered either neutralizing antibodies or maternally transferred antibodies.[148–150] Viral replication is reduced, but not eliminated, in the nasal passageways of these cotton rats.[148,149]

HRSV infection in mice results in a high level of peribronchiolar and perivascular mononuclear cell infiltrates composed primarily of lymphocytes and macrophages.[151] Unlike humans, minimal recruitment of neutrophils to the lung in HRSV-infected mice is observed, with a high number of recruited effector lymphocytes instead.[141,152] A type I immune response predominates following an acute RSV infection.[153] NK T cells are recruited early to the lung and produce a high level of interferon-γ, which in turn promotes the RSV-specific CD8 T-cell response following an acute RSV infection.[154] Development of a CD8 T cell response is required for viral clearance following RSV infection in mice.[135] In addition, preexisting neutralizing antibodies, either through passive administration or acquired immunity to previous infection, inhibits virus replication in the lungs.[135,155] However, during a primary HRSV infection virus is usually cleared before the development of a neutralizing antibody response.

HRSV-infected neonatal lambs exhibit increased numbers of neutrophils recruited to the bronchoalveolar space, similar to children with HRSV-induced disease.[133,156–158] However, the antibody response to HRSV infection and its ability to neutralize virus upon reinfection in neonatal lambs still needs to be determined.

8.7.4 Animal Viruses to Model Human Disease

Bovine RSV (BRSV) infects the respiratory tract of cattle inducing pulmonary disease.[159] BRSV infection in cattle is similar to HRSV infection in humans in that both induce acute disease, elicit an incompetent immune response permitting subsequent infections, exhibit an age-dependency and cause epidemic disease. BRSV induces severe URTD and LRTD in neonates and calves with clinical symptoms of nasal discharge, coughing, tachypnea, wheezing, hypercapnia, and hypoxemia.[139,160–165] The histopathological changes in the lung tissue in calves following BRSV infection is similar to HRSV-infected humans, with bronchiolitis, interstitial pneumonia, focused areas of consolidation, air trapping, and death of pulmonary epithelial cells observed.[160,165–172] In addition, LRTD in calves induced the recruitment of neutrophils and macrophages into the lung tissue and airways with limited lymphocytic infiltration, which is similar to the cellular infiltrates observed of HRSV-infected humans.[156–158,160,165,167] Like HRSV infection of humans, disease in neonates and calves can be inhibited by the passive administration of high levels of maternal antibodies.[164] However, unlike HRSV infection of humans, BRSV infection in calves is often associated with bacterial and mycoplasma coinfections.[161,173,174]

Pneumonia virus of mice (PVM) is a natural respiratory pathogen of mice with robust replication in the epithelial cells of the upper and lower respiratory tracts.[175] Following PVM infection, mice develop clinical signs of disease, as measured by weight loss, and LRTD, with development of tachypnea.[175] PVM-induced disease in mice is similar to severe HRSV-induced bronchiolitis in humans resulting in severe morbidity and mortality, edema, hemorrhaging, epithelial cell death, and fibrin depositions observed in the lung by histology.[168,169,171,172,176–179]

8.8 PARAMYXOVIRIDAE: METAPNEUMOVIRUS

8.8.1 Infection

Like HRSV, HMPV is most commonly associated with upper respiratory tract infections in children. However, in some instances the virus induces lower respiratory tract disease. Rhesus macaques infected intranasally or intratracheally with HMPV permitted very low viral replication in the upper respiratory tract with no detectable virus in the lower respiratory tract.[180] However, African green monkeys supported moderate HMPV replication in the upper and lower respiratory tracts with virus shed for 7–11 days p.i.[180]

Golden Syrian hamsters and ferrets support replication of HMPV in the upper and lower respiratory tracts following intranasal infection.[180] Hamsters clear the virus by day 6 p.i.[180] Unlike hamsters and ferrets, BALB/c mice do not support HMPV replication as well with a 1–2 log decrease in the viral load detected in the upper and lower respiratory tracts on day 4 p.i.[180] However, the peak viral titer for HMPV in the lungs of BALB/c mice occurs later during infection at approximately days 5–7 p.i.[181,182] An initial study reported that cotton rats were not permissive to HMPV replication following intranasal infection.[180] Another study observed minimal HMPV replication in the lungs of cotton rats with a peak viral titer at day 5 p.i., but still two logs lower than the HMPV peak titer observed in BALB/c mice.[182] In contrast, an additional study reported HMPV replication to be increased in the nasal passage and lung as compared to any mouse strain analyzed.[183] However, it is important to note that these investigators used different strains of HMPV at various infectious doses. Therefore if using cotton rats as a model for HMPV infection, it is important to take these factors into consideration when examining the effect of viral replication.

12. Palmenberg AC, Spiro D, Kuzmickas R et al. Sequencing and analyses of all known human rhinovirus genomes reveal structure and evolution. *Science* 2009; 324(5923): 55–59.
13. Greve JM, Davis G, Meyer AM et al. The major human rhinovirus receptor is ICAM-1. *Cell* 1989; 56(5): 839–847.
14. Mosser AG, Brockman-Schneider R, Amineva S et al. Similar frequency of rhinovirus-infectible cells in upper and lower airway epithelium. *J Infect Dis* 2002; 185(6): 734–743.
15. Dick EC. Experimental infections of chimpanzees with human rhinovirus types 14 and 43. *Proc Soc Exp Biol Med* 1968; 127(4): 1079–1081.
16. Pinto CA, Haff RF. Experimental infection of gibbons with rhinovirus. *Nature* 1969; 224(5226): 1310–1311.
17. Kisch AL, Webb PA, Johnson KM. Further properties of five newly recognized picornaviruses (rhinoviruses). *Am J Hygiene* 1964; 79: 125–133.
18. Yin FH, Lomax NB. Establishment of a mouse model for human rhinovirus infection. *J Gen Virol* 1986; 67 (Pt 11): 2335–2340.
19. Bartlett NW, Walton RP, Edwards MR et al. Mouse models of rhinovirus-induced disease and exacerbation of allergic airway inflammation. *Nat Med* 2008; 14(2): 199–204.
20. Johnston SL, Pattemore PK, Sanderson G et al. Community study of role of viral infections in exacerbations of asthma in 9–11 year old children. *BMJ* 1995; 310(6989): 1225–1229.
21. Corne JM, Marshall C, Smith S et al. Frequency, severity, and duration of rhinovirus infections in asthmatic and non-asthmatic individuals: A longitudinal cohort study. *Lancet* 2002; 359(9309): 831–834.
22. Cate TR, Couch RB, Johnson KM. Studies with rhinoviruses in volunteers: Production of illness, effect of naturallly acquired antibody, and demonstration of a protective effect not associated with serum antibody. *J Clin Invest* 1964; 43: 56–67.
23. Couch RB, Cate TR, Douglas RG, Jr., Gerone PJ, Knight V. Effect of route of inoculation on experimental respiratory viral disease in volunteers and evidence for airborne transmission. *Bacteriol Rev*1966; 30(3): 517–529.
24. Douglas RG, Jr., Cate TR, Gerone PJ, Couch RB. Quantitative rhinovirus shedding patterns in volunteers. *Am Rev Respir Dis* 1966; 94(2): 159–167.
25. Miller EK, Edwards KM, Weinberg GA et al. A novel group of rhinoviruses is associated with asthma hospitalizations. *J Allergy Clin Immunol* 2009; 123(1): 98–104 e1.
26. Bizzintino J, Lee WM, Laing IA et al. Association between human rhinovirus C and severity of acute asthma in children. *Eur Respir J* 2011; 37(5): 1037–1042.
27. Kirchberger S, Majdic O, Stockl J. Modulation of the immune system by human rhinoviruses. *Int Arch Allergy Immunol* 2007; 142(1): 1–10.
28. Levandowski RA, Weaver CW, Jackson GG. Nasal-secretion leukocyte populations determined by flow cytometry during acute rhinovirus infection. *J Med Virol* 1988; 25(4): 423–432.
29. D'Alessio DJ, Meschievitz CK, Peterson JA, Dick CR, Dick EC. Short-duration exposure and the transmission of rhinoviral colds. *J Infect Dis* 1984; 150(2): 189–194.
30. Fox JP, Cooney MK, Hall CE. The Seattle virus watch. V. Epidemiologic observations of rhinovirus infections, 1965–1969, in families with young children. *Am J Epidemiol* 1975; 101(2): 122–143.
31. Fox JP, Cooney MK, Hall CE, Foy HM. Rhinoviruses in Seattle families, 1975–1979. *Am J Epidemiol* 1985; 122(5): 830–846.
32. Edlmayr J, Niespodziana K, Popow-Kraupp T et al. Antibodies induced with recombinant VP1 from human rhinovirus exhibit cross-neutralisation. *Eur Respir J* 2011; 37(1): 44–52.
33. Alper CM, Doyle WJ, Skoner DP et al. Prechallenge antibodies: Moderators of infection rate, signs, and symptoms in adults experimentally challenged with rhinovirus type 39. *Laryngoscope*1996; 106(10): 1298–1305.
34. Grodzicker T, Anderson C, Sharp PA, Sambrook J. Conditional lethal mutants of adenovirus 2-simian virus 40 hybrids. I. Host range mutants of Ad2 + ND1. *J Virol* 1974; 13(6): 1237–1244.
35. Baum SG, Horwitz MS, Maizel JV, Jr. Studies of the mechanism of enhancement of human adenovirus infection in monkey cells by simian virus 40. *J Virol* 1972; 10(2): 211–219.
36. Klessig DF, Anderson CW. Block to multiplication of adenovirus serotype 2 in monkey cells. *J Virol* 1975; 16(6): 1650–1668.
37. Klessig DF, Grodzicker T. Mutations that allow human Ad2 and Ad5 to express late genes in monkey cells map in the viral gene encoding the 72 K DNA binding protein. *Cell* 1979; 17(4): 957–966.
38. Lewis AM, Jr., Levin MJ, Wiese WH, Crumpacker CS, Henry PH. A nondefective (competent) adenovirus-SV40 hybrid isolated from the AD.2-SV40 hybrid population. *Proc Natl Acad Sci USA* 1969; 63(4): 1128–1135.

39. Rabson AS, O'Conor GT, Berezesky IK, Paul FJ. Enhancement of adenovirus growth in African Green monkey kidney cell cultures by Sv40. *Proc Soc Exp Biol Med* 1964; 116: 187–190.
40. Tjian R, Fey G, Graessmann A. Biological activity of purified simian virus 40 T antigen proteins. *Proc Natl Acad Sci USA* 1978; 75(3): 1279–1283.
41. Prince GA, Porter DD, Jenson AB, Horswood RL, Chanock RM, Ginsberg HS. Pathogenesis of adenovirus type 5 pneumonia in cotton rats (*Sigmodon hispidus*). *J Virol* 1993; 67(1): 101–111.
42. Ginsberg HS, Moldawer LL, Sehgal PB et al. A mouse model for investigating the molecular pathogenesis of adenovirus pneumonia. *Proc Natl Acad Sci USA* 1991; 88(5): 1651–1655.
43. Kajon AE, Gigliotti AP, Harrod KS. Acute inflammatory response and remodeling of airway epithelium after subspecies B1 human adenovirus infection of the mouse lower respiratory tract. *J Med Virol* 2003; 71(2): 233–244.
44. Sparer TE, Tripp RA, Dillehay DL, Hermiston TW, Wold WS, Gooding LR. The role of human adenovirus early region 3 proteins (gp19 K, 10.4 K, 14.5 K, and 14.7 K) in a murine pneumonia model. *J Virol* 1996; 70(4): 2431–2439.
45. Harrod KS, Hermiston TW, Trapnell BC, Wold WS, Whitsett JA. Lung-specific expression of adenovirus E3-14.7 K in transgenic mice attenuates adenoviral vector-mediated lung inflammation and enhances transgene expression. *Hum Gene Ther* 1998; 9(13): 1885–1898.
46. Harrod KS, Mounday AD, Whitsett JA. Adenoviral E3-14.7 K protein in LPS-induced lung inflammation. *Am J Physiol Lung Cell Mol Physiol* 2000; 278(4): L631–L639.
47. Eggerding FA, Pierce WC. Molecular biology of adenovirus type 2 semipermissive infections. I. Viral growth and expression of viral replicative functions during restricted adenovirus infection. *Virology* 1986; 148(1): 97–113.
48. Brandt CD, Kim HW, Vargosko AJ et al. Infections in 18,000 infants and children in a controlled study of respiratory tract disease. I. Adenovirus pathogenicity in relation to serologic type and illness syndrome. *Am J Epidemiol* 1969; 90(6): 484–500.
49. Murtagh P, Cerqueiro C, Halac A, Avila M, Kajon A. Adenovirus type 7 h respiratory infections: A report of 29 cases of acute lower respiratory disease. *Acta Paedr* 1993; 82(6–7): 557–561.
50. Simila S, Linna O, Lanning P, Heikkinen E, Ala-Houhala M. Chronic lung damage caused by adenovirus type 7: A ten-year follow-up study. *Chest* 1981; 80(2): 127–131.
51. Simila S, Ylikorkala O, Wasz-Hockert O. Type 7 adenovirus pneumonia. *J Pediatr* 1971; 79(4): 605–611.
52. Becroft DM. Histopathology of fatal adenovirus infection of the respiratory tract in young children. *J Clin Pathol*1967; 20(4): 561–569.
53. Kolavic-Gray SA, Binn LN, Sanchez JL et al. Large epidemic of adenovirus type 4 infection among military trainees: Epidemiological, clinical, and laboratory studies. *Clin Infect Dis* 2002; 35(7): 808–818.
54. Barraza EM, Ludwig SL, Gaydos JC, Brundage JF. Reemergence of adenovirus type 4 acute respiratory disease in military trainees: Report of an outbreak during a lapse in vaccination. *J Infect Dis* 1999; 179(6): 1531–1533.
55. Dingle JH, Langmuir AD. Epidemiology of acute, respiratory disease in military recruits. *Am Rev Respir Dis* 1968; 97(6): Suppl:1–65.
56. Dudding BA, Top FH, Jr., Winter PE, Buescher EL, Lamson TH, Leibovitz A. Acute respiratory disease in military trainees: The adenovirus surveillance program, 1966–1971. *Am J Epidemiol* 1973; 97(3): 187–198.
57. Gray GC, Goswami PR, Malasig MD et al. Adult adenovirus infections: Loss of orphaned vaccines precipitates military respiratory disease epidemics. For the Adenovirus Surveillance Group. *Clin Infect Dis* 2000; 31(3): 663–670.
58. Hilleman MR, Gauld RL, Butler RL et al. Appraisal of occurrence of adenovirus-caused respiratory illness in military populations. *Am J Hygiene* 1957; 66(1): 29–41.
59. Hilleman MR, Werner JH, Dascomb HE, Butler RL. Epidemiologic investigations with respiratory disease virus RI-67. *Am J Public Health Nation's Health* 1955; 45(2): 203–210.
60. Chany C, Lepine P, Lelong M, Le TV, Satge P, Virat J. Severe and fatal pneumonia in infants and young children associated with adenovirus infections. *Am J Hygiene* 1958; 67(3): 367–378.
61. Zahradnik JM, Spencer MJ, Porter DD. Adenovirus infection in the immunocompromised patient. *Am J Med* 1980; 68(5): 725–732.
62. Brundage JF, Gunzenhauser JD, Longfield JN et al. Epidemiology and control of acute respiratory diseases with emphasis on group A beta-hemolytic streptococcus: A decade of U.S. Army experience. *Pediatrics*1996; 97(6 Pt 2): 964–970.
63. Gooch WM, 3rd, Mogabgab WJ. Simultaneous oral administration of live adenovirus types 4 and 7 vaccines. Protection and lack of emergence of other types. *Arch Environ Health* 1972; 25(6): 388–394.

64. Griffin JP, Greenberg BH. Live and inactivated adenovirus vaccines. Clinical evaluation of efficacy in prevention of acute respiratory disease. *Arch Internal Med* 1970; 125(6): 981–986.
65. Top FH, Jr., Dudding BA, Russell PK, Buescher EL. Control of respiratory disease in recruits with types 4 and 7 adenovirus vaccines. *Am J Epidemiol* 1971; 94(2): 142–146.
66. Chirmule N, Propert K, Magosin S, Qian Y, Qian R, Wilson J. Immune responses to adenovirus and adeno-associated virus in humans. *Gene Ther* 1999; 6(9): 1574–1583.
67. McKeon C, Samulski RJ. NIDDK workshop on AAV vectors: Gene transfer into quiescent cells. *Hum Gene Ther* 1996; 7(13): 1615–1619.
68. Yang Y, Li Q, Ertl HC, Wilson JM. Cellular and humoral immune responses to viral antigens create barriers to lung-directed gene therapy with recombinant adenoviruses. *J Virol* 1995; 69(4): 2004–2015.
69. van Boheemen S, de Graaf M, Lauber C et al. Genomic characterization of a newly discovered coronavirus associated with acute respiratory distress syndrome in humans. *mBio* 2012; 3(6).
70. Lassnig C, Sanchez CM, Egerbacher M et al. Development of a transgenic mouse model susceptible to human coronavirus 229E. *Proc Natl Acad Sci USA* 2005; 102(23): 8275–8280.
71. van der Hoek L, Pyrc K, Jebbink MF et al. Identification of a new human coronavirus. *Nat Med* 2004; 10(4): 368–373.
72. Woo PC, Lau SK, Chu CM et al. Characterization and complete genome sequence of a novel coronavirus, coronavirus HKU1, from patients with pneumonia. *J Virol* 2005; 79(2): 884–895.
73. Ding Y, He L, Zhang Q et al. Organ distribution of severe acute respiratory syndrome (SARS) associated coronavirus (SARS-CoV) in SARS patients: Implications for pathogenesis and virus transmission pathways. *J Pathol* 2004; 203(2): 622–630.
74. Farcas GA, Poutanen SM, Mazzulli T et al. Fatal severe acute respiratory syndrome is associated with multiorgan involvement by coronavirus. *J Infect Dis* 2005; 191(2): 193–197.
75. Guan Y, Zheng BJ, He YQ et al. Isolation and characterization of viruses related to the SARS coronavirus from animals in southern China. *Science* 2003; 302(5643): 276–278.
76. Li W, Zhang C, Sui J et al. Receptor and viral determinants of SARS-coronavirus adaptation to human ACE2. *EMBO J* 2005; 24(8): 1634–1643.
77. Qu XX, Hao P, Song XJ et al. Identification of two critical amino acid residues of the severe acute respiratory syndrome coronavirus spike protein for its variation in zoonotic tropism transition via a double substitution strategy. *J Biol Chem* 2005; 280(33): 29588–29595.
78. Song HD, Tu CC, Zhang GW et al. Cross-host evolution of severe acute respiratory syndrome coronavirus in palm civet and human. *Proc Natl Acad Sci USA* 2005; 102(7): 2430–2435.
79. Fouchier RA, Kuiken T, Schutten M et al. Aetiology: Koch's postulates fulfilled for SARS virus. *Nature* 2003; 423(6937): 240.
80. Kuiken T, Fouchier RA, Schutten M et al. Newly discovered coronavirus as the primary cause of severe acute respiratory syndrome. *Lancet* 2003; 362(9380): 263–270.
81. Qin C, Wang J, Wei Q et al. An animal model of SARS produced by infection of *Macaca mulatta* with SARS coronavirus. *J Pathol* 2005; 206(3): 251–259.
82. Greenough TC, Carville A, Coderre J et al. Pneumonitis and multi-organ system disease in common marmosets (*Callithrix jacchus*) infected with the severe acute respiratory syndrome-associated coronavirus. *Am J Pathol* 2005; 167(2): 455–463.
83. Glass WG, Subbarao K, Murphy B, Murphy PM. Mechanisms of host defense following severe acute respiratory syndrome-coronavirus (SARS-CoV) pulmonary infection of mice. *J Immunol* 2004; 173(6): 4030–4039.
84. Subbarao K, McAuliffe J, Vogel L et al. Prior infection and passive transfer of neutralizing antibody prevent replication of severe acute respiratory syndrome coronavirus in the respiratory tract of mice. *J Virol* 2004; 78(7): 3572–3577.
85. Roberts A, Deming D, Paddock CD et al. A mouse-adapted SARS-coronavirus causes disease and mortality in BALB/c mice. *PLoS Pathogens* 2007; 3(1): e5.
86. Martina BE, Haagmans BL, Kuiken T et al. Virology: SARS virus infection of cats and ferrets. *Nature* 2003; 425(6961): 915.
87. Roberts A, Vogel L, Guarner J et al. Severe acute respiratory syndrome coronavirus infection of golden Syrian hamsters. *J Virol* 2005; 79(1): 503–511.
88. Ebihara T, Endo R, Ma X, Ishiguro N, Kikuta H. Detection of human coronavirus NL63 in young children with bronchiolitis. *J Med Virol* 2005; 75(3): 463–465.
89. Fouchier RA, Hartwig NG, Bestebroer TM et al. A previously undescribed coronavirus associated with respiratory disease in humans. *Proc Natl Acad Sci USA* 2004; 101(16): 6212–6216.

90. Jacomy H, Talbot PJ. Vacuolating encephalitis in mice infected by human coronavirus OC43. *Virology*2003; 315(1): 20–33.
91. Nie QH, Luo XD, Zhang JZ, Su Q. Current status of severe acute respiratory syndrome in China. *World J Gastroenterol: WJG* 2003; 9(8): 1635–1645.
92. Tsui PT, Kwok ML, Yuen H, Lai ST. Severe acute respiratory syndrome: Clinical outcome and prognostic correlates. *Emerg Infect Dis* 2003; 9(9): 1064–1069.
93. Weiss SR, Navas-Martin S. Coronavirus pathogenesis and the emerging pathogen severe acute respiratory syndrome coronavirus. *Microbiol Mol Biol Rev: MMBR* 2005; 69(4): 635–664.
94. Hwang DM, Chamberlain DW, Poutanen SM, Low DE, Asa SL, Butany J. Pulmonary pathology of severe acute respiratory syndrome in Toronto. *Mod Pathol: An Off J US Can Acad Pathol, Inc* 2005; 18(1): 1–10.
95. Nicholls JM, Poon LL, Lee KC et al. Lung pathology of fatal severe acute respiratory syndrome. *Lancet* 2003; 361(9371): 1773–1778.
96. Rowe T, Gao G, Hogan RJ et al. Macaque model for severe acute respiratory syndrome. *J Virol* 2004; 78(20): 11401–11404.
97. McAuliffe J, Vogel L, Roberts A et al. Replication of SARS coronavirus administered into the respiratory tract of African Green, rhesus and cynomolgus monkeys. *Virology* 2004; 330(1): 8–15.
98. Roberts A, Paddock C, Vogel L, Butler E, Zaki S, Subbarao K. Aged BALB/c mice as a model for increased severity of severe acute respiratory syndrome in elderly humans. *J Virol* 2005; 79(9): 5833–5838.
99. Cui W, Fan Y, Wu W, Zhang F, Wang JY, Ni AP. Expression of lymphocytes and lymphocyte subsets in patients with severe acute respiratory syndrome. *Clin Infect Dis* 2003; 37(6): 857–859.
100. Li T, Qiu Z, Zhang L et al. Significant changes of peripheral T lymphocyte subsets in patients with severe acute respiratory syndrome. *J Infect Dis* 2004; 189(4): 648–651.
101. Wong RS, Wu A, To KF et al. Haematological manifestations in patients with severe acute respiratory syndrome: Retrospective analysis. *BMJ* 2003; 326(7403): 1358–1362.
102. He Y, Zhu Q, Liu S et al. Identification of a critical neutralization determinant of severe acute respiratory syndrome (SARS)-associated coronavirus: Importance for designing SARS vaccines. *Virology* 2005; 334(1): 74–82.
103. Li T, Xie J, He Y et al. Long-term persistence of robust antibody and cytotoxic T cell responses in recovered patients infected with SARS coronavirus. *PLoS One* 2006; 1: e24.
104. Enjuanes L, Smerdou C, Castilla J et al. Development of protection against coronavirus induced diseases. A review. *Adv Exp Med Biol* 1995; 380: 197–211.
105. Saif LJ. Animal coronaviruses: What can they teach us about the severe acute respiratory syndrome? *Rev Sci Tech* 2004; 23(2): 643–660.
106. Saif LJ. Animal coronavirus vaccines: Lessons for SARS. *Dev Biol* 2004; 119: 129–140.
107. Cavanagh D. Severe acute respiratory syndrome vaccine development: Experiences of vaccination against avian infectious bronchitis coronavirus. *Avian Pathol: J WVPA* 2003; 32(6): 567–582.
108. Addie DD. Feline coronavirus—That enigmatic little critter. *Veterinary J* 2004; 167(1): 5–6.
109. De Albuquerque N, Baig E, Ma X et al. Murine hepatitis virus strain 1 produces a clinically relevant model of severe acute respiratory syndrome in A/J mice. *J Virol* 2006; 80(21): 10382–10394.
110. Khanolkar A, Hartwig SM, Haag BA et al. Protective and pathologic roles of the immune response to mouse hepatitis virus type 1: Implications for severe acute respiratory syndrome. *J Virol* 2009; 83(18): 9258–9272.
111. Karron RA, Collins PL. Parainfluenza viruses. In: Knipe DM, Howley PM, eds. *Fields Virology*. 5th ed. Philadelphia, USA: Wolters Kluwer Lippincott Williams & Wilkins; 2007: 1497–1526.
112. Durbin AP, Elkins WR, Murphy BR. African green monkeys provide a useful nonhuman primate model for the study of human parainfluenza virus types-1, -2, and –3 infection. *Vaccine* 2000; 18(22): 2462–2469.
113. Hawthorne JD, Lorenz D, Albrecht P. Infection of marmosets with parainfluenza virus types 1 and 3. *Infect Immunity*1982; 37(3): 1037–1041.
114. Ottolini MG, Porter DD, Hemming VG, Hensen SA, Sami IR, Prince GA. Semi-permissive replication and functional aspects of the immune response in a cotton rat model of human parainfluenza virus type 3 infection. *J Gen Virol* 1996; 77(Pt 8): 1739–1743.
115. Clements ML, Belshe RB, King J et al. Evaluation of bovine, cold-adapted human, and wild-type human parainfluenza type 3 viruses in adult volunteers and in chimpanzees. *J Clin Microbiol* 1991; 29(6): 1175–1182.
116. Hall SL, Sarris CM, Tierney EL, London WT, Murphy BR. A cold-adapted mutant of parainfluenza virus type 3 is attenuated and protective in chimpanzees. *J Infect Dis* 1993; 167(4): 958–962.

117. Murphy TF, Dubovi EJ, Clyde WA, Jr. The cotton rat as an experimental model of human parainfluenza virus type 3 disease. *Exp Lung Res* 1981; 2(2): 97–109.
118. Ray R, Glaze BJ, Moldoveanu Z, Compans RW. Intranasal immunization of hamsters with envelope glycoproteins of human parainfluenza virus type 3. *J Infect Dis* 1988; 157(4): 648–654.
119. Brownstein DG, Smith AL, Johnson EA. Sendai virus infection in genetically resistant and susceptible mice. *Am J Pathol*1981; 105(2): 156–163.
120. Mazanec MB, Lamm ME, Lyn D, Portner A, Nedrud JG. Comparison of IgA versus IgG monoclonal antibodies for passive immunization of the murine respiratory tract. *Virus Res* 1992; 23(1–2): 1–12.
121. Orvell C, Grandien M. The effects of monoclonal antibodies on biologic activities of structural proteins of Sendai virus. *J Immunol* 1982; 129(6): 2779–2787.
122. Capraro GA, Johnson JB, Kock ND, Parks GD. Virus growth and antibody responses following respiratory tract infection of ferrets and mice with WT and P/V mutants of the paramyxovirus Simian Virus 5. *Virology* 2008; 376(2): 416–428.
123. Lemen RJ, Quan SF, Witten ML, Sobonya RE, Ray CG, Grad R. Canine parainfluenza type 2 bronchiolitis increases histamine responsiveness in beagle puppies. *Am Rev Respir Dis* 1990; 141(1): 199–207.
124. Wagener JS, Minnich L, Sobonya R, Taussig LM, Ray CG, Fulginiti V. Parainfluenza type II infection in dogs. A model for viral lower respiratory tract infection in humans. *Am Rev Respir Dis* 1983; 127(6): 771–775.
125. Folkerts G, Verheyen AK, Geuens GM, Folkerts HF, Nijkamp FP. Virus-induced changes in airway responsiveness, morphology, and histamine levels in guinea pigs. *Am Rev Respir Dis* 1993; 147(6 Pt 1): 1569–1577.
126. Belshe RB, Richardson LS, London WT et al. Experimental respiratory syncytial virus infection of four species of primates. *J Med Virol* 1977; 1(3): 157–162.
127. Hemming VG, Prince GA, Horswood RL et al. Studies of passive immunotherapy for infections of respiratory syncytial virus in the respiratory tract of a primate model. *J Infect Dis* 1985; 152(5): 1083–1087.
128. Dreizin RS, Vyshnevetskaia LO, Bagdamian EE, Iankevich OD, Tarasova LB. [Experimental RS virus infection of cotton rats. A viral and immunofluorescent study]. *Voprosy Virusologii* 1971; 16(6): 670–676.
129. Prince GA, Jenson AB, Horswood RL, Camargo E, Chanock RM. The pathogenesis of respiratory syncytial virus infection in cotton rats. *Am J Pathol* 1978; 93(3): 771–791.
130. Boukhvalova MS, Yim KC, Kuhn KH et al. Age-related differences in pulmonary cytokine response to respiratory syncytial virus infection: Modulation by anti-inflammatory and antiviral treatment. *J Infect Dis* 2007; 195(4): 511–518.
131. Curtis SJ, Ottolini MG, Porter DD, Prince GA. Age-dependent replication of respiratory syncytial virus in the cotton rat. *Exp Biol Med* 2002; 227(9): 799–802.
132. Prince GA, Horswood RL, Berndt J, Suffin SC, Chanock RM. Respiratory syncytial virus infection in inbred mice. *Infect Immunity*1979; 26(2): 764–766.
133. Olivier A, Gallup J, de Macedo MM, Varga SM, Ackermann M. Human respiratory syncytial virus A2 strain replicates and induces innate immune responses by respiratory epithelia of neonatal lambs. *Int J Exp Pathol* 2009; 90(4): 431–438.
134. Sow FB, Gallup JM, Olivier A et al. Respiratory syncytial virus is associated with an inflammatory response in lungs and architectural remodeling of lung-draining lymph nodes of newborn lambs. *Am J Physiol Lung Cell Mol Physiol* 2011; 300(1): L12–L24.
135. Collins PL, Crowe JE, Jr. Respiratory syncytial virus and metapneumovirus. In: Knipe DM, Howley PM, eds. *Fields Virology*. 5th ed. Philadelphia, PA 19106 USA: Wolters Kluwer Lippincott Williams & Wilkins; 2007: 1601–1646.
136. Jafri HS, Chavez-Bueno S, Mejias A et al. Respiratory syncytial virus induces pneumonia, cytokine response, airway obstruction, and chronic inflammatory infiltrates associated with long-term airway hyperresponsiveness in mice. *J Infect Dis* 2004; 189(10): 1856–1865.
137. DeVincenzo JP, Wilkinson T, Vaishnaw A et al. Viral load drives disease in humans experimentally infected with respiratory syncytial virus. *Am J Respir Crit Care Med* 2010; 182(10): 1305–1314.
138. Aung S, Rutigliano JA, Graham BS. Alternative mechanisms of respiratory syncytial virus clearance in perforin knockout mice lead to enhanced disease. *J Virol* 2001; 75(20): 9918–9924.
139. Bem RA, Domachowske JB, Rosenberg HF. Animal models of human respiratory syncytial virus disease. *Am J Physiol Lung Cell Mol Physiol* 2011; 301(2): L148–L156.
140. Miller AL, Bowlin TL, Lukacs NW. Respiratory syncytial virus-induced chemokine production: Linking viral replication to chemokine production *in vitro* and *in vivo*. *J Infect Dis* 2004; 189(8): 1419–1430.
141. Rutigliano JA, Graham BS. Prolonged production of TNF-alpha exacerbates illness during respiratory syncytial virus infection. *J Immunol* 2004; 173(5): 3408–3417.

142. Collins PL, Purcell RH, London WT, Lawrence LA, Chanock RM, Murphy BR. Evaluation in chimpanzees of vaccinia virus recombinants that express the surface glycoproteins of human respiratory syncytial virus. *Vaccine* 1990; 8(2): 164–168.
143. Crowe JE, Jr., Bui PT, Davis AR, Chanock RM, Murphy BR. A further attenuated derivative of a cold-passaged temperature-sensitive mutant of human respiratory syncytial virus retains immunogenicity and protective efficacy against wild-type challenge in seronegative chimpanzees. *Vaccine* 1994; 12(9): 783–790.
144. Crowe JE, Jr., Bui PT, Firestone CY et al. Live subgroup B respiratory syncytial virus vaccines that are attenuated, genetically stable, and immunogenic in rodents and nonhuman primates. *J Infect Dis* 1996; 173(4): 829–839.
145. Crowe JE, Jr., Collins PL, London WT, Chanock RM, Murphy BR. A comparison in chimpanzees of the immunogenicity and efficacy of live attenuated respiratory syncytial virus (RSV) temperature-sensitive mutant vaccines and vaccinia virus recombinants that express the surface glycoproteins of RSV. *Vaccine* 1993; 11(14): 1395–1404.
146. Hancock GE, Smith JD, Heers KM. Serum neutralizing antibody titers of seropositive chimpanzees immunized with vaccines coformulated with natural fusion and attachment proteins of respiratory syncytial virus. *J Infect Dis* 2000; 181(5): 1768–1771.
147. Teng MN, Whitehead SS, Bermingham A et al. Recombinant respiratory syncytial virus that does not express the NS1 or M2-2 protein is highly attenuated and immunogenic in chimpanzees. *J Virol* 2000; 74(19): 9317–9321.
148. Prince GA, Hemming VG, Horswood RL, Chanock RM. Immunoprophylaxis and immunotherapy of respiratory syncytial virus infection in the cotton rat. *Virus Research* 1985; 3(3): 193–206.
149. Prince GA, Horswood RL, Camargo E, Koenig D, Chanock RM. Mechanisms of immunity to respiratory syncytial virus in cotton rats. *Infect Immunity* 1983; 42(1): 81–87.
150. Prince GA, Horswood RL, Chanock RM. Quantitative aspects of passive immunity to respiratory syncytial virus infection in infant cotton rats. *J Virol* 1985; 55(3): 517–520.
151. Taylor G, Stott EJ, Hughes M, Collins AP. Respiratory syncytial virus infection in mice. *Infect Immunity* 1984; 43(2): 649–655.
152. Hussell T, Openshaw PJ. Intracellular IFN-gamma expression in natural killer cells precedes lung CD8+ T cell recruitment during respiratory syncytial virus infection. *J Gen Virol* 1998; 79 (Pt 11): 2593–2601.
153. Peebles RS, Jr., Graham BS. Pathogenesis of respiratory syncytial virus infection in the murine model. *Proc Am Thorac Soc* 2005; 2(2): 110–115.
154. Johnson TR, Hong S, Van Kaer L, Koezuka Y, Graham BS. NK T cells contribute to expansion of CD8(+) T cells and amplification of antiviral immune responses to respiratory syncytial virus. *J Virol* 2002; 76(9): 4294–4303.
155. Graham BS, Bunton LA, Rowland J, Wright PF, Karzon DT. Respiratory syncytial virus infection in anti-mu-treated mice. *J Virol* 1991; 65(9): 4936–4942.
156. Bem RA, Bos AP, Bots M et al. Activation of the granzyme pathway in children with severe respiratory syncytial virus infection. *Pediatr Res* 2008; 63(6): 650–655.
157. Everard ML, Swarbrick A, Wrightham M et al. Analysis of cells obtained by bronchial lavage of infants with respiratory syncytial virus infection. *Arch Dis Childhood* 1994; 71(5): 428–432.
158. McNamara PS, Ritson P, Selby A, Hart CA, Smyth RL. Bronchoalveolar lavage cellularity in infants with severe respiratory syncytial virus bronchiolitis. *Arch Dis Childhood* 2003; 88(10): 922–926.
159. Paccaud MF, Jacquier C. A respiratory syncytial virus of bovine origin. *Arch Gesamte Virusforsch* 1970; 30(4): 327–342.
160. Antonis AF, de Jong MC, van der Poel WH et al. Age-dependent differences in the pathogenesis of bovine respiratory syncytial virus infections related to the development of natural immunocompetence. *J Gen Virol* 2010; 91(Pt 10): 2497–2506.
161. Belknap EB, Ciszewski DK, Baker JC. Experimental respiratory syncytial virus infection in calves and lambs. *J Veterinary Diagn Invest: Off Publ Am Assoc Veterinary Lab Diagn, Inc* 1995; 7(2): 285–298.
162. Gershwin LJ. Bovine respiratory syncytial virus infection: Immunopathogenic mechanisms. *Anim Health Res Rev/Conf Res Workers in Anim Dis* 2007; 8(2): 207–213.
163. Grell SN, Riber U, Tjornehoj K, Larsen LE, Heegaard PM. Age-dependent differences in cytokine and antibody responses after experimental RSV infection in a bovine model. *Vaccine* 2005; 23(26): 3412–3423.
164. Van der Poel WH, Brand A, Kramps JA, Van Oirschot JT. Respiratory syncytial virus infections in human beings and in cattle. *J Infect* 1994; 29(2): 215–228.

165. Viuff B, Tjornehoj K, Larsen LE et al. Replication and clearance of respiratory syncytial virus: Apoptosis is an important pathway of virus clearance after experimental infection with bovine respiratory syncytial virus. *Am J Pathol* 2002; 161(6): 2195–2207.
166. Bryson DG, McFerran JB, Ball HJ, Neill SD. Observations on outbreaks of respiratory disease in housed calves— (2) Pathological and microbiological findings. *Veterinary Record*1978; 103(23): 503–509.
167. McInnes E, Sopp P, Howard CJ, Taylor G. Phenotypic analysis of local cellular responses in calves infected with bovine respiratory syncytial virus. *Immunology* 1999; 96(3): 396–403.
168. Reed JL, Brewah YA, Delaney T et al. Macrophage impairment underlies airway occlusion in primary respiratory syncytial virus bronchiolitis. *J Infect Dis* 2008; 198(12): 1783–1793.
169. Welliver TP, Garofalo RP, Hosakote Y et al. Severe human lower respiratory tract illness caused by respiratory syncytial virus and influenza virus is characterized by the absence of pulmonary cytotoxic lymphocyte responses. *J Infect Dis* 2007; 195(8): 1126–1136.
170. Welliver TP, Reed JL, Welliver RC, Sr. Respiratory syncytial virus and influenza virus infections: Observations from tissues of fatal infant cases. *Pediatr Infect Dis J* 2008; 27(10 Suppl): S92–S96.
171. Aherne W, Bird T, Court SD, Gardner PS, McQuillin J. Pathological changes in virus infections of the lower respiratory tract in children. *J Clin Pathol* 1970; 23(1): 7–18.
172. Johnson JE, Gonzales RA, Olson SJ, Wright PF, Graham BS. The histopathology of fatal untreated human respiratory syncytial virus infection. *Mod Pathol: Off J US Can Acad Pathol, Inc* 2007; 20(1): 108–119.
173. Srikumaran S, Kelling CL, Ambagala A. Immune evasion by pathogens of bovine respiratory disease complex. *Anim Health Res Rev/Conf Res Workers Anim Dis* 2007; 8(2): 215–229.
174. Viuff B, Uttenthal A, Tegtmeier C, Alexandersen S. Sites of replication of bovine respiratory syncytial virus in naturally infected calves as determined by *in situ* hybridization. *Veterinary Pathol* 1996; 33(4): 383–390.
175. Bonville CA, Bennett NJ, Koehnlein M et al. Respiratory dysfunction and proinflammatory chemokines in the pneumonia virus of mice (PVM) model of viral bronchiolitis. *Virology* 2006; 349(1): 87–95.
176. Bem RA, van Woensel JB, Lutter R et al. Granzyme A- and B-cluster deficiency delays acute lung injury in pneumovirus-infected mice. *J Immunol* 2010; 184(2): 931–938.
177. Domachowske JB, Bonville CA, Easton AJ, Rosenberg HF. Differential expression of proinflammatory cytokine genes *in vivo* in response to pathogenic and nonpathogenic pneumovirus infections. *J Infect Dis* 2002; 186(1): 8–14.
178. Garvey TL, Dyer KD, Ellis JA et al. Inflammatory responses to pneumovirus infection in IFN-alpha beta R gene-deleted mice. *J Immunol* 2005; 175(7): 4735–4744.
179. Rosenberg HF, Domachowske JB. Pneumonia virus of mice: Severe respiratory infection in a natural host. *Immunol Lett*2008; 118(1): 6–12.
180. MacPhail M, Schickli JH, Tang RS et al. Identification of small-animal and primate models for evaluation of vaccine candidates for human metapneumovirus (hMPV) and implications for hMPV vaccine design. *J Gen Virol* 2004; 85(Pt 6): 1655–1663.
181. Alvarez R, Tripp RA. The immune response to human metapneumovirus is associated with aberrant immunity and impaired virus clearance in BALB/c mice. *J Virol* 2005; 79(10): 5971–5978.
182. Hamelin ME, Yim K, Kuhn KH et al. Pathogenesis of human metapneumovirus lung infection in BALB/c mice and cotton rats. *J Virol* 2005; 79(14): 8894–8903.
183. Williams JV, Tollefson SJ, Johnson JE, Crowe JE, Jr. The cotton rat (*Sigmodon hispidus*) is a permissive small animal model of human metapneumovirus infection, pathogenesis, and protective immunity. *J Virol* 2005; 79(17): 10944–10951.
184. Higa HH, Rogers GN, Paulson JC. Influenza virus hemagglutinins differentiate between receptor determinants bearing N-acetyl-, N-glycollyl-, and N,O-diacetyineuraminic acids. *Virology* 1985; 144(1): 279–282.
185. Shinya K, Ebina M, Yamada S, Ono M, Kasai N, Kawaoka Y. Avian flu: Influenza virus receptors in the human airway. *Nature*2006; 440(7083): 435–436.
186. Ibricevic A, Pekosz A, Walter MJ et al. Influenza virus receptor specificity and cell tropism in mouse and human airway epithelial cells. *J Virol* 2006; 80(15): 7469–7480.
187. Hale BG, Randall RE, Ortín J, Jackson D. The multifunctional NS1 protein of influenza A viruses. *J Gen Virol* 2008; 89(10): 2359–2376.
188. Knipe DM, Howley PM, eds. *Feilds Virology*5ed. Philadelphia: Lippincott Williams & Wilkins; 2007.
189. Hayden FG, Fritz R, Lobo MC, Alvord W, Strober W, Straus SE. Local and systemic cytokine responses during experimental human influenza A virus infection. Relation to symptom formation and host defense. *J Clin Invest* 1998; 101(3): 643–649.

190. Richman DD, Murphy BR, Baron S, Uhlendorf C. Three strains of influenza A virus (H3N2): Interferon sensitivity *in vitro* and interferon production in volunteers. *J Clin Microbiol*1976; 3(3): 223–226.
191. Barnard DL. Animal models for the study of influenza pathogenesis and therapy. *Antiviral Res* 2009; 82(2): A110–A122.
192. Reeve P. Growth of some attenuated influenza A viruses in hamsters. *Med Microbiol Immunol* 1978; 166(1–4): 133–139.
193. Eichelberger MC, Prince GA, Ottolini MG. Influenza-induced tachypnea is prevented in immune cotton rats, but cannot be treated with an anti-inflammatory steroid or a neuraminidase inhibitor. *Virology*2004; 322(2): 300–307.
194. Huang SS, Banner D, Fang Y et al. Comparative analyses of pandemic H1N1 and seasonal H1N1, H3N2, and influenza B infections depict distinct clinical pictures in ferrets. *PLoS One* 2011; 6(11): e27512.
195. Svitek N, Rudd PA, Obojes K, Pillet S, von Messling V. Severe seasonal influenza in ferrets correlates with reduced interferon and increased IL-6 induction. *Virology* 2008; 376(1): 53–59.
196. Rimmelzwaan GF, Baars M, van Beek R et al. Induction of protective immunity against influenza virus in a macaque model: Comparison of conventional and iscom vaccines. *Journal of General Virology* 1997; 78(4): 757–765.
197. Boonnak K, Paskel M, Matsuoka Y, Vogel L, Subbarao K. Evaluation of replication, immunogenicity and protective efficacy of a live attenuated cold-adapted pandemic H1N1 influenza virus vaccine in non-human primates. *Vaccine*2012; 30(38): 5603–5610.
198. Kilbourne ED. Future influenza vaccines and the use of genetic recombinants. *Bull World Health Organ* 1969; 41(3): 643–645.
199. Chotpitayasunondh T, Ungchusak K, Hanshaoworakul W et al. Human disease from influenza A (H5N1), Thailand, 2004. *Emerg Infect Dis* 2005; 11(2): 201–209.
200. Peiris JSM, Yu WC, Leung CW et al. Re-emergence of fatal human influenza A subtype H5N1 disease. *The Lancet* 2004; 363(9409): 617–619.
201. To KF, Chan PK, Chan KF et al. Pathology of fatal human infection associated with avian influenza A H5N1 virus. *J Med Virol* 2001; 63(3): 242–246.
202. Shinya K, Hatta M, Yamada S et al. Characterization of a human H5N1 influenza A virus isolated in 2003. *J Virol*2005; 79(15): 9926–9932.
203. Govorkova EA, Rehg JE, Krauss S et al. Lethality to ferrets of H5N1 influenza viruses isolated from humans and poultry in 2004. *J Virol* 2005; 79(4): 2191–2198.
204. Maines TR, Lu XH, Erb SM et al. Avian influenza (H5N1) viruses isolated from humans in Asia in 2004 exhibit increased virulence in mammals. *J Virol*2005; 79(18): 11788–11800.
205. Van Hoeven N, Belser JA, Szretter KJ et al. Pathogenesis of 1918 pandemic and H5N1 influenza virus infections in a guinea pig model: Antiviral potential of exogenous alpha interferon to reduce virus shedding. *J Virol* 2009; 83(7): 2851–2861.
206. Chen Y, Deng W, Jia C et al. Pathological lesions and viral localization of Influenza A (H5N1) virus in experimentally infected Chinese rhesus macaques: Implications for pathogenesis and viral transmission. *Arch Virol*2009; 154(2): 227–233.
207. Shinya K, Makino A, Tanaka H et al. Systemic Dissemination of H5N1 influenza A viruses in ferrets and hamsters after direct intragastric inoculation. *J Virol* 2011; 85(10): 4673–4678.
208. CDC. Update: Estimates of deaths associated with seasonal influenza—United States, 1976–2007. *MMWR Morb Mortal Wkly Rep* 2012; 61(48): 990–993.
209. Barroso L, Treanor J, Gubareva L, Hayden FG. Efficacy and tolerability of the oral neuraminidase inhibitor peramivir in experimental human influenza: Randomized, controlled trials for prophylaxis and treatment. *Antivir Ther* 2005; 10(8): 901–910.
210. Carrat F, Vergu E, Ferguson NM et al. Time lines of infection and disease in human influenza: A review of volunteer challenge studies. *Am J Epidemiol* 2008; 167(7): 775–785.
211. Kim YH, Kim HS, Cho SH, Seo SH. Influenza B virus causes milder pathogenesis and weaker inflammatory responses in ferrets than influenza A virus. *Viral Immunol* 2009; 22(6): 423–430.
212. Ottolini MG, Blanco JCG, Eichelberger MC et al. The cotton rat provides a useful small-animal model for the study of influenza virus pathogenesis. *J Gen Virol* 2005; 86(10): 2823–2830.
213. Pica N, Chou Y-y, Bouvier NM, Palese P. Transmission of influenza B viruses in the guinea pig. *J Virol* 2012; 86(8): 4279–4287.
214. Reeve P, Pibermann M, Gerendas B. Studies with some influenza B viruses in cell cultures, hamsters and hamster tracheal organ cultures. *Med Microbiol Immunol* 1981; 169(3): 179–186.
215. Oliphant JW, Perrin TL. The histopathology of type B (Lee strain) influenza in mice. *Public Health Rep (1896–1970)* 1942; 57(22): 809–814.

216. Price DA, Postlethwaite RJ, Longson M. Influenzavirus A2 infections presenting with febril convulsions and gastrointestinal symptoms in young children. *Clin Pediatr (Phila)* 1976; 15(4): 361–367.
217. Hien TT, Liem NT, Dung NT et al. Avian Influenza A (H5N1) in 10 Patients in Vietnam. *New England J Med* 2004; 350(12): 1179–1188.
218. Matrosovich MN, Matrosovich TY, Gray T, Roberts NA, Klenk HD. Human and avian influenza viruses target different cell types in cultures of human airway epithelium. *Proc Natl Acad Sci USA* 2004; 101(13): 4620–4624.
219. Tran TH, Nguyen TL, Nguyen TD et al. Avian influenza A (H5N1) in 10 patients in Vietnam. *New Engl J Med* 2004; 350(12): 1179–1188.
220. Kugel D, Kochs G, Obojes K et al. Intranasal administration of alpha interferon reduces seasonal influenza A virus morbidity in ferrets. *J Virol* 2009; 83(8): 3843–3851.
221. Matsuoka Y, Lamirande EW, Subbarao K. The ferret model for influenza. *Curr Protoc Microbiol* 2009; Chapter 15: Unit 15G 2.
222. Rimmelzwaan GF, Kuiken T, van Amerongen G, Bestebroer TM, Fouchier RAM, Osterhaus ADME. Pathogenesis of influenza a (H5N1) virus infection in a primate model. *J Virol* 2001; 75(14): 6687–6691.
223. Kuiken T, Rimmelzwaan GF, Van Amerongen G, Osterhaus ADME. Pathology of human influenza A (H5N1) virus infection in cynomolgus macaques (*Macaca fascicularis*). *Veterinary Pathol Online* 2003; 40(3): 304–310.
224. Baskin CR, Bielefeldt-Ohmann H, Tumpey TM et al. Early and sustained innate immune response defines pathology and death in nonhuman primates infected by highly pathogenic influenza virus. *Proc Natl Acad Sci* 2009; 106(9): 3455–3460.
225. Kwon YK, Lipatov AS, Swayne DE. Bronchointerstitial pneumonia in guinea pigs following inoculation with H5N1 high pathogenicity avian influenza virus. *Veterinary Pathol Online* 2009; 46(1): 138–141.
226. Lu X, Tumpey TM, Morken T, Zaki SR, Cox NJ, Katz JM. A mouse model for the evaluation of pathogenesis and immunity to influenza A (H5N1) viruses isolated from humans. *J Virol* 1999; 73(7): 5903–5911.
227. Fukushi M, Ito T, Oka T et al. Serial histopathological examination of the lungs of mice infected with influenza A virus PR8 strain. *PLoS One* 2011; 6(6): e21207.
228. Julander JG, Hagloch J, Latimer S et al. Use of plethysmography in assessing the efficacy of antivirals in a mouse model of pandemic influenza A virus. *Antiviral Res* 2011; 92(2): 228–236.
229. Maines TR, Belser JA, Gustin KM et al. Local innate immune responses and influenza virus transmission and virulence in ferrets. *J Infect Dis* 2012; 205(3): 474–485.
230. Staeheli P, Grob R, Meier E, Sutcliffe JG, Haller O. Influenza virus-susceptible mice carry Mx genes with a large deletion or a nonsense mutation. *Mol Cell Biol* 1988; 8(10): 4518–4523.
231. Lee BO, Rangel-Moreno J, Moyron-Quiroz JE et al. CD4 T cell-independent antibody response promotes resolution of primary influenza infection and helps to prevent reinfection. *J Immunol* 2005; 175(9): 5827–5838.
232. Kris RM, Yetter RA, Cogliano R, Ramphal R, Small PA. Passive serum antibody causes temporary recovery from influenza virus infection of the nose, trachea and lung of nude mice. *Immunology* 1988; 63(3): 349–353.
233. Ennis F, Beare AS, Riley D et al. Interferon induction and increased natural killer-cell activity in influenza infections in man. *The Lancet* 1981; 318(8252): 891–893.
234. Stein-Streilein J, Guffee J. *In vivo* treatment of mice and hamsters with antibodies to asialo GM1 increases morbidity and mortality to pulmonary influenza infection. *J Immunol* 1986; 136(4): 1435–1441.
235. Eichelberger MC, Bauchiero S, Point D, Richter BWM, Prince GA, Schuman R. Distinct cellular immune responses following primary and secondary influenza virus challenge in cotton rats. *Cell Immunol*2006; 243(2): 67–74.
236. Mandelboim O, Lieberman N, Lev M et al. Recognition of haemagglutinins on virus-infected cells by NKp46 activates lysis by human NK cells. *Nature* 2001; 409(6823): 1055–1060.
237. He XS, Draghi M, Mahmood K et al. T cell-dependent production of IFN-gamma by NK cells in response to influenza A virus. *J Clin Invest* 2004; 114(12): 1812–1819.
238. Hofmann P, Sprenger H, Kaufmann A et al. Susceptibility of mononuclear phagocytes to influenza A virus infection and possible role in the antiviral response. *J Leukoc Biol* 1997; 61(4): 408–414.
239. Dawson TC, Beck MA, Kuziel WA, Henderson F, Maeda N. Contrasting effects of CCR5 and CCR2 deficiency in the pulmonary inflammatory response to influenza A virus. *Am J Pathol* 2000; 156(6): 1951–1959.
240. Tumpey TM, Garcia-Sastre A, Taubenberger JK et al. Pathogenicity of influenza viruses with genes from the 1918 pandemic virus: Functional roles of alveolar macrophages and neutrophils in limiting virus replication and mortality in mice. *J Virol* 2005; 79(23): 14933–14944.

241. Peper RL, Van Campen H. Tumor necrosis factor as a mediator of inflammation in influenza A viral pneumonia. *Microb Pathog* 1995; 19(3): 175–183.
242. La Gruta NL, Kedzierska K, Stambas J, Doherty PC. A question of self-preservation: Immunopathology in influenza virus infection. *Immunol Cell Biol* 2007; 85(2): 7.
243. Sealy R, Surman S, Hurwitz JL, Coleclough C. Antibody response to influenza infection of mice: Different patterns for glycoprotein and nucleocapsid antigens. *Immunology* 2003; 108(4): 431–439.
244. Couch RB, Kasel JA. Immunity to influenza in man. *Ann Rev Microbiol* 1983; 37: 529–549.
245. Geiss GK, Salvatore M, Tumpey TM et al. Cellular transcriptional profiling in influenza A virus-infected lung epithelial cells: The role of the nonstructural NS1 protein in the evasion of the host innate defense and its potential contribution to pandemic influenza. *Proc Natl Acad Sci* 2002; 99(16): 10736–10741.
246. Smith GL, Murphy BR, Moss B. Construction and characterization of an infectious vaccinia virus recombinant that expresses the influenza hemagglutinin gene and induces resistance to influenza virus infection in hamsters. *Proc Natl Acad Sci* 1983; 80(23): 7155–7159.

9 Clinical and Laboratory Diagnosis of Human Respiratory Viral Infections

Cristina Costa, Francesca Sidoti, and Rossana Cavallo

CONTENTS

9.1 INTRODUCTION

The diagnostic approaches to respiratory viral infections have evolved substantially in the last decades. The reasons for this change are the advances in detection methods, the emergence of new pathogens, and the increase in potentially susceptible population, taking into account the increasing number of immunocompromised and critical patients. Overall, these factors have led to a relevant improvement in terms of types and operating characteristics of diagnostic methods (including sensitivity and specificity), as well as turn-around-time. On the other hand, important issues of costs and clinical significance of detecting multiple viruses in a single specimen or novel and poorly defined agents are emerged.

In this chapter, clinical and laboratory approaches to the diagnosis of respiratory viruses are presented, in particular specimen collection and detection methods are revised and discussed taking into account performance and limitations.

9.2 EPIDEMIOLOGY, ETIOLOGY, AND CLINICAL PRESENTATION

Respiratory viral infections play a relevant role in human diseases and have a major impact on health with direct and indirect costs.

Acute respiratory illnesses are mostly caused by viral pathogens and represent the most common disease experienced by otherwise healthy children and adults worldwide, irrespective of any other demographic characteristic.

Upper respiratory tract infections (URTIs), such as common colds, are highly prevalent in pediatric populations (including infants and young children) and contribute with a relevant epidemiological impact to illnesses in older children and adults.

In pediatric populations up to eight episodes of cold per year can occur and number arises when taking into consideration individuals who attend day care centers.[1–4] URTIs can lead to severe complications, including otitis media and sinusitis, asthma exacerbations, and lower respiratory tract infections (LRTIs).

Although, in most of the cases hospitalization is not required for URTIs and the diagnosis is only clinical, the social and economic impact on healthcare is relevant. This is attributed to morbidity (e.g., medical consultation when it occurs, therapy, assistance), absence from school or work (also including parents of affected children), and abuse of antibiotics (e.g., costs and emergence of resistant bacterial strains).

LRTIs include pneumonia, bronchitis, and bronchiolitis. Although LRTIs occur much less frequently in comparison to URTIs, they have a high impact in terms of morbidity and mortality and imply greater healthcare costs. In hospitalized patients, LRTIs represents the third cause of nosocomial infections (following urinary tract infections and surgical site infections). Pneumonia is the first infectious cause of death and is the sixth among all causes of death.

Considering pediatric populations, approximately one third of children develop an infection involving the lower respiratory tract during the first year of life. Subsequently, the incidence decreases to 5–10% during school period, and further decreases in the following period.

Pneumonia is usually divided into community-acquired pneumonia (CAP) and healthcare-associated pneumonia (HCAP), including hospital-acquired pneumonia (HAP) and ventilator-associated pneumonia. Approximately 90% of the patients hospitalized for pneumonia present a CAP, with some clinical scores used for assessing the severity of CAP and deciding the need for admission to intensive care unit.[5–7] Both CAP and nosocomial pneumonia can progress to acute respiratory distress syndrome (ARDS) and acute lung injury, these entities are associated to a mortality rate higher than 50%.[8]

Three particular groups of patients must be considered in the evaluation of acute respiratory infections: immunocompromised patients, mainly solid organ and hematopoietic stem cell transplant recipients; critical patients in intensive care unit; and patients with asthma or chronic obstructive pulmonary disease. In these groups of individuals, URTIs may frequently lead to LRTIs with severe outcomes in terms of morbidity and mortality, being one of the most common causes of death.

Among transplant recipients, lung transplant patients present specific risk factors for infections, including potent immunosuppression regimens, direct exposure of the transplanted organ to the environment with airborne agents, impaired mucociliary clearance, poor cough reflex due to denervation of the allograft, and abnormal lymphatic drainage. In addition to direct consequences of infections with progression to organ disease, accumulating data, primarily from retrospective studies, indicate that viruses may determine severe indirect effects. In particular, it has been hypothesized that viruses may act as triggers for a cascade of immunological events, including upregulation of alloreactive cells, leading to the development of acute and chronic rejection.[9]

In critical patients, beside the relevant role played by bacterial pathogens, with severe clinical entity such as ventilator-associated pneumonia, viral agents may present as infections or more frequently coinfections and the clinical significance of their detection may be challenging.

In patients with asthma or chronic obstructive pulmonary disease, respiratory tract infection and particular URTIs may represent a trigger for severe episodes of exacerbations, thus impacting importantly on their clinical management.

Etiology of acute respiratory infections is largely affected by the type of available data and study population. For example, most of the studies have been performed on pediatric patients, in which prevalence of viral etiology is higher. On the other hand, when considering adults, bacterial account for at least 50% of the cases with defined etiology. However, it has to be taken into account that many cases may be underdiagnosed and the type and wideness of diagnostic tools with limited panels probably representing disadvantages in terms of sensitivity and, on the other hand, excessively wide panels being responsible for the finding of agents with unknown clinical significance.

Considering viral agents, the most common etiologies include influenza A and B, respiratory syncytial virus (RSV) A and B, parainfluenza virus (PIV) types 1–3, adenovirus, rhinovirus, human metapneumovirus (hMPV), and coronavirus types OC43 and 229E.

Less common respiratory viruses include (PIV) type 4, influenza virus C, some types of enteroviruses, whereas the impact of severe acute respiratory syndrome (SARS) coronavirus has been greatly resized following the relevant epidemiological role played in 2003 in concomitance with its discovery.

The clinical significance of more recently discovered viruses such as coronavirus types NL63 and HKU1, MImivirus, human bocavirus, parvovirus 4 and 5, polyomaviruses KIV, and WUV remains to be elucidated.[10–15]

In immunocompromised patients and critical patients, a role may be played by herpesviruses such as cytomegalovirus, varicella-zoster virus, Epstein-Barr virus, human herpesvirus-6, and herpes simplex virus type 1, mainly due to reactivation from latency sites, including the lungs; however, the potential clinical impact may be difficult to be extrapolated, particularly in patients with coinfections.[16]

Clinical presentation of respiratory viral infections is greatly overlapping among those caused by different viruses. For example, symptoms such as rhinitis, flu-like syndrome, laryngitis, or pneumonia are common. Moreover, clinical features may mimic those of bacterial infections. As a result of this, in the absence of further diagnostic evaluations, antibiotics are often used, in most of the cases unnecessarily. In the presence of an LRTI, hospitalization is often required. Specific antiviral treatment for respiratory viral infections is available for only few agents, mainly influenza virus and RSV. Therefore, accurate diagnosis of a specific viral infection allows for the knowledge of the underlying disease, for the initiation of a tailored treatment and the discontinuation of unnecessary antibiotics, for avoiding the secondary spread of infection, for a reduction of the costs related to unnecessary investigations, and of the duration of hospital stay. In a study on paediatric patients, the rapid detection of respiratory viruses determined a reduction of approximately 50% of hospital stays, 52% of use of antibiotics, and 28% of variable costs.[17] In another study on adults, there is evidence of a reduction of approximately 11% in the use of antibiotics as a consequence of a rapid detection of viral and atypical bacterial pathogens, although it has to be underlined that most of the clinicians did not discontinue antibiotic therapy only on the basis of respiratory virus detection.[18]

The presence of viral epidemics in the population, age of the patient, type and time of onset of the illness, symptoms, biomarkers, radiographic modifications, and response to therapy can help in the differential diagnosis of bacterial and viral pneumonia. However, no clinical algorithm exists that allows for a clear definition of the cause of pneumonia and an unclear consensus exists on the therapeutic approach.[19]

To summarize, an accurate diagnosis of respiratory viral infections must take into account the clinical appropriateness, the performance characteristics, the costs, and the need for quality, efficiency, and efficacy. These relay onto the specimen collection, the choice of adequate diagnostic methods and panels, and the interpretation of the results.

9.3 SPECIMENS

The collection of an adequate specimen is fundamental for a correct diagnosis and for avoiding costs and useless investigations. The specimen must be collected from an appropriate site: swabs, aspirates, and washes for URTIs; tracheo-bronchial aspirates, bronco-alveolar lavages, and lung biopsy for LRTIs.[20] The specimen must be collected as early as possible in the presence of a suggestive clinical presentation, taking into account the acute phase and the duration of viral shedding. The specimen must be stored in adequate conditions (i.e., at 4°C; in case of specimen collected from

>24 h, at −80°C), in idoneous containers and, preferably, sent to the laboratory as soon as possible. It is a good practice to contact the laboratory for conservation and sending information and to concur them, as well as to report complete information regarding the patient (age, underlying pathologies and comorbidities, life habits, clinical suspect, therapies, and previous lab investigations) and specimen collection (time and temperature). Time and temperature are critical issue for specimen collection, this is particularly relevant for viral-isolation techniques and for detection of RNA viruses by molecular methods because of RNA degradation. For example, RSV1 virus looses up to 90% of infectivity after 2 h at 24°C, PIV exhibits 80% decrease of infectivity after 5 h at 25°C; whereas adenovirus resists up to 10 h at room temperature. This should be taken into account as it may result in false negatives.

9.4 UPPER RESPIRATORY TRACT SPECIMENS

Nasopharyngeal and oropharyngeal (throat) aspirates, washes, and swabs are among the most used specimens for sampling the upper respiratory tract (URT). In the context of URT, aspirates and washes have been long considered the sample of choice. Nevertheless, an important advancement made in recent years is the introduction of novel swabs types such as flocked swabs. These consist of nylon fibers that are perpendicular to the swab shaft. These fibers act like a brush in collecting respiratory epithelial cells and efficiently release them in transport medium, unlike standard woven rayon swabs that trap sample material.[21] The sensitivity of flocked swabs is at least equivalent to nasal aspirates for the detection of different respiratory viruses in pediatric patients,[22,23] whereas studies are needed to compare flocked swabs to woven rayon swabs in adults. Also polyurethane foam is a novel material used for swabs and, in a recent study, this resulted better than flocked swabs for detection of influenza virus in anterior nares in children by rapid antigen test.[24] Swabs are usually collected and sent to a laboratory in a viral transport medium, however viral RNA stability has been evidenced also on dry respiratory swabs, with a higher sensitivity in comparison to those collected traditionally for detection of viruses by nucleic acid sequence-based amplification (NASBA, see below).[25] Although nasal washes and aspirates have been considered superior to swabs for detecting respiratory viruses by traditional methods (i.e., viral isolation and rapid antigen detection), the introduction of flocked swabs has impacted on this, as it has been demonstrated for influenza virus and RSV.[26,27] Specimens should be kept cold at refrigerator temperature in transit (2–8°C).

9.5 LOWER RESPIRATORY TRACT SPECIMENS

These include bronchoalveolar lavage, tracheal aspirate, and sputum. Expectorated sputum is collected by coughing up from the lower respiratory tract; the risk of saliva contamination is high and the specimen is always contaminated to some degree with oropharyngeal microorganisms. Salivary contamination is assessed by evaluating a Gram stain of the sample: the finding of more than 10 squamous epithelial cells/low power fields indicates salivary contamination. Tracheal aspirate is collected through tracheostomy from intubated patients; these patients are rapidly colonized with bacteria and other nosocomial pathogens that can be aspirated into the lungs and cause pneumonia, thus complicating the identification of the true etiological agent of pneumonia. Although the problem of oral contamination is more relevant in the evaluation of bacterial pathogens, it should be taken into consideration also for viruses potentially causing LRTIs that present salivary shedding (e.g., herpes simplex virus).

Invasive sampling methods for the lower respiratory tract include bronchoalveolar lavage, protected specimen brushing, and mini-bronchoalveolar lavage (this is also referred as nonbronchoscopic or blind and is performed using special catheters via the tracheal tube). Bronchoalveolar lavage is collected by bronchoscopy; in particular, a bronchoscope is wedged into a subsegment bronchus and 150–200 mL of saline solution is instilled in order to recover epithelial lining fluid. The risk of oral contamination is very low. The specimen is idoneous in the presence of >10 cells/500× field and <1% of epithelial cells.[28] Although respiratory viruses are usually evaluated by qualitative assays, the method of epithelial lining fluid sampling by bronchoalveolar lavage can result in very high differences in terms of fluid dilution by the saline solution.

More rarely, transbronchial lung biopsy may be used for evaluation of respiratory viral infections; for example, in lung transplant recipients in which lung biopsy is performed for the evaluation of graft rejection.[29]

9.6 TRADITIONAL DIAGNOSTIC METHODS

Diagnostic approaches to respiratory viral infections include direct methods such as techniques to detect viral infectivity (i.e., viral isolation on cell cultures) and methods to detect virions or their components (i.e., antigen detection and nucleic acid detection); as well as indirect methods for the evaluation of virus-specific serological response. In Table 9.1, a summary of the main features of diagnostic approaches is reported.

A number of serological tests including hemagglutination inhibition (HAI) test, microneutralization, complement fixation, and enzyme immunoassay (EIA) have been used for testing paired acute and convalescent phase sera to identify either seroconversion or a fourfold rise in antibody titer. However, serology exhibits limited clinical usefulness in consideration of the interval between the two samplings and the duration of the disease. The evaluation of IgG response usually has a limited impact on patient management, whereas assays for IgM antibodies can detect acute infection, but sensitivity is reduced because antibody levels are often low due to repeated exposure to vaccine or circulating virus. Similarly, for viruses characterized by latency such as herpesviruses that may reactivate in immunocompromised conditions, the role of serology remains merely epidemiological in consideration of the high seroprevalence in general population. HAI assays have been also used for subtyping influenza virus (H1 or H3). Recently, novel microagglutination assays that detect and measure antibody titers to novel influenza A virus subtypes H1, H3, and H5 have been developed. These assays utilize engineered reporter viruses, specifically a lentiviral vector pseudotyped to contain the influenza H protein for detection of neutralizing antibodies. The pseudotyped lentiviral particles express the H protein, but are replication deficient. Microneutralization assays employing with infectious or noninfectious reporter viruses are performed primarily for retrospective studies, epidemiologic surveys, and vaccine trials and have limited implications for routine diagnostics.

Viral isolation has been long considered as the gold standard for the detection of respiratory viruses for the excellent sensitivity for most respiratory viruses when performed on fresh specimens, despite relevant limitations such as the turn-around time of conventional methods in tubes being too long to be clinically relevant (up to 5–10 days depending on the virus). Viral isolation on tube cultures was traditionally used to identify the viral cytopathic effect (CPE) following inoculation of the clinical specimen onto the cell monolayer. This method requires the maintenance of idoneous

TABLE 9.1
Main Features of Diagnostic Approaches to Respiratory Viral Infections

	Viral Isolation	Antigen Detection	Nucleic Acid Testing
Viruses detected	Wide range	Limited range	Very wide range, including identification of novel pathogens
Turn-around time	5–10 days (traditional method) 24–48 h (shell vial method)	30 min	2–6 h
Technical expertise	High	Low	High
Sensitivity	Good (specimen collection and storage important)	Low (higher in pediatric patients)	High

H5N1, and A(H1N1)pdm09, has caused much anxiety, reflecting the need for greater preparedness. The ability of these emerging respiratory viruses to cross the species barrier from their natural animal reservoirs, acquire the ability to transmit between humans, and cause severe disease presents a formidable threat to global public health. Despite the burden of disease of respiratory viruses, there is a dearth of both prophylaxis and therapeutics against most respiratory viruses. Current therapies mainly manage disease symptoms and are limited in preventing complications [4]. Pathogen-specific interventions are largely limited to Palivizumab for infant respiratory syncytial virus (RSV) [5] and vaccines and antivirals against seasonal IAV. However, IAV vaccines and antivirals are rendered useless when new pandemic IAV or antiviral-resistant strains emerge, respectively. Consequently, both common and emerging respiratory viruses continue to pose a strain on health systems and the economy, and there remains an urgent need for the development of effective interventions.

Antibody-based therapies offer the promise of meeting this need since antibodies play an important role in recognizing and eliminating invading microbial pathogens during the natural course of an infection. In naïve individuals, specific antibody response to primary microbial exposure takes 1–2 weeks to fully develop. During this time, disease outcome is dependent on innate immunity, which eventually leads to a strong adaptive antibody response that clears the infection. During subsequent infection with the same pathogen, memory B cells are rapidly activated and a heightened antibody response ensues, resulting in more efficient pathogen clearance. The antibody response is polyclonal in nature, targeting multiple immunogenic epitopes of the invading pathogen (discussed in Section 10.2).

Both vaccination and passive immunotherapy eventually mimic secondary immune responses and confer protection against disease. Vaccination strategies rely on the endogenous production of antibodies by means of challenging individuals with inactivated or attenuated virus particles. While vaccines exist for some respiratory viruses and can induce lasting immunity to certain viruses (see Table 10.1), vaccines are only effective in disease prevention. Furthermore, the antigenic variation within each of the respiratory viruses coupled with the time required to develop vaccines severely hampers vaccine strategy, particularly during pandemic situations. Respiratory viruses with pandemic potential are highly contagious due to their ability to spread via airborne droplets. Taken together with an increasingly globalized world, it is likely that during the pandemic, the causative pathogen will spread to most parts of the world before a vaccine specific for the pandemic strain becomes widely available.

On the other hand, passive immunotherapy involves the direct transfer of pre-made antibodies and has been used in both disease prevention and treatment. Unlike vaccination, the application of pre-made antibodies could also be particularly useful for protecting immune-compromised individuals who may not respond to vaccination. Passive immunotherapy was first described by von Behring and Kitasato in the early 1890s [6] and was used to treat many infectious diseases until the early 1930s. This initial form of passive immunotherapy was known as serum therapy as it involved the use of crude antiserum preparations obtained from immunized animals to confer protection in humans. As such, essentially all patients developed serum sickness as they mounted an immune response against foreign proteins present in the animal antisera [7]. Convalescent sera from humans as a source of polyclonal antibodies reflect the natural immune response in totality and reduce the incidence of serum sickness; however, its production is limited to the availability of immune donors and is highly variable in terms of antibody specificity and quantity. This leads to significant batch-to-batch variation and variable pharmacokinetics [8].

Although improvements to antibody purification by the 1930s reduced the toxicity of serum therapy [9], its application in infectious disease management dwindled with the introduction of antimicrobial agents and vaccine development [10]. In 1975, a key milestone in antibody therapy was achieved with the discovery of a method to produce mouse monoclonal antibodies (mAbs) *in vitro* [11]. This method eliminated the toxicity associated with the use of blood products and allowed for the generation of an unlimited supply of homogeneous mAbs against any antigen that could be recognized as being immunogenic in mice. Together with the advent of recombinant DNA technology, many developments have since been made to enable the generation of mouse–human chimeric or humanized antibodies. Further technological advances made from the mid-1980s to early 2000s

TABLE 10.1
Examples of Viruses Indicated in Severe Respiratory Infections

Family Respiratory Virus	Type of Infection	Vaccine Availability	Evidence Supporting Utility of Antibody Therapy [Reference]
Arenaviridae			
Lymphocytic choriomeningitis virus	Systemic	No	Yes [143]
Lassa fever virus	Systemic	No	Yes [144]
Junin virus	Systemic	Yes	Yes [145]
Bunyaviridae			
Hantavirus	Systemic	No	Yes [146]
Coronaviridae			
Newly emergent CoV	Systemic	No	Yes (see Section 10.4)
Filoviridae			
Marburg	Systemic	No	Yes [147]
Herpesviridae			
Epstein–Barr virus	Systemic	No	In combination [148]
Cytomegalovirus	Systemic	No	In combination [149]
Orthomyxoviridae			
IAV	Localized/systemic	Mainly for seasonal IAV	Yes (see Section 10.4)
Paramyxoviridae			
Respiratory syncytial virus	Localized	No	Yes (see Section 10.4)
Hendra virus	Systemic	No	Yes [150]
Metapneumovirus	Localized	No	Yes [151]
Poxviridae			
Variola	Systemic	Yes	Yes [152]

now enable us to produce fully human mAbs to almost any antigen. In 1998, Palivizumab was the first mAb approved by the Food and Drug Administration (FDA) for the treatment of RSV infection in infants [5]. These developments led to a renewed interest in antibody-based therapies for acute respiratory infections. Table 10.1 provides examples of viruses that can cause severe respiratory disease in man. The potential for antibody therapy for some of these viruses, particularly those that cause disseminated disease, have been reported in animal models or humans. The continual refinement of these technologies forms the basis to propel antibody therapy from potential to reality and will be discussed in detail in Section 10.3.

10.2 UNDERSTANDING THE IMMUNE RESPONSE TO SEVERE RESPIRATORY VIRUS INFECTIONS: A PRIMER FOR ANTIBODY THERAPY STRATEGY AND DESIGN

Despite these technological advances, the development of mAbs for the treatment of infectious diseases has progressed slowly and Palivizumab remains the only mAb available for the treatment of an infectious disease. The main reason accounting for this slow progress may be that a clearer understanding of disease pathogenesis and antibody mechanisms has only recently become available. Furthermore, in order for antibody therapy of respiratory viruses to become economically feasible, the candidate mAb should confer cross-protection across the different antigenic variants within each virus. This concept is well demonstrated by modeling studies on seasonal IAV vaccination. During an IAV season where the vaccine does not match the circulating strain, the net societal cost of vaccination is estimated at US$65.59 per person. This was drastically higher than US$11.17 per person, binding and slower clearance, respectively. However, human B cells are not readily available in many instances. Thus, most mAbs to date are derived from nonhuman sources and may be humanized (Section 10.3.7) to improve tolerance when applied in humans.

10.3.3 Animal Hybridoma

Mouse hybridoma technology is an established method involving the fusion of mouse antibody-secreting B cells (harvested from mouse spleen) with nonsecreting B cells from an immortal cell line to produce an antibody-secreting mouse hybridoma. Prior to this, the mouse is immunized with a specific antigen to stimulate an antibody response that is specific against the initial antigen [11]. The method results in a collection of hybridoma clones that is then screened for the antibody of interest, which can be subsequently purified (Figure 10.4).

While this method remains the most commonly used in the generation of mAbs, there are a few critical limitations. It is not uncommon for hybridomas to produce a proportion of nonspecific mAbs and the method also gives rise to clones that lose the ability to produce mAbs over time. As such, a large number of hybridomas have to be screened and tested before the desired clone is identified, thus requiring great investment of time and labor. To overcome these limitations, improved methodologies have been developed. One technique, termed as B cell targeting, involves the use of antigen to select the desired B cells and bring them into contact with myeloma cells before they are fused together by electrical pulses. This method can be used to obtain mAbs for multiple antigens by using multitargeting or conformation-specific mAbs through the use of stereospecific targeting [40].

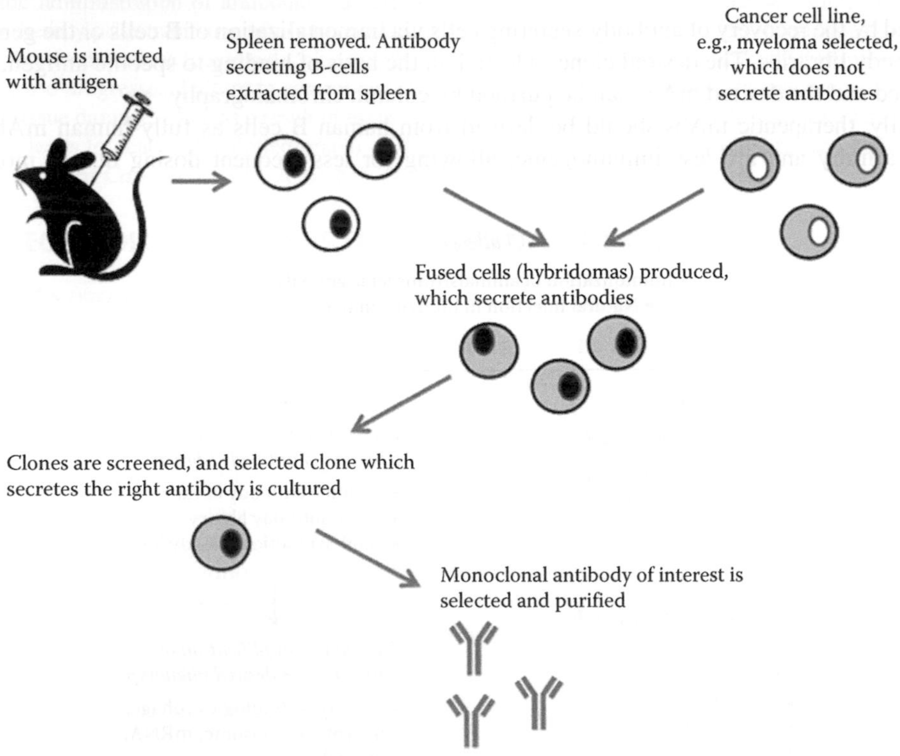
Mouse is injected with antigen
Spleen removed. Antibody secreting B-cells extracted from spleen
Cancer cell line, e.g., myeloma selected, which does not secrete antibodies
Fused cells (hybridomas) produced, which secrete antibodies
Clones are screened, and selected clone which secretes the right antibody is cultured
Monoclonal antibody of interest is selected and purified

FIGURE 10.4 Hybridoma production of monoclonal antibodies. A mouse is stimulated with the antigen of interest to produce antibody-secreting B cells in its spleen. These B cells are then fused to a nonsecreting myeloma to produce a monoclonal antibody-secreting hybridoma. The desired antibody is then selected and purified.

Besides the mouse, other mammals such as the rat, hamster, and rabbit can also be used for hybridoma-derived mAb production. However, some difficulty remains in producing hamster mAbs due to fibroblast overgrowth and hybridoma instability. Some sublines also do not fuse well due to mycoplasma contamination or genetic variation [41]. Much interest is focused on rabbits due to their natural ability to produce a wider repertoire of antibodies, even surpassing that of humans [42]. Rabbit antibodies also have simpler features and are therefore easier to clone and engineer [43]. In addition, recent advances in technology enable the rapid production of rabbit mAbs. For example, the rabbit immunospot array assay on a chip (ISAAC) method allows the production of high-affinity mAbs within a week. These antibodies display high specificity and are able to recognize slight epitope changes, including amino acid substitution, acetylation, or glycosylation [44].

10.3.4 Human Hybridoma

The concept of replacing mouse spleen-derived B cells with EBV-immortalized human B cells from peripheral blood cells was initiated by Steinitz et al. in 1977, as a method to produce human–human hybridomas [45]. This hinges on the discovery that EBV infects human B cells and transforms them after about a week in culture. First, EBV derived from the culture supernatant of the B95-8 marmoset cell line is used to transform peripheral blood mononuclear cells (PBMCs) that contain B cells [46]. The EBV-transformed B cells are then fused with a myeloma cell line via polyethylene glycol (PEG) or electrofusion. Unwanted products (e.g., fused B cell–B cell, fused myeloma–myeloma, and transformed but unfused PBMCs) are removed by screening with hypoxanthine–aminopterin–thymidine media and ouabain, and the remaining human–human hybridomas are then screened for the antibody of interest using methods such as enzyme-linked immunosorbent assay (ELISA) [47]. The main limitation of this method is that EBV-transformed cells are difficult to yield and typically produce low levels of antibody [41] although more recent studies have shown that transformation efficiency can be enhanced by CpG activation [48] or IL-2 treatment [49].

10.3.5 Generation of Antibody Libraries

As an alternative to B cell immortalization, specific mAbs may be obtained by screening from recombinant antibody libraries that constitute the genetic diversity of the human antibody repertoire. In the human immune system, diversity in antibody binding is achieved by the combinatorial assembly of germline segments (V(D)J recombination). This produces a naïve B cell repertoire, each expressing a unique antibody-binding site on their surface. Exposure to antigen selects from this repertoire and affinity for the particular antigen is achieved by somatic hypermutations (SHM) in the CDR regions of the variable antibody chains (a process also known as affinity maturation). Additional mechanisms such as (i) nonstandard recombinations, (ii) SHM-associated genetic insertions and deletions, and (iii) affinity maturation and direct antigen contact by non-CDR antibody regions also contribute to the diversity within the antibody repertoire [50].

Recombinant antibody libraries can be categorized into four main types, namely naïve, immune, semisynthetic, and synthetic. Naïve libraries are derived from hosts with no prior exposure to the antigen of interest and reflect diversity as a result of mainly V(D)J recombination. Heavy-chain diversity is mainly attributed to the CDR3 region, while light-chain diversity is equally attributed to all three CDR regions. The probability of obtaining mAb for a particular antigen is thus heavily dependent on the complexity of the library, which can be increased by combining the B cells from multiple donors. Immune antibody libraries are derived from the lymphocyte RNA of hosts previously exposed to the antigen of interest and reflects diversity as a result of V(D)J recombination and SHM. As both heavy and light chains have already undergone *in vivo* affinity maturation, the library is more likely to contain mAbs that bind the antigen strongly. Semisynthetic libraries involve the artificial alteration of CDR3 in the variable regions of the heavy chain. Synthetic libraries involve mutations in the CDR3 of both the heavy chain and the light chain. Both semisynthetic and synthetic libraries are used to increase the diversity of antibody libraries [51].

10.3.6 mAb Display Technologies

Following the creation of an antibody library, selection of the desired mAb is the next important step and mAb display technologies offer speed and accuracy in the screening process. At present, *in vitro* display technologies such as bacterial, yeast, or mammalian display offer libraries of much greater diversity due to fewer limitations in transformation and screening compared to *in vivo* technologies such as ribosomal display and the traditional phage display [52]. Generally, display platforms producing libraries of much greater diversity are used for antibody isolation while display platforms producing libraries of lesser diversity are used to fine-tune existing antibodies [53].

Most display technologies share four key steps: cloning of genotypic diversity, coupling of genotype with phenotype, selective pressure (bio-panning), and amplification. Some of the commonly used display technologies are covered in the subsections below, with screening methodologies for *in vivo* techniques (ribosome or mRNA display and phage display) broadly similar, and *in vitro* techniques (bacterial display, yeast display, and mammalian cell display) utilizing flow cytometry as a main screening tool (Figure 10.5).

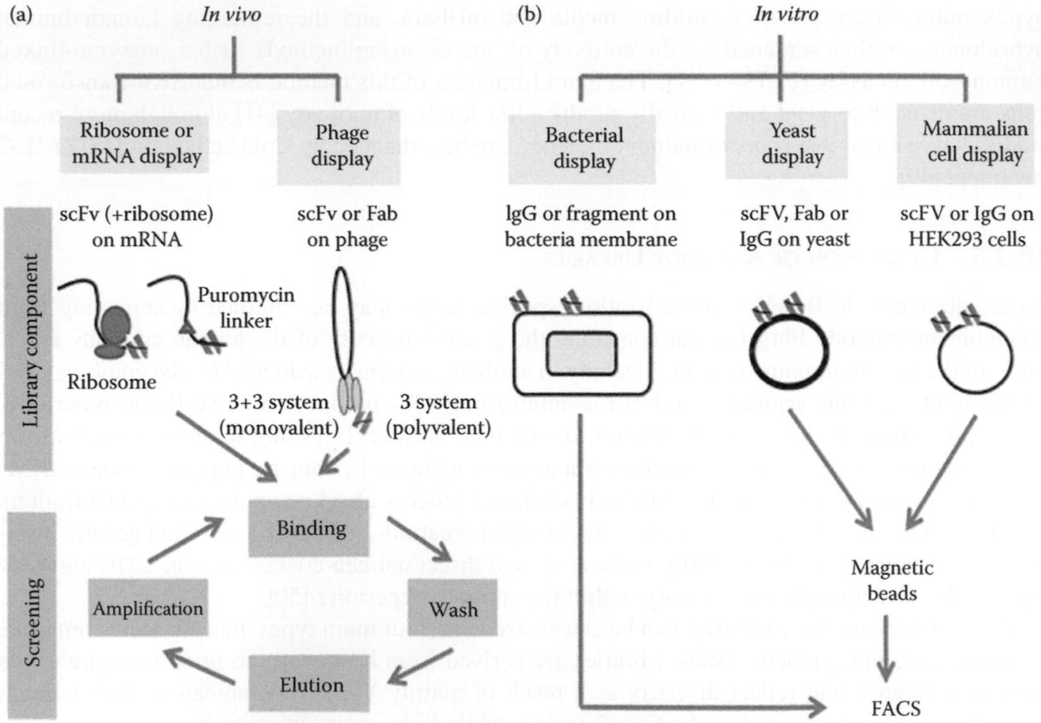

FIGURE 10.5 Display technologies—library creation and screening of clones. Conventional display technologies involve the presentation of libraries of antibody or antibody fragments on various cells or cell components, which are then screened for desired clones. At present, display technologies can be classified into *in vivo* or *in vitro* technologies. (a) *In vivo* technologies comprise of ribosome or mRNA display and phage display, which have a common screening step involving binding, washing, elution, and amplification. (b) *In vitro* technologies comprise bacterial, yeast, and mammalian display, which have a common flow cytometry screening step.

10.3.6.1 Phage Display

Phage display is the cornerstone of display technologies and is based on the concept of creating libraries of protein fragments presented on the surface of phages, which can then be screened for the fragment of interest. Millions of DNA coding for proteins, peptides, antibodies, or antibody fragments are batch-cloned to produce a protein fused to a phage coat protein (pVIII or pIII), which results in the protein or fragment being displayed on the surface of the phage. This generates a library of up to 10^{11} clones, which is then screened for interaction with specific targets. Phages that have bound to the target substance of interest are then isolated through washing (removal of unbound phages) and elution. This first round of selected phages can then be amplified via bacterial transformation. The selection can be enriched by regrowing the transformed bacteria, and the phage-bound fragments can be then be analyzed before the mAbs are finally eluted [54]. This cyclical screening process is often referred to as bio-panning and mimics the naturally occurring SHM, thus resulting in antibodies with higher affinity.

The affinity of selected mAbs may be further enhanced by modifications of this method. For example, both heavy- and light-chain fragments of Fv are expressed as scFv and then optimized via mutagenesis, after which the V_H and V_L domains can be cloned into heavy- and light-chain expression vectors and transfected into hybridoma cells for whole antibody expression with increased affinity [55].

Human single-domain phage libraries can also be constructed from human V_H3 and kappa domains, with single-strand mutagenesis to introduce diversity at variable regions [56].

There are however problems in phage library panning, which include the risk of high-affinity binders not being eluted, low expression in *Escherichia coli* possibly causing good binders to be lost during panning, and a general difficulty in achieving high throughput [57]. Another issue is that antibody or antibody fragments derived from eukaryotic cells may be difficult to express in a prokaryotic cell [58].

10.3.6.2 Ribosome or mRNA Display

Offering one of the largest libraries of up to 10^{14} clones, ribosome or mRNA display can be performed in both eukaryotic and prokaryotic cells [53,59]. The process involves the formation of a stable complex of mRNA and antibody (or fragment) in a similar concept of fragment display. In ribosome display, a ribosome that has been halted by chloramphenicol or cycloheximide (in prokaryotic or eukaryotic cells, respectively) is also linked to the stable complex. In mRNA display, the antibody fragment is linked to the mRNA via a puromycin linker [53,60]. Thereafter, it follows the same screening concepts as phage display, with the use of a mild eluting step (EDTA) to destabilize the mRNA and the addition of an RT-PCR amplifying step [53,61]. Ribosome display may prove more challenging to accomplish compared to traditional phage display due to RNA or ribosomal instability, and is limited to single-chain formats such as scFv [62].

10.3.6.3 Bacterial Display

Bacterial display first emerged in the late 1990s and involved fusing the desired antibody library to a surface protein on Gram-negative bacteria such as *E. coli.* This was mainly using the Lpp-Omp A′ system, a chimeric surface protein coding for part of the *E. coli* lipoprotein (Lpp) and the major outer membrane protein A (Omp A) [63]. A few years later, an alternative anchored periplasmic expression method (APEx system) was introduced, involving the periplasmic display of antibody fragments on the inner membrane of *E. coli* [64]. Further permutations of bacterial display revolve around the fusion of library fragments to variants of outer membrane proteins, with the aim of displaying the fragment in a manner that does not affect its folding properties, as it was postulated that a terminally fused fragment would closely represent the freely soluble form [65,66].

However, considerable difficulty was found in displaying large proteins on the terminal end of the outer membrane of *E. coli* as the recombinant protein has to traverse across both the inner and outer membranes of Gram-negative bacteria. This was eventually alleviated by the autotransporter display

TABLE 10.3
Examples of Neutralizing mAbs against IAV HA

Antibody	Mode of Action	Antigen Source	Method of mAb Generation	Type of Protection	Reference
(-o-) S139/1	Inhibits attachment	Seasonal virus	Mouse hybridoma	Heterosubtypic Mainly Group 1	[156]
(-xi-) VN04-2 (-xi-) VN04-3	Not reported	Attenuated reverse genetics H5N1 virus	Mouse hybridoma	Homosubtypic	[157]
(-o-) 9F4	Inhibits fusion	Baculovirus-expressed purified H5	Mouse hybridoma	Homosubtypic	[158]
(-o-) DPJY01[a]	Inhibits attachment	Attenuated H5N1 virus	Mouse hybridoma	Homosubtypic	[30]
(-o-) C179	Inhibits fusion	H2N2 virus	Mouse hybridoma	Yes Group 1 only	[159,160]
(-u-) AVFluIgG01	Inhibits attachment	H5N1 convalescent patient	Recombinant baculovirus expression	Homosubtypic	[161]
(-u-) 65C6 (-u-) 100F4 (-u-) 3C11	Inhibits attachment	H5N1 convalescent patient	EBV immortalization of memory B cells	Homosubtypic	[162]
(-u-) PN-SIA49	Inhibits fusion	H1N1 patient	EBV transformation of plasma B cells	Heterosubtypic Group 1 only	[163]
(-u-) PN-SIA28	Inhibits fusion			Heterosubtypic Group 1 and 2	
(-u-) CR6261	Inhibits fusion	Healthy donors	ScFv library constructed from IgM+ memory B cells	Heterosubtypic Group 1 only	[164,165]
(-u-) CR8020	Inhibits fusion	Seasonal influenza vaccinated donor	Immortalization of IgM+ memory B cells by genetic programming	Heterosubtypic Group 2 only	[166]
(-u-) FI6	Inhibits fusion	A(H1N1)pdm09 patient/vaccinated donor	RT-PCR of Ig genes from selected plasma cells	Heterosubtypic All 16 HA	[103]

[a] With the exception of DPJY01, all mAbs are of the IgG isotype. (-o-), (-xi-), and (-u-) denotes mouse, chimeric, and human mAbs, respectively.

these mAbs are generally homologous or homosubtypic and are unlikely to be heterosubtypic. On the other hand, the stem region is less exposed to the extracellular matrix compared to the globular head and is thought to be more conserved. Conservation of the stem domain is also attributed to the structural confines of the fusion machinery. As such, mAbs targeting this region display some degree of cross-specificity and neutralize viruses by preventing fusion of host and viral membranes (see Table 10.3).

Many studies of neutralizing mAbs were generated from mouse hybridoma technology; however, there is an increasing trend toward obtaining therapeutic antibody leads directly from humans. Human antibody leads are thought to be superior to antibodies derived from animals as they are indicative of the human response to pathogens. The strategy of screening for heterosubtypic human antibody leads prior to their selection and stable production also allows efforts to be focused on mAbs with the greatest possibility of success. This strategy was recently employed successfully in the identification of the first mAb, designated FI6, which neutralizes both group 1 and group 2 HA. In this study, the authors screened a total of 100,000 plasma cells from eight A(H1N1)pdm09 exposed or vaccinated donors. Only four plasma cells from a single donor were selected based on their ability to bind to group 1 and group 2 HA. These four plasma cells were then found to produce the identical FI6 mAb, highlighting the scarcity of naturally occurring broadly heterosubtypic antibodies after infection or vaccination [103].

The extracellular domain of the M2 ion channel protein (M2e) is another popular target for antibody therapies against IAV. Compared to the other two surface proteins, M2e is highly conserved between both human and avian influenza viruses [104,105] and is, therefore, thought to be an attractive "universal" influenza vaccine candidate. Indeed, several anti-M2e mAbs are heterosubtypic [106–109]. However, M2e is poorly immunogenic [110] with detectable M2e specific long-lasting humoral responses found in less than 20% of healthy donors [111]. This curtails M2e's development as a "universal" vaccine, leading some groups to focus on the production of anti-M2e mAbs as a potential "universal" passive immunotherapeutic instead.

Although M2 plays a role in viral entry, very few M2 particles are incorporated into IAV virions. Additionally, the M2e domain is a short peptide of 23 amino acids and is shielded from the extracellular millieu by HA and NA. As a result, neutralizing antibodies against M2 are presumably rare and all human and mouse anti-M2e mAbs characterized to date are nonneutralizing. M2 proteins are highly expressed on the surface of infected host cells; consequently, most anti-M2e mAbs target infected cells and mediate protection by ADCC or CDC [107]. This has been demonstrated directly in experiments involving Fc or C3 knockdown mice [106]. Such mAbs do not prevent infection but rather reduce viral replication and can confer protection against lethal IAV challenge when administered in mice either prophylactically or therapeutically. One notable mAb is TCN-032, which binds to the first five amino acids at the extreme N terminus of M2e. As a result, TCN-032 can bind directly to virus particles in addition to M2 expressed on infected host cell surfaces. This property is thought to contribute to direct viral clearance via opsonophagocytosis or virolysis, leading to enhanced *in vivo* protection compared to other anti-M2e mAbs that recognize epitopes proximal to the viral membrane [111]. TCN-032 is marketed by Theraclone and is undergoing phase II clinical trials [112].

10.4.3 Neutralizing Antibodies against Newly Emergent Coronavirus

Newly emergent coronaviruses (CoV) cross the species barrier to animals and humans from their natural bat reservoirs and have the potential to cause severe disease in man. SARS-CoV caused a pandemic in 2002–2003 and affected more than 8000 people with a case fatality rate of 10% [113]. The current Middle East Respiratory Syndrome CoV (MERS-CoV) epidemic was first detected in April 2012 and although the virus is currently less well adapted for human-to-human transmission, it is associated with a high case fatality rate of 60% [114].

The major target for neutralizing antibodies is the spike (S) protein due to its roles in viral attachment and fusion of host and viral membranes through its S1 and S2 domains, respectively. Several groups have developed potent neutralizing mAbs against the S protein and many of these studies utilized phage display technologies to produce mAbs from naïve, semisynthetic, or immune libraries (see Table 10.4). As the recovery from SARS is associated with potent and specific anti-S1- receptor binding domain (RBD) antibodies [115], most well-characterized mAbs were found to bind this domain and interfere with its interaction with host cell receptor angiotensin converting enzyme 2 (ACE2). However, the RBD displays high mutation rates, providing a way for viruses to escape neutralization and in some cases, a single amino acid mutation is sufficient to completely abolish antibody neutralization [116]. For this reason, clinical SARS isolates from the second SARS outbreak in 2003–2004 have been reported to resist neutralization by mAbs 80R and S3.1, which were previously found to be highly potent against viral isolates from the first outbreak (displaying 50% neutralization at 55.5 and 300 ng/mL against original SARS isolates, respectively). Furthermore, MERS-CoV differs extensively in its S1 domain compared to SARS and uses a different receptor, dipeptidyl peptidase-4 (DPP4) for its binding and entry into the target cell [117]. It is therefore unsurprising that anti-SARS-CoV-S1 or anti-SARS-CoV-RBD mAbs do not bind

TABLE 10.4
Examples of Neutralizing mAbs against SARS-CoV S Protein

Antibody	Mode of Action	Antigen Source	Method of mAb Generation	Reference
(-u-) CR3022	Binds S1, interferes with RBD	SARS patient	Immune ScFv phage display	[18,167]
(-u-) CR3014	Binds S1, interferes with RBD	SARS patient	Semisynthetic ScFv phage display	
(-o-) 341C (-o-) 534C	Binds S1, interferes with RBD	Inactivated purified SARS-CoV (Urbani strain)	Mouse hybridoma	[168]
(-u-) S3.1	Binds S1, interferes with RBD	SARS patient	EBV immortalization of plasma and memory B cells	[48,119]
(-u-) 80R	Binds S1, interferes with RBD Prevents fusion at higher concentrations	None	Naïve human ScFv phage display	[169]
(-u-) m396	Binds S1, interferes with RBD	None	Naïve human Fab phage display	[119,170]
(-u-) S230.15	Binds S1, interferes with RBD	SARS patient	EBV immortalization of plasma and memory B cell	[48,119]
(-u-) 201	Binds S1, interferes with RBD	Recombinant S protein ectodomain	Transgenic mouse hybridoma	[171]
(-u-) 68	Binds S1 but does not bind RBD			
(-u-) B1	Binds S2 domain	SARS patients	Immune ScFv phage display	[122]

to MERS-CoV [118]. Anti-SARS-S1-RBD mAbs are therefore typically homologous, and only a small number of homosubtypic mAbs binding to SARS isolates from the two outbreaks have been reported [119]. Naturally occurring heterosubtypic anti-CoV neutralizing antibodies are even more rare, as evidenced by no or low anti-SARS-CoV antibodies detected even in regions with high human CoV seroprevalence [120].

However, surprisingly, high cross-reactive neutralizing antibodies were found against MERS-CoV in a small number of archived SARS patients' sera and it is hypothesized that these antibodies may target the S2 domain [121]. The S2 domain contains the fusion peptide and is more conserved among SARS isolates compared to the S1 domain and can also elicit neutralizing antibodies [122,123]. mAbs specific for either of the two heptad repeats (HR1 and HR2) downstream of the fusion peptide were also found to broadly neutralize various clinical isolates of SARS-CoV [123]. Bioinformatic prediction of B cell epitopes revealed an immunogenic region that overlapped in both MERS- and SARS Co-V. This region coincides with the HR2 region and could account for the observed heterosubtypic protection [121], although this remains to be validated experimentally.

10.4.4 Antibodies Targeting Host Receptors

As an alternative strategy for targeting virus–host receptor interactions, mAbs have also been produced against host receptors and have been described for SARS-CoV [124] and human rhinoviruses [125]. This strategy involves host receptors that are more stable and less likely to mutate. Consequently, the chance of escape mutants in humans is likely to be reduced. However, these antibodies may induce side effects on receptor expressing cells and toxicity experiments in animal models are required.

10.5 ANTIBODIES: LOOKING TO THE FUTURE

10.5.1 Next-Generation Antibodies

Once lead antibodies have been validated, alterations to either the variable or constant antibody domains may be made to improve the affinity for target antigen and to improve pharmacological activity of the antibody (see Figure 10.7). Improvements to first-generation antibodies may be achieved through humanization of regions flanking the CDR domains or affinity maturation of the CDR domains, yielding second-generation antibodies with higher affinity for target antigen. These are then succeeded by third-generation antibodies, which have improved Fc functions in addition to improved variable domains. Many of these next-generation antibodies have been developed for use in noninfectious immune conditions with varying degrees of success and have been reviewed elsewhere [126]. We focus our discussion on the development of next-generation Palivizumab as an example of both the potential and challenges of antibody-based therapy for respiratory viruses.

In an attempt to improve the clinical potency of Palivizumab, Fab variants were created by introducing point mutations in the CDR regions and selecting for beneficial mutations using ELISA-based screening methods based on improved binding recombinant RSV F protein. Combinatorial Fab libraries that included the beneficial mutations were created and subjected to a subsequent round of screening [127]. Eventually, after conversion of Fab to IgG format, A4b4 was selected based on its ability to increase binding affinity to F protein by >100-fold compared to Palivizumab, mainly due to decreased antibody dissociation rate [127]. A4b4 was also found to be 44 times more potent in neutralizing RSV in tissue culture. However, these outstanding *in vitro* results failed to translate into significant improvement in *in vivo* efficacy and A4b4 only conferred a twofold improvement in the prevention of RSV in cotton rats. This was later attributed to poor serum pharmacokinetics and poor bioavailability of antibodics in lung tissue. Bioavailability and serum pharmacokinetics was partially restored by back-mutation of certain Fab residues to Palivizumab, giving rise to the eventual second-generation antibody, Motavizumab, with improved *in vitro* and *in vivo* neutralization abilities compared to Palivizumab [128]. Although Motavizumab proved noninferior to Palivizumab in clinical trials, FDA approval of Motavizumab was declined on the basis that observed increase in hypersensitivity reactions did not justify its use over Palivizumab [129].

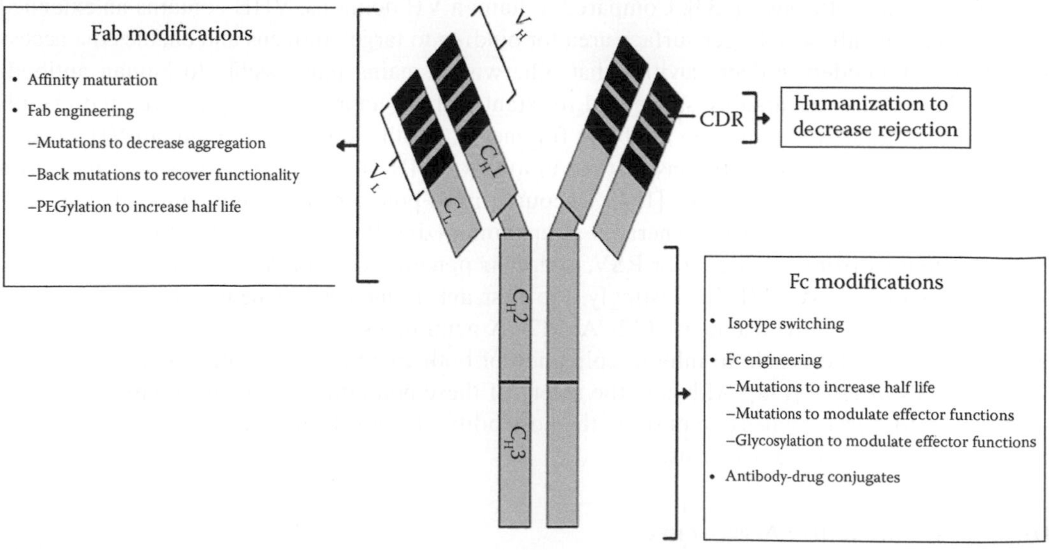

FIGURE 10.7 Creation of "bio-betters" through antibody engineering. Examples of alterations that can be made to the Fab, CDR, and Fc regions of the antibody are listed. (Adapted from Beck, A. et al., *Nat Rev Immunol*, 2010. 10(5): 345–352.)

This example illustrates that despite convincing *in vitro* data, improved antibody design does not necessarily translate to improvements in clinical potency and can adversely affect the safety profile of the antibody by increased immunogenicity.

As Motavizumab has a circulation half-life of about 3 weeks, a monthly injection schedule is required during the RSV season to ensure complete protection of high-risk infants [129]. In an attempt to improve the half-life of Motavizumab, Fc engineering was employed to enhance binding to the neonatal Fc receptor (FcRn) at pH 6. IgGs in circulation enter cells by pinocytosis and are degraded by proteases unless they bind to FcRn within the acidic environment of late endosomes. This allows IgGs to be recycled back to the cell surface, where restoration to neutral pH disrupts FcRn–IgG interaction, releasing bound IgGs back into the circulation. Using random mutagenesis, Fc libraries were constructed and mutations that conferred improved binding to FcRn at pH 6 were selected by phage display [130]. Using this method, the third-generation antibody Numax-YTE (MEDI-524-YTE) was engineered, consisting of a triple substitution in the C_H2 region of Motavizumab. Compared to Motavizumab, Numax-YTE retains its ability to neutralize RSV but showed a fourfold increase in serum half-life in cynomolgus monkeys, resulting in a fourfold increase in lung bioavailability [131].

10.5.2 Antibody Fragments as Therapeutics

Whole antibodies may be converted into smaller recombinant fragments (see Section 10.3.1) to reduce toxicity associated with Fc effector functions, improve biodistribution, or to reduce cost of production. Fab and ScFv fragments in monovalent or multivalent formats have limited success in therapeutic applications in the fields of noninfectious conditions [132]. However, they have been less successful in infectious diseases due to decreased avidity and consequently, a loss in potency or neutralizing ability compared to parental antibody. Antibody fragments are also prone to aggregation, which leads to insolubility. In recent years, the interest in antibody fragments for the treatment of viral diseases has been renewed after the discovery of naturally occurring antibodies that do not contain light chains and lacks the C_H1 domain. These single-domain antibodies are produced by the Camelidae family and the antigen-binding variable domain (VHH) may be engineered into other recombinant forms (nanobodies) that can be easily expressed within prokaryotic or eukaryotic hosts [133]. Compared to human VH domains, VHH contains an extended CDR3 loop. This allows a larger surface area for binding to target antigens and enables the access to epitopes embedded in deep cavities that otherwise remains inaccessible to human antibodies. VHHs are also remarkably stable and resistant to high temperatures, pressure, and chemical unfolding compared to human antibody fragments. Finally, compared to human VH, several hydrophilic amino acid substitutions that are unique to VHH prevents aggregation of nanobodies and enable them to remain soluble [134]. Encouragingly, potent neutralizing nanobodies against IAV H5N1 and RSV have been generated after immunizing llamas with either the recombinant H5 or F proteins from IAV H5N1 or RSV, and their potential development as therapeutic agents is being explored [135–137]. Interestingly, the first anti-influenza M2 neutralizing antibody to be described is the VHH fragment, M2-7A. M2-7A neutralizes IAVs by interfering with M2 ion channel function and is able to inhibit replication of both amantadine-sensitive and amantadine-resistant IAVs *in vitro* [138]. Although the safety of these nonhuman antibody fragments has not been validated, these studies demonstrate the possibility of a novel source and class of therapeutic antibodies against respiratory viruses.

10.5.3 Combination Approaches

As discussed in Section 10.4, a single type of mAb can protect against disease and binding is sufficient for viral neutralization. However, the intrinsic antigenic heterogenicity of each respiratory virus and their ability to mutate makes therapeutic strategies based on single mAb formulations impractical. Several groups have shown that a combination of noncompeting mAbs can be used synergistically to confer broader protection while preventing emergence of escape variants. This concept of "selective polyclonality" requires the characterization of epitope sites of individual mAbs and has been demonstrated for SARS-CoV [18,123], RSV [20], and IAV [19].

The progression of disease during viral respiratory infections is complex and the interaction between host and expressed viral proteins has been implicated in virulence and pathogenesis. This could account for the decreased efficiency of Palivizumab as the disease progresses (see Section 10.2) as an established disease is more dependent on host responses rather than sheer viral titers. It is therefore also prudent to consider antibodies that engage the cellular arms of the immune response to eliminate virus-infected cells. In this regard, the use of nonneutralizing mAbs should also be considered in combination with neutralizing mAbs, the balance of which has been reported to be crucial in determining the type of T cell response, with nonneutralizing antibodies contributing to a stronger cytotoxic T lymphocyte (CTL) response [139]. Nonneutralizing antibodies also contribute to ADCC by NK cells and have been linked to the cross-protection of IAV subtypes [140].

As an alternative to multiple antibodies, a single bispecific antibody (BsAb) may be used. These recombinant molecules have Fab domains that are independent of each other and can be used to direct target protein to particular immune cells. For example, BsAbs that bind the TCR receptor through one Fab domain and a viral protein through the other Fab domain have been generated to direct infected cells for lysis through CTL response [141,142].

10.6 CONCLUSION AND FUTURE PERSPECTIVES

The continual burden of disease caused by current and emerging respiratory viruses provides the impetus for research into novel therapeutic options. Much interest has been placed on antibody approaches due to their natural role in the immune response and their high target specificity. In addition, technological advances now permit the development of mAbs against virtually any antigen and the overall functionality may be improved through antibody engineering techniques. Many potently neutralizing mAbs have been generated against clinically important respiratory viruses and an impressive amount of preclinical data exists for many of these mAbs. Elaborate screening techniques have also been described for the generation of fully human heterosubtypic mAbs. The possibility of these "universal" mAbs against emerging respiratory viruses has garnered much interest in the use of mAbs for pandemic preparedness.

However, despite the promising preclinical data, Palivizumab remains the only mAb approved for prophylaxis of children at risk of severe RSV infection and its use in treatment is generally only effective if given during early onset of disease. Further, as exemplified by Motavizumab, improving the *in vitro* activity of first-generation mAbs by antibody engineering does not guarantee improvements in clinical efficiency. The ability of many of these respiratory viruses to mutate and evade binding by mAbs also presents a major problem.

As reviewed in this chapter, most studies have focused on potently neutralizing antibodies. However, because of the complex biology underlying disease progression as well as the continual antigenic evolution of these viruses, single mAb formulations based only on neutralizing activity may not be practical. Nonneutralizing antibodies mediating protection through ADCC and CTL should also be considered. Conceptually, the "sum of all" is more important than the "sum of one" in conferring protection and a shift toward a more polyclonal response may be necessary for antibody therapy to fulfil its potential in the treatment of respiratory infection. Additionally, to overcome the limited window of administration and symptoms due to pathogen–host interactions, antibody therapy needs to be multifunctional, linking cellular immunity to target infected cells in addition to virus particles. In this regard, the development of high-throughput methods to screen and characterize the diverse antibody repertoire would greatly facilitate and propel the selection and validation of antibody leads for combination antibody therapy.

110. Feng, J. et al., Influenza A virus infection engenders a poor antibody response against the ectodomain of matrix protein 2. *Virol J*, 2006. 3: 102.
111. Grandea, A.G., 3rd et al., Human antibodies reveal a protective epitope that is highly conserved among human and nonhuman influenza A viruses. *Proc Natl Acad Sci USA*, 2010. 107(28): 12658–12663.
112. Theraclone Sciences. Available from: http://theraclone-sciences.com/programs.php.
113. Skowronski, D.M. et al., Severe Acute Respiratory Syndrome (SARS): A year in review. *Annu Rev Med*, 2004. 56(1): 357–381.
114. de Groot, R.J. et al., Middle East Respiratory Syndrome Coronavirus (MERS-CoV); Announcement of the coronavirus study group. *J Virol*, 2013. 15: 15.
115. Cao, Z. et al., Potent and persistent antibody responses against the receptor-binding domain of SARS-CoV spike protein in recovered patients. *Virol J*, 2010. 7(299): 7–299.
116. Rockx, B. et al., Escape from human monoclonal antibody neutralization affects in vitro and in vivo fitness of severe acute respiratory syndrome coronavirus. *J Infect Dis*, 2010. 201(6): 946–955.
117. Raj, V.S. et al., Dipeptidyl peptidase 4 is a functional receptor for the emerging human coronavirus-EMC. *Nature*, 2013. 495(7440): 251–254.
118. Du, L., C. Ma, and S. Jiang, Antibodies induced by receptor-binding domain in spike protein of SARS-CoV do not cross-neutralize the novel human coronavirus hCoV-EMC. *J Infect*. 2013. pii: S0163-4453(13)00111-4. doi: 10.1016/j.jinf.2013.05.002.
119. Zhu, Z. et al., Potent cross-reactive neutralization of SARS coronavirus isolates by human monoclonal antibodies. *Proc Natl Acad Sci USA*, 2007. 104(29): 12123–12128.
120. Woo, P.C. et al., Relative rates of non-pneumonic SARS coronavirus infection and SARS coronavirus pneumonia. *Lancet*, 2004. 363(9412): 841–845.
121. Chan, K.H. et al., Cross-reactive antibodies in convalescent SARS patients' sera against the emerging novel human coronavirus EMC (2012) by both immunofluorescent and neutralizing antibody tests. *J Infect*, 2013. 10(13): 00071–00076.
122. Duan, J. et al., A human SARS-CoV neutralizing antibody against epitope on S2 protein. *Biochem Biophys Res Commun*, 2005. 333(1): 186–193.
123. Elshabrawy, H.A. et al., Human monoclonal antibodies against highly conserved HR1 and HR2 domains of the SARS-CoV spike protein are more broadly neutralizing. *PLoS One*, 2012. 7(11): 21.
124. Li, W. et al., Angiotensin-converting enzyme 2 is a functional receptor for the SARS coronavirus. *Nature*, 2003. 426(6965): 450–454.
125. Fang, F. and M. Yu, Viral receptor blockage by multivalent recombinant antibody fusion proteins: Inhibiting human rhinovirus (HRV) infection with CFY196. *J Antimicrob Chemother*, 2004. 53(1): 23–25.
126. Beck, A. et al., Strategies and challenges for the next generation of therapeutic antibodies. *Nat Rev Immunol*, 2010. 10(5): 345–352.
127. Wu, H. et al., Ultra-potent antibodies against respiratory syncytial virus: Effects of binding kinetics and binding valence on viral neutralization. *J Mol Biol*, 2005. 350(1): 126–144.
128. Wu, H. et al., Development of motavizumab, an ultra-potent antibody for the prevention of respiratory syncytial virus infection in the upper and lower respiratory tract. *J Mol Biol*, 2007. 368(3): 652–665.
129. FDA. Advisory Committee Briefing Document Motavizumab (Rezield™) 2010 25/5/2013]; Available from: http://www.fda.gov/downloads/AdvisoryCommittees/CommitteesMeetingMaterials/Drugs/AntiviralDrugsAdvisoryCommittee/UCM213827.pdf.
130. Dall'Acqua, W.F. et al., Increasing the affinity of a human IgG1 for the neonatal Fc receptor: Biological consequences. *J Immunol*, 2002. 169(9): 5171–5180.
131. Dall'Acqua, W.F., P.A. Kiener, and H. Wu, Properties of human IgG1s engineered for enhanced binding to the neonatal Fc receptor (FcRn). *J Biol Chem*, 2006. 281(33): 23514–23524.
132. Holliger, P. and P.J. Hudson, Engineered antibody fragments and the rise of single domains. *Nat Biotechnol*, 2005. 23(9): 1126–1136.
133. van der Linden, R.H. et al., Improved production and function of llama heavy chain antibody fragments by molecular evolution. *J Biotechnol*, 2000. 80(3): 261–270.
134. Vincke, C. and S. Muyldermans, Introduction to heavy chain antibodies and derived Nanobodies. *Methods Mol Biol*, 2012. 911: 15–26.
135. Ibanez, L.I. et al., Nanobodies with in vitro neutralizing activity protect mice against H5N1 influenza virus infection. *J Infect Dis*, 2011. 203(8): 1063–1072.
136. Schepens, B. et al., Nanobodies(R) specific for respiratory syncytial virus fusion protein protect against infection by inhibition of fusion. *J Infect Dis*, 2011. 204(11): 1692–1701.
137. Hultberg, A. et al., Llama-derived single domain antibodies to build multivalent, superpotent and broadened neutralizing anti-viral molecules. *PLoS One*, 2011. 6(4): 0017665.

138. Wei, G. et al., Potent neutralization of influenza A virus by a single-domain antibody blocking M2 ion channel protein. *PLoS One*, 2011. 6(12): 2.
139. Kruijsen, D. et al., Serum antibodies critically affect virus-specific CD4+/CD8+ T cell balance during respiratory syncytial virus infections. *J Immunol*, 2010. 185(11): 6489–6498.
140. Jegaskanda, S. et al., Cross-reactive influenza-specific antibody-dependent cellular cytotoxicity antibodies in the absence of neutralizing antibodies. *J Immunol*, 2013. 190(4): 1837–1848.
141. Staerz, U.D., J.W. Yewdell, and M.J. Bevan, Hybrid antibody-mediated lysis of virus-infected cells. *Eur J Immunol*, 1987. 17(4): 571–574.
142. Moran, T.M. et al., Inhibition of multicycle influenza virus replication by hybrid antibody-directed cytotoxic T lymphocyte lysis. *J Immunol*, 1991. 146(1): 321–326.
143. Seiler, P. et al., Enhanced virus clearance by early inducible lymphocytic choriomeningitis virus-neutralizing antibodies in immunoglobulin-transgenic mice. *J Virol*, 1998. 72(3): 2253–2258.
144. Frame, J.D. et al., The use of Lassa fever convalescent plasma in Nigeria. *Trans R Soc Trop Med Hyg*, 1984. 78(3): 319–324.
145. Blejer, J.L. et al., Protection conferred against Junin virus infection in rats. *Intervirology*, 1984. 21(3): 174–177.
146. Klingstrom, J. et al., Passive immunization protects cynomolgus macaques against Puumala hantavirus challenge. *Antivir Ther*, 2008. 13(1): 125–133.
147. Hevey, M., D. Negley, and A. Schmaljohn, Characterization of monoclonal antibodies to Marburg virus (strain Musoke) glycoprotein and identification of two protective epitopes. *Virology*, 2003. 314(1): 350–357.
148. Oettle, H. et al., Treatment with ganciclovir and Ig for acute Epstein-Barr virus infection after allogeneic bone marrow transplantation. *Blood*, 1993. 82(7):2257–2258.
149. Gutierrez, C.A. et al., Cytomegalovirus viremia in lung transplant recipients receiving ganciclovir and immune globulin. *Chest*, 1998. 113(4): 924–932.
150. Guillaume, V. et al., Acute Hendra virus infection: Analysis of the pathogenesis and passive antibody protection in the hamster model. *Virology*, 2009. 387(2): 459–465.
151. Alvarez, R. and R.A. Tripp, The immune response to human metapneumovirus is associated with aberrant immunity and impaired virus clearance in BALB/c mice. *J Virol*, 2005. 79(10): 5971–5978.
152. Crickard, L. et al., Protection of rabbits and immunodeficient mice against lethal poxvirus infections by human monoclonal antibodies. *PLoS One*, 2012. 7(11): 2.
153. Woof, J.M. and D.R. Burton, Human antibody-Fc receptor interactions illuminated by crystal structures. *Nat Rev Immunol*, 2004. 4(2): 89–99.
154. Klimovich, V.B., IgM and its receptors: Structural and functional aspects. *Biochemistry*, 2011. 76(5): 534–549.
155. Schroeder Jr, H.W. and L. Cavacini, Structure and function of immunoglobulins. *J Allergy Clinical Immunol*, 2010. 125(2, Supplement 2): S41–S52.
156. Yoshida, R. et al., Cross-protective potential of a novel monoclonal antibody directed against antigenic site B of the hemagglutinin of influenza A viruses. *PLoS Pathogens*, 2009. 5(3): 20.
157. Hanson, B.J. et al., Passive immunoprophylaxis and therapy with humanized monoclonal antibody specific for influenza A H5 hemagglutinin in mice. *Respir Res*, 2006. 7: 126.
158. Oh, H.L. et al., An antibody against a novel and conserved epitope in the hemagglutinin 1 subunit neutralizes numerous H5N1 influenza viruses. *J Virol*, 2010. 84(16): 8275–8286.
159. Okuno, Y. et al., A common neutralizing epitope conserved between the hemagglutinins of influenza A virus H1 and H2 strains. *J Virol*, 1993. 67(5): 2552–2558.
160. Smirnov, Y.A. et al., An epitope shared by the hemagglutinins of H1, H2, H5, and H6 subtypes of influenza A virus. *Acta Virol*, 1999. 43(4): 237–244.
161. Sun, L. et al., Generation, characterization and epitope mapping of two neutralizing and protective human recombinant antibodies against influenza A H5N1 viruses. *PLoS One*, 2009. 4(5): 7.
162. Hu, H. et al., A human antibody recognizing a conserved epitope of H5 hemagglutinin broadly neutralizes highly pathogenic avian influenza H5N1 viruses. *J Virol*, 2012. 86(6): 2978–2989.
163. Burioni, R. et al., Monoclonal antibodies isolated from human B cells neutralize a broad range of H1 subtype influenza A viruses including swine-origin Influenza virus (S-OIV). *Virology*, 2010. 399(1): 144–152.
164. Ekiert, D.C. et al., Antibody recognition of a highly conserved influenza virus epitope. *Science*, 2009. 324(5924): 246–251.
165. Throsby, M. et al., Heterosubtypic neutralizing monoclonal antibodies cross-protective against H5N1 and H1N1 recovered from human IgM+ memory B cells. *PLoS One*, 2008. 3(12): 16.

TABLE 11.1
Ten WHO Recommendations for Infection Prevention and Control of Acute Respiratory Infections

Recommendations	Overall Ranking
1. Use clinical triage for early identification of patients with ARIs to prevent the transmission of ARI pathogens to health care workers (HCWs) and other patients	Strong
2. Respiratory hygiene (i.e., covering the mouth and nose during coughing or sneezing with a medical mask, tissue, or a sleeve or flexed elbow followed by hand hygiene) should be used in persons with ARIs to reduce the dispersal of respiratory secretions containing potentially infectious particles	Strong
3. Maintain spatial separation (distance of at least 1 m) between each ARI patient and others, including HCWs (without the use of PPE), to reduce the transmission of ARI	Strong
4. Consider the use of patient cohorting (i.e., the placement of patients infected or colonized with the same laboratory-identified pathogens in the same designated unit, zone, or ward). If cohorting is not possible apply special measures (i.e., the placement of patients with the same suspected diagnosis—similar epidemiological and clinical information—in the same designated unit, zone or ward) within a healthcare setting to reduce transmission of ARI pathogens to HCWs and other patients	Conditional
5. Use appropriate PPE as determined by risk assessment (according to the procedure and suspected pathogen). Appropriate PPE when providing care to patients presenting with ARI syndromes may include a combination of the following: medical mask (surgical or procedure mask), gloves, long-sleeved gowns, and eye protection (goggles or face shields)[a]	Strong
6. Use PPE, including gloves, long-sleeved gowns, eye protection (goggles or face shields), and facial mask (surgical or procedure mask, or particulate respirators) during aerosol-generating procedures that have been consistently associated with an increased risk of transmission of ARI pathogens.[a] The available evidence suggests that performing or being exposed to endotracheal intubation either by itself or combined with other procedures (e.g., cardiopulmonary resuscitation or bronchoscopy) is consistently associated with increased risk of transmission	Conditional
7. Use adequately ventilated single rooms when performing aerosol-generating procedures that have been consistently associated with increased risk of ARI transmission	Conditional
8. Vaccinate HCWs caring for patients at high risk of severe or complicated influenza disease, to reduce illness and mortality among these patients	Strong
9. Considerations for ultraviolet germicidal irradiation—no recommendations possible	–
10. Implement additional infection, prevention, and control (IPC) precautions at the time of admission and continue for the duration of symptomatic illness, and modify according to the pathogen and patient information.[b] Always use standard precautions. There is no evidence to support the routine application of laboratory tests to determine the duration of IPC precautions	Conditional

[a] When a novel ARI is identified and the mode of transmission is unknown, it may be prudent to implement the highest level of IPC precautions whenever possible, including the use of fit tested particulate respirators, until the mode of transmission is clarified.

[b] Patient information (e.g., age, immune status, and medication) should be considered in situations where there is concern that a patient may be infectious for a prolonged period.

It is evident now that this is not the case. When infected, the cough would in fact produce large droplets of >5 μm, as the lungs would be highly congested with fluids and these large droplets would generally fall to ground within 1 m of the patient [8]. This distance of 1 m for viral droplets has been confirmed by a study by Hall et al. [9]. Consequently, infection control precautions will only be necessary when the health care worker come within 1 m of the patient. This is the theoretical concept behind the recommendations under "droplet precautions" which will be discussed below.

Some of these respiratory viral diseases, viz: RSV, parainfluenza virus, and adenoviruses emit a vast amount of viruses with their secretions. These can lead to extensive contamination of the patient's environment and infection control precautions will have to extend beyond the 1 m perimeter [10]. The isolation measure for these diseases is designated "contact precautions," which will also be discussed below. Nevertheless, the patient generally will not cough out droplets nuclei of <5 μm and, therefore, infectious material will not be disseminated for long distance through the air. Thus, "airborne precautions" are generally not necessary. There is no precise clinical data on transmission of metapneumovirus, but because of its similarity to RSV, it is generally recognized that "contact precautions" will be required for these infections [11]. Presently, none of these acute respiratory viral pathogens is classified as airborne [12].

However, it should be noted that these respiratory virus infections may spread by the airborne route under special circumstances. This is described as "opportunistic airborne infections" by Roy et al. [13] who also stressed that such diseases will not require "airborne infection isolation." Rather one should be alert to aerosol-generating procedures to be discussed below where airborne precautions will be needed.

11.2.1 Administrative Controls and Measures for Early Recognition and Isolation

Infection control measures can only be effectively implemented in healthcare facilities when administrative controls are in place. These include establishing sustainable infrastructures and activities to maintain infection control practices, clear policies on early recognition of ARVIs of potential concern, and access to prompt laboratory testing for identification of the etiologic agents. The healthcare facilities should also have adequate patient-to-staff ratio, provide staff training, and establish appropriate staff vaccination and prophylaxis programs [7].

As the spread of viral infections are now of international concern, the WHO has released a guideline, namely "infection prevention and control of epidemic- and pandemic-prone acute respiratory infections in health care" [7]. It will be referred to as the ARI guideline in subsequent discussions. The guideline recommends that in all hospitals, administrative measures should be taken to set up a system for patients with acute respiratory illness (ARI) so that they are managed in a coordinated manner with timely reports to the public health authorities. The workflow is shown in Figure 11.1 [7].

When a patient is first seen in the hospital, usually in an outpatient setting, a system should be set up for clinical triage where patients are screened for specific signs and symptoms of ARI. The moment these are detected, the infection control measures for these patients are shown in the upper box of Figure 11.1. They are basically the general infection control measures described above, but include accommodating the patient at least 1 m away from other patients [9].

Both epidemiological and clinical clues should be obtained from patients. The emergence of severe novel viral infections of public health concern such as when a new pandemic influenza strain is announced globally by the WHO and other health authorities and so the travel and occupational history should be obtained to ensure that they are not affected. Then their contact history with any known case or cluster of ARVIs of public health concern should be evaluated. Clinical clues may also be important such as the patient having severe respiratory illness after exposure to a cluster of ARI of unknown diagnosis but with a high mortality rate. If these clues suggest that the patient is having an ARVI of public health concern, then as shown in Figure 11.1, he should be isolated if possible in a single, well-ventilated room. However, if it is a new virus and the mode of transmission is still unclear, an airborne precaution room is recommended. The information may also be reported to the health authorities depending on local policies.

The relevant specimens should be submitted to the laboratory and once a specific diagnosis is made as shown in Figure 11.1, the specific infection control measures, as recommended in guidelines or in Table 11.2, should be followed.

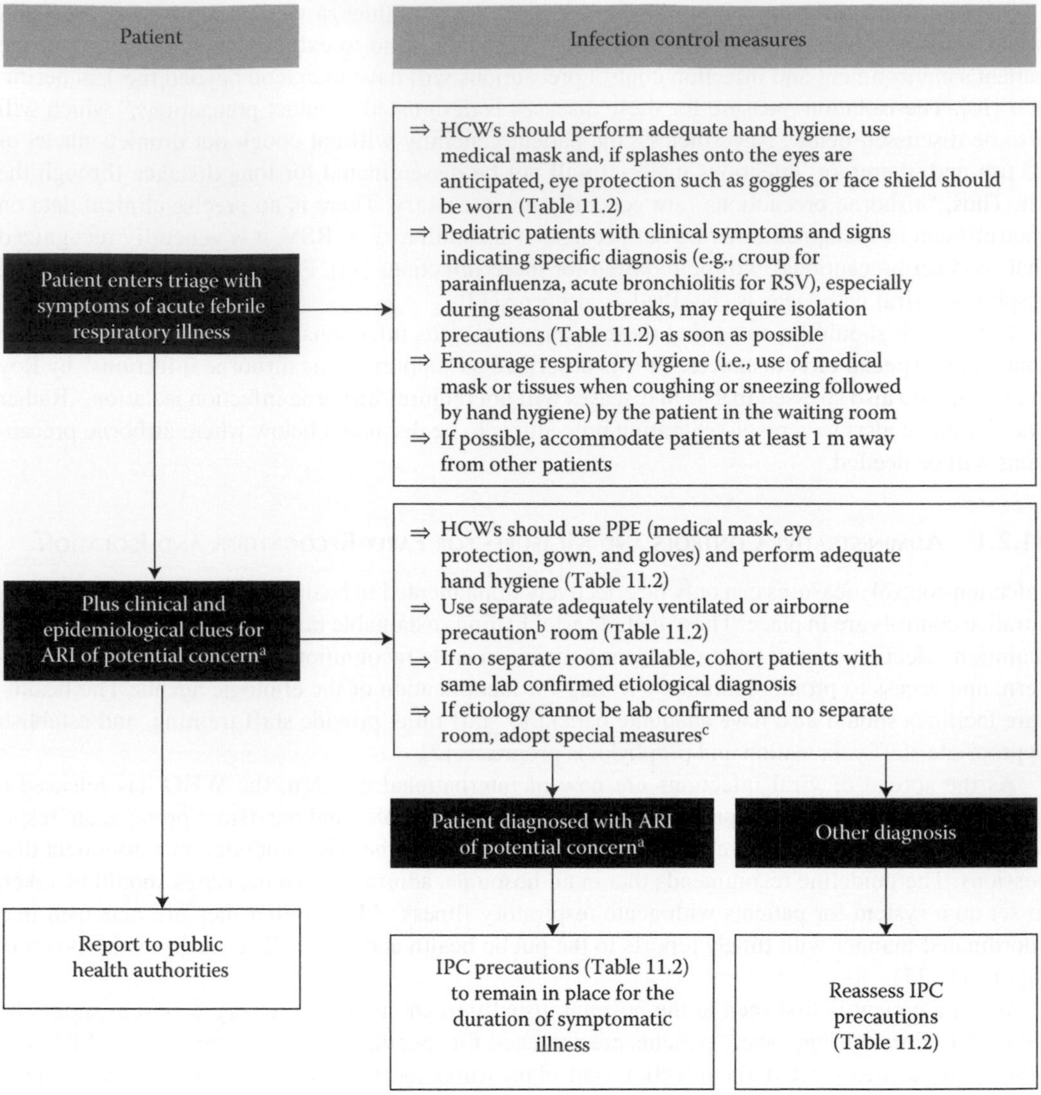
Patient
Infection control measures
⇒ HCWs should perform adequate hand hygiene, use medical mask and, if splashes onto the eyes are anticipated, eye protection such as goggles or face shield should be worn (Table 11.2)
⇒ Pediatric patients with clinical symptoms and signs indicating specific diagnosis (e.g., croup for parainfluenza, acute bronchiolitis for RSV), especially during seasonal outbreaks, may require isolation precautions (Table 11.2) as soon as possible
⇒ Encourage respiratory hygiene (i.e., use of medical mask or tissues when coughing or sneezing followed by hand hygiene) by the patient in the waiting room
⇒ If possible, accommodate patients at least 1 m away from other patients
Patient enters triage with symptoms of acute febrile respiratory illness
⇒ HCWs should use PPE (medical mask, eye protection, gown, and gloves) and perform adequate hand hygiene (Table 11.2)
⇒ Use separate adequately ventilated or airborne precaution[b] room (Table 11.2)
⇒ If no separate room available, cohort patients with same lab confirmed etiological diagnosis
⇒ If etiology cannot be lab confirmed and no separate room, adopt special measures[c]
Plus clinical and epidemiological clues for ARI of potential concern[a]
Patient diagnosed with ARI of potential concern[a]
Other diagnosis
Report to public health authorities
IPC precautions (Table 11.2) to remain in place for the duration of symptomatic illness
Reassess IPC precautions (Table 11.2)

[a] For the purpose of this document, ARIs of potential concern include: SARS, new influenza virus causing human infection (e.g., human cases of avian influenza), and novel organism causing ARIs that can cause outbreaks with high morbidity and mortality. Clinical and epidemiologic clues: e.g., severe disease in a previously healthy host, exposure to household member or close contact with severe ARI, cluster of cases, travel, exposure to ill animals or laboratory.

[b] Airborne precaution rooms include both mechanically and naturally ventilated rooms with ≥12 ACH and controlled direction of airflow.

[c] The term "special measures" means allowing patients with epidemiological and clinical information suggestive of a similar diagnosis to share a room, but with a spatial separation of at least 1 m.

FIGURE 11.1 Decision tree for IPC measures for patients with known or suspected acute respiratory infections. (Adapted from World Health Organization. *Infection prevention and control of epidemic- and pandemic-prone acute respiratory diseases in health care-WHO Interim Guideline*. June 2007. With permission.)

TABLE 11.2
IPC Precautions for HCWs and Caregivers Providing Care for Patients with ARIs according to a Sample of Pathogens

	Pathogen							
Precaution	**No Pathogen Identified, No Risk Factor for ARI of Potential Concern (e.g., Influenza-Like Illness without Risk Factor for ARI of Potential Concern)**	**Bacterial ARI[a], Including Plague**	**Tuberculosis**	**Parainfluenza RSV and Adenovirus**	**Influenza Virus with Sustained Human-to-Human Transmission (e.g., Seasonal Influenza, Pandemic Influenza)**	**New Influenza Virus with No Sustained Human-to-Human Transmission (e.g., Avian Influenza)**	**SARS**	**Novel ARI[b]**
Hand hygiene[c]	Yes	Yes	Yes	Yes	Yes	Yes	Yes	Yes
Gloves	Risk assessment[d]	Risk assessment[d]	Risk assessment[d]	Yes	Risk assessment[d]	Yes	Yes	Yes
Gown[e]	Risk assessment[d]	Risk assessment[d]	Risk assessment[d]	Yes	Risk assessment[d]	Yes	Yes	Yes
Eye protection	Risk assessment[f]	Risk assessment[f]	Risk assessment[f]	Risk assessment[f]	Risk assessment[f]	Yes	Yes	Yes
Medical mask on HCWs and caregivers	Yes	Risk assessment[f]	No	Yes	Yes	Yes[g]	Yes[h]	Not routinely[b]
Particulate respirator on HCWs and caregivers								
For room entry	No	No	Yes	No	No	Not routinely[g]	Not routinely[h]	Yes
Within 1 m of patient	No	No	Yes	No	No	Not routinely[g]	Not routinely[h]	Yes
For aerosol-generating procedures[i]	Yes	Not routinely[j]	Yes	Not routinely[j]	Yes	Yes	Yes	Yes
Medical mask on patient when outside isolation areas[k]	Yes	Yes	Yes	Yes[l]	Yes	Yes	Yes	Yes

(continued)

TABLE 11.2 (continued)
IPC Precautions for HCWs and Caregivers Providing Care for Patients with ARIs according to a Sample of Pathogens

	Pathogen							
Precaution	**No Pathogen Identified, No Risk Factor for ARI of Potential Concern (e.g., Influenza-Like Illness without Risk Factor for ARI of Potential Concern)**	**Bacterial ARI[a], Including Plague**	**Tuberculosis**	**Parainfluenza RSV and Adenovirus**	**Influenza Virus with Sustained Human-to-Human Transmission (e.g., Seasonal Influenza, Pandemic Influenza)**	**New Influenza Virus with No Sustained Human-to-Human Transmission (e.g., Avian Influenza)**	**SARS**	**Novel ARI[b]**
Adequately ventilated separate room	Yes, if available[m]	No	No	Yes, if available[m]	Yes, if available[n]	Yes	Yes	Not routinely[b]
Airborne precaution room[n]	No	No	Yes or cohort	No	No	Not routinely[o]	Not routinely[o]	Yes
Summary of IPC precautions for routine patient care, excluding aerosol-generating procedures	Standard	Standard	Standard	Standard	Standard	Standard	Standard	Standard
	Droplet	—	—	Droplet	Droplet	Droplet	Droplet	—
	—	—	—	Contact	—	Contact	Contact	Contact
	—	—	Airborne	—	—	—	—	Airborne

[a] Bacterial ARD refers to common bacterial respiratory infections caused by organisms such as *Streptococcus pneumoniae, Haemophilus influenzae, Chlamydia* spp., and *Mycoplasma pneumoniae.*

[b] When a novel ARD is newly identified, the mode of transmission is usually unknown, Implement the highest available level of infection control precautions, until the situation and mode of transmission is clarified.

[c] Perform hand hygiene in accordance with Standard Precautions (see Annex C).

[d] Gloves and gowns should be worn in accordance with Standard Precautions (see Annex C). If glove demand is likely to exceed supply, glove use should always be prioritized for contact with blood and body fluids (nonsterile gloves), and contact with sterile sites (sterile gloves).

[e] If splashing with blood or other body fluids is anticipated and gowns are not fluid-resistant, a waterproof apron should be worn over the gown.

[f] Facial protection (medical masks and eye protection) should be used in accordance with Standard Precautions by HCWs if activities are likely to generate splashes or sprays of blood, body fluids, secretions and excretions on the mucosa of eyes, nose, or mouth; or if in close contact with a patient with respiratory symptoms (e.g. coughing/sneezing) and sprays of secretions may reach the mucosa of eyes, nose, or mouth.

[g] As of the date of this document, no sustained efficient human-to-human transmission of avian influenza A is known to have occurred, and the available evidence does not suggest airborne transmission from humans to humans. Therefore, a medical mask is adequate for routine care.

[h] The current evidence suggests that SARS transmission in health-care settings occurs mainly by droplet and contact routes. Therefore, a medical mask is adequate for routine care.

[i] See Section 11.2.3, Page 213.

[j] Some aerosol-generating procedures have been associated with increased risk of transmission of SARS and tuberculosis (Table 6). To date, the infectious risk associated with aerosol-generating procedures in patients with bacterial ARDs, ARDs caused by rhinovirus, parainfluenza, RSV and adenovirus is not defined. As a minimum, a tightly-fitted medical mask should be used.

[k] If medical masks are not available, use other methods for source control (e.g. handkerchiefs, tissues, or hands) when coughing and sneezing.

[l] There are common pathogens in children, who may not be able to comply with this recommendation.

[m] Cohort patients with the same diagnosis. If this is not possible, place patient beds at least 1 m apart.

[n] Airborne precaution rooms can be naturally or mechanically ventilated, with adequate air change rate of at least 12 ACH and controlled direction of air flow.

[o] Airborne precaution rooms, if available, should be prioritized for patients with airborne infections (e.g. pulmonary tuberculosis, chickenpox, measles) and for those with novel organisms causing ARD.

this can occur. In the case of SARS, a previously undescribed coronavirus SARS-CoV was the cause,[6] probably originating in bats in southern China.[7] Why SARS-CoV suddenly became a human pathogen is unclear, but it may have been due to spontaneous mutation as it clearly did not arise due to recombination with other coronaviruses.[8] The more recent coronavirus (hCoV-EMC/2012) causing concern in the Middle East and Europe also appears to have only been very distantly related to previously known organisms.[9]

An entirely different picture of evolution appears to be typical for influenza viruses, including H1N1 09. As has been the case with the previous influenza pandemics, there was a recombination of several existing influenza strains. In the case of H1N1 09, there were identifiable elements of swine, human, and avian, almost certainly occurring initially in Mexico.[10] The novel H1N1 strain that resulted from this recombination was sufficiently different than other strains, which most of the human population had no adaptive immunity from exposure to the previous influenza strains or vaccination. Interestingly, some adults over 65 years of age had some serological immunity to H1N1 09, possibly due to the previous infection with H1N1 influenza circulating prior to 1950,[11] or possibly greater exposure to prior influenza vaccines that provided some level of coverage.[12]

In both SARS and H1N1 09, it is thought that close contact between an animal reservoir and humans facilitated the transmission of the novel pathogen into human hosts. So, while in theory, it may be possible to reduce the human–animal proximity that facilitates the zoonotic transfer of new pathogens, in practice, this may be impossible with the level of overcrowding and poverty in much of the developing world along with the relentless spread of human dwellings into wildlife habitats. Modernization of farming techniques enabling high-density animal farming may also be accelerating the development of new pathogens by increasing the level of contact between human and animal hosts.[13]

12.3 SURVEILLANCE AND LIMITING INITIAL SPREAD

If we cannot stop new pathogens arising, then the next best option is to identify them as soon as possible and limit the spread from the primary site. Again, in practice, this is very difficult to do as both SARS and H1N1 09 have demonstrated. It is, however, probably the only real opportunity to stop the global spread of a new pathogen unless it has an extremely low transmissibility from person to person.[14]

SARS originated in the south of the People's Republic of China (PRC) late in 2002 and became a global threat due to an infected physician traveling to Hong Kong in February 2003.[15] International criticism was leveled against authorities in the PRC for not revealing the extent of the epidemic earlier, prior to SARS spreading internationally when it could have potentially been contained.[16] While political considerations within the PRC clearly contributed to the delay in communicating with the international community,[16] significant deficiencies in the structure of its public health service severely limited its ability to recognize and track potential epidemics.[17,18]

As part of the global public health response after the SARS epidemic, the World Health Organization (WHO) established the international health regulations in 2005 (IHR 2005).[19] These internationally binding regulations require all countries to report all cases of human influenza caused by new viral subtypes to the WHO.[20] The international community also directed additional funding for improved surveillance of influenza and other respiratory infections in China and Southeast Asia post-SARS, with additional resources allocated after the increase in H5N1 avian influenza between 2003 and 2006.[21]

Post SARS, the consensus of international opinion was that the next viral pandemic would most likely arise in the Asia-Pacific region.[22] Continued concern over avian H5N1 influenza and whether it would evolve into a pathogen capable of sustained human-to-human transmission kept the focus on the Asia-Pacific region.

On April 21st 2009, the U.S. Centers for Disease Control and Prevention (CDC) reported the first two cases in California of what became known as H1N109.[23] By the time of the report from the United States, Mexico was experiencing a surge in cases of respiratory infection subsequently shown to be also due to H1N1 09.[24] It quickly became clear that H1N1 09 was already well established in

Mexico and the United States and on June 11th of 2009, despite significant internal politics about the merit of the decision, WHO declared a phase 6 pandemic based on the global spread of the virus.[25]

With H1N1 09, like SARS, our surveillance systems failed to identify the virus fast enough to prevent the spread beyond the initial country of origin. While additional funding was directed to the Asia-Pacific region post-SARS for enhanced surveillance, H1N1 09 has demonstrated that new viral threats can arise anywhere and that we still have much to do if we are going to achieve the goal of detecting emerging pathogens before they disseminate.[26] Whether sufficient resources will be made available to enable early detection next time, particularly in the current global economic climate, and for how long these resources will be maintained, remains to be seen.

12.4 CONTAINMENT AT INTERNATIONAL BORDERS

For emerging epidemics, as with both H1N1 09 and SARS, while more than one country is likely to have active infection at the time the threat is recognized, the vast majority of governments and public health authorities in the world will be trying to prevent it from entering and infecting their population. The two principal strategies employed are quarantine and screening at points of entry into the country, neither of which is recommended by the WHO[27] for reasons that will be outlined below. Exit screening, however, preventing infected individuals from leaving until they are noninfective, is widely acknowledged to be important in slowing the rate of spread,[28,29] even if it cannot realistically prevent it indefinitely. Unfortunately, and perhaps understandably, many countries are much more focused on preventing new cases of infection from entering their borders rather than preventing established cases from leaving. This is tacitly acknowledged by WHO as it is suggested that entry screening should be considered by passengers arriving from countries where there are concerns about the presence or thoroughness of exit screening.[27] Substantial difficulties also arise when neighboring countries have substantially different public health approaches and public health laws.[30]

While perhaps politically expedient to make the attempt, as already mentioned, there is substantial evidence of how ineffective quarantine and entry screening at international borders is for controlling influenza and other epidemics.[14,27] For example, during the SARS epidemic, Canada screened over 45 million travelers with questionnaires and detected only four cases of SARS. Thermal imaging was even less effective, with not a single case detected for over 35 million travelers screened.[31] Multiple studies have demonstrated that thermal imaging is both ineffective and inaccurate,[32] including H1N1 09.[33]

Although SARS did spread to 28 countries,[34] exit screening with quarantine has been credited with helping to contain the epidemic.[27] H1N1 09, in contrast, quickly bypassed almost all international borders. In Australia, for example, just 20 days after quarantine measures were enacted for H1N1 09, the public health authorities conceded defeat in the face of widespread infection in the general population.[35] The difference in effectiveness of control measures in containing SARS and H1N1 09 are due to the differences in the infectivity of the viruses and the speed of onset of infectivity after initial exposure. The fact that SARS continued to be viewed as a serious mortality threat, whereas H1N1 09 rapidly became regarded as a predominantly nonlethal disease, may also have reduced public compliance with public health measures for the latter.[36,37]

SARS had an incubation of 2–10 days and a maximum infectivity in the second week of symptoms.[38,39] Unlike most viral infections, asymptomatic or subclinical infection, if it occurred at all with SARS, was also extremely rare.[40,41] In contrast to SARS, influenza typically has an incubation period of 2–4 days with maximal infectivity in the first few days of symptoms. This short incubation time greatly reduces the window of opportunity that public health authorities have to identify contacts of confirmed cases and institute appropriate quarantine and preventative measures (such as oseltamivir or zanamivir). Asymptomatic or subclinical infections are also common with influenza, and are particularly so with H1N1 09.[42] To compound the difficulties with the much shorter incubation time with H1N1 09, it appears to be much more contagious than normal influenza,[43] possibly due to much higher viral loads in the lung and gut.[44] Some hosts may also be much more infective than others, such as the "supper shedders" identified during the SARS epidemic.[45]

Quarantine and entry screening at international borders comes not only at a substantial economic cost, but in some countries, it has created considerable debate about the legality and ethical basis for this approach.[46–49] The IHR 2005 specifically addresses issues of human rights related to quarantine and travel restrictions,[19] although compliance with these sections was far from universal.[26] The cost and time taken for additional screening measures are also predicably not popular with airlines.[50]

Despite the pessimism about entry screening and quarantine stopping the spread of epidemics, some modeling suggests it can still delay the spread of influenza and save lives.[51] During the H1N1 09 pandemic, New Zealand was initially able to contain and stop the spread of the virus due to diligent public health measures.[52] There were also notable successes during the 1918 influenza pandemic with some small countries with limited international travel such as Madagascar, American Samoa, and New Caledonia, delaying or completely preventing the infection from their populations.[27] With strict maritime quarantine, Australia delayed the arrival of the 1918 pandemic by about 3 months,[27] a delay that in the H1N1 09 pandemic could have been long enough to allow for the vaccine to be available, something that may be critical if we are ever faced with an epidemic that is both highly contagious and highly virulent.

One of the interesting and controversial areas with viral epidemics is the extent to which air travel itself is responsible for infecting passengers. There will undoubtedly be differences between pathogens depending on their innate infectivity; however, even for a highly contagious virus such as H1N1 09, there is considerable argument. Modeling based on a single infective individual by Wagner and colleagues suggests that in long haul, flights anywhere from 7 to 17 people may be infected during flight.[53] Modern high efficiency particulate air filters in aircraft recirculate air within very localized cabin areas,[50] in theory, containing most of the risk to within two rows of the infective individual. Analysis of a group of students exposed to H1N1 09 in flight found the risk to be approximately 3.5% for those seated within two rows of the index case.[54] It is not safe, however, to assume that there is no risk beyond the two-row limit, with one case of SARS leading to infection of 22 of 120 passengers and the crew dispersed throughout the aircraft.[55]

Clearly, effective exit screening combined with passengers being responsible and not traveling when they are symptomatic should significantly reduce the risk to passengers. However, in practice, as many frequent flyers will attest, many people fly while actively infected with respiratory tract infections and airlines seldom refuse to allow them to board, possibly, in part, due to many practical and potentially legal issues that would ensure over complex issues such as who has the responsibility for their care, who pays for additional accommodation, canceled flights, medical expenses, and so on. Again, the extent to which airlines and airline crew are prepared to act to prevent passengers with active respiratory tract infections from boarding is likely to be highly influenced by the level of threat they perceive the circulating epidemic poses to them. In the event of a highly lethal infection, we can expect substantial reductions in airline traffic, including the possible complete prohibition of travel between countries. In the event of infections of a lesser perceived threat, such as with H1N1 09, there was virtually no limitation placed on air travel.

Recent research has indicated that complete closure of air travel may not be needed and that alternative strategies such as closure of high-transmission risk routes may be more cost-effective and much less disruptive to air travelers.[56] Whether such an approach is truly practical when the primary driver of behavior is likely to be the public (and therefore political) perception of risk, remains to be seen.

12.5 CONTROL AT A NATIONAL AND LOCAL LEVEL IN ESTABLISHED EPIDEMICS

Despite all the discussion up to this point, and some evidence that increased investment in global surveillance and notification systems did produce a faster response to H1N1 09;[57] by far, the most likely scenario in any new epidemic is that it will not be contained and all countries will need to combat it based on the resources available to them. While some responses to each emerging threat are generic, some measures will need to be tailored to the characteristics of each pathogen.

An early and clear understanding of the severity of illness that is likely to be seen, including mortality, is essential for accurate public health planning.[58] For this reason, it is critical to collate and disseminate clinical data on the emerging epidemic as fast and widely as possible, which was one of the aims of the IHR 2005. With SARS, it became obvious that the health-care setting, and especially procedures such as nebulization and intubation were associated with extremely high risks of disseminating the infection,[15] leading to significant alterations in clinical approach.

Unfortunately, in the case of H1N1 09, marked differences between initial reports and subsequent clinical experience led to a significant amount of confusion and subsequently complaints over how WHO responded.[59–61] The initial population data from in and around Mexico City[62] examining 899 patients reported a high hospitalization rate (6.5%) and relatively high 60-day mortality (2.7%). Inpatient mortality was a disturbing 41%.[62] In hindsight, we know that H1N1 09 was actually a very mild infection in most patients, and the overall mortality was in the order of only 0.05–0.15%,[63,64] certainly no worse than the usual seasonal influenza.[65]

The WHO has been criticized for not paying enough attention to discrepancies in the Mexican data that indicated early on that H1N1 09 was not as virulent as was being reported.[66] There has been significant debate in the WHO over declaring a phase 6 pandemic and the subsequent implications across the international community,[25] with the director general of WHO acknowledging that its response was far from optimal, including being hampered by a lack of definitions of a pandemic and an inflexible approach.[67] However, high inpatient mortality rates were also reported from the United States and Canada,[68,69] and it is known that emerging viruses can become less virulent as they pass through serial human hosts.[70] Clearly, we need to understand why there was such a difference between the initial and subsequent experience with H1N1 09 so that the same thing does not occur next time.

Regardless of the projected mortality rate, trying to limit the spread of infection until a vaccine becomes available is the cornerstone of managing emerging epidemics. The key to limiting the spread at all stages is quickly and accurately diagnosing infection and then limiting the spread from that individual through nonpharmacological approaches combined with pharmacological therapy. Diagnosis may be readily apparent from obvious clinical features (e.g., smallpox, Ebola), but in the vast majority, the presentation is likely to be nonspecific enough that it cannot be clearly differentiated from other serious lower respiratory tract infections. One of the major lessons from H1N1 09 is that rapid microbiological testing is essential,[71] and that in most areas, there was a major lack of capacity to meet demand. The slower the ability to make a diagnosis, the more problematic it is to manage issues such as quarantine advice, contact tracing, and the use of medications, which may reduce the risk of transmission.

Another lesson from H1N1 09 is that our pandemic plans need to be flexible and the public health response needs to be able to adapt quickly to nuances of individual pathogens. Virtually, all pandemic influenza plans were based on an assumption that the vast majority of infected individuals would be febrile, leading to initiatives such as fever clinics and quarantine of febrile patients until a diagnosis was established.[72] With H1N1 09, many infected individuals were not febrile, and nor were there any specific clinical characteristics that made it possible to define infected versus noninfected patients. Well after it was recognized by clinicians that fever was often not present with H1N1 09, public health officials were still discussing on establishing fever clinics in Australia. These types of communication breakdowns between clinicians and public health officials are another area that needs to be improved and response to epidemics should be made more flexible.[71]

SARS highlighted the central role of health-care facilities as hubs of dissemination. Most cases of SARS outside the PRC were acquired in a health-care setting,[73] health-care workers representing 21% of cases with a mortality rate of 9.6%.[34] In the hospital setting, it is critical to treat all patients with respiratory tract infections as contagious and have the appropriate protective measures in place to protect staff and other patients. The psychological impact on health-care workers of dealing with an epidemic should not be underestimated and needs to be addressed as part of any response plan.[74]

While SARS severely tested the quarantine capacity of most hospitals, H1N1 09 overwhelmed them. Few, if any, hospitals have been built with the capacity to isolate all patients individually, which leads to cohorting of suspected cases and potentially spread between them to originally uninfected individuals. Again the facility to be able to rapidly make a diagnosis is critical to managing the quarantine situation. The basic measures such as limiting or preventing visitors, keeping the number of hospital staff having contact with infected patients to a minimum, and strict infection control including basic measures such as hand washing and proper fitting masks that are fit for purpose are critical.[28,75]

All public health pandemic plans advise that, where possible, infected individuals should be kept at home. Infected individuals need to be told not to go to work (or school) and employers need to be educated to enforce these guidelines. This is particularly important with hospital staff, with some health authorities instigating regular temperature checks of staff during the SARS epidemic.[76] School closures are likely to be highly effective when there is an epidemic that is severe and highly transmissible,[77] as school-age children have been shown to amplify the spread of epidemics.[28] However, school closures can be unpopular with working parents who need to find emergency child care or take time off work and therefore, this measure is subject to significant political control.

Other activities where large groups of people congregate should also be canceled or postponed during an epidemic.[28] The rate of spread of H1N1 09 was substantially accelerated in Australia by public health authorities and governments failing to stop national school sporting carnivals during the early stages of the pandemic.[78] Again, all these measures are likely to be unpopular with parts of the general public and therefore, with some politicians. It is very important that both groups are educated about the need for these measures as public support is critical for public health measures to be effective.[79]

With H1N1 09, we were fortunate in that neuraminidase inhibitors have been shown to reduce the transmission of influenza and at least for the majority of the pandemic, resistance rates were quite low. These drugs were clearly effective in reducing the spread of H1N1 09; however, diagnostic delays reduced the potential impact.[80] Most developed countries had sufficient stocks of these drugs to meet the demand, but this was not the case in many developing countries despite significant efforts over the past 5 years to improve the situation.[81] However, as with SARS, novel noninfluenza pathogens are unlikely to be affected by the existing antiviral drugs.

Ultimately, there is no substitute for individual responsibility. The experience in Hong Kong during the SARS epidemic shows how effective basic measures such as hand washing and cough hygiene can be, with substantial drops observed for all respiratory infections during the period of increased public vigilance.[82] Communication and education are clearly important in obtaining maximum compliance with public health measures;[83] however, the reality is that without a high level of perceived threat, most individuals stop being vigilant about personal protection measures.[82,84–86]

12.6 VACCINE DEVELOPMENT AND DISTRIBUTION

A significant positive result from the H1N1 09 pandemic was the speed in which an effective vaccine was developed.[87] A major factor in the quick success with the H1N1 09 vaccine is that it was a relatively straightforward adaptation of the usual seasonal influenza vaccine production process. While there is no reason to think that there will be any more problems with future influenza pandemics than with H1N1 09, the same may not be true of novel viruses, as has been shown with the lack of a current vaccine for SARS.[88]

With H1N1 09, there were problems with the uptake of the vaccine, driven by a variety of factors, including perceptions about the likelihood of developing a severe illness if infected and problems with the H1N1 vaccine in the 1970s.[89–91] These factors, however, are not likely to be an issue if we are faced with a highly virulent pandemic. What is a much more significant problem is the production and distribution of the vaccine,[92,93] particularly to developing countries.[93,94] These logistic issues remain a priority for the WHO to address ahead of future epidemics.

The existence of established protocols for manufacturing the influenza vaccine was clearly an advantage with H1N1 09. Much more problematic is the production of a safe and effective vaccine in the setting of a novel, noninfluenza pathogen, such as the recent coronavirus infections such as SARS. Indeed, nearly a decade later, research is still defining the appropriate vaccine targets for SARS.[95,96] Again, it should be acknowledged that the amount of resources allocated to the development of a coronavirus vaccine is much lower than it would be if there was a high perception of threat by governments; however, no amount of investment is guaranteed to produce a potent and safe vaccine in a quick time frame.

12.7 CONCLUSION

Both SARS and H1N1 09 challenged our global responses to emerging epidemics. With SARS, we were lucky in that it was contained due to a relatively low infectivity of the virus and good public health measures. With H1N1 09, we completely failed to contain the virus; however, again, we were lucky as it had a relatively low virulence contrary to initial reports.

We cannot prevent new pathogens arising, as has been shown recently with hCoV-EMC/2012 and H7N5 influenza, and our ability to contain highly infective pathogens is very limited. Enhanced surveillance is critical; the sooner we detect emerging threats, the more potential there is to contain them and the more time we gain to develop an effective vaccine. Accurate clinical information on the severity of the disease and infectivity is critical to planning the response and it is important that the reason for the discrepancy between the early reports of H1N1 09 and the subsequent experience must be fully understood.

Both H1N1 09 and SARS have highlighted health-care institutions as the major foci of disease transmission and all institutions need to have the facility to isolate infected patients as well as have maximal protection for the staff. There is no doubt that personal protective measures such as hand washing and avoidance behaviors are effective, and the general public also needs to be educated to act responsibly by staying at home when unwell and not traveling when potentially infective.

A key finding of the H1N1 09 epidemic was the crucial role of a rapid diagnosis when there is no clear clinical phenotype and many institutions concluded that they needed more diagnostic resources to meet their needs, especially during the peak period of the pandemic. The need for public health planning to be more flexible is also clear, right up to the international strategy level of the WHO. The most positive aspect of the H1N1 09 pandemic was the speed at which an effective vaccine was developed. However, whether this can be achieved for noninfluenza threats is highly questionable.

Overall, SARS taught us how much of an impact a virulent pathogen can have on health-care institutions and workers. H1N1 09 has taught us how quickly a new pathogen can spread and how even the one with a relatively low virulence can test our health-care resources. Whether we can respond fast enough to contain a highly infectious, highly virulent pathogen when it does arise remains highly questionable.

REFERENCES

1. Blair PJ, Putnam SD, Krueger WS, Chum C, Wierzba TF, Heil GL et al. Evidence for avian H9N2 influenza virus infections among rural villagers in Cambodia. *J Infect Public Health*. 2013; 6(2): 69–79.
2. Manabe T, Tran TH, Doan ML, Do TH, Pham TP, Dinh TT et al. Knowledge, attitudes, practices and emotional reactions among residents of avian influenza (H5N1) hit communities in Vietnam. *PLoS One*. 2012; 7(10): e47560.
3. Centers for Disease C, Prevention. Notes from the field: Highly pathogenic avian influenza A (H7N3) virus infection in two poultry workers—Jalisco, Mexico, July 2012. *MMWR Morb Mortal Wkly Rep*. 2012; 61(36): 726–727.
4. Wise J. Two more cases of novel coronavirus are confirmed in UK. *BMJ*. 2013; 346: f1030.

84. Lau JT, Tsui HY, Kim JH, Chan PK, Griffiths S. Monitoring of perceptions, anticipated behavioral, and psychological responses related to H5N1 influenza. *Infection*. 2010; 38(4): 275–283.
85. Wong LP, Sam IC. Behavioral responses to the influenza A(H1N1) outbreak in Malaysia. *J Behav Med*. 2010; 34(1): 23–31.
86. Van D, McLaws ML, Crimmins J, MacIntyre CR, Seale H. University life and pandemic influenza: Attitudes and intended behaviour of staff and students towards pandemic (H1N1) 2009. *BMC Public Health*. 2010; 10: 130.
87. Greenberg ME, Lai MH, Hartel GF, Wichems CH, Gittleson C, Bennet J et al. Response after one dose of a monovalent influenza A (H1N1) 2009 vaccine—Preliminary report. *N Engl J Med*. 2009; 361(25): 2405–2413.
88. Woodland DL. Progress towards a SARS vaccine. *Viral Immunol*. 2010; 23(5): 455.
89. Bone A, Guthmann JP, Nicolau J, Levy-Bruhl D. Population and risk group uptake of H1N1 influenza vaccine in mainland France 2009–2010: Results of a national vaccination campaign. *Vaccine*. 2010; 28(51): 8157–8161.
90. Maurer J, Uscher-Pines L, Harris KM. Perceived seriousness of seasonal and A(H1N1) influenzas, attitudes toward vaccination, and vaccine uptake among U.S. adults: Does the source of information matter? *Prev Med*. 2010; 51(2): 185–187.
91. Seale H, Heywood AE, McLaws ML, Ward KF, Lowbridge CP, Van D et al. Why do I need it? I am not at risk! Public perceptions towards the pandemic (H1N1) 2009 vaccine. *BMC Infect Dis*. 2010; 10: 99.
92. Rambhia KJ, Watson M, Sell TK, Waldhorn R, Toner E. Mass vaccination for the 2009 H1N1 pandemic: Approaches, challenges, and recommendations. *Biosecur Bioterror*. 2010; 8(4): 321–330.
93. Hessel L. Pandemic influenza vaccines: Meeting the supply, distribution and deployment challenges. *Influenza Other Respir Viruses*. 2009; 3(4): 165–170.
94. Enserink M. Swine flu pandemic. Developing countries to get some H1N1 vaccine—But when? *Science*. 2009; 326(5954): 782.
95. Li J, Ulitzky L, Silberstein E, Taylor D, Viscidi R. Immunogenicity and protection efficacy of monomeric and trimeric recombinant SARS coronavirus spike protein subunit vaccine candidates. *Viral Immunol*. 2013; 26(2): 126–132.
96. Jiang S, Bottazzi M, Du L, Lustigman S, Tseng C, Curti E et al. Roadmap to developing a recombinant coronavirus S protein receptor-binding domain vaccine for severe acute respiratory syndrome. *Expert Rev Vaccines*. 2012; 11(12): 1405–1413.

Section II

Common Viral Infections of Human Respiratory System

immune system) and proceed to discuss the clinical manifestations of RT infections in both children and adults. In addition, influenza virus, respiratory syncytial virus (RSV), and human rhinovirus (HRV) infections are discussed in more detail. Finally, we report on the latest developments focusing on the newly emerging global threats, Middle East respiratory syndrome coronavirus (MERS-CoV), and avian influenza viruses (H5N1 and H7N9).

13.2 HUMAN RESPIRATORY TRACT

The human RT is in direct contact with the external environment. Therefore, it is the port of entry for many pathogens. Fortunately, many hurdles need to be taken by the pathogen before it can cause disease. The RT is structured to prevent pathogens from entering and with the additional help of the systemic and local immune responses, disease can be usually prevented after exposure. In this chapter, we will divide the RT into the upper respiratory tract (URT) and the lower respiratory tract (LRT). This division is arbitrarily chosen as being above and under the laryngo-tracheal transition, respectively.

13.2.1 Anatomy of the Upper and Lower Respiratory Tract

The URT consists of the nasal vestibule, nasal septum, nasal concha (together; the nasal cavity), nasopharynx, oropharynx, paranasal sinuses, and larynx (Figure 13.1). The ears, especially the middle ear, are part of the aerated system (including the nares, the eustachian tube, and mastoid air cells) and are lined with the respiratory mucosa. Indeed, respiratory viruses can enter the middle

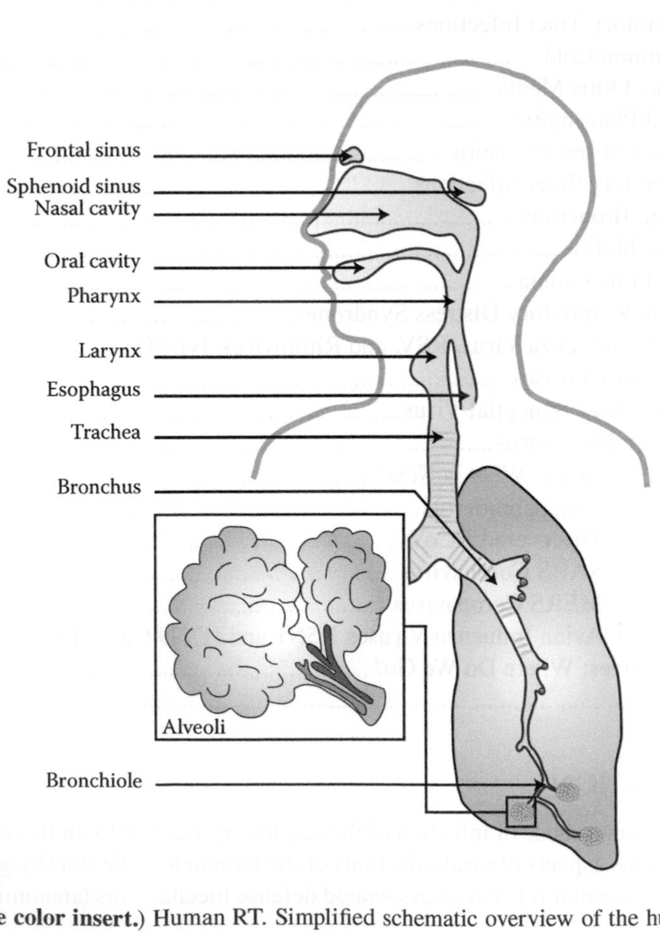

FIGURE 13.1 **(See color insert.)** Human RT. Simplified schematic overview of the human RT. (Courtesy of J.Y. Siegers.)

ear, and give rise to disease.[1] Therefore, we have incorporated the middle ear in our overview of URT infections. The cell types lining the different structures of the URT are nonciliated squamous epithelial cells, ciliated columnar epithelial cells, goblet cells, and olfactory epithelial cells.[1,2]

The LRT consists of the trachea, bronchi, bronchioles, and alveoli (Figure 13.1).[1] In comparison to the URT, different cell types are present, depending on the anatomical site. Ciliated columnar epithelial cells and goblet cells are lined at the trachea and bronchi. The bronchioles are covered with ciliated columnar epithelial cells, goblet cells, and in the smallest division, nonciliated cuboid cells are present. The RT tree finally branches into small alveoli, containing two types of pneumocytes: type 1 pneumocytes, forming the structure over which gas exchange can occur, and type 2 pneumocytes, which have several important functions.[2,3] First, they are the progenitor cells for type 1 pneumocytes, while in addition, they produce and secrete surfactant, a substance reducing alveolar surface tension that keeps the alveoli open during expiration.[1,2,4] The close contact between alveoli and capillaries required for O_2 and CO_2 exchange renders the LRT susceptible to invasive disease. Clearly, a robust barrier function is impossible for protection. Therefore, when a pathogen escapes the defense mechanism of the URT, the defense at the level of the alveoli consists of the immune system, including defensive proteins such as the surfactant (see the next section). However, this may also be detrimental to the host. In case of infection, an overly robust immune response of the host may also cause severe lung inflammation and jeopardize gas exchange.[5]

13.2.2 Defense Mechanisms of the Upper and Lower Respiratory Tract

At the entrance of the RT (via the oral route), a potential pathogen first faces saliva. Saliva is a mucous substance predominantly consisting of water, but it also contains enzymes, and antibacterial compounds such as secretory immunoglobulins (sIgA) and lysozyme. Together with the gingival crevicular fluid, secreted between the transition site of the teeth and the gingiva, it contributes to the defense mechanisms of the host via both mucosal (sIgA) and systemic (e.g., plasma IgG) immunity.

The RT is covered with an epithelial lining, which by itself is an important defense mechanism. In addition, the epithelial cells of the RT are covered with mucus secreted continuously by intraepithelial goblet cells and by mucous cells of submucosal glands, to the surface of the epithelium.[6,7] This sticky mucus can trap pathogens and eventually clear them from the airways with the help of continuously beating cilia (mucus-coated hairs).[1] The airway mucus is a viscoelastic gel with a complex composition in which almost 200 different proteins have been identified, mostly mucins, and also antimicrobial substances (lysozyme and defensins), sIgA, cytokines, and antioxidant proteins.[8]

Infection of epithelial cells provokes immediate host defense responses that include the production of proinflammatory cytokines, which recruit and activate other mucosal innate immune cells and initiate mechanisms of adaptive immunity (see below). The airway epithelial cells regulate both innate and adaptive immunity through the production of functional molecules and physical interactions with cells of the immune system.

The innate immune response is the first immune reaction of the body toward an invading antigen, mostly directed toward a broad range of pathogens.[9] The adaptive immune response consists of B-cell (Ig-mediated, or humoral) and T-cell-mediated (T-lymphocyte-mediated, cellular) immune responses and is capable of forming a pathogen-specific memory.[9,10] The antibody response plays an important role in protection from repetitive infections by the same virus, whereas the T-cell response is pivotal for the control of an already-established infection. The respective players of the innate immune response and the antigen-specific adaptive immune response have a strong interplay and function in harmony (for a review, see References 9,11).

Many lymphoid organs are localized throughout the body. In the URT, an important site is Waldeyer's ring, consisting of adenoids, paired palatine tonsils, tubal tonsils, and one or more lingual tonsils.[12,13] Furthermore, throughout the RT, mucosa-associated lymphoid tissues (MALTs) contribute to B- and T-cell-mediated responses.[9] Over the last few years, it has become increasingly clear that immune tissues continue to develop *de novo* locally during life. The so-called tertiary lymphoid organs, or inducible bronchus-associated lymphoid tissue (iBALT), are found in the lungs.[14–16] A study in mice showed that during and after influenza virus infection, dendritic cells (DCs) (part of the innate immune system) play an important role in the formation of iBALTs.[17] iBALTs are involved in Ig-class switching in germinal centers and support B- and T-cell proliferation during a viral infection.[17]

13.3 COMMON KNOWLEDGE OF RESPIRATORY VIRUSES

Transmission of respiratory viruses can occur through aerosols, or respiratory droplets, or via indirect contact with infected secretions, or contaminated environmental surfaces.[18] Annually, many people get infected with a respiratory virus. It is perfectly normal for a child under the age of five to suffer up to six acute respiratory tract infection (ARTI) episodes per year.[19–21] In addition, for children <1 year of age, ARTIs are the most frequent reason for emergency department visits.[22–25] Moreover, in the population at large, ARTIs are among the leading infectious diseases worldwide.[21] A recent study measuring the global burden of disease showed that RTIs come second to ischemic heart disease, in reducing worldwide disability-adjusted life years (DALYs).[26] Owing to the frequent occurrence of respiratory pathogens, ARTIs are associated with a high disease and economic burden.[26–30]

13.4 VIRUSES ASSOCIATED WITH ARTIs

Viruses commonly associated with ARTIs include influenza virus types A and B, RSV types A and B, human metapneumovirus (HMPV) types A and B, parainfluenza virus (PIV) types 1–4, HRV, adenovirus (AdV), and human coronaviruses (HCoVs) OC43 and 229E (Figures 13.2 and 13.3).[31–33] During the past two decades, a number of not previously discovered respiratory viruses were identified for the first time (e.g., HMPV).[19,34] In most cases, there was a direct link between the discovered virus and respiratory disease (e.g., severe acute respiratory syndrome coronavirus [SARS-CoV] and MERS-CoV), while for other viruses, this association is still less well established (e.g., human bocavirus [HBoV], Karolinska Institute [KI], and Washington University [WU] polyomaviruses [PyVs]).

In the following section, we will describe the major viral ARTIs resulting in upper respiratory tract infection (URTI) and lower respiratory tract infection (LRTI), their clinical manifestations, and the currently available intervention strategies.

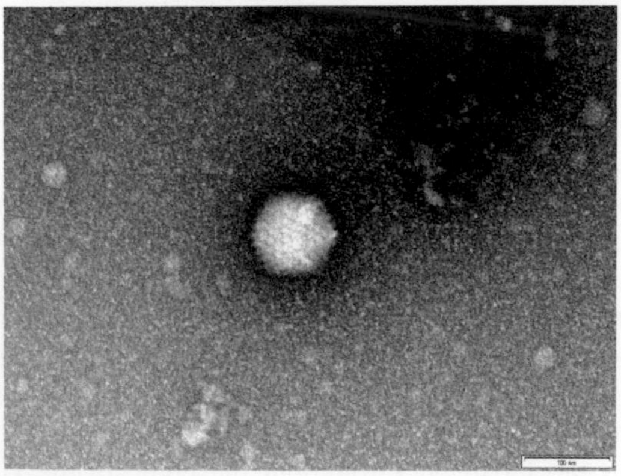

FIGURE 13.2 Adenovirus. Electron micrograph of a human AdV. Virions are nonenveloped and have a capsid with pseudoicosahedral symmetry. The capsid diameter is about 70–90 nm and the capsid shell consists of 720 hexon subunits arranged as 240 trimers and 12 vertex penton capsomers, each with a fiber protruding from the surface. (Courtesy of G.I. Aron and J.L. Murk; viralzone.expasy.org.)

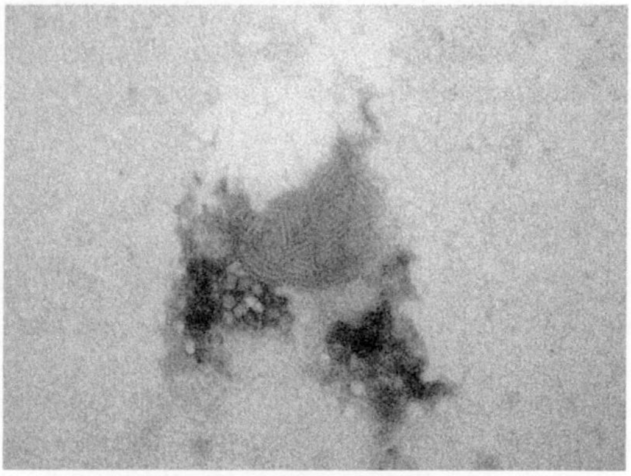

FIGURE 13.3 Human PIV type 3. Electron micrograph of a particle of an isolate of human PIV type 3. PIV-3 is an enveloped virus and spherical, with a diameter of about 150 nm (varying between 90 and 300 nm). With nucleoprotein, helix structures are clearly visible here as the stripped pattern (size 15–19 nm). (Courtesy of G.I. Aron and J.L. Murk.)

13.5 UPPER RESPIRATORY TRACT INFECTIONS

13.5.1 Common Cold

Common cold is characterized by a combination of the following signs and symptoms: rhinorrhea, nasal congestion, sneezing, sore throat, and coughing. This may sometimes be accompanied with (mild) fever, headache, muscle ache, and malaise.[35–37] Less-specific complaints are fatigue and loss of appetite. There is a wide variety of causative agents, including over 200 subtypes of viruses, which among others include rhinoviruses (including >100 serotypes), RSV, AdV, (para-) influenza virus, coronavirus, HMPV, and HBoV.[31,37] Because of the seasonal pattern of some viruses (e.g., RSV, HMPV, and (para-) influenza viruses), the incidence of common cold varies during the year, with a peak outbreak during autumn and winters in temperate climate zones.[35,37,38] The disease is normally self-limiting and diagnosed on the basis of the clinical presentation and is of limited clinical consequence in otherwise healthy individuals.[35,37] However, common cold can be a serious problem in very young infants. This is because they are dependent on nasal breathing and thus easily develop breathing and feeding difficulties upon congestion of their nose.[38]

13.5.2 Acute Otitis Media

Acute otitis media (AOM) can develop as part, or complication, of ARTI. It is a common ear infection in children, and arises because of infection of the middle ear mucosa. Most cases of AOM are caused by viral infections.[31,35,39] The symptoms include fever, earache, irritability, vomiting, and/or acute otorrhea. Diagnosis is based on the clinical presentation and visualization of the tympanic membrane, which is often bulging with erythema.[35,39,40] Earaches can cause severe pain and require antipyretics/analgesia. Currently, for the majority of viral infections, no specific treatment options are available. Nasal rinsing with saltwater can relieve symptoms. In case of possible bacterial involvement (depending on severity of illness, age, and recurrent infection), treatment with antibiotics should be started.[35,40,41]

13.5.3 Viral Pharyngitis

Patients with pharyngitis present with the following complaints: sore throat, difficulty in swallowing, mild fever, and sometimes, enlarged lymph nodes in the neck (lymphadenopathy). Headache and malaise may accompany these complaints.[35,42,43] In most cases, pharyngitis is associated with other URTI complaints.[42] Parainfluenza viruses, influenza viruses, AdV, enteroviruses, and rhinoviruses are the common causes of the disease.[35,38,44,45] When a viral pathogen is involved, the disease is usually self-limiting. Additional testing is suggested in patients with an atypical presentation or suspected bacterial coinfection.[35,42]

13.5.4 Viral Laryngotracheitis

Laryngotracheitis is a condition in which the mucosa is inflamed and swollen up in the area of the larynx and the vocal cords, sometimes extending to the trachea and even to the bronchi. An almost pathognomonic symptom of viral laryngotracheitis (VLT) in young children is the "seal-like" barking cough.[35,46] In older children and adults, this distinct cough is less pronounced or may not occur at all.[46] Other important symptoms are inspiratory stridor, and hoarseness, accompanied by fever and malaise. Parainfluenza type 3 and influenza viruses are the most frequent causes of VLT,[35,38,46] although other viruses, such as HMPV and RSV, may also be involved.[47,48] Inflammation of the larynx and trachea is usually mild and self-limiting, but considering the location, life-threatening airway obstructions can occur.[35,46] Patient management should focus on safeguarding the airway passage. The treatment consists of the reduction of local edema by means of using corticosteroids (including dexamethasone) and sometimes nebulized epinephrine.[49–53] On the basis of population-based studies, fewer than 5% of children with VLT are admitted to the hospital, although in severe cases, intensive care treatment may be required.[35,46,54]

It is important to set VLT aside from bacterial epiglottitis. Patients with bacterial epiglottitis present with acute onset of symptoms, including upper airway obstruction (caused by thick, purulent exudate), fever, and an overall severely ill child. Furthermore, lower airway symptoms, such as rales and wheezing, can also be present in these patients.[38,46] This severe and usually life-threatening affliction is primarily caused by *Haemophilus influenza* type B (HiB), and fortunately HiB immunization has led to a major decrease in the prevalence of this disease.[44,46]

13.6 LOWER RESPIRATORY TRACT INFECTIONS

13.6.1 Acute Bronchitis

Acute bronchitis is characterized by coughing for more than 5 days and excessive sputum production.[55] On the basis of clinical presentation, it is difficult to distinguish acute bronchitis from bronchiolitis in young infants. Fever is unusual in patients with acute bronchitis, which may be caused by a variety of respiratory viruses including influenza virus, parainfluenza virus, coronavirus, rhinovirus, RSV, and human metapneumovirus. The disease is often self-limiting and its duration should not exceed 3 months. If this is the case, chronic bronchitis should be considered and treatment options such as the administration of antihistamines or antibiotics should be regarded.[55]

13.6.2 Bronchiolitis

In temperate climate zones, young children, especially those under 2 years of age, are at risk of developing bronchiolitis during annual epidemics.[56] Bronchiolitis occurs when viruses infect the terminal bronchiolar epithelial cells, causing direct damage and inflammation in the small bronchi and bronchioles. Edema, excessive mucus production, and sloughed epithelial cells lead to obstruction of small airways and may cause atelectasis. Usually, signs and symptoms start 3–6 days after initial coryzal (common-cold-like) symptoms. Upon examination, children can have a sharp and dry cough, tachypnea, tachycardia, nasal flaring, subcostal and intercostal retractions, cyanosis, or pallor look. Upon auscultation, fine end-inspiratory crackles (rales and crepitation) and wheezing can be heard. Chest x-rays might show hyperinflation with flattening of the diaphragm, although this is rarely helpful in diagnosing bronchiolitis.[57] Hyperinflation is the result of air trapping, which is an abnormal retention of air in the lungs where it is difficult to exhale completely. Although less common than in children, bronchiolitis does occur in adult patients as well.[58] Most of the RT viruses have been found to cause bronchiolitis, including RSV, HMPV, (para-) influenza viruses, coronaviruses, rhinovirus, AdV, and HBoV.[57]

Treatment of bronchiolitis patients is supportive. In addition, current evidence suggests that nebulized 3% saline may significantly reduce the length of hospital stay and improve the clinical severity score in infants with acute viral bronchiolitis.[59] In severe cases, mechanical ventilation may be necessary, and in rare cases, extracorpal membranous oxygenation (ECMO) must be initiated.[60] These severe cases arise especially in prematurely born infants and very young healthy neonates.[35]

Wheezing as a result of viral infection mimics the signs and symptoms of asthma, especially in young infants. With the increase in body size, this distinction is more easily made, although viral infections are an important trigger for asthma exacerbations. Studies show that early viral infection (especially with RSV or HMPV) may predispose for the development of asthma later in life.[61–63]

13.6.3 Viral Pneumonia

In infancy, there is a relatively high incidence of pneumonia, which decreases toward adulthood, but increases again in the elderly with progressing age.[32,64] Both viruses and bacteria are known causes of pneumonia.[65] Signs and symptoms of pneumonia include fever, coughing, sputum production, pleuritic chest pain, dyspnea, and malaise, and coarse crackles can be heard upon auscultation.[32,66] A chest x-ray may confirm the diagnosis by revealing consolidations. However, viral or bacterial infection cannot be differentiated based on the radiologic findings. In addition, early in the course of pneumonia, a chest x-ray may reveal no abnormalities at all.[67] Hospitalization may be necessary and viral and bacterial testing should be considered to identify the causative agent, and to help in choosing the appropriate treatment.[35,67,68] All previously mentioned viral pathogens may be associated with viral pneumonia, although especially influenza viruses, RSV, HMPV, SARS-CoV, MERS-CoV, and hantavirus may be implicated.[69]

13.6.4 Acute Respiratory Distress Syndrome

ARDS (acute respiratory distress syndrome) is a consequence of alveolar injury and can be caused by a variety of insults, including sepsis, aspiration, trauma, and pneumonia. Virus infections causing pneumonia may lead to ARDS. Therefore, a variety of viruses can result in ARDS; however, it has predominantly been linked to infection with avian or pandemic influenza viruses, SARS-CoV, and MERS-CoV.[70,71]

It is a life-threatening disease, characterized by dyspnea, cyanosis (due to hypoxemia), tachypnea, use of accessory muscles for respiration, excessive sweating, and tachycardia. ARDS has been defined based on the following criteria (Berlin definitions): rapid disease onset (<1 week) and imaging (chest x-ray or computerized tomography [CT] scan), revealing bilateral opacities consistent with pulmonary edema. For differential diagnosis, cardiac disorders or fluid overload should be excluded. Among the most important criteria is the calculated ratio of arterial oxygen tension to the fraction of inspired oxygen (PaO_2/FiO_2). This ratio indicates severe impairment of oxygenation of the blood.[43]

13.7 MAJOR PLAYERS: INFLUENZA VIRUS, RSV, AND RHINOVIRUS TYPE C

13.7.1 Influenza Viruses

There are three types of influenza viruses causing disease in humans: influenza A, B, and C viruses.[56] Influenza viruses are negatively charged (sense) single-stranded RNA (ribonucleic acid) viruses and belong to the family Orthomyxoviridae (Figures 13.4 and 13.5).[72] The surface (envelop) of influenza viruses contains two important glycoproteins (antigens), hemagglutinin (HA) and neuraminidase

self-limiting or predominantly in high-risk patients, causes severe and life-threatening disease. RSV is notorious in pediatric patients, especially in prematurely born children and young infants, who may develop apnea as a severe complication of RSV infection.[23,78,79] Moreover, recent studies suggest an association between RSV infection and wheezing later in life, although more follow-up studies are needed to confirm this relationship.[80] RSV also may severely affect individuals at the other extreme of the age spectrum: the elderly.[81,82] For several years, passive immunization is possible for infants at risk for developing severe infection, with a humanized monoclonal antibody called palivizumab (Synagis®) that is used predominantly in prematurely born infants. A recent meta-analysis of three randomized trials comparing palivizumab with placebo in 2831 high-risk infants (e.g., preterm, bronchopulmonary dysplasia [BPD], and congenital heart disease) found that palivizumab reduced RSV hospitalizations (from 101 to 50 per 1000, relative risk [RR] 0.49 95% CI 0.37–0.64) and intensive care unit (ICU) admissions from 34 to 17 per 1000 (RR 0.5 95% CI 0.3–0.81 in two studies with 2789 patients) without increasing the risk of adverse events.[80,83,84] Still, it is important to realize that complete protection is not possible and monthly administration of the monoclonal antibody is necessary.[85] Unfortunately, many attempts to develop an RSV vaccine have failed. The most striking example is a clinical trial in the early 1960s. In this study, whole, inactivated virus-vaccinated children developed more severe and even fatal disease, compared to placebo.[86] This was a major setback to the RSV vaccine field. However, recently, new promising vaccine candidates are being developed. It may be expected that these will enter the clinical practice within the next few decades.

13.7.3 Human Rhinovirus

HRV is a small single-stranded RNA virus and is the most important cause of common cold, but is also found in the deeper areas of the RT, causing moderate to severe disease.[36,87–89] It is a member of the picornavirus family and belongs to the enterovirus genus.[72] There are three HRV species all with numerous subtypes: 77 HRV-A, 26 HRV-B, and 63 HRV-C subtypes have been identified.[89] A problem with the diagnosis of HRV-associated disease is the high detection rate by PCR (polymerase chain reaction) in healthy individuals, indicating that the presence of HRV RNA is not always associated with clinical symptoms. Currently, the detection of HRV RNA by PCR is the gold standard for HRV diagnosis.[90,91] In patients with an underlying disease such as chronic obstructive pulmonary disease (COPD) and asthma, HRV infections have been shown to be a major cause of exacerbations.[89] However, other respiratory virus infections as well as bacterial and viral coinfections may play a role in such exacerbations.[92,93] Recent data show that infection with HRV-C, which is phylogenetically distinct from the two other HRV species, is associated with more severe respiratory disease than infection with HRV-A or HRC-B viruses.[89] Indeed, HRV-C mono-infection was found to be associated with severe disease in otherwise healthy children <3 years of age.[89]

13.8 NEW KIDS ON THE BLOCK: WHAT IS NEW?

13.8.1 Human Metapneumovirus

In 2001, a not previously recognized paramyxovirus (negative single-stranded RNA virus) was isolated from children with bronchiolitis symptoms reminiscent of RSV infection, who tested negative for RSV infection. The virus was characterized as a metapneumovirus and was named HMPV (Table 13.1 and Figure 13.6).[93,94] The virus must have spilled over from an avian reservoir about 200 years ago to become a major human pathogen that affects humans mainly in the winter months.[94] The disease caused by HMPV is a relatively mild and self-limiting common cold in most cases, although a variety of complications may arise. As with RSV infection, the most striking is bronchiolitis. HMPV- and RSV-associated bronchiolitis cases are very similar although infants infected with HMPV tend to be slightly older than those infected with RSV.[95–97] Severe disease is predominantly seen in the young infants, immunocompromised, and elderly patients.[96] Although HMPV has been found to

TABLE 13.1
Discovered Respiratory Viruses over the Last 20 Years

Discovered Virus	Virus Abbreviation	Virus Family	First Description in Humans	Pandemic Potential
Avian influenza viruses (A subtypes)	H5N1	Orthomyxoviridae	1997[129]	Yes
	H7N7		2003[130,131]	Yes
	H7N9		2013[132]	Yes
Hendra virus	HeV	Paramyxoviridae	1994[133,134]	Outbreaks HeV since 1994 and ongoing
Nipah virus	NiV		1999[135]	Outbreaks NiV since 1999 and ongoing
Human metapneumovirus	HMPV[a]	Paramyxoviridae	2001[136]	Ubiquitous
Severe acute respiratory syndrome coronavirus	SARS-CoV[a]	Coronaviridae	2003[137,138]	Starting pandemic stopped in 2003
Human coronavirus Netherlands 63	HCoV-NL63[a]	Coronaviridae	2004[139,140]	Ubiquitous
Human coronavirus Hong Kong 1	HCoV-HKU1	Coronaviridae	2005[141]	Ubiquitous
Human bocavirus	HBoV	Parvoviridae	2005[142]	Ubiquitous
Human rhinovirus type C	HRV	Picornaviridae	2006[143]	Ubiquitous
Karolinska Institute, Washington University polyomavirus	KI/WU-PyV	Polyomaviridae	2007[144,145]	Unknown
Kampar (Melaka) virus	KamV(MelV)	Orthoreovirus	2007[146]	Unknown
Pandemic influenza A virus	H1N1p	Orthomyxoviridae	2009[147]	Pandemic 2009
Middle East respiratory syndrome coronavirus	MERS-HCoV[a]	Coronaviridae	2012[148]	Yes

[a] Viruses discovered at the Viroscience Lab, Erasmus MC Rotterdam, the Netherlands.

cause severe disease in the latter risk groups, it is not frequently tested for. Therefore, the true burden of the disease as a result of HMPV infection may currently be largely underestimated.[96]

No antiviral treatment or vaccinations are available for HMPV infection to date. However, promising developments have recently taken place. For instance, a cross-neutralizing antibody showed protection against several paramyxoviruses (RSV, HMPV, pneumonia virus of mice, and bovine RSV) in animals, which may form the basis for prophylaxis and/or therapy for human RSV and HMPV infections.[98] This monoclonal antibody also identified a new candidate antigenic site that could be included in a vaccine (pre-F-fusion protein). In addition, ongoing studies testing HMPV candidate vaccines recently revealed a promising way toward a live-attenuated vaccine.[99]

13.8.2 Recently Discovered HCoVs

13.8.2.1 SARS Coronavirus

Recent studies revealed a plethora of new coronaviruses in bats and other animals.[100,101] The scientific interest in these animals and their viruses was triggered by a large epidemic in humans caused by the introduction of a new coronavirus, SARS-CoV, from the animal world in the human population in 2002 (Table 13.1). Although the virus must have originated from bats, it was probably transmitted to humans initially by carnivores sold at live animal markets in China, before it further adapted to effective transmission in humans.[102] After it had started in China, the epidemic spread to other countries and continents in 2003, mainly through infected air travelers, and it rapidly became a pandemic threat.[103] An unprecedented well-coordinated and collaborative response by scientists from all over the world led to the rapid identification of SARS-CoV as the causative agent, and by a quick and well-coordinated public health response, an emerging pandemic was stopped in its wake for the first time in human history.[104–107] A total number of 8096 cases had been reported with a mortality rate of 9.6%, with a strong skewing toward higher age ranges.[103] Treatment options were limited, with supportive care as the main focus. However, interferon-α therapy proved to be beneficial in macaque studies, and was successfully practiced at the end stage of the epidemic in Canada.[108,109]

13.8.2.2 MERS Coronavirus

More recently, another coronavirus spilled over from the animal world, again causing severe and often fatal RT infections in humans. It was named after the region where the first case was described in 2012: the Middle East Respiratory Syndrome-coronavirus (MERS-CoV)[71] (Table 13.1). Like SARS-CoV, MERS-CoV most likely has its origin in bats. A potential intermediate host, such as the carnivores for SARS, has not yet been discovered for MERS-CoV although the dromedary camel has been suggested as a possible candidate.[110] Currently, more than 100 laboratory-confirmed cases have been reported, including more than 50 fatal cases.[111] Most cases so far have been reported in Saudi Arabia, although other Middle East countries and several imported cases in Europe have been described as well.[112] So far, limited human-to-human transmission of MERS-CoV has been reported upon close contact.[113] The overall median age of reported cases is about 50 years and immune-compromised individuals appear to have an increased risk.[111] Treatment options are currently based on supportive care. As was the case for SARS, recent data from macaque experiments suggest that interferon-α therapy may have beneficial effects.[114]

13.8.2.3 Avian Influenza Viruses H5N1 and H7N9 Cause Disease in Humans

In 1997, a highly pathogenic avian influenza A (H5N1) virus (HPAI-H5N1) was transmitted from birds to humans in Hong Kong, killing six of the 18 hospitalized patients identified[115] (Table 13.1). Apparently, the virus directly spilled over from birds and was not transmitted from human to human. To control the outbreak, live poultry markets were cleared and about a million birds were culled to stamp out the infection. This unexpected event clearly showed that avian influenza viruses continue to pose a global health threat. HPAI-H5N1 has become largely endemic in bird populations in Asia since this event, causing disease outbreaks with high mortality in poultry from time to time.[116,117] Since 2003, human infections with this virus continued to occur and until now, over 600 human cases have been reported from 15 countries with a case fatality rate over 50%.[118] This high death toll is a frightening perspective for what may happen if sustained human-to-human infection with this virus were to occur. Recent experimental transmission studies in ferrets suggest that this may happen in the future considering that only a limited number of mutations would allow the virus to become transmissible.[18,119]

In May 2013, another introduction of an avian influenza virus—H7N9—in the human population was reported.[120] Unlike HPAI-H5N1, this virus is not highly pathogenic but low pathogenic for poultry (LPAI-H7N9) and is therefore more difficult to track.[121] To date, more than 130 severe human cases of LPAI-H7N9 infection have been confirmed of which more than 40 have died (www.who.int). So far, only one isolated case of human-to-human transmission with this virus has been identified.[122] The age distribution of the LPAI-H7N9-affected patients is quite different from that of HPAI-H5N1-infected patients. Strikingly, most patients appear to be older than 50 years.[123] The reason for this is so far not known. Again, live poultry markets were cleared and birds were culled, to control the epidemics in China.[124] Indeed, the number of avian-to-human transmissions has gone down this summer, but climatological factors may have also played a role here.

13.9 FUTURE PERSPECTIVES: WHERE DO WE GO?

Respiratory viruses are there to stay and will continue to cause ARTIs. However, new vaccines and antiviral medication may in the near future reshape their clinical impact and management. In addition to the currently known respiratory viruses, newly emerging and reemerging viruses will continue to pose a threat to the global human population.[19,22,125] Many recently discovered human respiratory viruses arose from the animal world, and once they have crossed the species barrier to humans, may adapt to the new species, eventually resulting in efficient human-to-human infection.[101,126,127] In our modern globalizing world, a complex mix of factors may predispose for the emergence of these viruses, including social, technological, and ecological changes. Changes, which may contribute to an increase in viral spread, are changes in human behavior, the ever-increasing worldwide mobility of humans, demographic changes, human exploitation of the environment, and the globalized trade of goods. Moreover, an increase in contact between wild or feral animals and humans may contribute to viral spread, as is the ability of the virus to rapidly adapt to a changing environment.[128]

Since it is hard to influence these largely interconnected factors, early detection of newly emerging infectious disease threats by combining syndrome surveillance and laboratory- based monitoring of wild and domestic animal populations as well as human communities is crucial for the implementation of an early response when eradication of newly emerging infections is still an option. Genomics tools such as new-generation sequencing, transcriptomics, and microarray analyses of single-nucleotide polymorphisms have created novel molecular ways to analyze genomes of emerging pathogens and the associated host responses in an unprecedented manner. The rapid development of medical treatment options can also make optimal use of integrated host and virus genomics data, leading to novel therapeutic interventions based on in-depth molecular knowledge and understanding of the pathogenic pathways followed by the newly emerged infection. Finally, the development of novel generations of preventive and therapeutic vaccines against newly emerging pathogen threats also benefits from the rapidly emerging novel antigen expression and presentation technologies as well as from our molecular understanding of the respective arms of the immune system that combat invading pathogens.

REFERENCES

1. Marieb EN, Hoehn K. Chapter 22. The Respiratory System. In: Becker W, Jones A, Holmes DA, Hardin J, eds. *Human Anatomy and Physiology*, 7th ed. San Francisco, Pearson Education Inc., 2007: 789–90, 830–81.
2. Van Riel DA. Thesis: A critical role of cell tropism for the pathogenesis of influenza. PhD Dissertation. Rotterdam, 2010: 11–4.
3. Herzog EL, Brody AR, Colby TV, Mason R, Williams MC. Knowns and unknowns of the alveolus. *Proceedings of the American Thoracic Society* 2008; **5**: 778–82.
4. Castranova V, Rabovsky J, Tucker JH, Miles PR. The alveolar type II epithelial cell: A multifunctional pneumocyte. *Toxicology and Applied Pharmacology* 1988; **93**: 472–83.
5. Guilliams M, Lambrecht BN, Hammad H. Division of labor between lung dendritic cells and macrophages in the defense against pulmonary infections. *Mucosal Immunology* 2013; **6**: 464–73.
6. Wine JJ, Joo NS. Submucosal glands and airway defense. *Proceedings of the American Thoracic Society* 2004; **1**: 47–53.
7. Society for Mucosal Immunology, Smith PD, MacDonald TT, Blumberg RS. Chapter 20. The nasopharyngeal and oral immune system. In: *Principles of Mucosal Immunology*, First ed. New York, Garland Science, 2012: 1–529.
8. Vareille M, Kieninger E, Edwards MR, Regamey N. The airway epithelium: Soldier in the fight against respiratory viruses. *Clinical Microbiology Reviews* 2011; **24**: 210–29.
9. Murphy K. *Janeway's Immunobiology*, 8th ed., New York, Garland Science, 2011.
10. Geurts van Kessel C. Thesis: Division of labor between dendritic cell subsets in the lung during influenza virus infection. PhD Dissertation. Rotterdam, 2009; 1–141.
11. Yoo J-K, Kim TS, Hufford MM, Braciale TJ. Viral infection of the lung: Host response and sequelae. *The Journal of Allergy and Clinical Immunology* 2013. doi:10.1016/j.jaci.2013.06.006.
12. Brandtzaeg P, Kiyono H, Pabst R, Russell MW. Terminology: Nomenclature of mucosa-associated lymphoid tissue. *Mucosal Immunology* 2008; **1**: 31–7.
13. Muramatsu T, Tanaka Y, Higure R, Iizuka M, Hata H, Shiono M. Thymic and pulmonary mucosa-associated lymphoid tissue lymphomas. *The Annals of Thoracic Surgery* 2013; **95**: e69–70.

14. Sminia T, Van Der Brugge-Gamelkoorn GJ, Jeurissen SH. Bronchus-associated lymphoid tissue (BALT) structure and function. *Advances in Immunology* 1989; **107**: 119–50.
15. Moyron-Quiroz JE, Rangel-Moreno J, Kusser K et al. Role of inducible bronchus associated lymphoid tissue (iBALT) in respiratory immunity. *Nature Medicine* 2004; **10**: 927–34.
16. Foo SY, Phipps S. Regulation of inducible BALT formation and contribution to immunity and pathology. *Mucosal Immunology* 2010; **3**: 537–44.
17. Geurts van Kessel CH, Willart MAM, Bergen IM et al. Dendritic cells are crucial for maintenance of tertiary lymphoid structures in the lung of influenza virus-infected mice. *The Journal of Experimental Medicine* 2009; **206**: 2339–49.
18. Herfst S, Schrauwen EJA, Linster M et al. Airborne transmission of influenza A/H5N1 virus between ferrets. *Science* 2012; **336**: 1534–41.
19. Ahout I, Ferwerda G, de Groot R. Elucidation and clinical role of emerging viral respiratory tract infections in children. *Advances in Experimental Medicine and Biology* 2013; **764**: 191–204.
20. Feigin RD, Cherry J, Demmler-Harrison K. Chapter 194. Respiratory Syncytial Virus. In: *Textbook of Pediatric Infectious Diseases*, 4th ed., Philadelphia, Saunders Elsevier, 2009: 1–3856.
21. WHO. WHO | Acute respiratory infections. 2012. http://www.who.int/vaccine_research/diseases/ari/en/.
22. Brodzinski H, Ruddy RM. Review of new and newly discovered respiratory tract viruses in children. *Pediatric Emergency Care* 2009; **25**: 352–60; quiz 361–3.
23. Iwane MK, Edwards KM, Szilagyi PG et al. Population-based surveillance for hospitalizations associated with respiratory syncytial virus, influenza virus, and parainfluenza viruses among young children. *Pediatrics* 2004; **113**: 1758–64.
24. Regamey N, Kaiser L, Roiha HL et al. Viral etiology of acute respiratory infections with cough in infancy: A community-based birth cohort study. *The Pediatric Infectious Disease Journal* 2008; **27**: 100–5.
25. Glezen WP, Paredes A, Allison JE, Taber LH, Frank AL. REF Feigin 126 RSV: Risk of respiratory syncytial virus infection for infants from low-income families in relationship to age, sex, ethnic group, and maternal antibody level. *The Journal of Pediatrics* 1981; **98**: 708–15.
26. Murray CJL, Lopez AD. Measuring the global burden of disease. *New England Journal of Medicine* 2013; **369**: 448–57.
27. WHO. WHO | Battle against respiratory viruses (BRaVe) initiative. www.who.int. 2012. http://www.who.int/influenza/patient_care/clinical/brave/en/.
28. Gaunt ER, Harvala H, McIntyre C, Templeton KE, Simmonds P. Disease burden of the most commonly detected respiratory viruses in hospitalized patients calculated using the disability adjusted life year (DALY) model. *Journal of Clinical Virology: The Official Publication of the Pan American Society for Clinical Virology* 2011; **52**: 215–21.
29. Robinson RF. Impact of respiratory syncytial virus in the United States. *American Journal of Healthsystem Pharmacy AJHP Official Journal of the American Society of Health System Pharmacists* 2008; **65**: S3–6.
30. Fraaij PLA, Heikkinen T. Seasonal influenza: The burden of disease in children. *Vaccine* 2011; **29**: 7524–8.
31. Ruohola A, Waris M, Allander T, Ziegler T, Heikkinen T, Ruuskanen O. Viral etiology of common cold in children, Finland. *Emerging Infectious Diseases* 2009; **15**: 344–6.
32. Ruuskanen O, Lahti E, Jennings LC, Murdoch DR. Viral pneumonia. *Lancet* 2011; **377**: 1264–75.
33. Allander T, Jartti T, Gupta S et al. Human bocavirus and acute wheezing in children. *Clinical Infectious Diseases: An Official Publication of the Infectious Diseases Society of America* 2007; **44**: 904–10.
34. Jartti T, Jartti L, Ruuskanen O, Söderlund-Venermo M. New respiratory viral infections. *Current Opinion in Pulmonary Medicine* 2012; **18**: 271–8.
35. Royal College of Pediatrics and Child Health and ESPID. *Manual of Childhood Infections, The Blue Book*, 3rd ed. Oxford, Oxford University Press, 2011.
36. Peltola V, Jartti T, Putto-Laurila A et al. Rhinovirus infections in children: A retrospective and prospective hospital-based study. *Journal of Medical Virology* 2009; **81**: 1831–8.
37. Sexton D, McCain M. The common cold in adults: Diagnosis and clinical features. Uptodate.com December 16 2012. http://www.uptodate.com/contents/the-common-cold-in-adults-diagnosis-and-clinical-features.
38. Feigin RD, Cherry J, Demmler-Harrison GJ, Kaplan SL. *Textbook of Pediatric Infectious Diseases*. Elsevier Health Sciences, 2009.
39. Heikkinen T, Chonmaitree T. Importance of respiratory viruses in acute otitis media. *Clinical Microbiology Reviews* 2003; **16**: 230–41.
40. Klein JO, Pelton S. Acute otitis media in children: Epidemiology, microbiology, clinical manifestations, and complications. Uptodate.com April 25 2013. http://www.uptodate.com/contents/acute-otitis-media-in-children-epidemiology-microbiology-clinical-manifestations-and-complications.

41. Klein JO, Pelton S. Acute otitis media in children: Treatment. Uptodate.com June 14 2013. http://www.uptodate.com/contents/acute-otitis-media-in-children-treatment.
42. Chow AW, Doron S. Evaluation of acute pharyngitis in adults. Uptodate.com August 27 2013. http://www.uptodate.com/contents/evaluation-of-acute-pharyngitis-in-adults.
43. Kenneth McIntosh M. Severe acute respiratory syndrome (SARS). Uptodate.com May 9 2012. http://www.uptodate.com/contents/severe-acute-respiratory-syndrome-sars.
44. Lissauer T, Clayden G. *Illustrated Textbook of Paediatrics*, 3rd ed. London, Mosby Elsevier, 2010.
45. Caroline Breese Hall M. Clinical features and diagnosis of seasonal influenza in children. 2012. http://www.uptodate.com/contents/clinical-features-and-diagnosis-of-seasonal-influenza-in-children.
46. Woods CR. Clinical features, evaluation, and diagnosis of croup. Uptodate.com November 6 2012. http://www.uptodate.com/contents/clinical-features-evaluation-and-diagnosis-of-croup.
47. Kroll JL, Weinberg A. Human metapneumovirus. *Seminars in Respiratory and Critical Care Medicine* 2011; **32**: 447–53.
48. Miller EK, Gebretsadik T, Carroll KN et al. Viral etiologies of infant bronchiolitis, croup, and upper respiratory illness during four consecutive years. *The Pediatric Infectious Disease Journal* 2013; **32**: 950–5.
49. Woods CR. Approach to the management of croup. Uptodate.com August 29 2013. http://www.uptodate.com/contents/approach-to-the-management-of-croup.
50. Fogel JM, Berg IJ, Gerber MA, Sherter CB. Racemic epinephrine in the treatment of croup: Nebulization alone versus nebulization with intermittent positive pressure breathing. *The Journal of Pediatrics* 1982; **101**: 1028–31.
51. Westley CR, Cotton EK, Brooks JG. Nebulized racemic epinephrine by IPPB for the treatment of croup: A double-blind study. *American Journal of Diseases of Children (1960)* 1978; **132**: 484–7.
52. Kairys SW, Olmstead EM, O'Connor GT. Steroid treatment of laryngotracheitis: A meta-analysis of the evidence from randomized trials. *Pediatrics* 1989; **83**: 683–93.
53. Johnson DW, Jacobson S, Edney PC, Hadfield P, Mundy ME, Schuh S. A comparison of nebulized budesonide, intramuscular dexamethasone, and placebo for moderately severe croup. *The New England Journal of Medicine* 1998; **339**: 498–503.
54. Bjornson CL, Johnson DW. Croup. *Lancet* 2008; **371**: 329–39.
55. File TM. Acute bronchitis in adults. Uptodate.com March 7 2013. http://www.uptodate.com/contents/acute-bronchitis-in-adults.
56. Fraaij PLA, Osterhaus ADME. The epidemiology of influenza viruses in humans. *Respiratory Medicine* 2010; **5**: 7–14.
57. Piedra P, Stark A. Bronchiolitis in infants and children: Clinical features and diagnosis. Uptodate.com September 11 2013. http://www.uptodate.com/contents/bronchiolitis-in-infants-and-children-clinical-features-and-diagnosis (accessed 13 September 2013).
58. King TE. Bronchiolitis in adults. Uptodate.com May 2 2013. http://www.uptodate.com/contents/bronchiolitis-in-adults.
59. Zhang L, Mendoza-Sassi RA, Wainwright C, Klassen TP. Nebulized hypertonic saline solution for acute bronchiolitis in infants. *The Cochrane Database of Systematic Reviews* 2008; **4**: CD006458.
60. Greenough A. Role of ventilation in RSV disease: CPAP, ventilation, HFO, ECMO. *Paediatric Respiratory Reviews* 2009; **10 Suppl 1**: 26–8.
61. Gern JE, Busse WW. Association of rhinovirus infections with asthma. *Clinical Microbiology Reviews* 1999; **12**: 9–18.
62. Proud D. Role of rhinovirus infections in asthma. *Asian Pacific Journal of Allergy Immunology* 2011; **29**: 201–8.
63. Tregoning JS, Schwarze J. Respiratory viral infections in infants: Causes, clinical symptoms, virology, and immunology. *Clinical Microbiology Reviews* 2010; **23**: 74–98.
64. WHO. World Health Organization, Pneumonia. Factsheet N 331. 2011. http://www.who.int/mediacentre/factsheets/fs331/en/index.html.
65. Honkinen M, Lahti E, Österback R, Ruuskanen O, Waris M. Viruses and bacteria in sputum samples of children with community-acquired pneumonia. *Clinical Microbiology and Infection: The Official Publication of the European Society of Clinical Microbiology and Infectious Diseases* 2012; **18**: 300–7.
66. Lahti E, Peltola V, Waris M et al. Induced sputum in the diagnosis of childhood community-acquired pneumonia. *Thorax* 2009; **64**: 252–7.
67. Bartlett JG. Diagnostic approach to community-acquired pneumonia in adults. Uptodate.com July 24 2013. http://www.uptodate.com/contents/diagnostic-approach-to-community-acquired-pneumonia-in-adults.

68. Mandell LA, Wunderink RG, Anzueto A et al. IDSA: Community-acquired pneumonia (CAP). www.idsociety.org. 2011; 1–46.
69. Marrie TJ, Bartlett JG. Epidemiology, pathogenesis, and microbiology of community-acquired pneumonia in adults. Uptodate.com August 5 2013. http://www.uptodate.com/contents/epidemiology-pathogenesis-and-microbiology-of-community-acquired-pneumonia-in-adults.
70. Kuiken T, Fouchier RAM, Schutten M et al. Newly discovered coronavirus as the primary cause of severe acute respiratory syndrome. *Lancet* 2003; **362**: 263–70.
71. Zaki AM, van Boheemen S, Bestebroer TM, Osterhaus ADME, Fouchier RAM. Isolation of a novel coronavirus from a man with pneumonia in Saudi Arabia. *The New England Journal of Medicine* 2012; **367**: 1814–20.
72. Wright P, Neumann G, Kawaoka Y, Knipe DM. *Field's Virology*, 5th ed., Philadelphia, Lippincott Williams & Wilkins, 2007.
73. Dawood FS, Chaves SS, Pérez A et al. Complications and associated bacterial co-infections among children hospitalized with seasonal or pandemic influenza, United States, 2003–2010. *The Journal of Infectious Diseases* 2013. doi:10.1093/infdis/jit473. [Epub ahead of print]
74. Jamieson AM, Pasman L, Yu S et al. Role of tissue protection in lethal respiratory viral–bacterial coinfection. *Science (New York, NY)* 2013; **340**: 1230–4.
75. Fraaij PL, Osterhaus ADSM. *European Manual of Clinical Microbiology. Chapter: Influenza Virus*, 1st ed. Paris, 2012.
76. Fiore AE, Fry A, Shay D, Gubareva L, Bresee JS, Uyeki TM. Antiviral agents for the treatment and chemoprophylaxis of influenza—Recommendations of the Advisory Committee on Immunization Practices (ACIP). *MMWR Recommendations and Reports: Morbidity and Mortality Weekly Report Recommendations and Reports/Centers for Disease Control* 2011; **60**: 1–24.
77. Parrott RH, Kim HW, Arrobio JO et al. REF FEIGIN 318 RSV: Epidemiology of respiratory syncytial virus infection in Washington, DC. II. Infection and disease with respect to age, immunologic status, race and sex. *American Journal of Epidemiology* 1973; **98**: 289–300.
78. Nair H, Nokes DJ, Gessner BD et al. Global burden of acute lower respiratory infections due to respiratory syncytial virus in young children: A systematic review and meta-analysis. *Lancet* 2010; **375**: 1545–55.
79. Houben ML, Bont L, Wilbrink B et al. Clinical prediction rule for RSV bronchiolitis in healthy newborns: Prognostic birth cohort study. *Pediatrics* 2011; **127**: 35–41.
80. Blanken MO, Rovers MM, Molenaar JM et al. Respiratory syncytial virus and recurrent wheeze in healthy preterm infants. *New England Journal of Medicine* 2013; **368**: 1791–9.
81. Falsey AR, Hennessey PA, Formica MA, Cox C, Walsh EE. Respiratory syncytial virus infection in elderly and high-risk adults. *The New England Journal of Medicine* 2005; **352**: 77.
82. Welliver RC, Checchia PA, Bauman JH, Fernandes AW, Mahadevia PJ, Hall CB. Fatality rates in published reports of RSV hospitalizations among high-risk and otherwise healthy children. *Current Medical Research and Opinion* 2010; **26**: 2175–81.
83. Village EG. Palivizumab, a humanized respiratory syncytial virus monoclonal antibody, reduces hospitalization from respiratory syncytial virus infection in high-risk infants. *Pediatrics* 1998; **102**: 531–7.
84. Wang D, Bayliss S, Meads C. Palivizumab for immunoprophylaxis of respiratory syncytial virus (RSV) bronchiolitis in high-risk infants and young children: A systematic review and additional economic modelling of subgroup analyses. *Health Technology Assessment (Winchester, England)* 2011; **15**: iii–iv, 1–124.
85. CDC. CDC—Prophylaxis and high-risk groups—RSV. www.cdc.gov. 2013. http://www.cdc.gov/rsv/clinical/prophylaxis.html.
86. Kim HW, Canchola JG, Brandt CD et al. Respiratory syncytial virus disease in infants despite prior administration of antigenic inactivated vaccine. *American Journal of Epidemiology* 1969; **89**: 422–34.
87. Greenberg SB. Update on rhinovirus and coronavirus infections. *Seminars in Respiratory and Critical Care Medicine* 2011; **32**: 433–46.
88. O'Callaghan-Gordo C, Bassat Q, Díez-Padrisa N et al. Lower respiratory tract infections associated with rhinovirus during infancy and increased risk of wheezing during childhood. A cohort study. *PloS One* 2013; **8**: e69370.
89. Lauinger IL, Bible JM, Halligan EP et al. Patient characteristics and severity of human rhinovirus infections in children. *Journal of Clinical Virology* 2013; **58**: 216–20.
90. Van den Bergh MR, Biesbroek G, Rossen JWA et al. Associations between pathogens in the upper respiratory tract of young children: Interplay between viruses and bacteria. *PloS One* 2012; **7**: e47711.
91. Spuesens EBM, Fraaij PLA, Visser EG et al. Carriage of mycoplasma pneumoniae in the upper respiratory tract of symptomatic and asymptomatic children: An observational study. *PLoS Medicine* 2013; **10**: e1001444.

92. Esposito S, Daleno C, Scala A et al. Impact of rhinovirus nasopharyngeal viral load and viremia on severity of respiratory infections in children. *European Journal of Clinical Microbiology and Infectious Diseases* 2013; 1–8. [Epub ahead of print, DOI 10.1007/s10096-013-1926-5].
93. Broberg E, Niemelä J, Lahti E, Hyypiä T, Ruuskanen O, Waris M. Human rhinovirus C—Associated severe pneumonia in a neonate. *Journal of Clinical Virology: The Official Publication of the Pan American Society for Clinical Virology* 2011; **51**: 79–82.
94. Litwin CM, Bosley JG. Seasonality and prevalence of respiratory pathogens detected by multiplex PCR at a tertiary care medical center. *Archives of Virology* 2013. doi:10.1007/s00705-013-1794-4. [Epub ahead of print.]
95. Feuillet F, Lina B, Rosa-Calatrava M, Boivin G. Ten years of human metapneumovirus research. *Journal of Clinical Virology: The Official Publication of the Pan American Society for Clinical Virology* 2012; **53**: 97–105.
96. Schildgen V, van den Hoogen B, Fouchier R et al. Human metapneumovirus: Lessons learned over the first decade. *Clinical Microbiology Reviews* 2011; **24**: 734–54.
97. James E, Crowe, Jr. M, Editors S, Martin S, Hirsch M, Sheldon L, Kaplan M, Editor D, Anna R, Thorner M. Human metapneumovirus infections. Uptodate.com. 2013; 1–10.
98. Corti D, Bianchi S, Vanzetta F et al. Cross-neutralization of four paramyxoviruses by a human monoclonal antibody. *Nature* 2013; **501**: 439–43.
99. Talaat KR, Karron RA, Thumar B et al. Experimental infection of adults with recombinant wild-type human metapneumovirus (rHMPV-SHs). *Journal of Infectious Diseases* 2013; **208**: 1669–78.
100. Smits SL, Raj VS, Oduber MD et al. Metagenomic analysis of the ferret fecal viral flora. *PloS One* 2013; **8**: e71595.
101. Corman VM, Rasche A, Diallo TD et al. Highly diversified coronaviruses in neotropical bats. *The Journal of General Virology* 2013; **94**: 1984–94.
102. Wang LF, Eaton BT. Bats, civets and the emergence of SARS. *Current Topics in Microbiology and Immunology* 2007; **315**: 325–44.
103. WHO. WHO | Summary of probable SARS cases with onset of illness from 1 November 2002 to 31 July 2003. http://www.who.int/csr/sars/country/table2004_04_21/en/index.html.
104. Peiris JSM, Guan Y, Yuen KY. Severe acute respiratory syndrome. *Nature Medicine* 2004; **10**: S88–97.
105. Pang X, Zhu Z, Xu F et al. Evaluation of control measures implemented in the severe acute respiratory syndrome outbreak in Beijing, 2003. *JAMA: The Journal of the American Medical Association* 2003; **290**: 3215–21.
106. Svoboda T, Henry B, Shulman L et al. Public health measures to control the spread of the severe acute respiratory syndrome during the outbreak in Toronto. *The New England Journal of Medicine* 2004; **350**: 2352–61.
107. Glassera JW, Huperta N, McCauleya MM, Hatchettc R. Modeling and public health emergency responses: Lessons from SARS. *Epidemics* 2011; **3**: 32–7.
108. Haagmans BL, Kuiken T, Martina BE et al. Pegylated interferon-alpha protects type 1 pneumocytes against SARS coronavirus infection in macaques. *Nature Medicine* 2004; **10**: 290–3.
109. Ward SE, Loutfy MR, Blatt LM et al. Dynamic changes in clinical features and cytokine/chemokine responses in SARS patients treated with interferon alfacon-1 plus corticosteroids. *Antiviral Therapy* 2005; **10**: 263–75.
110. Reusken CB, Haagmans BL, Müller MA et al. Middle East respiratory syndrome coronavirus neutralising serum antibodies in dromedary camels: A comparative serological study. *The Lancet Infectious Diseases* 2013; **13**: 859–66.
111. WHO. WHO | Middle East respiratory syndrome coronavirus (MERS-CoV)—Update. WHO. 2013. http://www.who.int/csr/don/2013_08_30/en/index.html.
112. Al-Tawfiq JA. Middle East respiratory syndrome-coronavirus infection: An overview. *Journal of Infection and Public Health* 2013; **6**: 319–22.
113. Assiri A, McGeer A, Perl TM et al. Hospital outbreak of Middle East respiratory syndrome coronavirus. *The New England Journal of Medicine* 2013; **369**: 407–16.
114. Falzarano D, de Wit E, Rasmussen AL et al. Treatment with interferon-α2b and ribavirin improves outcome in MERS-CoV-infected rhesus macaques. *Nature Medicine* 2013; **19**: 1313–7.
115. Claas EC, Osterhaus AD, van Beek R et al. Human influenza A H5N1 virus related to a highly pathogenic avian influenza virus. *Lancet* 1998; **351**: 472–7.
116. Theary R, San S, Davun H, Allal L, Lu H. New outbreaks of H5N1 highly pathogenic avian influenza in domestic poultry and wild birds in Cambodia in 2011. *Avian Diseases* 2012; **56**: 861–4.
117. Si Y, de Boer WF, Gong P. Different environmental drivers of highly pathogenic avian influenza H5N1 outbreaks in poultry and wild birds. *PloS One* 2013; **8**: e53362.

145. Gaynor AM, Nissen MD, Whiley DM et al. Identification of a novel polyomavirus from patients with acute respiratory tract infections. *PLoS Pathogens* 2007; 3: e64.
146. Chua KB, Voon K, Crameri G et al. Identification and characterization of a new orthoreovirus from patients with acute respiratory infections. *PloS One* 2008; 3: e3803.
147. Morbidity and mortality weekly report. Swine influenza A (H1N1) infection in two children—Southern California, March–April 2009. *MMWR Morbidity and Mortality Weekly Report* 2009; 58: 400–2.
148. Zaki AM, van Boheemen S, Bestebroer TM, Osterhaus ADME, Fouchier RAM. Isolation of a novel coronavirus from a man with pneumonia in Saudi Arabia. *The New England Journal of Medicine* 2012; 367: 1814–20.

14 Viral-Induced Asthma and Chronic Obstructive Pulmonary Disease

Lena Uller and Carl Persson

CONTENTS

14.1 INTRODUCTION

Asthma and chronic obstructive pulmonary disease (COPD) are chronic conditions with bronchial inflammation as key disease component. The prevalence of asthma is about 10% in the Western world. Only 5% of the asthmatic population develop severe disease. Yet, these cases account for more than half of the health care spending in asthma. COPD is currently moving toward the third leading cause of morbidity and death worldwide. Both are heterogeneous and complex diseases defined by clinical presentation characteristics and bronchial responsiveness to challenges and drugs rather than by pathogenic mechanisms. The lung parenchyma is seriously affected only in

COPD with breakdown of tissue, producing abnormal degrees of emphysema and contributing to the breathing difficulty. A further distinction is reversibility of the bronchial obstruction in asthma, whereas in COPD, there is limited reversibility even when these patients are treated with large doses of inhaled bronchodilator drugs. However, by and large, the same pharmacological principles are used in the treatment of both asthma and COPD. Although the drugs are considered nonspecific, this longstanding treatment tradition agrees with a significant overlap of bronchial immunopathology between the two diseases.

The search for "the asthma gene" may have demonstrated an increasing complexity rather than revealing what is causing the disease or how the disease may be subdivided.[1] Yet, with increasing molecular knowledge, endotypes of the diseases will likely emerge[2] and guide the use of specifically targeted immunological drugs.[3,4] Based on clinical–physiological–cellular features of asthma and COPD, several grossly defined phenotypes have been discerned. Within this observational development is the potential classification of exacerbation-prone individuals. Among his many contributions, Romain Pauwels highlighted the importance of exacerbations as a central feature of asthma and COPD and as an important target for improved drug treatment. His analyses of important issues have been instrumental for much of the current research activities in this clinical field.[5] A distinct exacerbation phenotype is supported by observations in either disease indicating that a history of previous exacerbations is the best prediction of risk of future exacerbations.[6] An exacerbation-prone phenotype would also overlap with a severe disease phenotype where exacerbations are relatively frequent.[2,6,7] By as yet little known mechanisms, exacerbations promote disease development.[2,6,8] Corticosteroids, the mainstay therapy, and other drugs used in either disease have insufficient effects on viral-induced exacerbations.[9,10] Hence, discovering ways of preventing exacerbations of asthma and COPD would meet major medical needs.

A development made possible by novel detection methods concerns revelations of the lung microbiome in health and disease.[11] The healthy lung is clearly not sterile as was believed until recently. It is now hypothesized that the local microbiota may be of importance for onset and establishment of the obstructive lung diseases. The focus is on occurrence of bacteria, but latent viral infections in stable disease have also been detected.[9–11] The novel molecular technology has further been instrumental in establishing respiratory tract viral infections as a major cause of exacerbations of severe asthma and COPD.[10,12] Hence, the interaction between viral infection mechanisms and the mechanisms of the two major bronchial diseases is a topical area of research. Activities in this field include epidemiology and clinical features, treatment options, experimental models of exacerbations, and, not least, cellular mechanisms of asthma and COPD with regard to superimposed viral infections.

In this chapter, we will provide an overview of viral-induced exacerbations, including a summary of current discussions of roles of viral infections in early onset of obstructive lung diseases. Select medical history aspects, so far little noticed but indicating major roles of viral infections, are highlighted. Rhinovirus (RV) infections now emerge as the main culprits causing exacerbations of asthma and COPD. The main RV target cell is the bronchial epithelium that also takes center stage as effector cell in current discourses on immunopathogenesis of asthma and COPD. We discuss virus-induced epithelial injury in part because epithelial repair mechanisms alone have multipotential roles in the development of asthma and COPD. Our focus is on such features of epithelial shedding–restitution processes, and their sequelae, that are not well covered in current reviews of the field. We then consider the eosinophilic nature of viral infection-induced exacerbations of asthma and COPD potentially involving synergistic epithelial injury-evoking effects of the infection acting together with eosinophil granule proteins. In this regard, there is a need to highlight the actual mode of degranulation of eosinophils in diseased airway tissues. It is further possible that viral infection impedes transepithelial migration of leucocytes, increasing inflammation and counteracting host defense. The final pages are devoted to effects of RV infection, or challenge with double-stranded RNA (dsRNA), on the ability of bronchial epithelial cells to produce cytokines. We particularly summarize a variety of experimental actions of a select hub cytokine. This approach is of interest because virally stimulated bronchial epithelial cells obtained from asthmatic as well as COPD donors overproduce our selected upstream cytokine, and it is overexpressed in severe stages of these diseases. The multipotential actions of a single viral stimulation-induced cytokine may also exemplify research activities in this topical field and their link to hypotheses of exacerbations and development of severe asthma and COPD.

14.2 VIRAL INFECTION AND ORIGIN OF OBSTRUCTIVE LUNG DISEASES

Henry Hyde Salter, a physician in London 150 years ago, made original and unsurpassed descriptions regarding many facets of asthma and its treatments.[13,14] Salter's book on asthma—its pathology and treatment—is crammed with important and intriguing information. Salter also remains a widely quoted author and his books are a source of inspiration for anyone interested in asthma. In the preparation of this chapter, we discovered that Salter had made important observations and analyses on roles of common cold in asthma, its inception and exacerbation.[15] We were surprised to find that Salter's amazing insight, predating current concepts of virology, had been overlooked in this highly topical field.

Salter reported nearly 100 cases where "taking cold" was considered the "original cause" of asthma.[13] We think his analyses of these cases are highly intriguing: "catarrhal bronchitis …, in a large number of cases, has been infantile bronchitis, or that of early childhood, in many ways slight, and seemed to be nothing more than a common cold on the chest, and in almost all was so completely recovered from that the cases afterward presented the characters of pure spasmodic asthma, and not that of bronchitic asthma"…. "this frequent association of asthma with an antecedent event implying organic, although apparently temporary, injury of the lung, must have a very important influence on our notions of the aetiology of the disease." Indeed, viral infections producing common cold are currently considered a major factor in the onset of asthma.[9,16]

14.2.1 Wheeze- and Asthma-Inducing Viral Infections (RSV and RV) in Infancy

In recent decades, there has been much focus on the role of respiratory syncytial virus (RSV) in the early inception of asthma. RSV belongs to the paramyxoviridae family and can cause severe bronchiolitis in infancy associated with the development of recurrent wheeze. This viral infection-induced event early in life has frequently been followed by diagnosis of asthma. A prospective study has thus linked severe wheeze-evoking RSV infections in infancy with established asthma at 18 years of age in nearly 40% of the examined cohort; this figure is to be compared to below 10% in the control group.[17] Interestingly, RSV infection-induced desquamation of bronchial epithelium, determined as Creola bodies in aspirated sputum in the affected infants, was predictive of the development of recurrent wheeze and asthma 5 years later.[18] The occurrence of Creola bodies may also predict the development of asthma independent of infection.[18] These findings agree with a significant contribution of epithelial injury–repair processes to the pathogenesis of obstructive bronchial disease[19] (discussed in more detail below).

With the development of culture-independent, molecular techniques for diagnosing respiratory pathogens, increasingly strong evidence has emerged for a role of human rhinovirus (RV) in the onset of asthma.[9,16] Human RV belongs to the picornaviridae family within the genus *Enterovirus*. A total exceeding 100 different strains of RV have been identified. Subclassification of RV has been advanced, distinguishing at least three genetically defined groups, A, B, and C. RV can be further subgrouped depending on their host receptors: intercellular adhesion molecule 1 (ICAM-1) for major group RV (about 90% of known RV serotypes) and low-density lipoprotein receptor (LDL-R) for minor group viruses.[20] In an 11-year prospective follow-up study, Hyvärinen MK et al.[21] demonstrated that severe RV-induced wheezing in early childhood was associated with asthma in about 40% of children entering teen age; the corresponding association with RSV infections was 20% in their cohort. Other investigators have confirmed such a predominance of RV over RSV. It is not interpretation of treatment effects. Yet, *Moraxella catarrhalis* and *Streptococcus pneumoniae*, for example, have been associated with exacerbations of COPD.[37] Antibiotics also remain a commonly used therapy and have been effective in exacerbations occurring in severe COPD.[8] A critical review of the use of antibiotics in COPD exacerbations could not find convincing evidence for clinical efficacy.[10] Indeed, neither subgrouping of patients nor employment of markers of bacterial infection had been helpful in identifying patients that would respond to antibiotics.[10] Variable responses to treatment with antibiotics may underscore the need to better assess roles and mechanisms of interactions between bacterial and viral infections in COPD.

Atypical bacterial infections in children and adults, involving *Mycoplasma pneumoniae* and *Chlamydia pneumoniae*, have been associated with increased risk for the development of exacerbations of asthma. It is of note, however, that atypical bacterial infections in association with asthma exacerbations have had high rates of virus detection (reviewed in Reference 9). The possibility of a role of bacterial infection in asthma has received attention by clinical trial demonstration of curative benefit of macrolide antibiotics in established exacerbations of asthma.[38] As discussed by the authors, macrolides have anti-inflammatory effects in addition to an anti-infective property, making interpretations of what is behind their limited clinical efficacy difficult. Quite recently, Bruselle et al.[39] have demonstrated that maintenance treatment with macrolides reduced exacerbations exclusively in noneosinophilic asthma.

It is increasingly realized that viral and bacterial coinfection could be an important causative factor in exacerbations. Interaction between influenza and bacterial infection is known to promote the development of pneumonia[40] and patients with asthma have a known risk of developing invasive pneumonia. Further, individuals with COPD co-infected with RV and *Haemophilus influenzae* have exhibited increased severity of exacerbations compared to those without coinfection.[41,42] Johnston and colleagues recently demonstrated that experimental inoculation–infection with RV in COPD was followed by secondary bacterial infection in more than half of the inoculated patients.[43] Thus, both influenza and RV infection may impede bacterial host defense mechanisms and increase the risk of exacerbations as well as secondary pneumonia. The potential importance of coinfection is reflected by increasing number of research approaches in the field with revelation of intriguing molecular mechanisms and clinical observations. For example, experimental data have identified a potential role of the transcription factor IRF3 in reduced antibacterial defense evoked by viral infection. Thus, inducement of IRF3 by dsRNA, produced by viral infection and acting on cytoplasmic RIG-I-like receptors, reduced toll-like receptor (TLR)-mediated antibacterial defense by the suppression of the expression of IL-12 and IL-23.[44] This finding increases the interest in the pharmacology of IRF3 inhibition.[45]

14.4 CURRENT TREATMENTS OF ASTHMA AND COPD

Glucocorticoids are used at increased doses in treatments of exacerbations. These drugs are mainstay therapy in asthma but their efficacy in preventing exacerbations, also when combined with bronchodilators, is incomplete.[8] Glucocorticoids are less efficacious in COPD than in asthma, but are increasingly used in both diseases. These drugs exert broad anti-inflammatory effects, but may to some extent spare host defense mechanisms.[19,46] However, the commonly inhaled glucocorticoids in asthma and COPD have been associated with an increased incidence of pneumonia[47] and nontuberculous mycobacterial pulmonary disease.[48]

During several decades, authors have interchangeably claimed that they have identified the important mechanism of the action of the airway steroids. However, it remains a major challenge to define in detail the crucial mechanism(s) that explain the clinical efficacy of glucocorticoids in asthma and COPD. Once found, "the key steroid mechanism" could be targeted by a novel class of compounds with reduced side effects. However, considering the limited efficacy of even high doses of the current glucocorticoids,[49] it appears that quite novel pharmacological principles will be required to effectively treat exacerbations of asthma and COPD.

14.5 BRONCHIAL EPITHELIUM: MAJOR RV TARGET, INJURY–REPAIR, FUNCTION, AND ROLE IN ASTHMA AND COPD

14.5.1 Epithelial Barrier Functions Affected by Virus

The major cell components of bronchial epithelium are little differentiated basal cells and superimposed columnar cells carrying cilia or mucus secretory cells. It is established that the columnar cells have desmosomal attachments to the basal cells that in turn are anchored on the basement membrane through hemidesmosomes. Unless the epithelium has undergone metaplastic changes, both basal and columnar cells have contact with the basement membrane. This arrangement defines the pseudostratified nature of the bronchial epithelial lining. Maintaining the functions of this lining is vital because it constitutes the interface between the environment and the internal tissue of the lower respiratory tract. The epithelial cells thus serve as a tight and reactive barrier to noxious factors that land on the respiratory mucosal surface. Together with the nasal and tracheal epithelium, the bronchial epithelial lining is also the primary respiratory tract viral infection target. The epithelial lining cells receive major attention not only regarding their role in host defense but also because they have a capacity to be leading effector cells governing pathogenic effects in asthma and COPD.

Viral infection will alter the epithelial lining barrier through effects on the airway surface liquid with its content of active solutes. The infection may further reduce the adhesion/attachments between epithelial lining cells and between epithelial cells and the epithelial basement membrane. Viral infection may produce necrosis of epithelial cells. However, quite distinct from such ultimate effects, the viral infection will induce epithelial-derived cytokines, chemokines, and interferons. Thus, three major facets of airway mucosal barrier functions are affected by viral infections:

- The thin fluid barrier covering the apical aspect of bronchial epithelium
- The physical tightness of the epithelial cell sheet
- Not least, the biologically active "barrier" created by epithelial cell production of immunoactive and inflammatory agents

The bronchial epithelium has received more attention in asthma than in COPD. This may in part be explained by demonstrations of an increased epithelial fragility (but not denudation) in the asthmatic bronchi that can be readily reached by biopsy procedures. A simple reasoning has been that asthma is caused by inhaled allergens: due to their size, they deposit in the more proximal large- to medium-sized bronchi, whereas cigarette smoke, the main culprit in COPD, will preferentially deposit in and injure more peripheral parts of the respiratory tree. Yet, small airways disease is also likely a major component of asthma. Likewise, inflammatory processes in COPD evidently also engage the main bronchi. Furthermore, whether it leads to epithelial metaplasia,[50] as often occurs in COPD and asthma, or epithelial fragility, as is known to occur in asthma, epithelial injury is considered a central mechanism in both diseases.[19,51–54]

14.5.2 Shedding of Infected Epithelial Cells, A Disease or Defense Mechanism?

At local bronchial insults of infection or other environmental noxious challenge, the columnar cells will take the initial blow. The desmosomal connection between basal cells and columnar epithelium, possibly involving a critical role of e-cadherin, may be resolved by influences of cell-derived cytokines such as TNFα and IFNγ,[55] known to occur in diseased bronchi at viral exacerbations. If this most superficial layer of cells become deranged and lost by shedding/death, there is still the basal cell layer left. The basal cells in the intact pseudostratified human bronchi constitute a pervious, cobbled layer with little cell-to-cell contact between them. However, this condition does not prevail when they lose the protection of their columnar cell cover. Erjefält and Persson[56] discovered

14.5.5 Multipotential Pathogenic Effects of Epithelial Injury–Repair

During the 1990s, *in vivo* events following nonsanguineous loss of epithelial cells from an intact epithelial basement membrane were unraveled. The new knowledge concerned the onset of epithelial restitution, participating repair cell phenotypes, participating plasma-derived proteins, and the speed by which a naked basement membrane became covered by a novel cell sheet.[51,69] Radical shedding of epithelial cells is commonly referred to as denudation since it leaves the basement membrane naked. This is a condition where a plasma-derived, fibrin-fibronectin-rich gel promptly covers the basement membrane. The gel provides a rather poor physical barrier. Yet, its continuous supply of plasma proteins from a profuse subepithelial microcirculation, together with recruited granulocytes and other cells, offer a prime milieu for a very speedy epithelial repair. All types of epithelial cells bordering the denuded area, including ciliated and secretory cells (that were previously considered end-differentiated cells), promptly dedifferentiate into poorly differentiated, flattened cells that migrate at a high speed to cover the basement membrane. Thus, basal cell-like repair cells will soon substitute the plasma-derived gel. Depending on the size of the denuded area, this initial epithelial restitution occurs within several minutes to a few hours. The repair cells may dominate the scene for several days during which time they proliferate and develop until they become a fully differentiated epithelium. The poorly differentiated repair epithelium is frequently confused with basal cells. However, the repair cells may share an increased sensitivity to viral infection with the basal cells.[58]

Shedding-like loss of epithelial cells and the ensuing restitution processes have produced a range of "pathogenic" effects that are also known to characterize obstructive bronchial diseases. Thus, simple shedding of epithelial cells evoked prompt and sustained plasma exudation (no bleeding!), increased mucosal secretion, and recruitment and activation of eosinophils and neutrophils. These innate inflammatory responses were soon followed by increased proliferation not only of the epithelial lining cells in the area of interest but also of subepithelial cells, including fibroblasts and smooth muscle cells. Hence, repeated epithelial shedding–restitution processes alone could be sufficient to produce a range of airway effects, which are considered defining inflammatory and remodeling features of obstructive bronchial diseases.[19,51] The proposal of shedding–restitution as a multipotent pathogenic process[19] preceded the current focus on epithelial cells as major producer of immunoactive defense and pathogenic molecules (discussed later). The concept was based on demanding *in vivo* approaches[69] that have not yet lent themselves to detailed exploration of involved molecular mechanisms. It is revisited here because it underscores the potential importance of viral infection-induced epithelial damage in bronchial airways.

14.5.6 RV Infection-Evoked Epithelial Injury

RV infection of otherwise healthy bronchial mucosae may not cause overt epithelial injury. Owing to a speedy restitution (discussed above) individual epithelial cells harboring replicating virus may be shed and die without leaving any hole in the epithelial lining. As evidenced by the occurrence of columnar epithelial cells in sputa, the less dramatic kind of epithelial shedding, that leaves the basal cells to account for a physical barrier, commonly occurs in obstructive bronchial diseases. In *in vitro* studies, it has been demonstrated that RV causes more clear damage if the exposed epithelial culture is neither differentiated nor confluent.[59] This observation may reflect the possibility that already injured epithelial linings are vulnerable. Further, viral infection of bronchial epithelia may act in synergy with other culprits to produce epithelial injury. For example, interaction between epithelial viral infection and cigarette smoke-induced oxidative stress and cell death[70] is likely. As suggested by little colocalization of virally infected cells and apoptotic indices,[71] respiratory tract viral infection *in vivo* may cause death of epithelial cells that are not infected. The mechanism behind such remote cell effects of viral infection has not been explored. Alternatively, viral infection causes cell necrosis rather than apoptosis.[60] Necrotic cells themselves can also constitute hotbeds spreading disease-like effects in the airways (see below).

14.5.7 Viral Infection Causes Eosinophilic Exacerbations of Asthma and COPD

For more than a century, the eosinophil has been considered a central inflammatory cell in asthma.[23] It is a biomarker of asthma and has successfully guided steroid treatment for some 40 years. Eagerly awaited eosinophil-targeted drugs (anti-IL-5 antibodies) became available toward the end of the twentieth century. Unexpectedly, these drugs failed to show clinical efficacy in mild to moderate, eosinophilic asthma. The eosinophil as the culprit in asthma fell into disrepute. This was largely transient because during the last decade, clinical efficacy of anti-IL-5 drugs has been demonstrated in severe asthma[6]. A meta-analysis of clinical trials has revealed a particular efficacy of these drugs in exacerbations of asthma.[72] There is also a rapidly growing interest in potential roles of the eosinophil in COPD. RV infection increases airway levels of eosinophil-active chemokines/cytokines, notably eotaxin,[73,74] and viral-induced exacerbations of COPD, as well as asthma, are associated with bronchial eosinophilia (reviewed in Reference 12). Eosinophil-derived toxic granule proteins have a capacity to produce bronchial epithelial injury.[75] Epithelial damage may reflect interaction between viral infection and the tissue-toxic granular proteins emanating from eosinophils.[76] Hence, modes of degranulation of eosinophils in diseased airways are of interest.

We have demonstrated that a major mode of degranulation of eosinophils in human diseased airway tissues is through primary cytolysis. This mechanism involves rupture of the eosinophil cell membrane and release of protein-laden granules in the tissue.[77,78] For a century, free eosinophil granules were largely ignored or considered unimportant artifacts of sample handling. However, the use of whole mount tissue preparation and deep tissue staining of granule proteins indicated that the free granules are real *in vivo* phenomena in diseased bronchi.[77] We learned that the free granules emanate from eosinophil necrosis in human diseased airway tissues, and that they correlate with disease severity.[23,79] Uller originally demonstrated that necrosis/lysis of eosinophils is a primary event in diseased airway tissue (not preceded by apoptosis).[78] Further, eosinophils undergoing necrosis/lysis exhibited little signs of prior piecemeal degranulation.[77,78,80] Most recently, necrosis/lysis of bronchial tissue eosinophils, but not eosinophil numbers, was demonstrated to be associated with lack of clinical control of asthma.[79,81] Hence, in many studies, notably involving bronchial biopsies from donors with severe asthma,[23,79] necrosis/lysis of eosinophils stands out as the dominant mode of activation of eosinophils. Necrotic eosinophils release active "danger-associated" molecules beyond the toxic proteins and cytokines contained in the specific granules. However, as yet, few studies have addressed immunopharmacological control of primary eosinophil necrosis/lysis. Eosinophil lysis/necrosis in infection has not been explored much. Investigators examining effects of *Staphylococcus aureus* on granulocytes have recently confirmed the observation by Uller[80] that cytolysis of eosinophils is a primary mechanism that is not preceded by apoptosis.[82] We have strong reasons to hypothesize that viral and bacterial infection may be causally involved in lysis/necrosis of eosinophils and that this mode of eosinophil activation is an important component of asthma and COPD exacerbations.

The focus on airway tissue eosinophils in viral infection puts the emphasis not only on recruitment, that is well reviewed,[83] but also on the elimination of these cells, that appears to be somewhat misunderstood. It is widely thought that the process of apoptosis, followed by phagocytosis, disposes of these cells. Unfortunately, *in vivo* observations in health and disease do not support this popular notion. Instead, it emerges that the bronchial tissue eosinophilia is resolved by transepithelial cell migration followed by final elimination through mucociliary transport.[78] This concept, which is largely based on observations in patients, brings many novel inferences.[78] For this chapter, it seems important to highlight the possibility that viral infections may impede the epithelial transmigration of eosinophils (reviewed in Reference 84). Such an effect could contribute to RV infection-evoked aggravation of inflammation in asthma and COPD; in stable conditions, leucocytes continuously traffic across the epithelial lining. We have suggested that inhibition of bronchial transepithelial exit of inflammatory cells should receive attention as a mechanism and strategy by which viruses can escape host immune surveillance and defense.[84]

100. Takai T. TSLP expression: Cellular sources, triggers, and regulatory mechanisms. *Allergol Int* 2012; **61**(1): 3–17.
101. Makris D, Lazarou S, Alexandrakis M et al. Tc2 response at the onset of COPD exacerbations. *Chest* 2008; **134**(3): 483–8.
102. Mjösberg JM, Trifari S, Crellin NK et al. Human IL-25- and IL-33-responsive type 2 innate lymphoid cells are defined by expression of CRTH2 and CD161. *Nat Immunol* 2011; **12**(11): 1055–62.
103. Brandelius A, Yudina Y, Calven J et al. dsRNA-induced expression of thymic stromal lymphopoietin (TSLP) in asthmatic epithelial cells is inhibited by a small airway relaxant. *Pulm Pharmacol Ther* 2011; **24**(1): 59–66.
104. Mahmutovic-Persson I, Johansson M, Brandelius A et al. Capacity of capsazepinoids to relax human small airways and inhibit TLR3-induced TSLP and IFNbeta production in diseased bronchial epithelial cells. *Int Immunopharmacol* 2012; **13**(3): 292–300.
105. Taylor KE, Mossman KL. Recent advances in understanding viral evasion of type I interferon. *Immunology* 2013; **138**(3): 190–7.
106. Gaajetaan GR, Bruggeman CA, Stassen FR. The type I interferon response during viral infections: A "SWOT" analysis. *Rev Med Virol* 2012; **22**(2): 122–37.
107. Contoli M, Message SD, Laza-Stanca V et al. Role of deficient type III interferon-lambda production in asthma exacerbations. *Nat Med* 2006; **12**(9): 1023–6.
108. Holt PG, Sly PD. Viral infections and atopy in asthma pathogenesis: New rationales for asthma prevention and treatment. *Nat Med* 2012; **18**(5): 726–35.
109. Miller EK, Hernandez JZ, Wimmenauer V et al. A mechanistic role for type III IFN-lambda1 in asthma exacerbations mediated by human rhinoviruses. *Am J Respir Crit Care Med* 2012; **185**(5): 508–16.
110. Bedke N, Haitchi HM, Xatzipsalti M, Holgate ST, Davies DE. Contribution of bronchial fibroblasts to the antiviral response in asthma. *J Immunol* 2009; **182**(6): 3660–7.
111. Oliver BG, Johnston SL, Baraket M et al. Increased proinflammatory responses from asthmatic human airway smooth muscle cells in response to rhinovirus infection. *Respir Res* 2006; **7**: 71.
112. Joubert P, Hamid Q. Role of airway smooth muscle in airway remodeling. *J Allergy Clin Immunol* 2005; **116**(3): 713–6.
113. Takeda N, Sumi Y, Prefontaine D et al. Epithelium-derived chemokines induce airway smooth muscle cell migration. *Clin Exp Allergy* 2009; **39**(7): 1018–26.

15 Pediatric Viral Pneumonia

Matti Korppi

CONTENTS

15.1 INTRODUCTION

Community-acquired pneumonia (CAP) remains a significant cause for childhood morbidity worldwide. In developed countries, CAP is commonly encountered in daily practice, and in developing countries, pneumonia is the leading infectious cause of death in children less than 5 years old.[1] In the studies conducted in western countries, about a third of CAP cases have been of viral origin, and another third of mixed viral–bacterial origin.[2] Viral etiology has been more common in young preschool-aged children than in older school-aged children. Respiratory syncytial virus (RSV) and rhinoviruses are the most often identified viruses.[3] In western countries, about half of the children younger than 5 years with CAP have needed treatment in hospital.[4]

15.2 EPIDEMIOLOGY OF PNEUMONIA

The prospective population-based studies on pediatric CAP in western countries are from the 1970s and 1980s.[2] The incidence rates, 35–40/1000 in <5 years old, about 20/1000 in 5–10 years old, and 10/1000 in >10-year-old children were rather similar in Finland and in the United States.[4,5] Half of the <5-year-old children, but only <20% of the 5–0 years old and <10% of the >10-year-old children were treated in hospital.[4] In the Finnish CAP studies, about 25% of the cases were viral, 25% were bacterial, 25% were mixed viral–bacterial infections, and 25% remained without a microbe-specific diagnosis.[5,6] Currently, when sensitive tests based on molecular biology are available, one or more microbes can be identified in most CAP cases. In later hospital-based register studies, the incidence figures have been only one-tenth, 0.15% for all children and 0.3% for children aged <5 years.[7] In hospital-based studies, the included cases represent more severe infections and more often bacterial infections.

In developing countries, the incidence of pneumonia may be 15 times higher than in developed countries. In children, 150 million pneumonia cases are annually recorded in developing countries compared with 5 million cases in developed countries.[1,3] In 2008, about 1.5 million <5-year-old children died from pneumonia, and nearly all fatal cases occurred in developing countries.[8] Only one death per year was recorded in Canadian children during a 9-year surveillance period including infections has been rather similar in PCR-based studies and in studies using more conventional methods of antibody assays and antigen detection.[3] In a prospective 3-year hospital-based study from Finland with PCR for rhino- and enteroviruses available, the etiology of CAP was found in 85% of the 254 cases, with viral infection in 62% and bacterial infection in 53%.[14] In a prospective 2-year CAP study in 338 less than 3-year-old Spanish children, modern methods were available for 14 viruses, and at least one virus was identified in 67% and viral co-infection in 27% of the cases.[17] RSV, rhinoviruses, human bocavirus, human metapneumovirus, and parainfluenza viruses were, in this order, the most common findings.

All respiratory viruses are capable to cause respiratory infections at all levels of the respiratory tract, including the lungs. The invasiveness of the disease depends on host factors, such as age and immune status, and viral factors. Primary infections in young children are usually more invasive than reinfections at a later age. In the CAP study from Spain, infants less than 12 months of age presented more than 1 to 3-year-old children with multiple viral findings, and those with dual viral–viral infections needed hospital care more often than those with single infections.[19] Among respiratory viruses in children, RSV, rhinoviruses and parainfluenza virus type 3 typically present with pneumonia in infants and young children. Correspondingly, among pneumonia cases, rhinovirus is the most commonly found virus presenting often as mixed infection with other agents, followed by RSV and adenoviruses in order. Adenoviruses, especially serotypes 3, 7, and 14, may cause invasive pneumonia cases with large tissue damage and severe sequelae.[3]

15.3.2 Newly Identified Viruses

Human metapneumovirus was recognized 10–15 years ago,[18] and shares many properties with RSV, including human beings as the only hosts, a similar seasonality, a similar age distribution, and nearly identical clinical and laboratory features.[19] Human metapneumovirus can be identified by culture, PCR and antibody assays. Sero-epidemiological studies have indicated that virtually all children are infected with human metapneumovirus by school age.[20] The clinical picture of human metapneumovirus infection has varied from mild common cold to severe pneumonia with high fever and generalized symptoms.[19] In the United States, pneumonia has been diagnosed in about 10% of infants admitted for human metapneumovirus infection.[18,19] Human metapneumovirus was identified by PCR in 8% of 1296 Israeli children with CAP,[21] and an antibody response to hMPV in paired sera was documented in 5% of 101 Italian children with CAP.[22] Without any doubt, human metapneumovirus is an etiological agent in pediatric CAP, but the prevalence is less than 10% of viral CAP, and the role is limited to infants and young children.

Human bocavirus was discovered 5–10 years ago by molecular virus screening,[23] and until now, the virus has not been cultured but it can be identified by electron microscopy. Available evidence suggests that nearly all children have produced antibodies to human bocavirus by school age.[24] Currently, the only diagnostic methods for human bocavirus pneumonia are PCR in respiratory samples and the recently developed enzyme immune assay in paired sera.[25] In different studies, pneumonia has been present in 10–75% of children positive by PCR for human bocavirus,[26] and the proportion of mixed infections has varied from 20% to 80%.[13,27] In a study from Thailand, human bocavirus was the third most common agent after RSV and rhinoviruses in 367 children admitted for CAP at age <5 years, accounting for 12% but some other virus was found in 91% of the cases.[28] Antibodies to human bocavirus were measured by enzyme immune assay in paired sera in 101 Italian children with CAP, and evidence for human bocavirus etiology was found in 12% of all cases.[29] In that study, 42% were mixed infections, 50% were found by rises in IgG antibodies and nearly all by IgM antibodies. The final clinical role of human bocavirus is still open, but recent evidence suggests that human bocavirus is a true causative agent if there is a high viral load by quantitative PCR in respiratory samples, viremia by PCR in blood samples or an antibody response between paired sera.[13,27]

15.3.3 Differentiation between Viral and Bacterial Pneumonia

The differentiation of bacterial from viral pneumonia, if only possible, would have important therapeutic implications. Diagnostic tests still fail to identify causative agents in many patients with pneumonia, and the microbe-specific diagnosis of bacterial pneumonia is even more difficult than the microbe-specific diagnosis of viral pneumonia.[2,30] An identification of viral etiology does not rule bacterial co-infection out.

Markers of host response, such as white blood cell counts, serum C-reactive protein and procalcitonin concentrations, and chest radiograph findings have been used to distinguish bacterial from viral pneumonia.[2,3] Respiratory viruses often follow seasonal patterns and are most likely to cause pneumonia during larger epidemics (RSV and influenza A or B virus), during local outbreaks (human metapneumo- and parainfluenza viruses), or during infection seasons in autumn and winter (rhinoviruses and human bocaviruses). In addition, the onset of the pneumonia symptoms, and response of the symptoms to antibiotics may be different in viral and bacterial pneumonia.[3] Compared with a rapid response in uncomplicated pneumococcal pneumonia,[31] viral pneumonia has usually a slow onset, and if treated with antibiotics, has a slow or no response.

In chest radiograph, presence of bilateral interstitial infiltrates suggests viral pneumonia, and presence of alveolar or mixed interstitial–alveolar infiltrates suggests bacterial pneumonia.[2] However, bacteria and viruses either alone or together can cause a broad range of chest radiographic changes with a limited value for an estimation of the etiology of CAP, even for a separation between viral and bacterial pneumonia.[32,33] In addition, young children often have patchy perihilar infiltrates in chest radiographs, originating from swelling in the small airways and enlarged lymph nodes, which should not be diagnosed at all as pneumonia.

Total white blood count <10 × 10 E9/L, C-reactive protein <20 mg/L and procalcitonin <0.1 ug/L, if the symptoms presumptive for pneumonia have continued for more than 12 h, usually means viral pneumonia,[3] and total white blood count >15 × 10 E9/L, C-reactive protein >60 mg/L or procalcitonin >0.5 μg/L evidence for bacterial pneumonia.[2,34,35]

According to British Thoracic Society guidelines, sudden onset of fever >38.5°C, respiratory rate >50/min, and chest recessions are suggestive for bacterial rather than viral pneumonia.[36] The guidelines are targeted to diagnose children with severe pneumococcal pneumonia and to start antibiotics without delay. On the other hand, respiratory rate >50/min and chest recessions are also typical features of viral bronchiolitis.

15.3.4 Mixed Infections

Before the development of PCR for viral identification, dual respiratory viral findings were rather rare, less than 5%, when findings by culture, antigen detection and antibody assays were combined.[15] When PCR has been in use, two or even three viruses have been detected in 10–20% of children with CAP.[3,17] Especially, human bocavirus has been detected in association with other respiratory viruses.[13] In a comprehensive virological study of CAP in children, two or more viruses were found 18% of the 338 cases, human bocavirus being involved in 69%, influenza viruses in 52% and RSV in 51% of the multiple viral cases.[27] The clinical relevance of detecting several viruses in pediatric CAP, and the possible association with more severe illness, is uncertain. Viral–viral interaction, as the interaction between viruses and immunity, including different signaling pathways of innate and adaptive immunity, are poorly understood.

Evidence of mixed viral–bacterial infection has been revealed in up to 45% of CAP cases in children.[3,15] The typical combination has been *Streptococcus pneumoniae* and some respiratory virus, usually RSV or rhinovirus.[14,16] In addition, *Streptococcus pyogenes* and *Staphycoccous aureus* may be present in developing countries.[3] Presuming that a preceding viral infection is needed to pave the way for bacterial infection, the true incidence of mixed viral–bacterial infections must be higher than reported. There is some evidence that mixed infections could induce a more severe

18. van den Hoogen BG, Osterhaus DM, Fouchier RA. Clinical impact and diagnosis of human meta pneumovirus infection. *Pediatr Infect Dis J.* 2004;23(1 Suppl):S25–32. Review.
19. Williams JV, Harris PA, Tollefson SJ et al. Human meta pneumovirus and lower respiratory tract disease in otherwise healthy infants and children. *N Engl J Med.* 2004;350:443–50.
20. Leung J, Esper F, Weibel C, Kahn JS. Seroepidemiology of human meta pneumovirus (hMPV) on the basis of a novel enzyme-linked immunosorbent assay utilizing hMPV fusion protein expressed in recombinant vesicular stomatitis virus. *J Clin Microbiol.* 2005;43:1213–9.
21. Wolf DG, Greenberg D, Shemer-Avni Y, Givon-Lavi N, Bar-Ziv J, Dagan R. Association of human metapneumovirus with radiologically diagnosed community-acquired alveolar pneumonia in young children. *J Pediatr.* 2010;156:115–20.
22. Don M, Korppi M, Valent F, Vainionpaa R, Canciani M. Human meta pneumovirus pneumonia in children: Results of an Italian study and mini-review. *Scand J Infect Dis.* 2008;40:821–6.
23. Allander T, Tammi MT, Eriksson M et al. Cloning of a human parvovirus by molecular screening of respiratory tract samples. *Proc Natl Acad Sci USA.* 2005;102:12891–6.
24. Kahn JS, Kesebir D, Cotmore SF et al. Seroepidemiology of human bocavirus defined using recombinant virus-like particles. *J Infect Dis.* 2008;198:41–50.
25. Söderlund-Venermo M, Lahtinen A et al. Clinical assessment and improved diagnosis of bocavirus-induced wheezing in children, Finland. *Emerg Infect Dis.* 2009;15:1423–30.
26. Schildgen O, Müller A, Allander T et al. Human bocavirus: Passenger or pathogen in acute respiratory tract infections? *Clin Microbiol Rev.* 2008;21:291–304. Review.
27. Christensen A, Nordbø SA, Krokstad S, Rognlien AG, Døllner H. Human bocavirus commonly involved in multiple viral airway infections. *J Clin Virol.* 2008;41:34–7.
28. Fry AM, Lu X, Chittaganpitch M, Peret T et al. Human bocavirus: A novel parvovirus epidemiologically associated with pneumonia requiring hospitalization in Thailand. *J Infect Dis.* 2007;195:1038–45.
29. Don M, Söderlund-Venermo M, Valent F et al. Serologically verified human bocavirus pneumonia in children. *Pediatr Pulmonol.* 2010;45:120–6
30. Korppi M, Leinonen M, Ruuskanen O. Pneumococcal serology in children's respiratory infections. *Eur J Clin Microbiol Infect Dis.* 2008;27:167–75.
31. Mertsola J, Waris M, Leinonen M, Ruuskanen O. Clinical response to antibiotic therapy for community-acquired pneumonia. *Eur J Pediatr.* 2004;163:140–4.
32. Korppi M, Kiekara O, Heiskanen-Kosma T, Soimakallio S. Comparison of radiological findings and microbial aetiology of childhood pneumonia. *Acta Paediatr.* 1993;82: 360–3
33. Virkki R, Juven T, Rikalainen H, Svedström E, Mertsola J, Ruuskanen O. Differentiation of bacterial and viral pneumonia in children. *Thorax.* 2002;57:438–41.
34. Korppi M, Heiskanen-Kosma T, Leinonen M. White blood cells, C-reactive protein and erythrocyte sedimentation rate in pneumococcal pneumonia in children. *Eur Respir J.* 1997;10:1125–9.
35. Schuetz P, Albrich W, Mueller B. Procalcitonin for diagnosis of infection and guide to antibiotic decisions: Past, present and future. *BMC Med.* 2011;9:107. Review.
36. Harris M, Clark J, Coote N et al. British Thoracic Society guidelines for the management of community acquired pneumonia in children: Update 2011. *Thorax* 2011;66(Suppl 2):ii1–23.
37. McCullersJA. Do specific virus–bacteria pairings drive clinical outcomes of pneumonia? *Clin Microbiol Infect.* 2013;19:113–8. Review.
38. Poggensee G, Gilsdorf A, Buda S et al. The first wave of pandemic influenza (H1N1) 2009 in Germany: From initiation to acceleration. *BMC Infect Dis.* 2010;10:155.
39. Shun-Shin M, Thompson M, Heneghan C, Perera R, Harnden A, Mant D. Neuraminidase inhibitors for treatment and prophylaxis of influenza in children: Systematic review and meta-analysis of randomised controlled trials. *BMJ.* 2009;339:b3172. Review.
40. Harper SA, Bradley JS, Englund JA et al. Seasonal influenza in adults and children—Diagnosis, treatment, chemoprophylaxis, and institutional outbreak management: Clinical practice guidelines of the Infectious Diseases Society of America. *Clin Infect Dis.* 2009;48:1003–32.
41. Heinonen S, Silvennoinen H, Lehtinen P, Vainionpää R, Ziegler T, Heikkinen T. Effectiveness of inactivated influenza vaccine in children aged 9 months to 3 years: An observational cohort study. *Lancet Infect Dis.* 2011;11:23–9.
42. American Academy Pediatrics. Policy statements—Modified recommendations for use of palivizumab for prevention of respiratory syncytial virus infections. *Pediatrics.* 2009;124:1694–701.

16 Pulmonary Bacterial Coinfection with Viral Respiratory Infection in Children

Kentigern Thorburn and Andrew Riordan

CONTENTS

16.1 INTRODUCTION

It has long been suspected that respiratory bacterial infections may be associated with preceding or concomitant viral infections. The recent experience with the influenza H1N1 pandemic has refocused attention on the role of bacterial coinfection in contributing to disease severity and death in children with viral respiratory tract infection. The experience with influenza A—H1N1 strain infection of 35 pediatric intensive care units (PICU) in the United States during the 2009–2010 influenza pandemic (838 children) was that bacterial coinfection/pneumonia was found in 33%.[1] This was in keeping with earlier findings during three influenza seasons (2004–2007) when bacterial coinfection increased consistently each season from 6% to 15% to 35% in the 166 influenza-associated pediatric deaths reported to the CDC in the United States.[2] Some experts suggest that presenting such data is unrepresentative, as it reflects the extreme end of the spectrum. The vast majority of children with influenza infection suffer a far milder illness, do not have bacterial coinfection, and need only symptomatic treatment not antibiotics.

Far outscoring infrequent influenza pandemics, there is a substantial volume of children with viral respiratory infections each and every year due to viral bronchiolitis—annually accounting for up to 90,000 hospitalizations in the United States, 20,000 in the United Kingdom, and at least 3.4 million hospital attendances or admissions worldwide every year.[3,4] Pulmonary bacterial coinfection may be more commonplace than previously appreciated in certain subsets of this sizable group of hospitalized children with viral respiratory tract infection.[5,6] However, this subject is confounded by the paucity of studies specifically addressing pulmonary bacterial coinfection in children with viral respiratory infections.

16.2 METHODOLOGY

To evaluate the role pulmonary bacterial coinfection plays in children (0–18 years) with viral respiratory infection, data were identified by searching Medline, PubMed, and the reference lists of the relevant published papers.

Search terms such as "coinfection," "bacterial coinfection," "secondary infection," "secondary pneumonia," "concomitant bacterial pneumonia," "superinfection," "bronchiolitis," "viral bronchiolitis," "viral pneumonia," "influenza," "H1N1," "parainfluenza," "respiratory syncytial virus," "adenovirus," and so on and "children," "infant," "paediatric/pediatric" were used to screen for relevant literature.

Only papers relating to the pediatric population (aged 0–18 years) were considered.

To make the chapter relevant and current, source data were restricted to more recent papers (published from 2000 onwards), unless they were relevant to background information. Cited papers were selected when pertinent to clinical aspects, rather than listing all the published data and duplicating established data.

Only papers in which pulmonary bacterial coinfection could be clearly differentiated from other sites of bacterial coinfection were utilized.

Studies that relied on nasopharyngeal cultures for identification of bacterial coinfection were excluded, as nasopharyngeal bacterial cultures reflect colonization not infection.

Viral bronchiolitis is a clinical diagnosis of a viral lower respiratory tract infection where the inflammatory process in the small/distal airways/bronchioles (i.e., bronchiolitis) results in pulmonary hyperinflation, areas of atelectasis, and wheezing due to small/distal airways obstruction. In this chapter "RSV bronchiolitis" is not differentiated from "RSV pneumonia" as informed clinicians generally appreciate the pneumonic aspects of severe viral bronchiolitis. "Viral bronchiolitis" is synonymous with "viral lower respiratory tract infection (LRTI)," "viral chest infection," and "viral pneumonia." We have not included viral pneumonitis, since this tends to occur in immunocompromised individuals.

In this chapter, the following questions will be addressed:

1. Does pulmonary bacterial coinfection occur in children with viral respiratory infections?
2. If so, what is its incidence?
3. Does the incidence of pulmonary bacterial coinfection depend on the primary viral pathogen?
4. What are the common bacterial (co)pathogens reported?
5. What are the mechanisms of predisposition to pulmonary bacterial coinfection?
6. Does pulmonary bacterial coinfection reflect or affect severity of illness?

7. When is antibiotic treatment (even prophylaxis) indicated or justified?
8. Might antiviral strategies impact on pulmonary bacterial coinfection?

16.3 DIAGNOSIS OF BACTERIAL PNEUMONIA

There is no widely accepted gold standard for the diagnosis of bacterial pneumonia in children, let alone pulmonary bacterial coinfection or secondary bacterial pneumonia.[7] In clinical studies the diagnosis is made using a variable combination of clinical, radiological, haematological, biochemical, microbiology, and virology criteria. Heterogeny of diagnostic criteria between studies confounds confident comparison. Additionally, it is difficult clinically to differentiate bacterial from viral causes of pneumonia.[7,8]

Purists will challenge the basic diagnosis of pulmonary bacterial coinfection. It is difficult to confidently diagnose pulmonary bacterial coinfection because: (a) serological assays may only reflect a nonspecific response to a previous infection or a response to colonizing bacteria during a viral infection; (b) nasopharyngeal cultures merely reflect colonization, not infection; (c) cultures of sputum samples in children are difficult to obtain, unreliable, inadequately validated and potentially contaminated by the upper respiratory tract flora; and (d) tracheal aspirate samples reflect upper respiratory tract bacteria pushed down by the suction catheter or endotracheal tube.

To further confound matters, the criteria used to make the diagnosis of bacterial coinfection/pneumonia (e.g., type of sample; timing of sampling; sampling technique; growth densities) are often not specified, especially in retrospective studies.

For this chapter it was therefore necessary to accept that laboratory confirmation of an infective agent (bacterial or viral) is essential for diagnosis, whether it is direct evidence (as in culture or PCR) or more indirect (as in serology). This introduces two major limitations. First, that most studies involved hospitalized children. Second, most publications originate from resource-rich countries, a bias suffered by much of the medical literature in this field. Thus, the majority of the world's children may not be adequately represented by the chapter's "evidence base." However, key messages can be inferred to this larger patient group.

16.4 DOES PULMONARY BACTERIAL COINFECTION OCCUR IN CHILDREN WITH VIRAL RESPIRATORY INFECTIONS?

The answer to this question is undoubtedly yes—as demonstrated by a selection of the larger studies below.

16.4.1 Pneumonia

Mixed viral/bacterial respiratory infections were identified in 36 (24%) of the 154 children hospitalized with pneumonia in a prospective North American study (median age 33 months; range 2 months–17 years).[9] In a prospective Brazilian study, mixed viral/bacterial respiratory infections were identified in 43 (23%) of the 184 children (median age 19 months; range 1 month–5 years) hospitalized with pneumonia.[10]

16.4.2 Respiratory Syncytial Virus Bronchiolitis

Pathogenic bacteria were identified in "good quality sputum samples" in 82 (44%) of 188 children hospitalized with confirmed RSV bronchiolitis/bronchopulmonary infection in a prospective Japanese study (median age 11 months; IQR 4–21 months; half were under 1 year of age).[11] Pulmonary bacterial coinfection was identified on admission bronchoalveolar lavage in 145 (38%) of 384 mechanically ventilated infants and children with confirmed RSV respiratory infection in a prospective British study (median age 2.8 months; IQR 1.3–11.5 months).[12,13]

TABLE 16.1 (continued)
Studies Reporting Pulmonary Bacterial Coinfection with Viral Respiratory Infection in Children

Study (Year)	Study Period/ Study Design	Study Group (Country)	Patients Studied for Coinfection[a]	Coinfection Incidence [Bacteriology Method]	Viral Pathogen(s) (in Entire Study Group)	Coinfection Bacteria
Randolph et al.[1] (2011)	2009–2010/ retrospective	Admitted to PICU with pandemic H1N1 infection (USA)	838	33% (bacterial diagnosis made at base PICU)	Influenza A -H1N1 838, RSV coinfection 14, Adenovirus 4	*S. aureus* 71, (MRSA 34 of 71), *Pseudomonas* 30, *S. pneumoniae* 15, *H. influenzae* 13, *S. pyogenes* 7, other bacteria 54
Spaeder et al.[42] (2013)	2010–2011/ retrospective	Admitted to PICU with human metapneumovirus infection (USA)	111	9% (tracheal aspirates-bacterial culture)	hMPV 111, Rhinovirus coinfection 6, RSV coinfection 4, H1N1 coinfection 1	*MRSA* 2, *M. catarrhalis* 2, *Enterobacter 2*, *S. pneumoniae* 1, *H. influenzae* 1, *Pseudomonas* 1, *E. coli 1*, *Serratia* 1

Source: Modified from Thorburn and Riordan, *Expert Rev. Anti Infect. Ther.* 10, 909–916, 2012. With permission.

[a] Number of patients in the study in whom pulmonary bacterial coinfection was assessed.

RSV = respiratory syncytial virus; hMPV = human metapneumovirus; PICU = pediatric intensive care unit; BAL = broncho-alveolar lavage sample.

S = Streptococcus: S. pneumoniae, S. pyogenes, S. agalactiae, S. group C.

S = Staphylococcus: S. aureus, S. milleri; MRSA = *methicillin-resistant Staphylococcus aureus;* CONS = *coagulase-negative Staphylococcus aureus.*

H = Haemophilus: H. influenzae, H. hemolyticus.

M = Moraxella: M. catarrhalis.

M = Mycoplasma: M. pneumoniae.

C = Chlamydia: C. pneumoniae, C. trachomatis.

E = Escherichia: E. coli

B = Bordertella: B. pertussis

P = Pneumocystis: P. jiroveci

M = Mycobacterium: M. tuberculosis

pathogen. However, pediatric studies of community-acquired pneumonia (CAP) show a variety of respiratory viruses in the group of mixed viral/bacterial pneumonias, without influenza dominating.[9,10] Furthermore, the RSV studies report similar or higher incidences of pulmonary bacterial coinfection (see Table 16.1). Then there is the phenomenon that even with the same viral pathogen coinfection rates may fluctuate between seasons, as demonstrated by the consecutive increase (6%, 15%, 35%) in bacterial coinfection during the three influenza seasons (2004–2007) in the influenza-associated pediatric deaths reported to the CDC in the United States.[2]

16.7 WHAT ARE THE COMMON BACTERIAL (CO)PATHOGENS REPORTED?

The bacterial pathogens reported in more recent pediatric papers are shown in Table 16.1.

Upper respiratory tract flora in children predominates—*Streptococcus pneumoniae, Staphylococcus aureus, Haemophilus influenzae, Moraxella catarrhalis.* Often the *Haemophilus influenzae* are reported as being nontypeable, although many studies have not specified typing data.

However, there is a wide variety of bacterial pathogens reported in the pediatric literature. Gram-negative bacteria, for example, *Pseudomonas* species, are often associated with underlying chronic illness or comorbidity.[1,12]

The recent influenza pandemic experience has certainly reinforced the association of *Staphylococcus aureus* (both methicillin-sensitive [MSSA] and especially methicillin-resistant *Staphylococcus aureus* [MRSA]) and *Streptococcus pneumoniae* with influenzal infections.[1,2,22]

16.8 WHAT ARE THE MECHANISMS OF PREDISPOSITION TO PULMONARY BACTERIAL COINFECTION?

Viral infection can predispose to bacterial coinfection in at least two ways—weakening of the body's physical barrier (the respiratory epithelium), thereby enhancing bacterial entry, and by altering immune responses.[23]

Viral-induced damage to the epithelial barrier and impairment of mucociliary function debilitate the respiratory tract defenses, promoting vulnerability to bacterial coinfection.[24] The neuraminidase activity of the influenza virus actively thins respiratory mucus, exposing receptors on the epithelial surface and enhancing bacterial adherence—especially staphylococci and pneumococci.[23–25] RSV, parainfluenza type 3, and rhinovirus infection have also been shown to enhance bacterial adherence to the respiratory epithelial cells (especially *Haemophilus influenzae* and *Streptococcus pneumoniae*).[24–26] Bacterial adherence with promotion of colonization by bacterial pathogens may be the first step in the pathogenesis of lower airways infection with potential pathogens carried first in the nasopharynx then migrating down the trachea into the lungs.

The influenza virus can suppress the respiratory burst response and phagocytic function of neutrophils and alveolar macrophages, facilitating secondary bacterial infection.[23–25] Continued viral replication with release of new viral particles damages the epithelial layer exposing it to bacterial adherence and infection. Other proposed mechanisms are viral infections enhancing expression of host receptors used by bacteria to gain entry into the epithelial cells (e.g., the upregulation of platelet-activating factor receptor); downregulation of pathogen sensing and dampening of immune responses permitting increased bacterial coinfection; inference with surfactant (especially surfactant protein A) production.[23,27]

16.9 DOES PULMONARY BACTERIAL COINFECTION REFLECT OR AFFECT SEVERITY OF RESPIRATORY ILLNESS?

The pediatric literature suggests that pulmonary bacterial coinfection impacts adversely on severity of respiratory viral illness.

To be convinced that pulmonary bacterial coinfection affects disease severity, one would expect to see a persistently higher incidence of coinfection in children with clinically more severe disease, that is, those requiring intensive care support. However, Table 16.1 demonstrates a nonspecific scatter of incidences when comparing hospitalized children to those with more severe disease requiring admission to PICU. Although high rates of chronic underlying illness or comorbidity in reported PICU study populations could confound severity of illness interpretations, a study of 384 children ventilated for RSV bronchiolitis found no difference in the incidence of pulmonary bacterial coinfection between children with comorbidity and those without.[12,13]

The most compelling arguments for pulmonary bacterial coinfection affecting disease severity (i.e., worse than viral infection alone) come from pediatric studies demonstrating increased mortality, increased risk of mechanical ventilation, increased duration of mechanical ventilation, and increased length of hospital stay in children with pulmonary bacterial coinfection.

16.9.1 Mortality

Pulmonary bacterial coinfection may increase the risk of mortality in influenza, but not RSV bronchiolitis. When assessing the associations with patient-related factors present before PICU admission in 838 children admitted to 35 USA PICU with influenza A–H1N1 infection during the 2009–2010 pandemic significant mortality risk factors were: bacterial pneumonia/coinfection (relative risk [RR] 1.8; 95%CI: 1.2–2.8; $p = 0.007$), *Staphylococcus aureus* lung coinfection (RR 2.3; 95%CI: 1.3–3.9; $p = 0.004$), and MRSA lung coinfection (RR 3.2; 95%CI: 1.8–5.9; $p = 0.0003$).[1] In multivariate analysis early MRSA lung coinfection continued as a significant mortality risk factor (RR 3.3; 95%CI: 1.7–6.4; $p = 0.0005$). Moreover, in the 251 previously healthy children, early MRSA lung coinfection remained the major mortality risk factor (RR 8; 95%CI: 3.1–20.6; $p < 0.0001$).[1] However, in children ventilated for RSV bronchiolitis, pulmonary bacterial coinfection does not confer enhanced mortality risk.[12,13,18] Comorbidity and nosocomial RSV infection have been shown to be the dominant mortality risk factors in this patient group with severe RSV bronchiolitis.[28]

16.9.2 Risk of Mechanical Ventilation

Pulmonary bacterial coinfection may increase the risk of mechanical ventilation in influenza. In 10,173 children hospitalized for seasonal influenza across 43 tertiary pediatric hospitals in the United States during 2006–2009, pulmonary bacterial coinfection/bacterial pneumonia was a significant risk factor for mechanical ventilation (univariate analysis odds ratio [OR] 6.47, 95%CI 5.36–7.81; multivariate logistic regression OR 5.8, 95%CI 5.36–6.29; $p < 0.001$ in both).[14]

16.9.3 Duration of Mechanical Ventilation

Pulmonary bacterial coinfection may increase the duration of ventilation in RSV bronchiolitis. In 384 British children ventilated for RSV bronchiolitis, the duration of ventilation was longer in those with pulmonary bacterial coinfection (median duration of ventilation 6 days, IQR 4–8 vs. 4 days, IQR 3–7; $p < 0.01$) than the children with RSV infection only.[12,13] A finding also borne out in a smaller North American study of previously healthy children ventilated for respiratory failure due to RSV bronchiolitis (mean duration of ventilation 10 days SEM $\pm$ 2 vs. 7 days SEM $\pm$ 1 for those without bacterial coinfection).[18]

16.9.4 Length of Stay

Pulmonary bacterial coinfection may increase the length of hospital stay of children with respiratory viral infections. In a study of children admitted to German PICU with severe influenza infection during the pre-pandemic influenza seasons 2005–2008, those with bacterial coinfection stayed twice as long in PICU as the other influenza patients.[22] A North American study of children hospitalized with CAP found that twice as many children with mixed viral/bacterial pathogens stayed more than 5 days in hospital than those with only viral pathogens (59% vs. 31%; $p = 0.001$).[9]

16.10 WHEN IS ANTIBIOTIC TREATMENT INDICATED OR JUSTIFIED?

The answer lies in the balance of the risk of pulmonary bacterial coinfection (or risk of not diagnosing it), severity of disease, and the patient setting.

Most children with respiratory viral infections do not need antibiotics. Prescribing antibiotics may indeed be harmful as they have adverse effects and may lead to an increase in antibiotic resistance. It can be difficult to identify which children with respiratory viral infections may benefit from antibiotics due to the challenges of diagnosing bacterial respiratory infections in children.

Some experts caution that the level of antibiotic prescribing in patients with influenza is seriously out of proportion to the number of bacterial infections that actually occur.[29] Reports show that prescription of antibiotics in children hospitalized with viral bronchiolitis is common—with incidences of 34–99% reported.[21] Studies show that in otherwise healthy infants admitted to PICU with RSV infection, bacteremia, urinary tract infection, and meningitis are uncommon. Although bacterial pneumonia in this cohort may be more prevalent, over-diagnosis is common.[17] Some are shocked by this indiscriminate antimicrobial use and state that avoiding unjustified antibiotic use is of paramount importance in order to decrease worldwide development of resistance.[30] So, the tug of war between the over-prescription of antibiotics and the potential sequelae associated with bacterial coinfection in children continues to stoke up debate.

For most children with viral respiratory tract infection or bronchiolitis the traditional doctrine against 'blind' antibiotics should hold fast, especially in resource-rich settings. In the resource-limited environment where experience and studies of CAP demonstrate a high incidence of mixed viral/bacterial pneumonia and the dire consequences of missing bacterial infections, the World Health Organization (WHO) guidelines recommend antibiotics for children with severe and very severe CAP (see Table 16.2).[31–33]

TABLE 16.2
World Health Organization Guidelines/Recommendations for Resource-Limited Countries for Antibiotic Treatment of Children with Severe and Very Severe CAP

Severe CAP	Benzylpenicillin IM or IV for at least 3 days—when improving switch to oral amoxicillin for a total treatment course of 5 days
	If not improved within 48 h or deteriorates—look for complications and treat (high-dose amoxicillin–clavulanic acid with or without a macrolide)
	If no complications—switch to chloramphenicol 75 mg/kg/day IM or IV until clinical improvement, then continue oral treatment for a total course of 10 days
Very severe CAP	Standard therapy: Ampicillin IM or IV and gentamicin IM or IV for 5 days
	If clinically the child responds well—complete treatment with oral amoxicillin plus IM gentamicin for an additional 5 days
	Alternative therapies: (i) Chloramphenicol IM or IV until clinical improvement, then continue orally for a total treatment course of 10 days; (ii) Ceftriaxone IM or IV once daily for 10 days
	Treatment if not improving after 48 h of standard or alternative therapies: gentamicin IM or IV and cloxacillin or dicloxacillin or flucloxacillin or oxacillin. When clinically improves—continue cloxacillin (or dicloxacillin) for a total treatment course of 3 weeks

Source: Adapted from World Health Organization. Pocket Book of Hospital Care for Children. Guidelines for the Management of Common Illnesses with Limited Resources. *WHO Press* 2005; 72–81; From Thorburn K, Riordan A. *Expert Rev. Anti Infect. Ther.* 2012; **10**: 909–16. With permission.

Note: IM = intramuscular; IV = intravenous.

In cases where there is clinical evidence (or suspicion) of pulmonary bacterial coinfection, it is generally accepted that antibiotic treatment is indicated as reflected in national guidelines.[8,34] Insightful clinicians will acknowledge the quandary and lack of diagnostic gold standards in clinically differentiating the solely viral, only bacterial, and mixed viral/bacterial coinfection respiratory tract infections.[7,33]

There is a paucity of pediatric studies on biochemical markers of bacterial infection to assist the clinician in this regard. It is suggested that in children with pneumonia and a C-reactive protein (CRP) greater than 60 mg/L, a bacterial cause is likely.[35] However, a CRP below this cut-off should not in itself be a reason to withhold antibiotics. Some pediatric studies have found CRP to be unhelpful in identifying/differentiating those with bacterial pulmonary coinfection in children ventilated with severe RSV bronchiolitis.[12,13,18] Adult studies have shown the usefulness of procalcitonin (PCT) in enabling rational antibiotic prescribing in CAP and on intensive care.[36] The adult studies found that PCT levels may give a clue as to etiology, as patients with typical bacterial infection have higher PCT levels than patients with atypical and viral etiologies. Similar studies of biochemical markers/indicators of bacterial infection in children are needed to help pediatricians identify children with respiratory infections who might benefit from antibiotics.[37]

For children in respiratory failure with a severe viral infection and/or severe viral bronchiolitis/pneumonia, especially those requiring PICU admission and mechanical ventilation, empirical antibiotic treatment would seem justified initially.[1,5,12,18,33,34]

Tracheobronchial sampling on PICU admission or intubation; commencing empirical antibiotic cover; then rationalizing their continuation or discontinuation after reviewing clinical progress, inflammatory markers, and subsequent microbiology results have been advocated. In Alder Hey Children's Hospital co-amoxiclav is used as the initial "empirical antibiotic" in this patient group as it would cover the common potential respiratory bacterial pathogens—*Streptococcus pneumoniae, Staphylococcus aureus, Haemophilus influenzae*, and *Moraxella catarrhalis*. Choice of empiric antibiotic regimens would be influenced by the local potential pathogen profile (e.g., to cover MRSA if locally prevalent), and risk factors like preexisting immunocompromise, chronic lung disease, or hospital-acquired infection.[8] The need for antibiotics should be reviewed 48 h after they are started to see whether continued use is justified.

Further prospective studies in this domain are needed. For example, a randomized controlled trial investigating the impact of empirical antibiotics in the subgroup of children with respiratory failure due to viral bronchiolitis would be informative and instructive. It certainly would influence PICU antibiotic practice internationally. To achieve the required sample size such a study would undoubtedly need to be multi-centered.

16.11 MIGHT ANTIVIRAL STRATEGIES IMPACT ON PULMONARY BACTERIAL COINFECTION?

The use of antiviral treatment might impact on the risk of bacterial infection in children with respiratory viral illness. However, this has not been shown in clinical practice. A retrospective study of children with chronic medical conditions who were given oseltamivir within 1 day of the diagnosis of influenza did not find a decrease in pneumonia nor otitis media. There was a significant reduction in the risks of other respiratory illnesses and hospitalization.[38]

An effective vaccination to prevent the primary viral infection that predisposes to the bacterial coinfection would be a desirable preventive approach. Seasonal influenza vaccination may help diminish influenza infections. Over the next 5–10 years, there may be a chance of ascertaining whether improved uptake of seasonal influenza vaccination decreases the number of severe cases. An effective RSV vaccine is still awaited, with clinical trials of RSV vaccines currently in progress.

16.12 CONCLUSIONS

- There is a general paucity of studies addressing the field of pulmonary bacterial coinfection with viral respiratory infections in children.
- The incidence of pulmonary bacterial coinfection in children hospitalized with a viral respiratory infection can vary widely from under 1% to 59%.
- For the same patient group admitted to PICU and/or requiring ventilatory support the reported incidence is 9–39%.
- There is not a widely accepted gold standard for the diagnosis of bacterial pneumonia in children, let alone pulmonary bacterial coinfection or secondary bacterial pneumonia.
- Viral infection can predispose to pulmonary bacterial coinfection on two fronts—weakening of the body's physical barrier (the respiratory epithelium), thereby enhancing bacterial entry and altering immune responses.
- Whether treatment (or empiric "cover") with antibiotics are indicated or justified lies in the balance of risk of pulmonary bacterial coinfection (or risk of not diagnosing it), severity of disease, and the patient setting.
- The benefit of antiviral treatment to decrease the risk of bacterial coinfection in children with respiratory viral illness has not been shown in clinical practice.
- Effective vaccination to prevent the primary viral infection prevents the disease that predisposes to bacterial coinfection, and is championed as the panacea.

REFERENCES

1. Randolph AG, Vaughn F, Sullivan R et al. Critically ill children during the 2009–2010 influenza pandemic in the United States. *Pediatrics* 2011; **128**: e1450–8.
2. Finelli L, Fiore A, Dhara R et al. Influenza-associated pediatric mortality in the United States: Increase of *Staphylococcus aureus* coinfection. *Pediatrics* 2008; **122**: 805–11.
3. Hall CB, Weinberg GA, Iwane MK et al. The burden of respiratory syncytial virus infection in young children. *N. Engl. J. Med.* 2009; **360**: 588–98.
4. Nair H, Nokes DJ, Gessner BD et al. Global burden of acute lower respiratory infections due to respiratory syncytial virus in young children: A systematic review and meta-analysis. *Lancet* 2010; **375**: 1545–55.
5. Yogev R. Respiratory syncytial virus, antibiotics, and the critical care dilemma. *Pediatr. Crit. Care Med.* 2011; **11**: 434–6.
6. Thorburn K, Riordan A. Pulmonary bacterial coinfection in infants and children with viral respiratory infection. *Expert Rev. Anti Infect. Ther.* 2012; **10**: 909–16.
7. Lynch T, Bialy L, Kellner JD et al. A systemic review on the diagnosis of pediatric bacterial pneumonia: When gold is bronze. *PLoS ONE* 2010; **5**: e11989.
8. Harris M, Clark J, Coote N et al. British Thoracic Society of Standards of Care Committee. British Thoracic Society guidelines for the management of community acquired pneumonia in childhood: Update. *Thorax* 2011; **56** (Suppl 2): ii1–23.
9. Michelow IC, Olsen K, Lozano J et al. Epidemiology and clinical characteristics of community-acquired pneumonia in hospitalized children. *Pediatrics* 2004; **113**: 701–7.
10. Nascimento-Carvalho CM, Ribeiro CT, Cardosa MR et al. The role of respiratory viral infections among children hospitalized for community-acquired pneumonia in a developing country. *Pediatr. Infect. Dis. J.* 2008; **27**: 939–41.
11. Hishiki H, Ishiwada N, Fukasawa C et al. Incidence of bacterial coinfection with respiratory syncytial virus bronchopulmonary infection in paediatric inpatients. *J. Infect. Chemother* 2011; **17**: pp.87–90.
12. Thorburn K, Harigopal S, Reddy V, Taylor N, van Saene HFK. High incidence of pulmonary bacterial co-infection in children with severe respiratory syncytial virus (RSV) bronchiolitis. *Thorax* 2006; **61**: 611–15.
13. Thorburn K, Shetty N, Darbyshire AP. Concomitant bacterial pneumonia and empirical antibiotics in severe respiratory syncytial virus infection. *Pediatr. Crit. Care Med.* 2011; **12**: 119.
14. Eriksson CO, Graham DA, Uyeki TM, Randolph AG. Risk factors for mechanical ventilation in U.S. children hospitalized with seasonal influenza and 2009 pandemic influenza A. *Pediatr. Crit. Care Med.* 2012; **13**: 625–31.

often in mixed infections than others, for example, HBoV1, which has been detected with other viruses in up to 78% of cases.[14] HRV seems to be of particular interest as it is the most prevalent virus in respiratory illnesses, even in the first years of life,[15,16] being associated with severe acute bronchiolitis.[17]

Concerning community-acquired pneumonia, several studies suggest that codetection with bacteria (most commonly *Streptococcus pneumoniae*) increases the morbidity and mortality of patients with influenza,[18] but viral coinfection has also been correlated with illness severity.[19,20] Recently, Marcos et al.[21] showed in their study that 12% of A/H1N1-positive adults with confirmed clinical pneumonia had evidence of coinfection with other respiratory viruses, correlating with a longer hospitalization, possibly reflecting a more severe clinical course. Prospective studies incorporating a more comprehensive prognostic assessment and cell cultures, in addition to quantitative polymerase chain reaction (PCR) to diagnose active codetections, will help to clarify the clinical relevance of multiple respiratory viral infections in children and adults.

The aims of this chapter are to summarize current knowledge on mixed viral infections regarding recent epidemiological studies and to describe the potential impact of coinfection on disease outcomes.

17.2 MAIN VIRAL CODETECTION

17.2.1 RSV AND HMPV

In 2001, HMPV was described as the third human pathogenic member of the *Paramyxovirinae* family, besides RSV and PIVs, causing respiratory disease.[2] HMPV and RSV infections occur worldwide with a broad clinical spectrum from a mild to severe and sometimes life-threatening infection.[22–29] Single infections of these two viruses are mostly related to bronchiolitis among children under 5 years of age, but they are also described in cases of otitis media, flu-like syndrome, asthma exacerbation, and recently in community-acquired pneumonia.[20,30–35] Several studies have acknowledged the possibility of multiple infections in RSV bronchiolitis.[36,37] The incidence of dual respiratory viral infections varies from 10% to 30% in hospitalized infants with bronchiolitis[7,38–43] and may have an impact on the severity of the disease.[7,44–46] A study performed in a pediatric hospital in France between 2003 and 2005 showed a significant correlation between dual viral infections and increased severity among 180 children hospitalized for bronchiolitis. Children coinfected with RSV and HRV were at a 2.7 times higher risk for admission to the pediatric intensive care unit than those singly infected.[7] This observation was confirmed in other clinical studies showing a correlation between coinfection and predisposition to severe infection and a higher risk of admission to the pediatric intensive care unit.[44–46] However, numerous studies describing coinfections of RSV/HMPV report no clinical differences among patients with single and multiple infections. Such differences include the severity of disease, clinical signs of infection, intensity, and duration of hospital stays.[42,43,47–53] In particular, the study by Woensel et al.[50] showed no coinfection with RSV and HMPV in 30 mechanically ventilated children hospitalized for severe bronchiolitis. Another study revealed that RSV monoinfected patients had longer hospitalization and higher hypoxia ($P < 0.001$) than HMPV coinfected children.[43] Further studies need to be carried out for a better understanding of the interaction between RSV and HMPV and the clinical differences between single and multiple respiratory viral infections. Some other respiratory viruses in association with HMPV or RSV have been described in the literature. The coinfection of HMPV and the severe acute respiratory syndrome (SARS) coronavirus is a recent example. In Canada, HMPVs were codetected in respiratory specimens from five out of nine patients with the severe acute respiratory syndrome coronavirus (SARS-CoV).[54] Another epidemiological study revealed that among 48 patients who had contracted SARS during the SARS outbreak in the Prince of Wales Hospital in Hong Kong in early March 2003, 25 (52.1%) were also infected with HMPV.[55] In one clinical case report, HMPV RNA was identified postmortem in the brain and lung tissue of a child infected with SARS CoV. This fatal encephalitis may have been correlated with HMPV infection[32] but the synergy between HMPV and SARS was not confirmed in the *in vivo* experimental study.[56] In addition to SARS-associated coronaviruses, four non-SARS-related HCoV (HCoV, 229EOC43, HKU1, and NL63) are recognized as common respiratory pathogens, but a recent study showed that they were not coinfected with HMPV or RSV.[57] In addition, several studies evaluated HMPV coinfections with other respiratory viruses, but no sufficient data were obtained to conclude on the epidemiology or the association with clinical disease (Table 17.1).[43,58,59]

17.2.2 Coronaviruses

Coronaviruses (HCoV) are large, enveloped RNA viruses of both human medical and veterinary importance.[60] Six human HCoVs are known to infect the human respiratory tract: HCoV-OC43, HCoV-229E,[56] SARS-CoV,[56] HCoV-NL63,[3,61] HCoV-HKU,[14] and the recently discovered HCoV-EMC.[62] Coronaviruses are mainly associated with bronchiolitis and pneumonia.[4,63,64] HCoV-NL63 and HCoV-OC43 infections frequently occur in early childhood, more often than HCoV-HKU1 and HCoV-229E infections.[65] The occurrence of coinfection with HCoV-NL[63] and other respiratory viruses, including other HCoV, RSV, PIV, influenza A and B viruses, and HMPV, has been reported among patients with LRTIs.[43,60,66–68] In 2005, Van der Hoek et al.[69] identified HCoV-NL63 in a considerable number of nasal aspirates of children under 3 years of age with LRTIs. With an overall occurrence of 5.2%, this virus is the third most-frequently detected pathogen in this patient group. It was also observed that HCoV-NL63 coinfection with RSV-A occurred predominantly in hospitalized patients, in contrast to HCoV-NL63 coinfections with PIV3 that were exclusively present in the outpatient group, suggesting an impact of HCoV-NL63 on disease severity during coinfection. This hypothesis correlated with the study of Dominguez et al. in 2009, showing retrospective data results from a 1-year study on the epidemiology and clinical associations of the four human non-SARS HCoV among children with LRTIs.[70] It was observed that HCoV-NL63-positive patients were nearly twice as likely to be hospitalized ($P = 0.02$) and to have an LRTI ($P = 0.04$) than HCoV-OC43-positive patients. This suggested the possibility that HCoV may play a role in gastrointestinal and central nervous system disease. HCoV-positive specimens were also PCR positive for other respiratory viruses, mainly HMPV, but none of them were positive for HBoV.

A recent study showed that coinfection of HCoV-OC43 and other respiratory viruses in children with LRTIs did not lead to increased rates of hospitalization, admission to intensive care unit, or death.[71] To further understand the epidemiology of ALRTIs in children, a 3-year study conducted in China among 810 children revealed that in 49 HCoV-HKU1- and HCoV-NL63-positive samples, 36 (73.47%) were coinfected with at least one other virus, most commonly HRV (14 cases) and RSV (11 cases).[72] With similar objectives, Kuypers et al. frequently detected coronaviruses in association with other respiratory viruses, particularly RSVs, both in healthy children and in children with ARIs. Similar findings of frequent viral coinfections have been reported for HCoV-NL63[73,74] and HKU1.[75] Similarly, Gaunt et al.[76] observed that in 42% and 38% of infections with HCoV-OC43 and HCoV-HKU1 among all age populations with either upper respiratory tract infections (URTIs) or LRTIs, other respiratory viruses were codetected, most commonly RSVs. In this study, no differences in clinical outcome were observed for those coinfected with RSV and coronavirus compared with those singly infected with either virus. This suggests that RSV presumably facilitates coronavirus infections (or vice versa) without exacerbating morbidity.

In September 2012, a novel coronavirus was isolated from a patient in Saudi Arabia who had died of an acute respiratory illness and renal failure. The clinical presentation was reminiscent of the outbreak caused by the SARS-CoV exactly 10 years ago that involved over 8000 cases.[77] Until now, no description of mixed viral respiratory infections involving HCoV-EMC has been described in the literature (Table 17.2).

TABLE 17.1
Recent Epidemiological Studies Highlighting HMPV or RSV in Mixed Viral Respiratory Infections

Reference	Country	Population	Tested Pathogens	Diagnostic Method	Observation (Codetection)	Correlation with Severity?
Semple et al.[44]	United Kingdom	196 infants under 2 years of age with bronchiolitis	HMPV, RSV	PCR	10% rate of detection of HMPV among RSV-infected infants admitted to the general ward. 72% rate of detection among RSV-infected infants admitted to the PICU	YES
Richard et al.[7]	France	180 hospitalized infants with bronchiolitis	IV-A/B,RSV-A/B,PIV-1/2/3/4,HCoV NL63,HRV,EV	PCR/virus antigen/virus culture	25.4% of total codetected pathogens. 34.1% codetection among children admitted to the PICU versus 15.4% among children in the short-term unit. The pathogens most involved in coinfections were RSV (81.8%) and RV (50%)	YES
Canducci et al.[43]	Italy	322 children with acute respiratory infections	HMPV, RSV, HCoV 229E/ OC43/ NL63/ HKU1,HBoV	PCR	6.5% of total codetected pathogens. RSV-HMPV codetections were observed in less severe cases than those RSV singly infected. The pathogens most involved in coinfections were RSV(23.3%) and HMPV (14.4%)	NO
Brand et al.[11]	The Netherlands	142 children under 2 years with bronchiolitis	IV-A/B, RSV, PIV-1/2/3/4, HMPV, HRV, HAdV, HCoV 229E/OC43, HBoV, EV, PV	PCR	41% of total codetected pathogens. Disease severity in children with bronchiolitis is not associated with mixed viral respiratory infections. The most associations were RSV-RV (41%) and RSV-HAdV (16%)	NO
Wolf et al.[48]	Israel	1296 children under 5 years of age with community-acquired alveolar pneumonia (CAAP)	IV-A/B, RSV, PIV-1/2/3/4, HMPV,HAdV	PCR/IF/viruses culture	3.2% of HMPV-negative children were coinfected by other respiratory viruses. 1.8% HMPV-positive samples were coinfected, mostly with RSV.	NO

TABLE 17.2
Recent Epidemiological Studies Highlighting Coronaviruses in Mixed Viral Respiratory Infections

Reference	Country	Population	Tested Pathogens	Diagnostic Method	Observation (Codetection)	Correlation with Severity?
van der Hoek et al.[3]	Germany	940 children under 3 years with LRTI	FluA, FluB, HPIV, RSV, HCoV NL63	PCR	59% of total coinfection, mostly represented by HCoV-NL63 in association with RSV-A. This codetection occurred predominantly in hospitalized patients (61%) rather than in the outpatient group (29%). In contrast, HCoV-NL63 coinfections with PIV3 were exclusively present in the outpatient group (16%)	N/A
Dare et al.[67]	Thailand	1156 patients with pneumonia, 513 outpatients, and 281 controls	IV-A/B, RSV, PIV-1/2/3, HRV, HAdV, HCoV 229E/OC43/NL63/HKU1,	qPCR	30.5% of all HCoV-positive samples were codetected with other respiratory viruses. Among the patients with pneumonia, 17 (26.6%) of the 64 who were infected with HCoV had a viral coinfection. Among the outpatients and control patients with HCoV infections, seven (58.3%) of 12 and one (16.7%) of six, respectively, were coinfected with another virus	N/A
Minosse et al.[60]	Italy	433 hospitalized adult patients with LRTI	IV-A/B, RSV, PIV-1/2/3, HMPV, HRV, HAdV, HCoV 229E/OC43/NL-63	PCR	6.5% of all positive samples were also positive for more than one virus. 33% were coinfected with NL63-HRV and 10% were coinfected with NL63-HADV	N/A
Gaunt et al.[76]	Scotland	11,661 patients of all ages	IV-A/B, RSV, PIV-1/2/3/4, HMPV, HRV, HAdV, HCoV 229E/OC43, HBoV, EV, PV	PCR	11–41% of coronavirus-positive samples tested positive for at least one other respiratory virus. In 42% and 38% of infections with HCoV-OC43 and HCoV-HKU1, other respiratory viruses were codetected, most commonly RSV	No
Jin et al.[72]	China	813 patients under 14 years of age with acute respiratory tract infections	IV-A/B, RSV, PIV-1/2/3, HMPV, HCoV HKU1/NL63	RT-PCR	34.4% of positive samples were coinfected with one other respiratory virus. Of all HCoV-HKU1- and HCoV-NL63-positive samples, 73.47% were coinfected with at least one other virus, most commonly HRV and RSV	N/A

17.2.3 Bocaviruses

Four species of HBoV1–4 have been identified since 2005 and classified in the *Bocavirus* genus (family *Parvoviridae*, subfamily *Parvovirinae*).[5,78–80] Several reports have documented that HBoV1 is prevalent in respiratory tract samples. Although many studies have reported HBoV1 asymptomatic carriers, this virus has been shown to cause respiratory tract diseases.[5,81,82] HBoV2 has mainly been detected in fecal samples, but it has also been linked to gastroenteritis.[79,83,84] HBoV3 and HBoV4 have also recently been detected in fecal samples,[79,80] although no link to the disease has been established for these two species. In a recent study performed in China between March 2008 and July 2010, nasal aspirates from 1238 hospitalized children with LRTI in Beijing Children's Hospital were tested for HBoV1–4 by nested PCR.[85] The clinical diagnoses of patients providing HBoV-positive samples included pneumonia (63.1%), bronchitis (14.9%), bronchopneumonia (12.8%), and acute asthmatic bronchopneumonia (9.2%). It was observed that 85.1% of the total HBoV-positive samples were coinfected with additional respiratory viruses. HRV (44.3%), RSV (32.1%), and PIV (18.3%) were the most predominant pathogens in HBoV-1-positive samples. Specifically, HBoV is commonly detected in association with other respiratory viruses,[86–88] both in symptomatic and asymptomatic subjects.[58,72,89–96] These controversial observations can be explained by prolonged HBoV DNA shedding in the respiratory tract.[92,97,98] Moreover, several studies have demonstrated that HBoV DNA identification in respiratory tract samples is not proof of a primary infection.[88,99–101] Observations of HBoV, both in asymptomatic and symptomatic patients, lead us to question the role of HBoV as a real pathogen, and the significance of a PCR-positive test.

Despite this challenging molecular diagnostic problem, difficulties remain to clearly correlate clinical observations with the impact of single or multiinfections with HBoV.[89,102–105] The implication of HBoV in pneumonia has been increasingly described. In a recent study, 64% of children with pneumonia had serological evidence of HBoV infection and coinfection with another virus. Children coinfected had more wheezing than children singly infected.[88] In a Thai pneumonia study, 40 (91%) out of 44 children younger than 5 years with pneumonia were infected with HBoV and coinfected with other respiratory viruses.[87] Moreover, in a comprehensive virological study of childhood pneumonia, HBoV was the main respiratory virus codetected in 33 (69%) out of 48 episodes, followed by influenza viruses (13/25; 52%) and RSV (34/67; 51%). Despite the results obtained from the study of Don et al.,[101] showing serological evidence of an acute HBoV infection in 12% of children with pneumonia, the clinical relevance of detection of several viruses in pneumonia, as well as the correlation with severe illness, remains uncertain (Table 17.3).[94,106,107]

17.2.4 Rhinoviruses

HRV has long been considered to be a benign virus causing mild URTIs, but although there is evidence that HRV is also involved in acute lower respiratory tract infections (ALRIs)[108] and more specifically in bronchiolitis,[7] its role in pneumonia has not yet been well established.[109,110] HRV is frequently found as an asymptomatic carriage.[17,111,112] It seems that the recently discovered and potentially more pathogenic HRV-C[113,114] is correlated with the severity of ARIs.[115,116] In HRV-C studies conducted so far, no clear clinical difference has been noted between patients with single or mixed HRV-C infections.[82,117,118] In a recent study on viral pneumonia etiologies, HRV was the most commonly identified virus (23.6%), followed by PIV (20.8%), HMPV (18.1%), influenza virus (16.7%), and RSV (13.9%).[119] Most HRV-C coinfections involve RSV.[117,120–122] However, in one large study, HRVs were statistically the least likely virus of 17 examined to be associated with coinfections (Table 17.4).[123]

17.2.5 Influenza Viruses

The term "influenza-like illnesses" is used by the scientific community, because influenza infections can be clinically indistinguishable from diseases caused by other respiratory viruses, such as

TABLE 17.3
Recent Epidemiological Studies Highlighting Bocaviruses in Mixed Viral Respiratory Infections

Reference	Country	Population	Tested Pathogens	Diagnostic Method	Observation (Codetection)	Correlation with Severity?
Christenson et al. [91]	Norway	376 children with LRTI and URTI	IV-A/B, RSV, PIV-1/2/3, HMPV, HRV, HAdV, HCoV 229E/OC43/NL63, HBoV, EV	qPCR	78% of the 376 samples tested were coinfected with one other respiratory virus. Coinfections were detected in 78% of the 45 HBoV-positive samples mostly with RSV	N/A
Wang et al.[103]	China	817 children with respiratory tract infection	IV-A/B, RSV, PIV-1/2/3, HMPV, HRV, HAdV, HCoV 229E/OC43/NL63/HKU1, HBoV	PCR	51% of the total positive samples were coinfected with one other respiratory virus. HBoV causes systemic infection, induces immune responses, and may play a crucial role in the respiratory disease of children, often being associated with coinfection	N/A
Don et al.[101]	Italy	124 children aged 1 month to 15 years with presumptive pneumonia	IV-A/B, RSV, PIV-1/2/3, HMPV, HAdV, HBoV	Serology	25% of the total PCR-positive samples were coinfected by one other respiratory pathogen. Single HBoV infections were related to more severe pneumonia	YES
Fry et al.[87]	Thailand	512 outpatients and 280 control patients	IV-A/B, RSV, PIV-1/2/3, HMPV, HRV, HAdV, HCoV 229E/OC43/NL63/HKU1, HBoV	Culture/PCR	83% of the HBoV-infected patients with pneumonia were coinfected with other viruses. HBoV-rhinovirus was the most common viral coinfection, with HBoV-RSV and HBoV-HPIVbeing the next most common ones	YES
Cilla et al.[19]	Spain	315 children less than 3 years of age with community-acquired pneumonia	IV-A/B/C, RSV A/B, PIV-1/2/3/4, HMPV, HRV, HAdV, HCoV NL63, HBoV	PCR	27% of the episodes of childhood community-acquired pneumonia PCR positive were coinfected with one other respiratory pathogen, a percentage that increased to 35% in the cold months of the year. They observed a greater severity in viral coinfections than in single viral infections due to the greater frequency of hospitalization in coinfected patients	YES

TABLE 17.4
Recent Epidemiological Studies Highlighting Rhinoviruses in Mixed Viral Respiratory Infections

Reference	Country	Population	Tested Pathogens	Diagnostic Method	Observation (Codetection)	Correlation with Severity?
Miller et al.[117]	United States	1123 children under 5 years of age	IV-A/B, RSV, PIV-1/2/3/4, HMPV, HRV group A/B/C,	PCR	15.6% of children infected with an HRV were coinfected with another virus. Other viruses included HRSV (7.8%), HMPV (3.6%), influenza (2.4%), and HPIV (2.4%). More coinfections were detected with HRV group A (23.4%) than with HRV group C (10.4%, $P = 0.037$). HRV group C might play an important role in asthma exacerbation	N/A
Choi et al.[119]	Korea	198 adult patients with CAP or with health-care CAP	IV-A/B, RSV A/B, PIV-1/2/3/4, HMPV, HRV, HAdV, HCoV 229E/OC43/NL63/HKU1, HBoV, EV	PCR Culture	12.5% of patients with identified viral pathogens were coinfected with another virus. HRV was the most codetected pathogen followed by influenza viruses and RSV	YES
Xiang et al.[121]	China	258 children (167 boys and 91 girls) who had lower acute RTIs	IV-A/B, RSV A/B, PIV-1/2/3/4, HMPV, HRV, HAdV, HCoV 229E/OC43/NL63/HKU1, HBoV, EV	PCR	HRV-C was singly detected in 14 patients. In the remaining 8-HRV-C-positive, seven were codetected with RSV and one with HPIV-3. HCoV NL63 was also codetected in one HRV-C-positive sample	N/A
Linsuwanon et al.[122]	Thailand	289 infants and young children for acute bronchiolitis or CAP	IV-A/B, RSV A/B, PIV-1/2/3/4, HMPV, HRV, HAdV, HBoV, WUPyV/KIPyV	PCR	The frequency of coinfection of HRV group C with other respiratory viral pathogens was approximately 40%. RSV was codetected with HRV (all species) in 13.8%	N/A
Greer et al.[123]	Australia	1247 children with symptoms of ARTI	IV-A, RSV, PIV-1/2/3/4, HMPV, HRV, HAdV, HCoV, HBoV, WUPyV/KIPyV	PCR	HRVs were the most commonly detected virus group and were involved in the highest total number of codetections, being found with another virus in 78 specimens (23.6% of HRV detections). However, a higher proportion of HBoV, RSV, HHAdV, HCoV, HEV, and PyV positives were involved in codetections (29.6–73.5%)	N/A

those that cause the common cold.[124] ILI can be related to seasonal A and B influenza viruses, to the pandemic influenza A/H1N1v virus strain, and to a large number of common or newly discovered respiratory viruses.[2,125–128] The predominant pathogens of ILI are typically influenza viruses, which annually cause recurring epidemics affecting an estimated 5–15% of the world's population with URTIs.[1,129] In a study by Renois et al.,[124] the use of RT-PCR DNA microarray systems resulted in demonstrating that 10.5% of the infections in the upper respiratory tracts of ILI patients were mixed, and of these, 50% implicated HRVs, followed by PIV and HCoVs. It has been hypothesized that picornaviruses may be a factor in promoting clinical illness, by functioning additively or synergistically in the pathogenesis of lower respiratory syndromes, such as bronchiolitis.[130] Therefore, the preexisting asymptomatic HRV airway infections may enhance the risk of ILI. The role of HRV as a cofactor was recently examined by Pascalis et al.[131] during the A/H1N1v epidemic in Reunion Island through a prospective population-based cohort study on 125 households, of which at least one member had developed symptoms of ILI. Out of the 194 individuals who tested positive for at least one respiratory virus, that is, pandemic A/H1N1 (pH1N1) or noninfluenza respiratory viruses (NIRVs), 31 had evidence of viral coinfection. Coinfection included pH1N1 for only 11 individuals, HRV in four, HCoV in five, and PIV in two. All these findings suggest a lack of interplay between NIRVs (especially HRV) and pH1N1, and suggest that competition may have played a role in the loss of transmission of the pandemic *Influenza* virus. Similar observations based on epidemiological data have been reported previously.[132–134] Only a few studies have investigated the full range of mixed respiratory viruses competing in ILIs during the pH1N1 pandemic.[124,133,135–138] Through a clinical and virological survey conducted in adult and pediatric patients with ILI, Schnepf et al.[135] highlighted a high frequency of noninfluenza viruses during the preepidemic period of a flu alert. Of the 413 endonasal swabs from patients with ILI, 68 samples (16.5%) were positive for H1N1v. Other respiratory pathogens were also detected in 19.1% of positive respiratory samples. The most prevalent viruses codetected with H1N1v were HRV (62.6%), followed by PIVs (24.2%) and adenovirus (5.3%) (Table 17.5).

17.2.6 Polyomaviruses

In 2007, two new human polyomaviruses, KI polyomavirus (KIPyV) and WU polyomavirus (WUPyV), were identified in respiratory specimens from patients with respiratory illnesses.[139,140] Since then, KIPyV and WUPyV have been frequently detected in respiratory specimens, especially those from children with respiratory symptoms and from patients coinfected with a respiratory virus.[141–151] The first retrospective studies of respiratory specimens in Sweden and Australia reported a KIPyV prevalence of 1% and 2.5%, respectively.[139,141] Studies conducted in Australia and the United States showed a WUPyV prevalence in respiratory specimens of 3% and 0.7%, respectively.[140] However, KIPyV and WUPyV were detected at similar rates in specimens from symptomatic patients and in persons without respiratory symptoms,[144,146,150,151] suggesting that these viruses might not cause respiratory illness in immunocompetent children. Although it has been suggested that KIPyV and WUPyV might be major pathogens in immunosuppressed patients,[141,152–154] recently, Kuypers et al.[155] did not discover a clear role for these viruses as respiratory pathogens that cause typical upper and lower respiratory tract symptoms. High rates of coinfection with other respiratory pathogens were described in several studies, leading to a lack of understanding of the implication of these viruses in respiratory tract infections.[139–142,144,148,154,156] In Southern China, a recent study among children with respiratory infection aimed at investigating the prevalence and clinical characteristics of WUPyV infection.[157] Of the specimens collected from 771 children with acute respiratory tract infection admitted for hospitalization, 15 tested positive for WUPyV. Four of these 15 were coinfected with RSV, one was coinfected with an adenovirus, and one was coinfected with an HRV, respectively. Patients with WUPyV infection predominantly displayed cough, moderate fever, and wheezing, and were diagnosed with pneumonia ($n = 8$), bronchiolitis ($n = 4$), URTIs ($n = 2$), and bronchitis ($n = 1$). One patient developed

TABLE 17.5
Recent Epidemiological Studies Highlighting Influenza Viruses in Mixed Viral Respiratory Infections

Reference	Country	Population	Tested Pathogens	Diagnostic Method	Observation (Codetection)	Correlation with Severity?
Renois et al.[124]	France	56 adults and 39 children with ILIs	IV-A/B/C, IV-A/H1N1pdm09, RSV-A/B, PIV-1/2/3/4A/4B, HMPV A/B, HRV A/B/C, HAdV, HCoV 229E, HBoV, EV	RT-PCR	They described a few viral codetections with the A/H1N1v virus: three associations with HRV, one with RSV A, and one with HCoV 229E. Noninfluenza viruses were more codetected in ILI patients such as HRV and HPIV-1	NO
Pascalis et al.[131]	La Reunion	335 individuals (corresponding to 125 households with at least one member who had ILI)	IV-A/B, IV-A/H1N1pdm09, RSV-A/B, PIV-1/2/3/4, HMPV A/B, HRV, HAdV, HCoV 229E/NL63/229E/HKU1, HBoV 1/2/3/4, EV	RT-PCR	A/H1N1v-positive patients were less coinfected than A/H1N1-negative individuals, suggesting that NIRV coinfections during influenza epidemics may act as cofactors that contribute to shape an outbreak and modulate the attack rate	NO
Razajanatovo et al. (2011)	Madagascar	313 children and adults with ILI symptoms	IV-A/B, RSV-A/B, PIV-1/2/3, HMPV A/B, HRV, HAdV, HCoV 229E/NL63/229E/OC43, HBoV	RT-PCR/virus culture	Among all positive specimens, a single infection occurred in 166 (70.6%) outpatients while coinfections were detected in 69 (29.4%) outpatients. Analyses of coinfection pairs showed that HRVs with RSV or FLUAV are the most common paired viruses with 15 and 14 cases, respectively, followed by FLUA with RSV (eight cases) or HCoV-OC43 (five cases)	NO
Schnepf et al. [135]	France	413 children and adults with ILI symptoms	IV-A/B, IV-A/H5N1, RSV-A/B, PIV-1/2/3/4, HMPV, HRV, HAdV, HCoV 229E/NL63/229E, HBoV	RT-PCR	The frequency of viral coinfection was slightly higher in samples positive for H1N1v as compared to samples positive for other respiratory pathogens, but without significance. RHV was the more frequent copathogen in H1N1v- positive patients (13.2% [9/68])	NO
Casalegno et al.[133]	France	1456 infants with ILI	IV-A, HRV	RT-PCR	Few coinfection rates were detected between A/H1N1 and HRV (0.7%). This represented a 4.6% and 25.9% H1N1-positive relative frequency, considering the HRV-positive and HRV-negative specimens, respectively	NO

encephalitis, suggesting that WUPyV infection can cause acute respiratory tract infections with atypical symptoms with severe complications in children. However, in a few cases, KIPyV and WUPyV were the sole pathogens detected, despite wide testing performed for viruses, bacteria, and fungi (Table 17.6).[144,152]

17.3 CONCLUSION

Virology is probably one of the fields of microbiology where diagnostic capacities have evolved most extensively over the past 15 years. Traditional methods for direct pathogen detection still remain the gold standards, but molecular diagnostics have been refined, and are now increasingly used in clinical and epidemiological settings. This improvement has directly impacted our knowledge of the viral and bacterial etiologies of respiratory infections, and has led to significant advancements in health care. Some of these traditional techniques have even been significantly adapted to become less time consuming, more specific, and more sensitive through the use of rapid culture techniques, immunoenzymatic reactions, and so on.

The diagnosis of viral infections pursues several objectives. Most often, in a clinical setting, it is to prove the viral etiology of a suspected disease. The accurate identification of the viral pathogen is important to the extent that it determines the choice of treatment, its duration, its follow-up, and management. In most epidemiological studies on respiratory infections, molecular diagnostics reveal a large range of viruses as possible etiological agents. However, the significance of multiple infections remains unclear. Indeed, data on mixed viral infections are still controversial due to difficulties in establishing a causal relationship with disease severity. In addition, most molecular diagnostic methods rely on nucleic acid amplification by PCR, whose significance also remains controversial. Indeed, nucleic acid identification in nasopharyngeal samples does not always reveal a current infection, as several prior studies on the HBoV have noted. The term "co-infection," widely used in the literature, is sometimes a misnomer, because it refers to the physical presence of several pathogens in biological samples during infection. When diagnosing with a PCR, mixed viral positive detection in biological samples from asymptomatic individuals must be interpreted with caution. On the other hand, in several epidemiological studies, specific pathogens, such asHMPV, for example, are mainly identified in samples from symptomatic individuals, suggesting their role as real pathogens in respiratory infections. Therefore, there is a need to better describe respiratory infections and also to correlate molecular diagnosis with clinical features. Some clinical studies have highlighted mixed viral infections as a potential risk factor for severe respiratory diseases, and conversely, other studies have shown no correlation. Therefore, it is important to join the data collected from both clinical and updated molecular diagnostic tests to clarify a possible correlation with disease severity, which in turn may allow, in the long term, to reduce the use of antibiotics and to mitigate antibody resistance and nosocomial infections. Early, fast, and comprehensive detection of respiratory etiological agents is in the interest of public health, particularly for the control of epidemics. Indeed, recent studies point to the cocirculation of respiratory pathogens that may have an impact on seasonal outbreaks. Such an impact was demonstrated in recent studies on the cocirculation of human HRVs and influenza viruses.

Another important aspect of viral mixed infection concerns the predisposition to a subsequent bacterial superinfection, which is thought to occur through diverse mechanisms that encompass the disruption of the epithelial barrier, virus-induced immunomodulation, and viral production of cytokines and chemokines. The mechanisms of synergy between the pneumococcus and influenza virus have been well described, but there are a few data on the impact of other viruses. As several types of viruses are identified in biological samples, it is important to study their impact on superinfections by examining virus-induced innate and adaptive immune responses. However, some viruses appear to infect the host asymptomatically, suggesting that other factors are involved in the induction of the disease. Environmental and ecological host factors seem to be particularly important to understand the impact of mixed viral infections on disease severity.

77. Khan G. A novel coronavirus capable of lethal human infections: An emerging picture. *Virol J* 2013; **10**: 66.
78. Kapoor A, Slikas E, Simmonds P et al. A newly identified bocavirus species in human stool. *J Infect Dis* 2009; **199**: 196–200.
79. Arthur JL, Higgins GD, Davidson GP, Givney RC, Ratcliff RM. A novel bocavirus associated with acute gastroenteritis in Australian children. *PLoS Pathog* 2009; **5**: e1000391.
80. Kapoor A, Simmonds P, Slikas E et al. Human bocaviruses are highly diverse, dispersed, recombination prone, and prevalent in enteric infections. *J Infect Dis* 2010; **201**: 1633–43.
81. Kesebir D, Vazquez M, Weibel C et al. Human bocavirus infection in young children in the United States: Molecular epidemiological profile and clinical characteristics of a newly emerging respiratory virus. *J Infect Dis* 2006; **194**: 1276–82.
82. Lau SKP, Yip CCY, Que T-L et al. Clinical and molecular epidemiology of human bocavirus in respiratory and fecal samples from children in Hong Kong. *J Infect Dis* 2007; **196**: 986–93.
83. Chow BDW, Ou Z, Esper FP. Newly recognized bocaviruses (HBoV, HBoV2) in children and adults with gastrointestinal illness in the United States. *J Clin Virol* 2010; **47**: 143–7.
84. Han T-H, Kim C-H, Park S-H, Kim E-J, Chung J-Y, Hwang E-S. Detection of human bocavirus-2 in children with acute gastroenteritis in South Korea. *Arch Virol* 2009; **154**: 1923–7.
85. Guo L, Gonzalez R, Xie Z et al. Bocavirus in children with respiratory tract infections. *Emerg Infect Dis* 2011; **17**: 1775–7.
86. Schildgen O, Müller A, Allander T et al. Human bocavirus: Passenger or pathogen in acute respiratory tract infections? *Clin Microbiol Rev* 2008; **21**: 291–304, table of contents.
87. Fry AM, Lu X, Chittaganpitch M et al. Human bocavirus: A novel parvovirus epidemiologically associated with pneumonia requiring hospitalization in Thailand. *J Infect Dis* 2007; **195**: 1038–45.
88. Söderlund-Venermo M, Lahtinen A, Jartti T et al. Clinical assessment and improved diagnosis of bocavirus-induced wheezing in children, Finland. *Emerg Infect Dis* 2009; **15**: 1423–30.
89. Allander T, Jartti T, Gupta S et al. Human bocavirus and acute wheezing in children. *Clin Infect Dis* 2007; **44**: 904–10.
90. Ghietto LM, Cámara A, Zhou Y et al. High prevalence of human bocavirus 1 in infants with lower acute respiratory tract disease in Argentina, 2007–2009. *Braz J Infect Dis* 2012; **16**: 38–44.
91. Christenson K, Thorén FB, Bylund J. Analyzing cell death events in cultured leukocytes. In: Ashman RB, ed. *Leucocytes*. Totowa, NJ, Humana Press, 2012: 65–86.
92. Martin ET, Fairchok MP, Kuypers J et al. Frequent and prolonged shedding of bocavirus in young children attending daycare. *J Infect Dis* 2010; **201**: 1625–32.
93. Manning A, Russell V, Eastick K et al. Epidemiological profile and clinical associations of human bocavirus and other human parvoviruses. *J Infect Dis* 2006; **194**: 1283–90.
94. Calvo C, García-García ML, Blanco C et al. Multiple simultaneous viral infections in infants with acute respiratory tract infections in Spain. *J Clin Virol* 2008; **42**: 268–72.
95. Liu W-K, Chen D-H, Liu Q et al. Detection of human bocavirus from children and adults with acute respiratory tract illness in Guangzhou, southern China. *BMC Infect Dis* 2011; **11**: 345.
96. Bezerra PGM, Britto MCA, Correia JB et al. Viral and atypical bacterial detection in acute respiratory infection in children under five years. *PLoS One* 2011; **6**: e18928
97. Blessing K, Neske F, Herre U, Kreth H-W, Weissbrich B. Prolonged detection of human bocavirus DNA in nasopharyngeal aspirates of children with respiratory tract disease. *Pediatr Infect Dis J* 2009; **28**: 1018–9.
98. Von Linstow M-L, Høgh M, Høgh B. Clinical and epidemiologic characteristics of human bocavirus in Danish infants: Results from a prospective birth cohort study. *Pediatr Infect Dis J* 2008; **27**: 897–902.
99. Kantola K, Hedman L, Allander T et al. Serodiagnosis of human bocavirus infection. *Clin Infect Dis* 2008; **46**: 540–6.
100. Hedman L, Söderlund-Venermo M, Jartti T, Ruuskanen O, Hedman K. Dating of human bocavirus infection with protein-denaturing IgG-avidity assays—Secondary immune activations are ubiquitous in immunocompetent adults. *J Clin Virol* 2010; **48**: 44–8.
101. Don M, Söderlund-Venermo M, Valent F et al. Serologically verified human bocavirus pneumonia in children. *Pediatr Pulmonol* 2010; **45**: 120–6.
102. Ruuskanen O, Lahti E, Jennings LC, Murdoch DR. Viral pneumonia. *Lancet* 2011; **377**: 1264–75.
103. Wang K, Wang W, Yan H et al. Correlation between bocavirus infection and humoral response, and co-infection with other respiratory viruses in children with acute respiratory infection. *J Clin Virol* 2010; **47**: 148–55.
104. Gerna G, Piralla A, Campanini G, Marchi A, Stronati M, Rovida F. The human bocavirus role in acute respiratory tract infections of pediatric patients as defined by viral load quantification. *New Microbiol* 2007; **30**: 383–92.

105. Dina J, Nguyen E, Gouarin S et al. Development of duplex real-time PCR for detection of two DNA respiratory viruses. *J Virol Methods* 2009; **162**: 119–25.
106. Jennings LC, Anderson TP, Werno AM, Beynon KA, Murdoch DR. Viral etiology of acute respiratory tract infections in children presenting to hospital: Role of polymerase chain reaction and demonstration of multiple infections. *Pediatr Infect Dis J* 2004; **23**: 1003–7.
107. Midulla F, Scagnolari C, Bonci E et al. Respiratory syncytial virus, human bocavirus and rhinovirus bronchiolitis in infants. *Arch Dis Child* 2010; **95**: 35–41.
108. Papadopoulos NG, Bates PJ, Bardin PG et al. Rhinoviruses infect the lower airways. *J Infect Dis* 2000; **181**: 1875–84.
109. Broberg E, Niemelä J, Lahti E, Hyypiä T, Ruuskanen O, Waris M. Human rhinovirus C-associated severe pneumonia in a neonate. *J Clin Virol* 2011; **51**: 79–82.
110. Tapparel C, L'Huillier AG, Rougemont A-L, Beghetti M, Barazzone-Argiroffo C, Kaiser L. Pneumonia and pericarditis in a child with HRV-C infection: A case report. *J Clin Virol* 2009; **45**: 157–60.
111. Mackay IM. Human rhinoviruses: The cold wars resume. *J Clin Virol* 2008; **42**: 297–320.
112. Mermond S, Zurawski V, D'Ortenzio E et al. Lower respiratory infections among hospitalized children in New Caledonia: A pilot study for the pneumonia etiology research for child health project. *Clin Infect Dis* 2012; **54**: S180–9.
113. Lamson D, Renwick N, Kapoor V et al. MassTag polymerase-chain-reaction detection of respiratory pathogens, including a new rhinovirus genotype, that caused influenza-like illness in New York State during 2004–2005. *J Infect Dis* 2006; **194**: 1398–402.
114. Kaiser L, Aubert J-D, Pache J-C et al. Chronic rhinoviral infection in lung transplant recipients. *Am J Respir Crit Care Med* 2006; **174**: 1392–9.
115. Renwick N, Schweiger B, Kapoor V et al. A recently identified rhinovirus genotype is associated with severe respiratory-tract infection in children in Germany. *J Infect Dis* 2007; **196**: 1754–60.
116. Brownlee JW, Turner RB. New developments in the epidemiology and clinical spectrum of rhinovirus infections. *Curr Opin Pediatr* 2008; **20**: 67–71.
117. Miller EK, Edwards KM, Weinberg GA et al. A novel group of rhinoviruses is associated with asthma hospitalizations. *J Allergy Clin Immunol* 2009; **123**: 98–104.e1.
118. Louie JK, Roy-Burman A, Guardia-Labar L et al. Rhinovirus associated with severe lower respiratory tract infections in children. *Pediatr Infect Dis J* 2009; **28**: 337–9.
119. Choi S-H, Hong S-B, Ko G-B et al. Viral infection in patients with severe pneumonia requiring intensive care unit admission. *Am J Respir Crit Care Med* 2012; **186**: 325–32.
120. Jin Y, Yuan X-H, Xie Z-P et al. Prevalence and clinical characterization of a newly identified human rhinovirus C species in children with acute respiratory tract infections. *J Clin Microbiol* 2009; **47**: 2895–900.
121. Xiang Z, Gonzalez R, Xie Z et al. Human rhinovirus group C infection in children with lower respiratory tract infection. *Emerg Infect Dis* 2008; **14**: 1665–7.
122. Linsuwanon P, Payungporn S, Samransamruajkit R et al. High prevalence of human rhinovirus C infection in Thai children with acute lower respiratory tract disease. *J Infect* 2009; **59**: 115–21.
123. Greer RM, McErlean P, Arden KE et al. Do rhinoviruses reduce the probability of viral co-detection during acute respiratory tract infections? *J Clin Virol* 2009; **45**: 10–5.
124. Renois F, Talmud D, Huguenin A et al. Rapid detection of respiratory tract viral infections and coinfections in patients with influenza-like illnesses by use of reverse transcription-PCR DNA microarray systems. *J Clin Microbiol* 2010; **48**: 3836–42.
125. Drosten C, Günther S, Preiser W et al. Identification of a novel coronavirus in patients with severe acute respiratory syndrome. *N Engl J Med* 2003; **348**: 1967–76.
126. Falsey AR, Walsh EE, Hayden FG. Rhinovirus and coronavirus infection-associated hospitalizations among older adults. *J Infect Dis* 2002; **185**: 1338–41.
127. Falsey AR, Erdman D, Anderson LJ, Walsh EE. Human metapneumovirus infections in young and elderly adults. *J Infect Dis* 2003; **187**: 785–90.
128. Zambon MC, Stockton JD, Clewley JP, Fleming DM. Contribution of influenza and respiratory syncytial virus to community cases of influenza-like illness: An observational study. *Lancet* 2001; **358**: 1410–6.
129. Monto AS. Epidemiology of viral respiratory infections. *Am J Med* 2002; **112 (Suppl 6A)**: 4S–12.
130. McMillan JA, Weiner LB, Higgins AM, Lamparella VJ. Pharyngitis associated with herpes simplex virus in college students. *Pediatr Infect Dis J* 1993; **12**: 280–4.
131. Pascalis H, Temmam S, Turpin M et al. Intense co-circulation of non-influenza respiratory viruses during the first wave of pandemic influenza pH1N1/2009: A cohort study in Reunion Island. *PLoS ONE* 2012; **7**: e44755.

been described in recipients of SOT recipients.[1,2,4,5] Further, influenza has been associated with the development of both acute and chronic rejection in SOT recipients as well as late onset airflow obstruction in stem cell transplant recipients.[4,6–10]

The timing of influenza outbreaks in the HSCT population and in patients with hematologic malignancy aligns with seasonal outbreaks in the general population.[11] Influenza typically causes infection in a small percentage of HSCT patients annually relative to other common respiratory viruses; however, rates of infection can be high during influenza outbreaks.[12] Risk factors for severe and progressive influenza infection complicating HSCT include presence of lymphopenia, onset early after HSCT, and pediatric transplant recipients; however donor type and cell source have not been found to be associated with an increased risk of infection.[11] In addition, there is a higher risk of superinfection with bacterial and fungal pathogens in HSCT recipients and in patients with lymphopenia.[13] Symptoms may include those of upper respiratory tract infection (URTI) and/or lower respiratory tract infection (LRTI), but mild to no clinical symptoms may occur.[11,14] Likewise, symptoms may last 1–2 weeks but prolonged viral shedding may occur with little to no symptoms.[11] A mortality rate of up to 28% in HSCT infected with influenza has been documented with reduced mortality noted in patients who receive early antiviral therapy.[11,12]

Influenza is less well studied in the SOT population; most studies have focused on lung transplant recipients. There are studies that have documented an association between influenza infection and SOT rejection.[7,15] An association has also been found between influenza infection and bronchiolitis obliterans in lung transplant recipients.[16] There were numerous studies published from data collected during the 2009 pandemic of influenza A/H1N1 that provided additional insight into the course among transplant patients. From a careful review of existing case series,[17–20] immune suppression is a risk factor for severe influenza requiring hospitalization and admission to the intensive care unit. The largest study to date reviewed 115 cases of novel influenza A/H1N1 among US and Canadian transplant recipients (38 kidney, 23 liver, 22 heart, 18 lung, and 14 other transplant recipients).[21] The median time since transplant was 3.8 years. Sixty-one percent were lymphopenic at the time of presentation and 65% required hospitalization.[21] Twenty-five percent developed pneumonia, typically viral pneumonia, while 13% required ICU-level care.[21] Most received oseltamivir monotherapy with early antiviral therapy being associated with improved clinical outcomes.[21]

To date, there have been no prospective studies of antiviral therapy in transplant recipients and as such, the optimal regimen and duration has been incompletely defined. Available data, though, does strongly suggest early therapy may be associated with improved outcomes.[3,21–27] As such, any transplant patient should be started on appropriate antiviral therapy if there is suspicion for influenza without waiting for diagnostic testing results;[21,22,24] therapy should be continued even if rapid antigen testing is negative because of the poor sensitivity of this class of tests.[21,22,24] Due to widespread M2 inhibitor resistance among all naturally circulating influenza viruses affecting humans, neuraminidase inhibitors are recommended as the first-line agents for the treatment of influenza.[28] The commercially available neuraminidase inhibitors, laninamivir, oseltamivir, peramivir, and zanamivir have been reviewed in detail elsewhere.[29] As a result of the data from stem cell transplant data and the limited data in SOT patients,[21,30,31] prolonged antiviral therapy may be of benefit in transplant patients.[22,24] Many experts recommend continuing treatment until viral replication has stopped which, given prolonged viral shedding in immunocompromised patients, is typically greater than the approved 5 day course.[30,31] In addition, some experts recommend using high-dose oseltamivir (renally adjusted equivalent of 150 mg twice daily) to increase the rate of viral clearance.[18,30]

From the available data, use of antiviral therapy is associated with a reduced rate of progression to pneumonia, a lower mortality rate, and overall improved clinical outcomes.[3,23,30–35] Antiviral therapy may also reduce risk of development of *de novo* or progression of existing chronic rejection among lung transplant recipients.[3] There is currently no published data on the safety, tolerability, or efficacy of inhaled zanamivir in transplant patients and zanamivir should be used with care in patients with underlying lung disease because of the enhanced risk of bronchospasm.[36]

Resistance to the neuraminidase inhibitors results from mutations in either the neuraminidase or the hemagglutinin and has been reviewed in great detail elsewhere.[37–39] Resistance to NAIs appears to emerge during treatment at the highest rate among immunocompromised patients.[28,38–48]

Influenza can be prevented through the use of vaccination or antiviral medications. Current guidelines suggest that all transplant recipients and their close contacts receive the inactivated, injectable influenza vaccine annually.[49–51] Influenza vaccination with the inactivated vaccine is recommended for HSCT and SOT recipients because of the risk of viral replication in immunosuppressed patients who receive the live attenuated intranasal vaccine. Response to vaccination posttransplant is variable given underlying immunosuppression related to antirejection medications.[52] Efficacy of influenza vaccination appears to be somewhat reduced in SOT and HSCT recipients compared to healthy controls.[52–54] Among HSCT recipients, exceptionally low rates of response to vaccination has been consistentlydemonstrated in the first 6–12 months posttransplant.[55] Further, even when recipients have a humoral response to influenza vaccination, peaks of antibody titers and duration of protective titers are reduced compared to healthy controls.[56] Despite the limitations of influenza vaccination, a recent meta-analysis clearly demonstrated that it was associated with reduced risk of influenza-like illness and laboratory-confirmed influenza SOT and cancer patients.[54] The optimal timing of vaccination has been investigated in SOT recipients, although most experts recommend providing influenza vaccine either before transplant or waiting 3–6 months following use of lymphocyte-depleting induction regimens.[49,57] Although influenza vaccination has been consistently found to be safe without a significant enhanced risk of inducing rejection,[52,54] utilization in transplant patients and their recipients remain low.

In patients predicted to have a poor response to inactivated vaccine, such as early posttransplant, or in periods where vaccine may not be available, such as early following the start of a pandemic, antiviral prophylaxis may be considered. One recent study of kidney, liver, kidney–liver, and HSCT patients were given 12 weeks of oseltamivir 75 mg QD (or the renally adjusted equivalent) or placebo for seasonal prophylaxis.[58] Statistically fewer patients who received antiviral prophylaxis developed culture (0.4% vs. 3.8%; 88% protective efficacy) or RT-PCR (1.7% vs. 8.4%; 74.9% protective efficacy) proven influenza.[58] The intervention was generally well tolerated. Of the patients who had breakthrough infection with influenza despite prophylaxis with oseltamivir, none had changes in IC_{50} suggestive of resistance emerging.[58] Since there is concern that the current regimen may be associated with a low but true risk of resistance emergences, all patients who develop symptoms on prophylaxis should be counseled to seek care immediately.

18.3 RESPIRATORY SYNCYTIAL VIRUS

Among respiratory viruses, RSV is particularly problematic given its high level of infectivity. Transmission can occur via fomites or droplet inhalation and nosocomial outbreaks of RSV have been documented.[59] RSV infection in immunocompromised adults can lead to a wide range of symptoms including mild upper respiratory infection, which can then progress to severe LRTI.[60] Mortality due to RSV infection is more likely to occur in HSCT and lung transplant recipients than other organ transplant recipients or immunocompromised patients.

RSV infection is a common pathogen in HSCT recipients typically affecting approximately 5% of HSCT recipients and is well-known to cause significant morbidity and mortality when infection leads to pneumonia.[61–63] The risk of progression to LRTI is greatest within the first month posttransplant or in patients who have not yet engrafted.[64] Bone marrow transplant recipients infected with RSV can have a mortality rate up to 78%.[59]

As in HSCT, RSV can lead to URTI or severe LRTI in SOT recipients. RSV in SOT is best studied in lung transplant recipients.[65] However, RSV infection in lung transplant recipients can lead to significant morbidity related to graft rejection and bronchiolitis obliterans.[66–68] Generally mortality is exceptionally rare in other transplant populations, although case reports of progressive and fatal cases have been described.[69,70]

81. Ghosh S, Champlin RE, Englund J, Giralt SA, Rolston K, Raad I et al. Respiratory syncytial virus upper respiratory tract illnesses in adult blood and marrow transplant recipients: Combination therapy with aerosolized ribavirin and intravenous immunoglobulin. *Bone Marrow Transplant*. 2000; **25**(7): 751–5.
82. Shah DP, Ghantoji SS, Shah JN, El Taoum KK, Jiang Y, Popat U et al. Impact of aerosolized ribavirin on mortality in 280 allogeneic haematopoietic stem cell transplant recipients with respiratory syncytial virus infections. *J Antimicrob Chemother*. 2013.
83. Whimbey E, Champlin RE, Englund JA, Mirza NQ, Piedra PA, Goodrich JM et al. Combination therapy with aerosolized ribavirin and intravenous immunoglobulin for respiratory syncytial virus disease in adult bone marrow transplant recipients. *Bone Marrow Transplant*. 1995; **16**(3): 393–9.
84. Shah JN, Chemaly RF. Management of RSV infections in adult recipients of hematopoietic stem cell transplantation. *Blood*. 2011; **117**(10): 2755–63.
85. Lewinsohn DM, Bowden RA, Mattson D, Crawford SW. Phase I study of intravenous ribavirin treatment of respiratory syncytial virus pneumonia after marrow transplantation. *Antimicrob Agents Chemother*. 1996; **40**(11): 2555–7.
86. Schleuning M, Buxbaum-Conradi H, Jager G, Kolb HJ. Intravenous ribavirin for eradication of respiratory syncytial virus (RSV) and adenovirus isolates from the respiratory and/or gastrointestinal tract in recipients of allogeneic hematopoietic stem cell transplants. *The Hematology Journal: The Official Journal of the European Haematology Association/EHA*. 2004; **5**(2): 135–44.
87. Sparrelid E, Ljungman P, Ekelof-Andstrom E, Aschan J, Ringden O, Winiarski J et al. Ribavirin therapy in bone marrow transplant recipients with viral respiratory tract infections. *Bone Marrow Transplant*. 1997; **19**(9): 905–8.
88. Dokos C, Masjosthusmann K, Rellensmann G, Werner C, Schuler-Luttmann S, Muller KM et al. Fatal human metapneumovirus infection following allogeneic hematopoietic stem cell transplantation. *Transplant Infectious Disease: An Official Journal of the Transplantation Society*. 2013; **15**:e97–e101.
89. Egli A, Bucher C, Dumoulin A, Stern M, Buser A, Bubendorf L et al. Human metapneumovirus infection after allogeneic hematopoietic stem cell transplantation. *Infection*. 2012; **40**(6): 677–84.
90. Franquet T, Rodriguez S, Martino R, Salinas T, Gimenez A, Hidalgo A. Human metapneumovirus infection in hematopoietic stem cell transplant recipients: High-resolution computed tomography findings. *J Comput Assist Tomogr*. 2005; **29**(2): 223–7.
91. Englund JA, Boeckh M, Kuypers J, Nichols WG, Hackman RC, Morrow RA et al. Brief communication: Fatal human metapneumovirus infection in stem-cell transplant recipients. *Ann Int Med*. 2006; **144**(5): 344–9.
92. Cane PA, van den Hoogen BG, Chakrabarti S, Fegan CD, Osterhaus AD. Human metapneumovirus in a haematopoietic stem cell transplant recipient with fatal lower respiratory tract disease. *Bone Marrow Transplantation*. 2003; **31**(4): 309–10.
93. Debur MC, Vidal LR, Stroparo E, Nogueira MB, Almeida SM, Takahashi GA et al. Human metapneumovirus infection in hematopoietic stem cell transplant recipients. *Transplant Infectious Disease: An Official Journal of the Transplantation Society*. 2010; **12**(2): 173–9.
94. Dare R, Sanghavi S, Bullotta A, Keightley MC, George KS, Wadowsky RM et al. Diagnosis of human metapneumovirus infection in immunosuppressed lung transplant recipients and children evaluated for pertussis. *J Clin Microbiol*. 2007; **45**(2): 548–52.
95. Larcher C, Geltner C, Fischer H, Nachbaur D, Muller LC, Huemer HP. Human metapneumovirus infection in lung transplant recipients: clinical presentation and epidemiology. *The Journal of Heart and Lung Transplantation: The Official Publication of the International Society for Heart Transplantation*. 2005; **24**(11): 1891–901.
96. Park SY, Baek S, Lee SO, Choi SH, Kim YS, Woo JH et al. Efficacy of oral ribavirin in hematologic disease patients with paramyxovirus infection: Analytic strategy using propensity scores. *Antimicrob Agents Chemother*. 2013; **57**(2): 983–9.
97. Shachor-Meyouhas Y, Ben-Barak A, Kassis I. Treatment with oral ribavirin and IVIG of severe human metapneumovirus pneumonia (HMPV) in immune compromised child. *Pediatr Blood & Cancer*. 2011; **57**(2): 350–1.
98. Raza K, Ismailjee SB, Crespo M, Studer SM, Sanghavi S, Paterson DL et al. Successful outcome of human metapneumovirus (hMPV) pneumonia in a lung transplant recipient treated with intravenous ribavirin. *The Journal of Heart and Lung Transplantation: The Official Publication of the International Society for Heart Transplantation*. 2007; **26**(8): 862–4.
99. Wyde PR, Chetty SN, Jewell AM, Boivin G, Piedra PA. Comparison of the inhibition of human metapneumovirus and respiratory syncytial virus by ribavirin and immune serum globulin in vitro. *Antiviral Res*. 2003; **60**(1): 51–9.

100. Wendt CH, Weisdorf DJ, Jordan MC, Balfour HH, Jr., Hertz MI. Parainfluenza virus respiratory infection after bone marrow transplantation. *New Engl J Med.* 1992; **326**(14): 921–6.
101. Reed G, Jewett PH, Thompson J, Tollefson S, Wright PF. Epidemiology and clinical impact of parainfluenza virus infections in otherwise healthy infants and young children <5 years old. *J Infect Dis.* 1997; **175**(4): 807–13.
102. Chakrabarti S, Collingham KE, Holder K, Oyaide S, Pillay D, Milligan DW. Parainfluenza virus type 3 infections in hematopoetic stem cell transplant recipients: response to ribavirin therapy. *Clinical Infectious Diseases: An Official Publication of the Infectious Diseases Society of America.* 2000; **31**(6): 1516–8.
103. Nichols WG, Corey L, Gooley T, Davis C, Boeckh M. Parainfluenza virus infections after hematopoietic stem cell transplantation: Risk factors, response to antiviral therapy, and effect on transplant outcome. *Blood.* 2001; **98**(3): 573–8.
104. Vilchez RA, McCurry K, Dauber J, Iacono A, Keenan R, Zeevi A et al. The epidemiology of parainfluenza virus infection in lung transplant recipients. *Clinical Infectious Diseases: An Official Publication of the Infectious Diseases Society of America.* 2001; **33**(12): 2004–8.
105. Dignan F, Alvares C, Riley U, Ethell M, Cunningham D, Treleaven J et al. Parainfluenza type 3 infection post stem cell transplant: High prevalence but low mortality. *J Hosp Infect.* 2006; **63**(4): 452–8.
106. Ghosh S, Champlin R, Couch R, Englund J, Raad I, Malik S et al. Rhinovirus infections in myelosuppressed adult blood and marrow transplant recipients. *Clinical infectious diseases: An official publication of the Infectious Diseases Society of America.* 1999; **29**(3): 528–32.
107. Ison MG, Hayden FG, Kaiser L, Corey L, Boeckh M. Rhinovirus infections in hematopoietic stem cell transplant recipients with pneumonia. *Clinical Infectious Diseases: An Official Publication of the Infectious Diseases Society of America.* 2003; **36**(9): 1139–43.
108. Milano F, Campbell AP, Guthrie KA, Kuypers J, Englund JA, Corey L et al. Human rhinovirus and coronavirus detection among allogeneic hematopoietic stem cell transplantation recipients. *Blood.* 2010; **115**(10): 2088–94.
109. Malcolm E, Arruda E, Hayden FG, Kaiser L. Clinical features of patients with acute respiratory illness and rhinovirus in their bronchoalveolar lavages. *Journal of Clinical Virology: The Official Publication of the Pan American Society for Clinical Virology.* 2001; **21**(1): 9–16.
110. Kaiser L, Aubert JD, Pache JC, Deffernez C, Rochat T, Garbino J et al. Chronic rhinoviral infection in lung transplant recipients. *Am J Respir Crit Care Med.* 2006; **174**(12): 1392–9.
111. Hayden FG, Herrington DT, Coats TL, Kim K, Cooper EC, Villano SA et al. Efficacy and safety of oral pleconaril for treatment of colds due to picornaviruses in adults: results of 2 double-blind, randomized, placebo-controlled trials. *Clinical Infectious Diseases: An Official Publication of the Infectious Diseases Society of America.* 2003; **36**(12): 1523–32.
112. Garnett CT, Pao CI, Gooding LR. Detection and quantitation of subgroup C adenovirus DNA in human tissue samples by real-time PCR. *Meth Mol Med.* 2007; **130**: 193–204.
113. Echavarria M. Adenoviruses in immunocompromised hosts. *Clin Microbiol Rev.* 2008; **21**(4): 704–15.
114. Ljungman P, Ribaud P, Eyrich M, Matthes-Martin S, Einsele H, Bleakley M et al. Cidofovir for adenovirus infections after allogeneic hematopoietic stem cell transplantation: a survey by the Infectious Diseases Working Party of the European Group for Blood and Marrow Transplantation. *Bone Marrow Transplant.* 2003; **31**(6): 481–6.
115. Hoffman JA, Shah AJ, Ross LA, Kapoor N. Adenoviral infections and a prospective trial of cidofovir in pediatric hematopoietic stem cell transplantation. *Biology of Blood and Marrow Transplantation: Journal of the American Society for Blood and Marrow Transplantation.* 2001; **7**(7): 388–94.
116. de Mezerville MH, Tellier R, Richardson S, Hebert D, Doyle J, Allen U. Adenoviral infections in pediatric transplant recipients: a hospital-based study. *Pediatr Infect Dis J.* 2006; **25**(9): 815–8.
117. Hofland CA, Eron LJ, Washecka RM. Hemorrhagic adenovirus cystitis after renal transplantation. *Transplant Proc.* 2004; **36**(10): 3025–7.
118. Humar A. Reactivation of viruses in solid organ transplant patients receiving cytomegalovirus prophylaxis. *Transplantation.* 2006; **82**(2 Suppl): S9–14.
119. Humar A, Kumar D, Mazzulli T, Razonable RR, Moussa G, Paya CV et al. A surveillance study of adenovirus infection in adult solid organ transplant recipients. *American Journal of Transplantation: Official Journal of the American Society of Transplantation and the American Society of Transplant Surgeons.* 2005; **5**(10): 2555–9.
120. Bridges ND, Spray TL, Collins MH, Bowles NE, Towbin JA. Adenovirus infection in the lung results in graft failure after lung transplantation. *J Thoracic Cardiovasc Surg.* 1998; **116**(4): 617–23.
121. Ohori NP, Michaels MG, Jaffe R, Williams P, Yousem SA. Adenovirus pneumonia in lung transplant recipients. *Hum Pathol.* 1995; **26**(10): 1073–9.

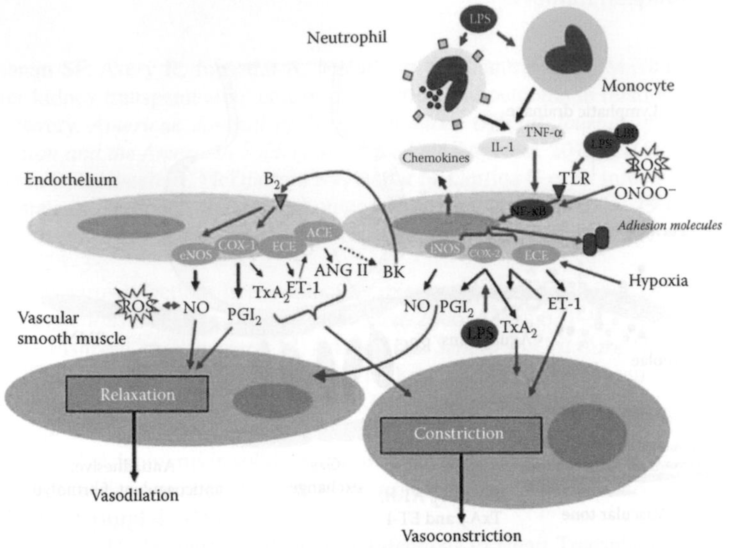

FIGURE 4.3 Schematic illustration of physiologic endothelial–smooth muscle interactions and EC response to inflammatory stimuli. Inflammatory stimuli induce the activation of nuclear factor-κB (NF-κB) or other transcription factors. NF-κB promotes the synthesis of vasoactive agents regulating vascular tone. TNF-α: tumor necrosis factor-α; IL-1: interleukin-1; NO: nitric oxide; $ONOO^-$: peroxynitrite; ET-1: endothelin-1; PGI_2: prostacyclin; TxA_2: thromboxane A_2; ANG II: angiotensin II; BK: bradykinin; ROS: reactive oxygen species; eNOS: endothelial NO synthase; iNOS: inducible NO synthase; COX-1: constitutive cyclooxygenase; COX-2: inducible cyclooxygenase; ACE: angiotensin-converting enzyme; ECE: endothelin-converting enzyme; B_2: B_2 kinin receptor. Red arrows action; black arrows synthesis (and uptake for ET-1); dotted arrow breakdown. (Reproduced from Orfanos SE et al. *Intensive Care Med* 2004; **30**(9): 1702–14. With permission.)

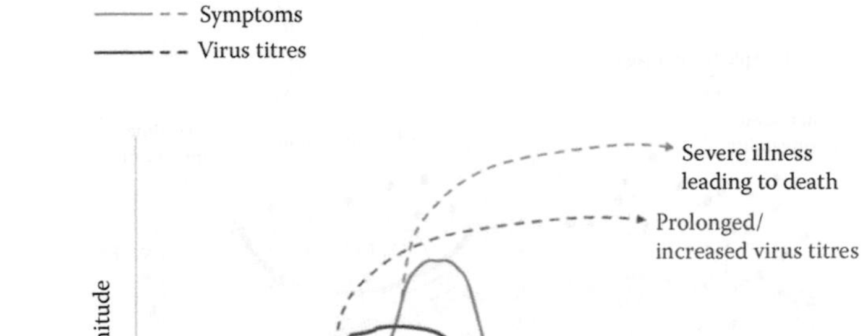

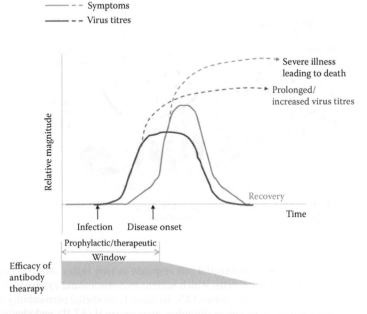

FIGURE 10.1 Window of administration of antibody therapy. Both prophylactic and therapeutic administration of antibodies can efficaciously protect against viral disease. Administration of antibody therapy prior to or soon after infection leads to the suppression of viral titers (continuous red graph) and recovery from disease (continuous blue graph). However, the effectiveness of antibody therapy is reduced as the disease progresses. Failure to control viral titers (red dotted graph) early in disease progression leads to severe tissue damage, often as a result of excessive host responses. This leads to disease complications and ultimately leads to death (blue dotted graph). (Adapted from Dubois, M.E., P. Yoshihara, and M.K. Slifka, *Semin Respir Crit Care Med*, 2005. 26(6): 635–642.)

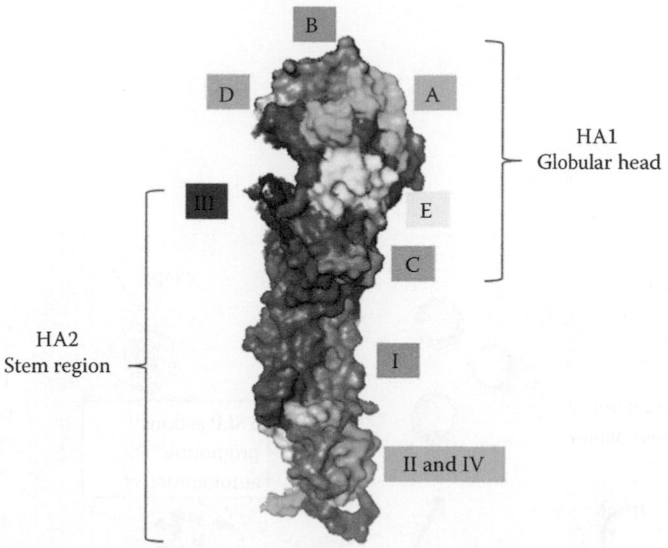

FIGURE 10.6 Major antigenic sites on HA. This space filled model of a H3 monomer (Protein Data Bank accession 1HGE) was generated using PyMol. Antigenic sites A to E on HA1 (dark gray) are indicated. Antigenic sites I through IV on HA2 (light gray) are also indicated. (Adapted from Ye, J., H. Shao, and D.R. Perez, *Immunotherapy*, 2012. 4(2): 175–186.)

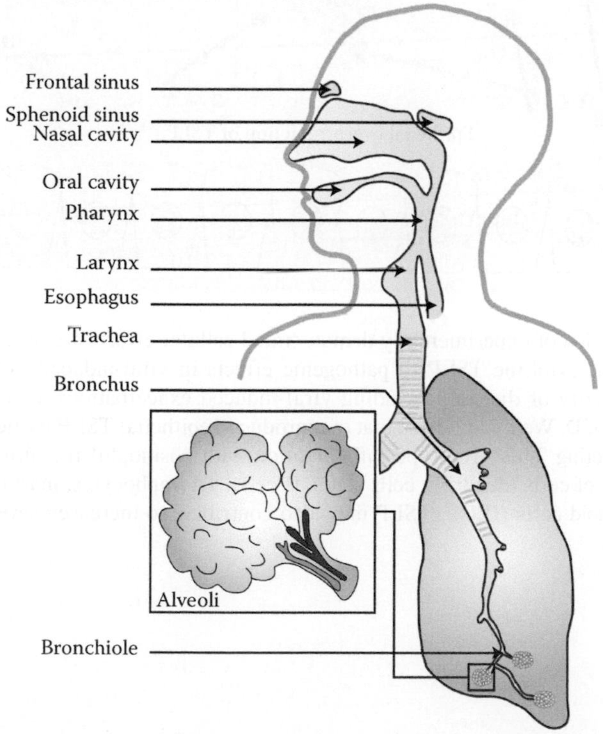

FIGURE 13.1 Human RT. Simplified schematic overview of the human RT. (Courtesy of J.Y. Siegers.)

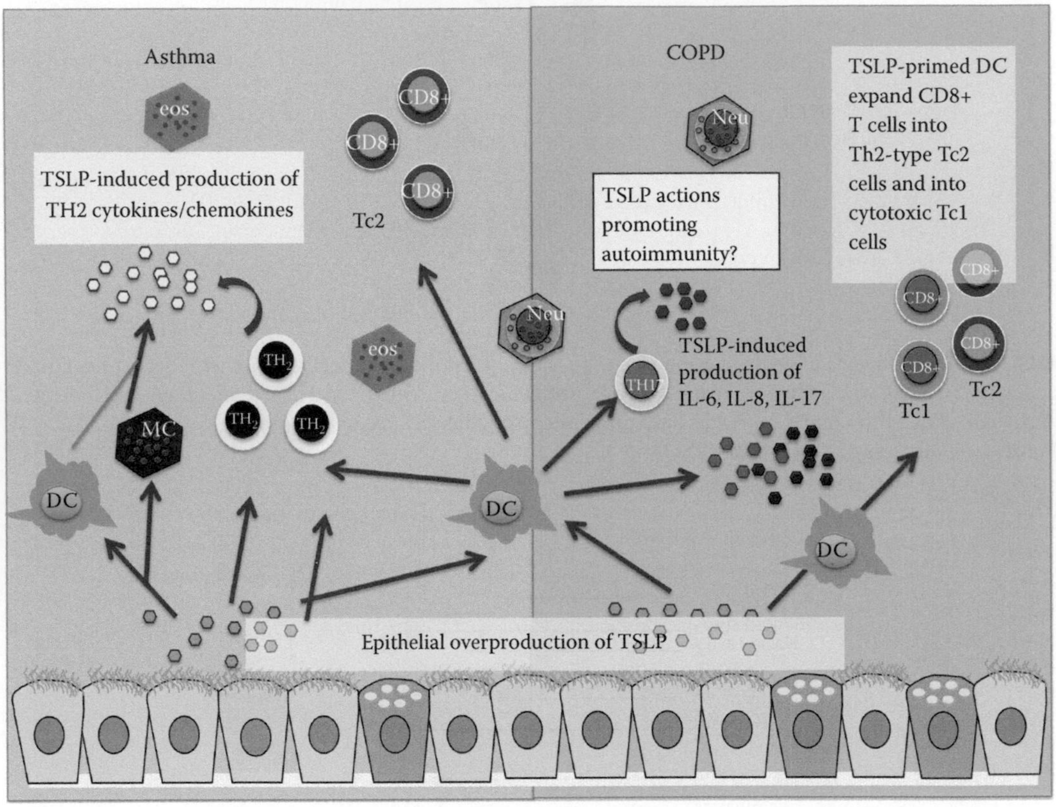

FIGURE 14.1 A selection of experimentally demonstrated cellular effects are used to illustrate the potential contributions by the cytokine TSLP to pathogenic effects in viral-induced asthma and COPD. With increasing age and severity of disease, including viral-induced exacerbations, there is significant overlap between asthma and COPD. We hypothesize that overproduced epithelial TSLP participates in viral-induced exacerbations by promoting Th2-, Tc2-type inflammation with eosinophil recruitment and activation. By its influence on a range of cells (dendritic cells (DC), B cells, T lymphocytes, mast cells (MC), eosinophils (eos), and innate lymphoid cells (ILC)), TSLP may also contribute to increased severity of chronic asthma and COPD.

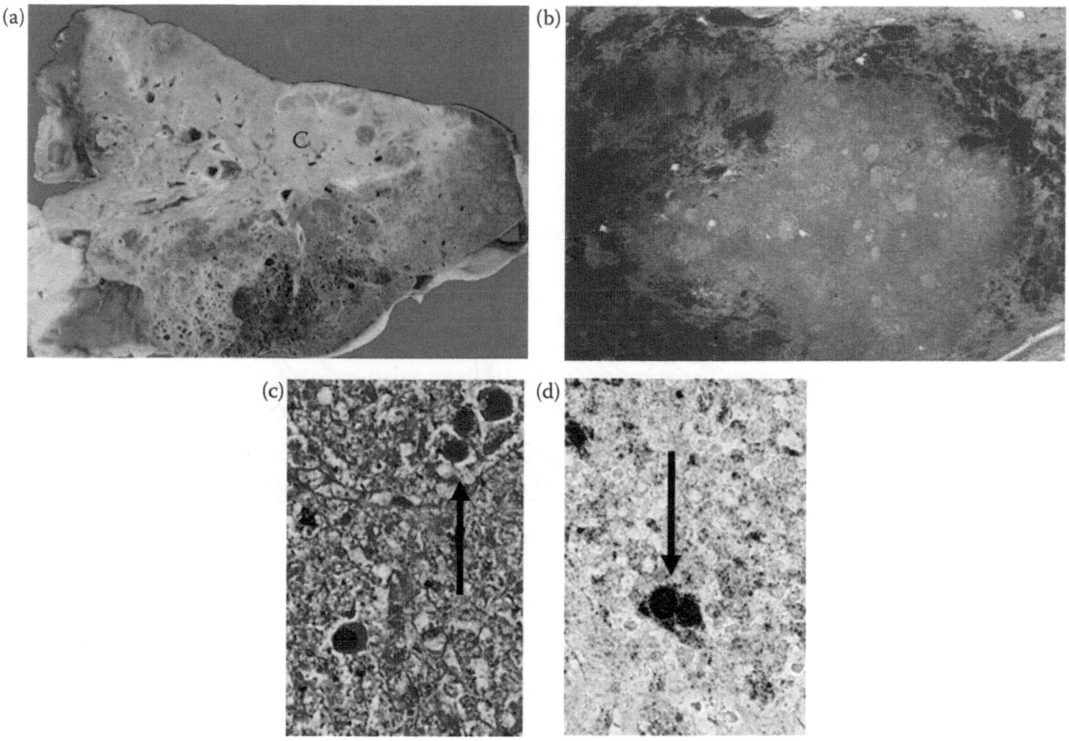

FIGURE 19.1 Fatal case of AdV pneumonia. (a) Gross lung with pale, consolidated region; (b) histopathology showing hemorrhagic necrotic lung tissue (H&E stain, ×40); (c) high magnification showing three cells with intranuclear inclusions (arrow) (H&E, ×400); and (d) immunohistochemical staining for AdV showing positive staining of the intranuclear inclusions in two cells (arrow) (immunoperoxidase, ×400). (Reproduced with permission from Lynch JP, III, Fishbein M, Echavarria M. *Seminars in Respiratory and Critical Care Medicine.* 2011; 32(4): 494–511.)

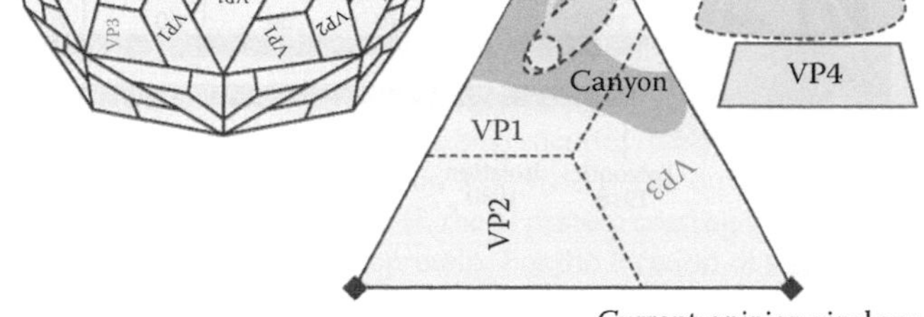

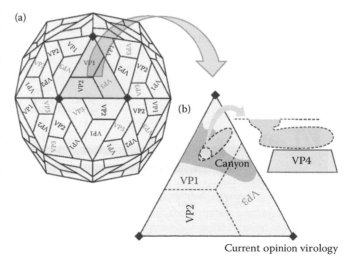

FIGURE 20.1 (a) Structure of Rhinovirus. Rhinovirus is a nonenveloped, spherical virus composed of a protein shell surrounding the naked RNA genome. The protein capsid consists of four polypeptides, viral capsid protein 1 (VP1), VP2, VP3, and VP4, in an icosahedral formation. (b) A hydrophobic pocket or "canyon" exists within VP1, which is the likely point of contact for ICAM-1. VP4 is located on the internal surface of the virus and is important in assembly of the virus during replication and infection of new cells. (Reprinted from *Current Opinion in Virology*, Vol. 2, JL Kennedy et al., Pathogenesis of rhinovirus infection, pp. 287–293, 2012, with permission from Elsevier.)

19.6.3 AdV Infections in Refugees and Aboriginal Populations

Epidemics of HAdV and other viral respiratory infections are common in international refugee settings, owing to malnutrition, high population density, and poor shelter conditions.[165,166] The incidence of HAdV and other viral respiratory infections has been documented to be up to 5 times higher in Aboriginal populations (e.g., Alaskan,[167] Canadian,[168] or Australian[169] native people).

19.6.4 HSCT Recipients

HAdV infections occur in 5–47% of HSCT recipients.[1,4,22–24,41,81,149–152,170–174] The incidence is 2–3.5 times higher in children (>20%) compared to <10% in adults.[83,171,172,175,176] Higher rates were observed when regular screening for HAdV DNA was performed in plasma by PCR.[149,177] Additional risk factors for HAdV infections among HSCT recipients include allogeneic HSCT,[83,172] human leukocyte antigen (HLA) mismatch,[83,178] severe T cell depletion,[83,138,179] myeloablative conditioning,[1] and graft versus host disease (GVHD).[1,22,24,149,150,152,172] Infection can reflect primary infection[89] or reactivation of latent infection.[4,89]

AdV infection in HSCT recipients is usually detected within 100 days of transplant.[83,138,139,180] In most patients, the disease is localized (e.g., urinary tract, gastroenteritis, or upper or lower RTIs) but dissemination occurs in 10–30% of cases.[83,171,175] Among 76 adult HSCT recipients with *symptomatic* HAdV infections, mortality rate was 26%.[172] Mortality rates were higher among patients with pneumonia (73%) and disseminated disease (61%).[172] Severe lymphopenia,[1,83] severe GVHD,[172] isolation from more than one site,[83] and high HAdV viral loads in plasma[179,181–183] correlate with higher mortality. However, the disease may be self-limited, particularly when the viral load is low.[42,180,183] A retrospective study in 42 pediatric HSCT recipients detected HAdV in blood (by PCR) in 11 patients (42%); viremia cleared in seven patients without antiviral therapy.[42] Cidofovir (CDV) (an antiviral agent with excellent *in vitro* activity against HAdV) has been used successfully in nonrandomized trials to treat HAdV infections,[184] but indications and efficacy of therapy are controversial (discussed later in the Section 19.10). Quantification of HAdV DNA load by real-time PCR in plasma of HSCT recipients and evaluation of their viral kinetics may identify patients at high risk for dissemination[175,179,181] or assess response to therapy.[175,181] However, *routine* screening for HAdV by PCR in low-risk patients is controversial.

19.6.5 SOT Recipients

The incidence of HAdV infections is 5–22% among SOT recipients.[1,83,152,185] AdV infections have been noted in liver,[186,187] renal,[142,148,157,188,189] intestinal,[131,190,191] heart,[185] and lung[192] transplant recipients. Among SOT recipients, risk factors for HAdV include pediatric age,[83,186,191] receipt of antilymphocyte antibodies,[83] and donor-positive/recipient-negative HAdV status.[83] In a prospective study, HAdV viremia (by PCR) was detected within 12 months of transplant in 19/263 (7.3%) SOT recipients, including liver, 10/121 (8.3%); kidney, 6/92 (6.5%); and heart, 3/45 (6.7%).[185] During viremia, 11/19 (58%) were asymptomatic. All 19 patients recovered spontaneously without sequela. In a retrospective review, 49/484 (10%) pediatric liver transplant recipients developed HAdV infections; 9/49 (18%) died of invasive HAdV infection.[186] In a retrospective review, 11/191 (5.8%) adult liver transplant recipients developed HAdV infections; two died.[187] Clinical manifestations of HAdV infection are protean, but HAdV exhibits a proclivity for the transplanted organ.[83] In liver transplant recipients, HAdV typically causes jaundice, hepatomegaly, and hepatitis.[83] Similarly, among 23 pediatric small bowel transplant recipients with clinical HAdV infections, the allograft was involved in 19 patients (82.6%).[131] In renal transplant patients, the principal symptom is HC; further, HAdV may target the renal allograft, leading to graft failure.[142,148,188,189] The cardinal pathological features of HAdV infection include granulomatous interstitial nephritis, intranuclear inclusions (Cowdry A), and macrophages.[193] In pediatric heart-transplant recipients, the presence of HAdV in posttransplant endomyocardial biopsies increased the risk for graft loss and posttransplant coronary artery disease.[194,195] In a cohort of 383 lung transplant recipients (LTRs), four (1.3%) developed HAdV infections.[192] The incidence was 3/40 (8%) among pediatric LTR and 1/268 (0.4%) among adult LTR. All four developed hemorrhagic, necrotizing HAdV pneumonia and died within 45 days of transplant.[192] In another study, eight of 19 pediatric LTRs developed HAdV infection, resulting in two early deaths.[188] A case of fatal AdV pneumonia in an adult LTR 4 years posttransplant was described.[196] Although HAdV may cause severe infections in SOT recipients, we do not recommend *routine* PCR surveillance in adult SOT recipients. The need for therapy for mild or asymptomatic cases is not clear.

19.6.6 HIV-Infected Patients

In one study, the risk for HAdV infection in patients with acquired immunodeficiency syndrome (AIDS) was 28% at one year (17% if CD4 count was >200/mm^3 and 38% if the CD4 count was <200/mm^3).[197] The GI tract is involved in >90%, but most patients are asymptomatic or have mild symptoms (e.g., diarrhea).[197] Asymptomatic shedding of HAdV from the GI tract may be common in HIV-infected populations.[87] UTIs may occur in up to 20% of AIDS patients, but bladder inflammation and bleeding are rare.[83] However, fatal HAdV infections (particularly serotypes 1, 2, and 3) have been cited in HIV-infected patients.[83] Since the availability of highly active antiretroviral therapy (HAART), HAdV disease is uncommon in HIV/AIDS patients until immune system deterioration occurs.[83]

19.6.7 Congenital Immunodeficiency Syndromes

AdV infections may complicate congenital immunodeficiency disorders such as severe combined immunodeficiency syndrome (SCID), common variable immunodeficiency, agammaglobulinemia, immunoglobulin A deficiency, and others.[83,198] Incidence data for HAdV in patients with congenital immunodeficiencies are limited.[83] In one review of 201 patients with Bruton's X-linked agammaglobulinemia, only one died as a result of HAdV infection.[198] Data from a registry of primary immunodeficiency disorders in Kuwait analyzed 176 patients observed from 2004 to 2011 (mean follow-up 3.5 years); two died as a result of HAdV-associated liver failure.[199]

19.7 IMPORTANCE OF SEROTYPES

Globally, serotypes 1–5, 7, 21, and 41 are most commonly associated with human disease (Table 19.1).

Different serotypes display different tissue trophisms, and correlate with clinical manifestations of infection.[1,23,28,30] Among children, the most common HAdV serotypes associated with RTI are types 1–7 and 11.[28,202] In adults (particularly military recruits), serotypes implicated in FRI include subspecies B1 (HAdV-3, -7, and -21), species B2 (HAdV-11 and -14), species C (HAdV-1, -2, -5, and -6), and species E (HAdV-4).[9,21,40,53] Historically, most infections among military recruits in the United States were due to HAdV strains 4 and 7.[13,14,95] Recently, HAdV-14 was implicated as a cause of severe FRI in both military and civilian populations in the United States.[15,21,30,203,204] and also in Canada[205] and Ireland.[206] Other B2 subspecies rarely cause FRI, but HAdV-11 was implicated in outbreaks of FRI in China,[102] Singapore,[43] the Middle East,[207] the United States,[18] and Latin America.[208] HAdV-11 may also cause UTI or HC in children or transplant recipients.[4,30,83] Other serotypes associated with HC include HAdV-33, -34, and -35.[4,30] Species D (HAdV-8, -19, and -37) usually cause conjunctivitis,[28,114] but more common serotypes (e.g., HAdV-3, -4, -7, and -11) can also cause conjunctivitis.[10] Gastroenteritis is associated with infection by enteric HAdV-40 and -41 (species F),[4] and HAdV-12, -18, and -31 (species A).[4] The only HAdV serotype classified within species G (HAdV-52) was isolated from stool specimens from a case of gastroenteritis.[29]

19.8.1.7 Emergence of AdV Serotype 14 in the United States

HAdV-14 was first isolated in the Netherlands in 1955 during an outbreak of acute respiratory disease (ARD) among military recruits.[30] HAdV-14 was subsequently isolated during outbreaks of ARD in Great Britain in 1955,[242] Uzbekistan in 1962,[30] and Czechoslovakia in 1963.[30] Apart from sporadic isolations in the Netherlands in the early 1970s, no cases of HAdV-14 infection were globally reported between the 1960s and 2004.[12,30] HAdV-14 had never been identified in North America prior to 2003.[30,40] Beginning in 2005, outbreaks of FRI due to HAdV-14 were noted in several military bases in the United States.[92,107,218,243] By 2007, HAdV-14 became a dominant serotype at several U.S. military bases[40,107,218] and was implicated in several outbreaks in civilian populations in multiple states.[21,30,203,204,244,245] Molecular studies confirmed that HAdV isolates from different geographic locations (both military and civilian populations) from 2003 to 2009 were identical and represented a new genomic type designated as HAdV-14p1 (formerly known as HAdV-14a).[21] The complete genetic sequence of HAdV-14p1 suggests recombination between HAdV-14 and HAdV-11 strains.[30,40] As a recently emerged virus, and with lack of herd immunity, HAdV-14p1 has an increased potential for high attack rates and rates of transmission.[40] Beginning in 2009–2010, cases of HAdV-14p1 infections (some fatal) were detected in Europe,[107] Ireland,[202,246] and China.[247]

19.8.1.8 AdV Serotype 21

The detection of HAdV-21 has only been sporadically reported in the literature but in association with severe pediatric pulmonary disease,[248,249] community infections,[250–252] and sporadic outbreaks in military populations.[218,253] HAdV-21 was associated with epidemics of FRIs in military recruits in the Netherlands and Germany from the 1960s to 1985,[253–255] but only sporadic cases were noted over the next two decades.[253] HAdV-21 may cause pharyngitis,[256] RTIs,[257] and conjunctivitis,[256] but is uncommon.[28] In the United States from 2004 to 2006, HAdV-21 accounted for 2.0% and 2.4% of HAdV RTI in civilians and military recruits, respectively.[200] In Toronto, Canada (2007–2008), HAdV-21 accounted for 5.5% of clinical respiratory HAdV isolates. In contrast, HAdV-21 was never isolated in 741 pediatric respiratory isolates from Korea from 1991 to 2007,[28] and was only detected in four out of 743 HAdV-positive specimens from pediatric patients hospitalized for acute LRTI (lower respiratory tract infections) from 1999 to 2010 in Buenos Aires, Argentina.[258]

19.8.1.9 AdV Serotype 31

HAdV-31 may cause gastroenteritis in healthy children, and has been associated with fatal infections in HSCT recipients.[25,259–262] Nosocomial transmission (seven cases) was noted in a pediatric SCT (stem cell transplantation) unit.[261]

19.8.1.10 AdV Serotype 36

Experimental infection of laboratory animals with HAdV-36 results in obesity as a result of increased adipogenesis.[254] Seroprevalence studies have shown an increased risk of obesity for individuals seropositive for HAdV-36.[263–265] The possible role of this otherwise extremely rare HAdV as a causative agent or cofactor in obesity warrants further investigation.

19.8.1.11 AdV Serotype 37

HAdV-37 accounts for <1% of HAdV infections,[5,28,110,200] but may cause EKC.[110,114,115,117,119–121]

19.8.1.12 AdV Species F (Serotypes 40 and 41)

Globally, HAdV-species F (serotypes 40 and 41) are endemic, and typically cause gastroenteritis and diarrheal illness in children.[69–79,266] Fatalities may occur as a result of dehydration in infants.[69,70] In immunocompromised hosts (particularly HSCT recipients), fatal dissemination may occur.[89,267] Epidemics have been cited in schools[74] and hospitals.[89] Nosocomial transmission may occur due to high HAdV levels in feces during diarrheal illnesses.[89] Shedding of these viruses may be prolonged in immunosuppressed patients.[89] Endogenous reactivation (probably originating from HAdV in mucosal lymphoid cells)[85] may occur.

19.8.1.13 AdV Types 53, 54, and 56

The detection of HAdV types 53, 54, and 56[33–36] in association with outbreaks of EKC was recently described in Japan.

19.9 DIAGNOSIS OF AdV INFECTION

HAdV can be detected in clinical specimens from affected sites (e.g., nasopharyngeal aspirates, swabs, washings, conjunctivae, bronchoalveolar lavage [BAL], urine, stool, blood, cerebrospinal fluid [CSF], and biopsies) by virus-specific direct or indirect immunofluorescence, conventional or shell vial cultures, or PCR.[4,28,38,268] Viral cultures by conventional techniques are the gold standard, but may take up to 28 days to detect the cytopathic effect.[1,4,28,38] However, cultures are insensitive to detect HAdV in blood.[269] Immunofluorescence is widely used to detect HAdV in respiratory samples but the sensitivity may be as low as 60%. Biopsy of involved tissues may reveal HAdV nuclear inclusions,[1] and immunohistochemical stains may identify the intranuclear HAdV hexon antigen.[148] PCR in plasma, urine, or other clinical specimens may establish the diagnosis,[1,38,181,270] and is highly sensitive for disseminated disease.[268,271,272] Quantification of the viral load using real-time PCR can be used to assess response to antiviral therapy (Figure 19.2).[175,271] Among transplant recipients, weekly screening of blood and stool may detect HAdV infection prior to the onset of symptoms, and may facilitate early "preemptive" therapy.[23,149,177,185] The overall impact of routine surveillance is controversial, although it has been increasingly used, especially in high-risk patients.[1]

The determination of serotype with the neutralization test is laborious and time consuming. Multiplex PCR-based techniques targeting the fiber genes[209] or hypervariable regions of the hexon[211] and/or amplification and sequencing of hexon genes allow definitive identification of the serotype/species.[26,28] Recently, a real-time qualitative PCR assay that detects 57 HAdV types was developed.[38] Serological tests may be useful in epidemiological investigations, but are of limited practical value in individual patients.[83]

19.10 THERAPY

Currently, no antiviral drug is FDA (Food and Drug Administration) approved to treat AdV infections,[83] as prospective randomized controlled trials are lacking. CDV, a cytosine nucleotide analog that inhibits the viral DNA polymerase, has the greatest *in vitro* activity against HAdV[184,273] and is

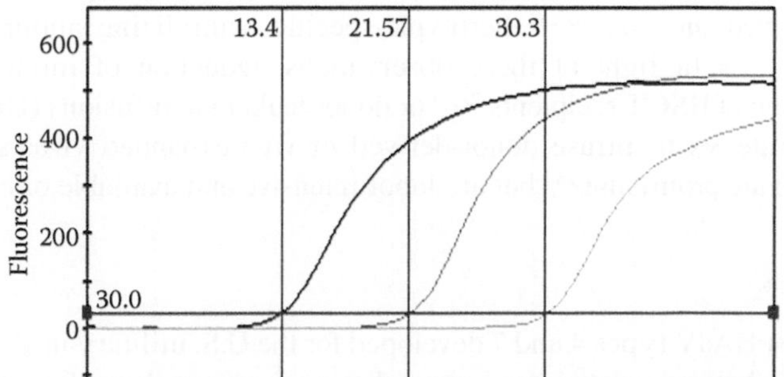

FIGURE 19.2 Detection of AdV by real-time PCR with a TaqMan probe. Follow-up in respiratory samples from a patient with acute respiratory infection.

the preferred therapeutic agent.[1] CDV is available only intravenously.[1] Regimens (dosing, frequency, and duration) are variable. The standard dose is 5 mg/kg every 1–2 weeks[83,177] or 1 mg/kg twice weekly.[83,177,274] The duration of the therapy is variable (weeks to months) and depends on clinical response and persistence or eradication of HAdV.[177,274] CDV is generally well tolerated,[149,177] but nephrotoxicity, myelosuppression, and uveitis may complicate its use.[1,83] Hydration and probenecid may minimize nephrotoxicity.[1,143,149,275] Careful monitoring of renal function (serum creatinine and proteinuria) is critical.

Numerous nonrandomized studies in HSCT and SOT recipients cited favorable responses to CDV.[22,23,25,149,177,178,274–278] In a multicenter trial in allogeneic HSCT recipients, CDV eradicated HAdV infection in 20/29 patients (69%).[277] Another study of 14 HSCT recipients with HAdV HC cited improvement with CDV in 10 patients (77%).[279] In a cohort of 10 pediatric HSCT recipients with severe HAdV infections, CDV was associated with clinical improvement in eight patients and viral clearance in nine patients.[178] Mori et al.[138] reported 26 HSCT recipients with HC due to HAdV; 22 patients were treated with CDV, resulting in complete ($n = 15$) or partial ($n = 6$) remissions in all but one case. Yusuf et al.[177] reported clinical and microbiological cure in 56/57 pediatric HSCT recipients with HAdV infections treated with CDV. However, another study of 13 pediatric HSCT recipients with HAdV infections cited no apparent benefit among 11 patients treated with CDV.[173] In another study of 14 adult HSCT recipients with adenoviremia, HAdV infection resolved in 13 patients, even though only five were treated with CDV.[174] The interpretation of these studies is confounded by heterogeneous patient populations, differing the extent and sites of disease, and degree of immunosuppression or immune reconstitution.[83] Given the lack of controlled trials, indications for and efficacy of CDV remain controversial.[24]

Given the potential for spontaneous resolution, not all patients with HAdV infections or viremia require treatment.[1,42] High mortality rates in retrospective studies in part reflect inclusion of patients with disseminated infections or severe impairments in immune defenses. Antiviral treatment should be considered for the following indications: disseminated (≥2 sites) disease, pneumonia, high viral loads in blood, virulence or trophism of the viral strain, and persistent severe lymphopenia or immune deficits. Further, "preemptive" therapy may have a role in viremic but *asymptomatic* organ transplant recipients at high risk for dissemination. Prospective, randomized trials are needed to elucidate indications for therapy in both symptomatic and asymptomatic patients with AdV infections.

A novel antiviral agent CMX001 (an oral analog of CDV) (Chimerix, Inc., Durham, NC), combined with mesenchymal stem cell infusion, was associated with eradication of disseminated HAdV infection in a pediatric HSCT recipient who had failed to respond to IV CDV.[280]

Immune reconstitution has been shown to play a critical role in controlling HAdV infection.[83] Increases in lymphocyte counts or CD4 counts were associated with clearance of HAdV infection[281,282] and improved survival.[282,283] Serotypic-specific neutralizing antibodies correlate with clearance of HAdV.[83,282] In light of these observations, reduction of immunosuppression,[148,149] immune reconstitution of HSCT recipients,[22,83] or donor leukocyte infusions (DLIs)[25,81,284] may have adjunctive roles. Strategies to infuse donor-derived *ex vivo* expanded virus-specific cytotoxic T lymphocytes (CTLs) are promising,[284] but are labor intensive and available only in a few centers.

19.11 VACCINES

Oral vaccines against HAdV types 4 and 7 developed for the U.S. military in 1971 successfully controlled the burden of AdV-associated respiratory disease for more than 25 years but were depleted by 1999.[17] New oral vaccines against HAdV-4 and HAdV-7 using the same original enteric-coated tablet formulation and virus strains as those implemented in 1971 were approved by the FDA in March 2011, but *only* for at-risk military populations (age 17–50). The AdV vaccination program for military recruits resumed in October 2011.[163] Importantly, antibodies to HAdV-4 and HAdV-7 may cross-protect against other serotypes (e.g., HAdV-3[107,218] and HAdV-14).[107,218,285]

REFERENCES

1. Ison MG. Adenovirus infections in transplant recipients. *Clinical Infectious Diseases: An Official Publication of the Infectious Diseases Society of America*. 2006; **43**(3): 331–9.
2. Chang SY, Lee CN, Lin PH, Huang HH, Chang LY, Ko W et al. A community-derived outbreak of adenovirus type 3 in children in Taiwan between 2004 and 2005. *Journal of Medical Virology*. 2008; **80**(1): 102–12.
3. Lynch JP, III, Fishbein M, Echavarria M. Adenovirus. *Seminars in Respiratory and Critical Care Medicine*. 2011; **32**(4): 494–511.
4. Kim Y-J, Boeckh M, Englund J. Community respiratory virus infections in immunocompromised patients: Hematopoietic stem cell and solid organ transplant recipients, and individuals with human immunodeficiency virus infection. *Seminars in Respiratory and Critical Care Medicine*. 2007; **28**: 222–42.
5. Yeung R, Eshaghi A, Lombos E, Blair J, Mazzulli T, Burton L et al. Characterization of culture-positive adenovirus serotypes from respiratory specimens in Toronto, Ontario, Canada: September 2007–June 2008. *Virology Journal*. 2009; **6**: 11.
6. Mitchell LS, Taylor B, Reimels W, Barrett FF, Devincenzo JP. Adenovirus 7a: A community-acquired outbreak in a children's hospital. *The Pediatric Infectious Disease Journal*. 2000; **19**(10): 996–1000.
7. Kojaoghlanian T, Flomenberg P, Horwitz MS. The impact of adenovirus infection on the immunocompromised host. *Reviews in Medical Virology*. 2003; **13**(3): 155–71.
8. Chemaly RF, Ghosh S, Bodey GP, Rohatgi N, Safdar A, Keating MJ et al. Respiratory viral infections in adults with hematologic malignancies and human stem cell transplantation recipients: A retrospective study at a major cancer center. *Medicine (Baltimore)*. 2006; **85**(5): 278–87.
9. Moura PO, Roberto AF, Hein N, Baldacci E, Vieira SE, Ejzenberg B et al. Molecular epidemiology of human adenovirus isolated from children hospitalized with acute respiratory infection in Sao Paulo, Brazil. *Journal of Medical Virology*. 2007; **79**(2): 174–81.
10. Lin KH, Lin YC, Chen HL, Ke GM, Chiang CJ, Hwang KP et al. A two decade survey of respiratory adenovirus in Taiwan: The reemergence of adenovirus types 7 and 4. *Journal of Medical Virology*. 2004; **73**(2): 274–9.
11. Li QG, Zheng QJ, Liu YH, Wadell G. Molecular epidemiology of adenovirus types 3 and 7 isolated from children with pneumonia in Beijing. *Journal of Medical Virology*. 1996; **49**(3): 170–7.
12. Chen HL, Chiou SS, Hsiao HP, Ke GM, Lin YC, Lin KH et al. Respiratory adenoviral infections in children: A study of hospitalized cases in southern Taiwan in 2001–2002. *Journal of Tropical Pediatrics*. 2004; **50**(5): 279–84.
13. Kolavic-Gray SA, Binn LN, Sanchez JL, Cersovsky SB, Polyak CS, Mitchell-Raymundo F et al. Large epidemic of adenovirus type 4 infection among military trainees: Epidemiological, clinical, and laboratory studies. *Clinical Infectious Diseases: An Official Publication of the Infectious Diseases Society of America*. 2002; **35**(7): 808–18.
14. Sanchez JL, Binn LN, Innis BL, Reynolds RD, Lee T, Mitchell-Raymundo F et al. Epidemic of adenovirus-induced respiratory illness among US military recruits: Epidemiologic and immunologic risk factors in healthy, young adults. *Journal of Medical Virology*. 2001; **65**(4): 710–8.
15. Kajon AE, Moseley JM, Metzgar D, Huong HS, Wadleigh A, Ryan MA et al. Molecular epidemiology of adenovirus type 4 infections in US military recruits in the postvaccination era (1997–2003). *The Journal of Infectious Diseases*. 2007; **196**(1): 67–75.
16. Ryan MA, Gray GC, Smith B, McKeehan JA, Hawksworth AW, Malasig MD. Large epidemic of respiratory illness due to adenovirus types 7 and 3 in healthy young adults. *Clinical Infectious Diseases: An Official Publication of the Infectious Diseases Society of America*. 2002; **34**(5): 577–82.
17. Russell KL, Hawksworth AW, Ryan MA, Strickler J, Irvine M, Hansen CJ et al. Vaccine-preventable adenoviral respiratory illness in US military recruits, 1999–2004. *Vaccine*. 2006; **24**(15): 2835–42.
18. Civilian outbreak of adenovirus acute respiratory disease—South Dakota, 1997. *MMWR Morbidity and Mortality Weekly Report*. 1998; **47**(27): 567–70.
19. Zarraga AL, Kerns FT, Kitchen LW. Adenovirus pneumonia with severe sequelae in an immunocompetent adult. *Clinical Infectious Diseases: An Official Publication of the Infectious Diseases Society of America*. 1992; **15**(4): 712–3.
20. Dudding BA, Wagner SC, Zeller JA, Gmelich JT, French GR, Top FH, Jr. Fatal pneumonia associated with adenovirus type 7 in three military trainees. *New England Journal of Medicine*. 1972; **286**(24): 1289–92.
21. Louie JK, Kajon AE, Holodniy M, Guardia-LaBar L, Lee B, Petru AM et al. Severe pneumonia due to adenovirus serotype 14: A new respiratory threat? *Clinical Infectious Diseases: An Official Publication of the Infectious Diseases Society of America*. 2008; **46**(3): 421–5.

22. Neofytos D, Ojha A, Mookerjee B, Wagner J, Filicko J, Ferber A et al. Treatment of adenovirus disease in stem cell transplant recipients with cidofovir. *Biology of Blood and Marrow Transplantation: Journal of the American Society for Blood and Marrow Transplantation*. 2007; **13**(1): 74–81.
23. Zheng X, Lu X, Erdman DD, Anderson EJ, Guzman-Cottrill JA, Kletzel M et al. Identification of adenoviruses from high risk pediatric stem cell transplant recipients and controls. *Journal of Clinical Microbiology*. 2008; **46**: 317–20.
24. Symeonidis N, Jakubowski A, Pierre-Louis S, Jaffe D, Pamer E, Sepkowitz K et al. Invasive adenoviral infections in T-cell-depleted allogeneic hematopoietic stem cell transplantation: High mortality in the era of cidofovir. *Transplant Infectious Disease: An Official Journal of the Transplantation Society*. 2007; **9**(2): 108–13.
25. Bordigoni P, Carret AS, Venard V, Witz F, Le Faou A. Treatment of adenovirus infections in patients undergoing allogeneic hematopoietic stem cell transplantation. *Clinical Infectious Diseases: An Official Publication of the Infectious Diseases Society of America*. 2001; **32**(9): 1290–7.
26. Lu X, Erdman DD. Molecular typing of human adenoviruses by PCR and sequencing of a partial region of the hexon gene. *Archives of Virology*. 2006; **151**(8): 1587–602.
27. Henquell C, Boeuf B, Mirand A, Bacher C, Traore O, Dechelotte P et al. Fatal adenovirus infection in a neonate and transmission to health-care workers. *Journal of Clinical Virology: The Official Publication of the Pan American Society for Clinical Virology*. 2009; **45**(4): 345–8.
28. Lee J, Choi EH, Lee HJ. Comprehensive serotyping and epidemiology of human adenovirus isolated from the respiratory tract of Korean children over 17 consecutive years (1991–2007). *Journal of Medical Virology*. 2010; **82**(4): 624–31.
29. Jones MS, 2nd, Harrach B, Ganac RD, Gozum MM, Dela Cruz WP, Riedel B et al. New adenovirus species found in a patient presenting with gastroenteritis. *Journal of Virology*. 2007; **81**(11): 5978–84.
30. Kajon AE, Lu X, Erdman DD, Louie J, Schnurr D, George KS et al. Molecular epidemiology and brief history of emerging adenovirus 14-associated respiratory disease in the United States. *The Journal of Infectious Diseases*. 2010; **202**(1): 93–103.
31. Aoki K, Kaneko H, Kitaichi N, Ohguchi T, Tagawa Y, Ohno S. Clinical features of adenoviral conjunctivitis at the early stage of infection. *Japanese Journal of Ophthalmology*. 2011; **55**(1): 11–5.
32. Seto D, Chodosh J, Brister JR, Jones MS. Using the whole-genome sequence to characterize and name human adenoviruses. *Journal of Virology*. 2011; **85**(11): 5701–2.
33. Walsh MP, Chintakuntlawar A, Robinson CM, Madisch I, Harrach B, Hudson NR et al. Evidence of molecular evolution driven by recombination events influencing tropism in a novel human adenovirus that causes epidemic keratoconjunctivitis. *PloS One*. 2009; **4**(6): e5635.
34. Akiyoshi K, Suga T, Fukui K, Taniguchi K, Okabe N, Fujimoto T. Outbreak of epidemic keratoconjunctivitis caused by adenovirus type 54 in a nursery school in Kobe City, Japan in 2008. *Japanese Journal of Infectious Diseases*. 2011; **64**(4): 353–5.
35. Hiroi S, Koike N, Nishimura T, Takahashi K, Morikawa S, Kase T. Genetic analysis of human adenovirus type 54 detected in Osaka, Japan. *Japanese Journal of Infectious Diseases*. 2011; **64**(6): 535–7.
36. Robinson CM, Seto D, Jones MS, Dyer DW, Chodosh J. Molecular evolution of human species D adenoviruses. *Infection, Genetics and Evolution: Journal of Molecular Epidemiology and Evolutionary Genetics in Infectious Diseases*. 2011; **11**(6): 1208–17.
37. Walsh MP, Seto J, Jones MS, Chodosh J, Xu W, Seto D. Computational analysis identifies human adenovirus type 55 as a re-emergent acute respiratory disease pathogen. *Journal of Clinical Microbiology*. 2010; **48**(3): 991–3.
38. Buckwalter SP, Teo R, Espy MJ, Sloan LM, Smith TF, Pritt BS. Real-time qualitative PCR for 57 human adenovirus types from multiple specimen sources. *Journal of Clinical Microbiology*. 2012; **50**(3): 766–71.
39. Aoki K, Benko M, Davison AJ, Echavarria M, Erdman DD, Harrach B et al. Toward an integrated human adenovirus designation system that utilizes molecular and serological data and serves both clinical and fundamental virology. *Journal of Virology*. 2011; **85**(11): 5703–4.
40. Houng HS, Gong H, Kajon AE, Jones MS, Kuschner RA, Lyons A et al. Genome sequences of human adenovirus 14 isolates from mild respiratory cases and a fatal pneumonia, isolated during 2006–2007 epidemics in North America. *Respiratory Research*. 2010; **11**: 116.
41. Ebner K, Rauch M, Preuner S, Lion T. Typing of human adenoviruses in specimens from immunosuppressed patients by PCR-fragment length analysis and real-time quantitative PCR. *Journal of Clinical Microbiology*. 2006; **44**(8): 2808–15.
42. Walls T, Hawrami K, Ushiro-Lumb I, Shingadia D, Saha V, Shankar AG. Adenovirus infection after pediatric bone marrow transplantation: Is treatment always necessary? *Clinical Infectious Diseases: An Official Publication of the Infectious Diseases Society of America*. 2005; **40**(9): 1244–9.

43. Kajon AE, Dickson LM, Metzgar D, Houng HS, Lee V, Tan BH. Outbreak of febrile respiratory illness associated with adenovirus 11a infection in a Singapore military training cAMP. *Journal of Clinical Microbiology*. 2010; **48**(4): 1438–41.
44. Wang H, Tuve S, Erdman DD, Lieber A. Receptor usage of a newly emergent adenovirus type 14. *Virology*. 2009; **387**(2): 436–41.
45. Gaggar A, Shayakhmetov DM, Liszewski MK, Atkinson JP, Lieber A. Localization of regions in CD46 that interact with adenovirus. *Journal of Virology*. 2005; **79**(12): 7503–13.
46. Arnberg N, Mei Y, Wadell G. Fiber genes of adenoviruses with tropism for the eye and the genital tract. *Virology*. 1997; **227**(1): 239–44.
47. Mei YF, Wadell G. Hemagglutination properties and nucleotide sequence analysis of the fiber gene of adenovirus genome types 11p and 11a. *Virology*. 1993; **194**(2): 453–62.
48. Mei YF, Lindman K, Wadell G. Two closely related adenovirus genome types with kidney or respiratory tract tropism differ in their binding to epithelial cells of various origins. *Virology*. 1998; **240**(2): 254–66.
49. Mei YF, Wadell G. Molecular determinants of adenovirus tropism. *Current Topics in Microbiology and Immunology*. 1995; **199 (Pt 3)**: 213–28.
50. Beatty MS, Curiel DT. Chapter two—Adenovirus strategies for tissue-specific targeting. *Advances in Cancer Research*. 2012; **115**: 39–67.
51. Arnberg N. Adenovirus receptors: Implications for targeting of viral vectors. *Trends in Pharmacological Sciences*. 2012; **33**(8): 442–8.
52. Wang H, Li ZY, Liu Y, Persson J, Beyer I, Moller T et al. Desmoglein 2 is a receptor for adenovirus serotypes 3, 7, 11 and 14. *Nature Medicine*. 2011; **17**(1): 96–104.
53. Erdman DD, Xu W, Gerber SI, Gray GC, Schnurr D, Kajon AE et al. Molecular epidemiology of adenovirus type 7 in the United States, 1966–2000. *Emerging Infectious Diseases*. 2002; **8**(3): 269–77.
54. Ariga T, Shimada Y, Shiratori K, Ohgami K, Yamazaki S, Tagawa Y et al. Five new genome types of adenovirus type 37 caused epidemic keratoconjunctivitis in Sapporo, Japan, for more than 10 years. *Journal of Clinical Microbiology*. 2005; **43**(2): 726–32.
55. Jin XH, Aoki K, Kitaichi N, Ariga T, Ishida S, Ohno S. Genome variability of human adenovirus type 8 causing epidemic keratoconjunctivitis during 1986–2003 in Japan. *Molecular Vision*. 2011; **17**: 3121–7.
56. Itakura S, Aoki K, Sawada H, Shinagawa M. Analysis with restriction endonucleases recognizing 4- or 5-base-pair sequences of human adenovirus type 3 isolated from ocular diseases in Sapporo, Japan. *Journal of Clinical Microbiology*. 1990; **28**(10): 2365–9.
57. Ariga T, Shimada Y, Ohgami K, Tagawa Y, Ishiko H, Aoki K et al. New genome type of adenovirus serotype 4 caused nosocomial infections associated with epidemic conjunctivitis in Japan. *Journal of Clinical Microbiology*. 2004; **42**(8): 3644–8.
58. Wadell G, Varsanyi TM. Demonstration of three different subtypes of adenovirus type 7 by DNA restriction site mapping. *Infection and Immunity*. 1978; **21**(1): 238–46.
59. Li QG, Wadell G. Analysis of 15 different genome types of adenovirus type 7 isolated on five continents. *Journal of Virology*. 1986; **60**(1): 331–5.
60. Wadell G, Cooney MK, da Costa Linhares A, de Silva L, Kennett ML, Kono R et al. Molecular epidemiology of adenoviruses: Global distribution of adenovirus 7 genome types. *Journal of Clinical Microbiology*. 1985; **21**(3): 403–8.
61. Li QG, Wadell G. Comparison of 17 genome types of adenovirus type 3 identified among strains recovered from six continents. *Journal of Clinical Microbiology*. 1988; **26**(5): 1009–15.
62. Kajon A, Wadell G. Genome analysis of South American adenovirus strains of serotype 7 collected over a 7-year period. *Journal of Clinical Microbiology*. 1994; **32**(9): 2321–3.
63. de Silva LM, Colditz P, Wadell G. Adenovirus type 7 infections in children in New South Wales, Australia. *Journal of Medical Virology*. 1989; **29**(1): 28–32.
64. Azar R, Varsano N, Mileguir F, Mendelson E. Molecular epidemiology of adenovirus type 7 in Israel: Identification of two new genome types, Ad7 k and Ad7d2. *Journal of Medical Virology*. 1998; **54**(4): 291–9.
65. Nakayama M, Miyazaki C, Ueda K, Kusuhara K, Yoshikawa H, Nishima S et al. Pharyngoconjunctival fever caused by adenovirus type 11. *The Pediatric Infectious Disease Journal*. 1992; **11**(1): 6–9.
66. James L, Vernon MO, Jones RC, Stewart A, Lu X, Zollar LM et al. Outbreak of human adenovirus type 3 infection in a pediatric long-term care facility—Illinois, 2005. *Clinical Infectious Diseases: An Official Publication of the Infectious Diseases Society of America*. 2007; **45**(4): 416–20.
67. Ishiko H, Aoki K. Spread of epidemic keratoconjunctivitis due to a novel serotype of human adenovirus in Japan. *Journal of Clinical Microbiology*. 2009; **47**(8): 2678–9.

68. Kaneko H, Aoki K, Ohno S, Ishiko H, Fujimoto T, Kikuchi M et al. Complete genome analysis of a novel intertypic recombinant human adenovirus causing epidemic keratoconjunctivitis in Japan. *Journal of Clinical Microbiology*. 2011; **49**(2): 484–90.
69. Filho EP, da Costa Faria NR, Fialho AM, de Assis RS, Almeida MM, Rocha M et al. Adenoviruses associated with acute gastroenteritis in hospitalized and community children up to 5 years old in Rio de Janeiro and Salvador, Brazil. *Journal of Medical Microbiology*. 2007; **56**(Pt 3): 313–9.
70. Madisch I, Wolfel R, Harste G, Pommer H, Heim A. Molecular identification of adenovirus sequences: A rapid scheme for early typing of human adenoviruses in diagnostic samples of immunocompetent and immunodeficient patients. *Journal of Medical Virology*. 2006; **78**(9): 1210–7.
71. Fukuda S, Kuwayama M, Takao S, Shimazu Y, Miyazaki K. Molecular epidemiology of subgenus F adenoviruses associated with pediatric gastroenteritis during eight years in Hiroshima Prefecture as a limited area. *Archives of Virology*. 2006; **151**(12): 2511–7.
72. Sdiri-Loulizi K, Gharbi-Khelifi H, de Rougemont A, Hassine M, Chouchane S, Sakly N et al. Molecular epidemiology of human astrovirus and adenovirus serotypes 40/41 strains related to acute diarrhea in Tunisian children. *Journal of Medical Virology*. 2009; **81**(11): 1895–902.
73. Magwalivha M, Wolfaardt M, Kiulia NM, van Zyl WB, Mwenda JM, Taylor MB. High prevalence of species D human adenoviruses in fecal specimens from Urban Kenyan children with diarrhea. *Journal of Medical Virology*. **82**(1): 77–84.
74. Goncalves G, Gouveia E, Mesquita JR, Almeida A, Ribeiro A, Rocha-Pereira J et al. Outbreak of acute gastroenteritis caused by adenovirus type 41 in a kindergarten. *Epidemiology and Infection*. 2011; **139**(11): 1672–5.
75. Li L, Shimizu H, Doan LT, Tung PG, Okitsu S, Nishio O et al. Characterizations of adenovirus type 41 isolates from children with acute gastroenteritis in Japan, Vietnam, and Korea. *Journal of Clinical Microbiology*. 2004; **42**(9): 4032–9.
76. Marie-Cardine A, Gourlain K, Mouterde O, Castignolles N, Hellot MF, Mallet E et al. Epidemiology of acute viral gastroenteritis in children hospitalized in Rouen, France. *Clinical Infectious Diseases: An Official Publication of the Infectious Diseases Society of America*. 2002; **34**(9): 1170–8.
77. Soares CC, Volotao EM, Albuquerque MC, da Silva FM, de Carvalho TR, Nozawa CM et al. Prevalence of enteric adenoviruses among children with diarrhea in four Brazilian cities. *Journal of Clinical Virology: The Official Publication of the Pan American Society for Clinical Virology*. 2002; **23**(3): 171–7.
78. Cunliffe NA, Booth JA, Elliot C, Lowe SJ, Sopwith W, Kitchin N et al. Healthcare-associated viral gastroenteritis among children in a large pediatric hospital, United Kingdom. *Emerging Infectious Diseases*. **16**(1): 55–62.
79. Iturriza Gomara M, Simpson R, Perault AM, Redpath C, Lorgelly P, Joshi D et al. Structured surveillance of infantile gastroenteritis in East Anglia, UK: Incidence of infection with common viral gastroenteric pathogens. *Epidemiology and Infection*. 2008; **136**(1): 23–33.
80. Kim Y-J, Boeckh M, Englund JA. Community respiratory virus infections in immunocompromised patients: Hematopoietic stem cell and solid organ transplant recipients, and individuals with human immunodeficiency virus infection. *Seminars in Respiratory and Critical Care Medicine*. 2007; **28**(2): 222–42.
81. Taniguchi K, Yoshihara S, Tamaki H, Fujimoto T, Ikegame K, Kaida K et al. Incidence and treatment strategy for disseminated adenovirus disease after haploidentical stem cell transplantation. *Annals of Hematology*. 2012; **91**(8): 1305–12.
82. King JC, Jr. Community respiratory viruses in individuals with human immunodeficiency virus infection. *American Journal of Medicine*. 1997; **102**(3A): 19–24; discussion 5–6.
83. Echavarria M. Adenoviruses in immunocompromised hosts. *Clinical Microbiology Review*. 2008; **21**(4): 704–15.
84. Barker JH, Luby JP, Sean Dalley A, Bartek WM, Burns DK, Erdman DD. Fatal type 3 adenoviral pneumonia in immunocompetent adult identical twins. *Clinical Infectious Diseases: An Official Publication of the Infectious Diseases Society of America*. 2003; **37**(10): e142–6.
85. Garnett CT, Erdman D, Xu W, Gooding LR. Prevalence and quantitation of species C adenovirus DNA in human mucosal lymphocytes. *Journal of Virology*. 2002; **76**(21): 10608–16.
86. Roy S, Calcedo R, Medina-Jaszek A, Keough M, Peng H, Wilson JM. Adenoviruses in lymphocytes of the human gastro-intestinal tract. *PloS One*. 2011; **6**(9): e24859.
87. Curlin ME, Huang ML, Lu X, Celum CL, Sanchez J, Selke S et al. Frequent detection of human adenovirus from the lower gastrointestinal tract in men who have sex with men. *PloS One*. 2010; **5**(6): e11321.
88. Bil-Lula I, Ussowicz M, Rybka B, Wendycz-Domalewska D, Ryczan R, Gorczynska E et al. Hematuria due to adenoviral infection in bone marrow transplant recipients. *Transplant Proceedings*. **42**(9): 3729–34.

89. Mattner F, Sykora KW, Meissner B, Heim A. An adenovirus type F41 outbreak in a pediatric bone marrow transplant unit: Analysis of clinical impact and preventive strategies. *The Pediatric Infectious Disease Journal*. 2008; **27**(5): 419–24.
90. Buffington J, Chapman LE, Stobierski MG, Hierholzer JC, Gary HE, Jr., Guskey LE et al. Epidemic keratoconjunctivitis in a chronic care facility: Risk factors and measures for control. *Journal of American Geriatric Society.* 1993; **41**(11): 1177–81.
91. Ersoy Y, Otlu B, Turkcuoglu P, Yetkin F, Aker S, Kuzucu C. Outbreak of adenovirus serotype 8 conjunctivitis in preterm infants in a neonatal intensive care unit. *The Journal of Hospital Infection*. 2012; **80**(2): 144–9.
92. Lessa FC, Gould PL, Pascoe N, Erdman DD, Lu X, Bunning ML et al. Health care transmission of a newly emergent adenovirus serotype in health care personnel at a military hospital in Texas, 2007. *The Journal of Infectious Diseases*. 2009; **200**(11): 1759–65.
93. Russell KL, Broderick MP, Franklin SE, Blyn LB, Freed NE, Moradi E et al. Transmission dynamics and prospective environmental sampling of adenovirus in a military recruit setting. *The Journal of Infectious Diseases*. 2006; **194**(7): 877–85.
94. McNeill KM, Ridgely Benton F, Monteith SC, Tuchscherer MA, Gaydos JC. Epidemic spread of adenovirus type 4-associated acute respiratory disease between U.S. Army installations. *Emerging Infectious Diseases*. 2000; **6**(4): 415–9.
95. Jeon K, Kang CI, Yoon CH, Lee DJ, Kim CH, Chung YS et al. High isolation rate of adenovirus serotype 7 from South Korean military recruits with mild acute respiratory disease. *European Journal of Clinical Microbiology Infectious Disease.* 2007; **26**(7): 481–3.
96. Finn A, Anday E, Talbot GH. An epidemic of adenovirus 7a infection in a neonatal nursery: Course, morbidity, and management. *Infectious Control of Hospital Epidemiology.* 1988; **9**(9): 398–404.
97. Sanchez MP, Erdman DD, Torok TJ, Freeman CJ, Matyas BT. Outbreak of adenovirus 35 pneumonia among adult residents and staff of a chronic care psychiatric facility. *The Journal of Infectious Diseases*. 1997; **176**(3): 760–3.
98. Klinger JR, Sanchez MP, Curtin LA, Durkin M, Matyas B. Multiple cases of life-threatening adenovirus pneumonia in a mental health care center. *American Journal of Respiratory Critical Care Medicine*. 1998; **157**(2): 645–9.
99. Gerber SI, Erdman DD, Pur SL, Diaz PS, Segreti J, Kajon AE et al. Outbreak of adenovirus genome type 7d2 infection in a pediatric chronic-care facility and tertiary-care hospital. *Clinical Infectious Diseases: An Official Publication of the Infectious Diseases Society of America*. 2001; **32**(5): 694–700.
100. Kandel R, Srinivasan A, D'Agata EM, Lu X, Erdman D, Jhung M. Outbreak of adenovirus type 4 infection in a long-term care facility for the elderly. *Infectious Control of Hospital Epidemiology*. 2010; **31**(7): 755–7.
101. Ghanaiem H, Averbuch D, Koplewitz BZ, Yatsiv I, Braun J, Dehtyar N et al. An outbreak of adenovirus type 7 in a residential facility for severely disabled children. *The Pediatric Infectious Disease Journal*. 2011; **30**(11): 948–52.
102. Zhu Z, Zhang Y, Xu S, Yu P, Tian X, Wang L et al. Outbreak of acute respiratory disease in China caused by B2 species of adenovirus type 11. *Journal of Clinical Microbiology*. 2009; **47**(3): 697–703.
103. Harris DJ, Wulff H, Ray CG, Poland JD, Chin TD, Wenner HA. Viruses and disease. 3. An outbreak of adenovirus type 7A in a children's home. *American Journal of Epidemiology.* 1971; **93**(5): 399–402.
104. Chany C, Lepine P, Lelong M, Le TV, Satge P, Virat J. Severe and fatal pneumonia in infants and young children associated with adenovirus infections. *American Journal of Hygiene.* 1958; **67**(3): 367–78.
105. Schmitz H, Wigand R, Heinrich W. Worldwide epidemiology of human adenovirus infections. *American Journal of Epidemiology*. 1983; **117**(4): 455–66.
106. Rubin BA. Clinical picture and epidemiology of adenovirus infections (a review). *Acta Microbiology Hungary*. 1993; **40**(4): 303–23.
107. Trei JS, Johns NM, Garner JL, Noel LB, Ortman BV, Ensz KL et al. Spread of adenovirus to geographically dispersed military installations, May–October 2007. *Emerging Infectious Diseases*. 2010; **16**(5): 769–75.
108. Singh-Naz N, Brown M, Ganeshananthan M. Nosocomial adenovirus infection: Molecular epidemiology of an outbreak. *The Pediatric Infectious Disease Journal*. 1993; **12**(11): 922–5.
109. Sauerbrei A, Sehr K, Brandstadt A, Heim A, Reimer K, Wutzler P. Sensitivity of human adenoviruses to different groups of chemical biocides. *The Journal of Hospital Infection*. 2004; **57**(1): 59–66.
110. Hong JY, Lee HJ, Piedra PA, Choi EH, Park KH, Koh YY et al. Lower respiratory tract infections due to adenovirus in hospitalized Korean children: Epidemiology, clinical features, and prognosis. *Clinical Infectious Diseases: An Official Publication of the Infectious Diseases Society of America.* 2001; **32**(10): 1423–9.

111. Hakim FA, Tleyjeh IM. Severe adenovirus pneumonia in immunocompetent adults: A case report and review of the literature. *European Journal of Clinical Microbiology Infectious Disease*. 2008; **27**(2): 153–8.
112. Cherry J. Adenoviruses. In: Feigin RD, Cherry JD, Demmler GJ, Kaplan SL, eds. *Textbook of Pediatric Infectious Diseases*, 5th ed. 2003; **2**(Saunders, Philadelphia, PA): 1843–56.
113. Murtagh P, Giubergia V, Viale D, Bauer G, Pena HG. Lower respiratory infections by adenovirus in children. Clinical features and risk factors for bronchiolitis obliterans and mortality. *Pediatric Pulmonology*. 2009; **44**(5): 450–6.
114. Tabbara KF, Omar N, Hammouda E, Akanuma M, Ohguchi T, Ariga T et al. Molecular epidemiology of adenoviral keratoconjunctivitis in Saudi Arabia. *Molecular Vision*. **16**: 2132–6.
115. Aoki K, Tagawa Y. A twenty-one year surveillance of adenoviral conjunctivitis in Sapporo, Japan. *International Ophthalmology Clinic*. 2002; **42**(1): 49–54.
116. Percivalle E, Sarasini A, Torsellini M, Bruschi L, Antoniazzi E, Grazia Revello M et al. A comparison of methods for detecting adenovirus type 8 keratoconjunctivitis during a nosocomial outbreak in a neonatal intensive care unit. *Journal of Clinical Virology: The Official Publication of the Pan American Society for Clinical Virology*. 2003; **28**(3): 257–64.
117. Hamada N, Gotoh K, Hara K, Iwahashi J, Imamura Y, Nakamura S et al. Nosocomial outbreak of epidemic keratoconjunctivitis accompanying environmental contamination with adenoviruses. *The Journal of Hospital Infection*. 2008; **68**(3): 262–8.
118. Ishiko H, Shimada Y, Konno T, Hayashi A, Ohguchi T, Tagawa Y et al. Novel human adenovirus causing nosocomial epidemic keratoconjunctivitis. *Journal of Clinical Microbiology*. 2008; **46**(6): 2002–8.
119. Chang CH, Lin KH, Sheu MM, Huang WL, Wang HZ, Chen CW. The change of etiological agents and clinical signs of epidemic viral conjunctivitis over an 18-year period in southern Taiwan. *Graefes Archives of Clinical Experimental Ophthalmology*. 2003; **241**(7): 554–60.
120. Matsui K, Saha S, Saitoh M, Mizuki N, Itoh N, Okada E et al. Isolation and identification of adenovirus from conjunctival scrapings over a two-year period (between 2001 and 2003) in Yokohama, Japan. *Journal of Medical Virology*. 2007; **79**(2): 200–5.
121. Jin XH, Ishiko H, Nguyen TH, Ohguchi T, Akanuma M, Aoki K et al. Molecular epidemiology of adenoviral conjunctivitis in Hanoi, Vietnam. *American Journal of Ophthalmology*. 2006; **142**(6): 1064–6.
122. Kaneko H, Suzutani T, Aoki K, Kitaichi N, Ishida S, Ishiko H et al. Epidemiological and virological features of epidemic keratoconjunctivitis due to new human adenovirus type 54 in Japan. *The British Journal of Ophthalmology*. 2011; **95**(1): 32–6.
123. Kaneko H, Ishiko H, Ohguchi T, Tagawa Y, Aoki K, Suzutani T et al. Nucleotide sequence variation in the hexon gene of human adenovirus type 8 and 37 strains from epidemic keratoconjunctivitis patients in Japan. *The Journal of General Virology*. 2009; **90**(Pt 9): 2260–5.
124. Nakamura M, Hirano E, Kowada K, Ishiguro F, Yamagishi Z, Adhikary AK et al. Surveillance of adenovirus D in patients with epidemic keratoconjunctivitis from Fukui Prefecture, Japan, 1995–2010. *Journal of Medical Virology*. 2012; **84**(1): 81–6.
125. Saitoh-Inagawa W, Aoki K, Uchio E, Itoh N, Ohno S. Ten years' surveillance of viral conjunctivitis in Sapporo, Japan. *Graefes Archives of Clinical Experimental Ophthalmology*. 1999; **237**(1): 35–8.
126. Sendra-Gutierrez JM, Martin-Rios D, Casas I, Saez P, Tovar A, Moreno C. An outbreak of adenovirus type 8 keratoconjunctivitis in a nursing home in Madrid. *Euro Surveillance: Bulletin Europeen sur les Maladies Transmissibles = European Communicable Disease Bulletin*. 2004; **9**(3): 27–30.
127. Kapelushnik J, Or R, Delukina M, Nagler A, Livni N, Engelhard D. Intravenous ribavirin therapy for adenovirus gastroenteritis after bone marrow transplantation. *Journal of Pediatric Gastroenterology Nutrition*. 1995; **21**(1): 110–2.
128. Wang WH, Wang HL. Fulminant adenovirus hepatitis following bone marrow transplantation. A case report and brief review of the literature. *Archives of Pathological Laboratort Medicine*. 2003; **127**(5): e246–8.
129. Hedderwick SA, Greenson JK, McGaughy VR, Clark NM. Adenovirus cholecystitis in a patient with AIDS. *Clinical Infectious Diseases: An Official Publication of the Infectious Diseases Society of America*. 1998; **26**(4): 997–9.
130. Bateman CM, Kesson AM, Shaw PJ. Pancreatitis and adenoviral infection in children after blood and marrow transplantation. *Bone Marrow Transplantation*. 2006; **38**(12): 807–11.
131. Florescu DF, Islam MK, Mercer DF, Grant W, Langnas AN, Freifeld AG et al. Adenovirus infections in pediatric small bowel transplant recipients. *Transplantation*. 2010; **90**(2): 198–204.
132. Yokose N, Hirakawa T, Inokuchi K. Adenovirus-associated hemorrhagic cystitis in a patient with plasma cell myeloma treated with bortezomib. *Leukocyte Research*. 2009; **33**(8): e106.

133. Bil-Lula I, De Franceschi N, Pawlik K, Wozniak M. Improved real-time PCR assay for detection and quantification of all 54 known types of human adenoviruses in clinical samples. *Medical Science Monitor: International Medical Journal of Experimental and Clinical Research*. 2012; **18**(6): BR221–8.
134. Akiyama H, Kurosu T, Sakashita C, Inoue T, Mori S, Ohashi K et al. Adenovirus is a key pathogen in hemorrhagic cystitis associated with bone marrow transplantation. *Clinical Infectious Diseases: An Official Publication of the Infectious Diseases Society of America*. 2001; **32**(9): 1325–30.
135. Teramura T, Naya M, Yoshihara T, Kanoh G, Morimoto A, Imashuku S. Adenoviral infection in hematopoietic stem cell transplantation: Early diagnosis with quantitative detection of the viral genome in serum and urine. *Bone Marrow Transplantation*. 2004; **33**(1): 87–92.
136. Miyamura K, Hamaguchi M, Taji H, Kanie T, Kohno A, Tanimoto M et al. Successful ribavirin therapy for severe adenovirus hemorrhagic cystitis after allogeneic marrow transplant from close HLA donors rather than distant donors. *Bone Marrow Transplantation*. 2000; **25**(5): 545–8.
137. Fanourgiakis P, Georgala A, Vekemans M, Triffet A, De Bruyn JM, Duchateau V et al. Intravesical instillation of cidofovir in the treatment of hemorrhagic cystitis caused by adenovirus type 11 in a bone marrow transplant recipient. *Clinical Infectious Diseases: An Official Publication of the Infectious Diseases Society of America*. 2005; **40**(1): 199–201.
138. Mori Y, Miyamoto T, Kato K, Kamezaki K, Kuriyama T, Oku S et al. Different risk factors related to adenovirus- or BK virus-associated hemorrhagic cystitis following allogeneic stem cell transplantation. *Biology of Blood and Marrow Transplantation: Journal of the American Society for Blood and Marrow Transplantation*. 2012; **18**(3): 458–65.
139. Gorczynska E, Turkiewicz D, Rybka K, Toporski J, Kalwak K, Dyla A et al. Incidence, clinical outcome, and management of virus-induced hemorrhagic cystitis in children and adolescents after allogeneic hematopoietic cell transplantation. *Biology of Blood and Marrow Transplantation: Journal of the American Society for Blood and Marrow Transplantation*. 2005; **11**(10): 797–804.
140. Hofland CA, Eron LJ, Washecka RM. Hemorrhagic adenovirus cystitis after renal transplantation. *Transplant Proceedings*. 2004; **36**(10): 3025–7.
141. Ferreira GF, Oliveira RA, Lucon M, de Paula FJ, Lucon AM, Ianhez LE et al. Hemorrhagic cystitis secondary to adenovirus or herpes simplex virus infection following renal transplantation: Four case reports. *Transplant Proceedings*. 2009; **41**(10): 4416–9.
142. Yagisawa T, Nakada T, Takahashi K, Toma H, Ota K, Yaguchi H. Acute hemorrhagic cystitis caused by adenovirus after kidney transplantation. *Urology International*. 1995; **54**(3): 142–6.
143. Keswani M, Moudgil A. Adenovirus-associated hemorrhagic cystitis in a pediatric renal transplant recipient. *Pediatric Transplant*. 2007; **11**(5): 568–71.
144. Koga S, Shindo K, Matsuya F, Hori T, Kanda S, Kanetake H. Acute hemorrhagic cystitis caused by adenovirus following renal transplantation: Review of the literature. *Journal of Urology*. 1993; **149**(4): 838–9.
145. Ito M, Hirabayashi N, Uno Y, Nakayama A, Asai J. Necrotizing tubulointerstitial nephritis associated with adenovirus infection. *Human Pathology*. 1991; **22**(12): 1225–31.
146. Bruno B, Zager RA, Boeckh MJ, Gooley TA, Myerson DH, Huang ML et al. Adenovirus nephritis in hematopoietic stem-cell transplantation. *Transplantation*. 2004; **77**(7): 1049–57.
147. Mori K, Yoshihara T, Nishimura Y, Uchida M, Katsura K, Kawase Y et al. Acute renal failure due to adenovirus-associated obstructive uropathy and necrotizing tubulointerstitial nephritis in a bone marrow transplant recipient. *Bone Marrow Transplantation*. 2003; **31**(12): 1173–6.
148. Sujeet K, Vasudev B, Desai P, Bellizzi J, Novoa-Takara L, He C et al. Acute kidney injury requiring dialysis secondary to adenovirus nephritis in renal transplant recipient. *Transplant Infectious Disease: An Official Journal of the Transplantation Society*. 2011; **13**: 174–7.
149. Sivaprakasam P, Carr TF, Coussons M, Khalid T, Bailey AS, Guiver M et al. Improved outcome from invasive adenovirus infection in pediatric patients after hemopoietic stem cell transplantation using intensive clinical surveillance and early intervention. *Journal of Pediatric Hematology Oncology*. 2007; **29**(2): 81–5.
150. Robin M, Marque-Juillet S, Scieux C, Peffault de Latour R, Ferry C, Rocha V et al. Disseminated adenovirus infections after allogeneic hematopoietic stem cell transplantation: Incidence, risk factors and outcome. *Haematologica*. 2007; **92**(9): 1254–7.
151. Kroes AC, de Klerk EP, Lankester AC, Malipaard C, de Brouwer CS, Claas EC et al. Sequential emergence of multiple adenovirus serotypes after pediatric stem cell transplantation. *Journal of Clinical Virology: The Official Publication of the Pan American Society for Clinical Virology*. 2007; **38**(4): 341–7.
152. de Mezerville MH, Tellier R, Richardson S, Hebert D, Doyle J, Allen U. Adenoviral infections in pediatric transplant recipients: A hospital-based study. *The Pediatric Infectious Disease Journal*. 2006; **25**(9): 815–8.

238. Tai FH, Chu S, Chi WH, Wei HY, Hierholzer JC. Epidemic haemorrhagic conjunctivitis associated with adenovirus type 11 in Taiwan. *Southeast Asian Journal of Tropical Medicine Public Health*. 1974; **5**(3): 342–9.
239. Yin-Murphy M, Lim KH, Chua PH. Adenovirus type 11 epidemic conjunctivitis in Singapore. *Southeast Asian Journal of Tropical Medicine Public Health*. 1974; **5**(3): 333–41.
240. Asim M, Chong-Lopez A, Nickeleit V. Adenovirus infection of a renal allograft. *American Journal of Kidney Disease*. 2003; **41**(3): 696–701.
241. Yang Z, Zhu Z, Tang L, Wang L, Tan X, Yu P et al. Genomic analyses of recombinant adenovirus type 11a in China. *Journal of Clinical Microbiology*. 2009; **47**(10): 3082–90.
242. Kendall EJ, Riddle RW, Tuck HA, Rodan KS, Andrews BE, McDonald JC. Pharyngo-conjunctival fever; school outbreaks in England during the summer of 1955 associated with adenovirus types 3, 7, and 14. *British Medical Journal*. 1957; **2**(5037): 131–6.
243. Tate JE, Bunning ML, Lott L, Lu X, Su J, Metzgar D et al. Outbreak of severe respiratory disease associated with emergent human adenovirus serotype 14 at a US air force training facility in 2007. *The Journal of Infectious Diseases*. 2009; **199**(10): 1419–26.
244. Lewis PF, Schmidt MA, Lu X, Erdman DD, Campbell M, Thomas A et al. A community-based outbreak of severe respiratory illness caused by human adenovirus serotype 14. *The Journal of Infectious Diseases*. 2009; **199**(10): 1427–34.
245. Vento TJ, Prakash V, Murray CK, Brosch LC, Tchandja JB, Cogburn C et al. Pneumonia in military trainees: A comparison study based on adenovirus serotype 14 infection. *The Journal of Infectious Diseases*. 2011; **203**(10): 1388–95.
246. O'Flanagan D, O'Donnell J, Domegan L, Fitzpatrick F, Connell J, Coughlan S et al. First reported cases of human adenovirus serotype 14p1 infection, Ireland, October 2009 to July 2010. *Euro Surveillance: Bulletin Europeen sur les Maladies Transmissibles = European Communicable Disease Bulletin*. 2011; **16**(8): pii:19801.
247. Zhang G, Hu Y, Wang H, Zhang L, Bao Y, Zhou X. High incidence of multiple viral infections identified in upper respiratory tract infected children under three years of age in Shanghai, China. *PloS One*. 2012; **7**(9): e44568.
248. Becroft DM. Bronchiolitis obliterans, bronchiectasis, and other sequelae of adenovirus type 21 infection in young children. *Journal of Clinical Pathology*. 1971; **24**(1): 72–82.
249. James AG, Lang WR, Liang AY, Mackay RJ, Morris MC, Newman JN et al. Adenovirus type 21 bronchopneumonia in infants and young children. *The Journal of Pediatrics*. 1979; **95**(4): 530–3.
250. Hierholzer JC, Torrence AE, Wright PF. Generalized viral illness caused by an intermediate strain of adenovirus (21/H21 + 35). *The Journal of Infectious Diseases*. 1980; **141**(3): 281–8.
251. Darougar S, Pearce R, Gibson JA, McSwiggan DA. Adenovirus type 21 keratoconjunctivitis. *The British Journal of Ophthalmology*. 1978; **62**(12): 836–7.
252. Wright J, Couchonnal G, Hodges GR. Adenovirus type 21 infection. Occurrence with pneumonia, rhabdomyolysis, and myoglobinuria in an adult. *JAMA: The Journal of the American Medical Association*. 1979; **241**(22): 2420–1.
253. van der Avoort HG, Adrian T, Wigand R, Wermenbol AG, Zomerdijk TP, de Jong JC. Molecular epidemiology of adenovirus type 21 in the Netherlands and the Federal Republic of Germany from 1960 to 1985. *Journal of Clinical Microbiology*. 1986; **24**(6): 1084–8.
254. Van Der Veen J, Dijkman JH. Association of type 21 adenovirus with acute respiratory illness in military recruits. *American Journal of Hygiene*. 1962; **76**: 149–59.
255. Rose HM, Lamson TH, Buescher EL. Adenoviral infection in military recruits. *Archives of Environmental Health*. 1970; **21**(3): 356–61.
256. Larsen RA, Jacobson JT, Jacobson JA, Strikas RA, Hierholzer JC. Hospital-associated epidemic of pharyngitis and conjunctivitis caused by adenovirus (21/H21 + 35). *The Journal of Infectious Diseases*. 1986; **154**(4): 706–9.
257. Wold W, Horwitz M. Adenoviruses. In: Knipe DM, Howley PM, eds., *Fields Virology*, 5th ed., Philadelphia: Lippincott, Williams & Wilkins, Inc. 2007: pp.2395–436.
258. Barrero PR, Valinotto LE, Tittarelli E, Mistchenko AS. Molecular typing of adenoviruses in pediatric respiratory infections in Buenos Aires, Argentina (1999–2010). *Journal of Clinical Virology: The Official Publication of the Pan American Society for Clinical Virology*. 2012; **53**(2): 145–50.
259. Seidemann K, Heim A, Pfister ED, Koditz H, Beilken A, Sander A et al. Monitoring of adenovirus infection in pediatric transplant recipients by quantitative PCR: Report of six cases and review of the literature. *American Journal of Transplantation: Official Journal of the American Society of Transplantation and the American Society of Transplant Surgeons*. 2004; **4**(12): 2102–8.

260. Kampmann B, Cubitt D, Walls T, Naik P, Depala M, Samarasinghe S et al. Improved outcome for children with disseminated adenoviral infection following allogeneic stem cell transplantation. *British Journal of Haematology*. 2005; **130**(4): 595–603.
261. Leruez-Ville M, Chardin-Ouachee M, Neven B, Picard C, Le Guinche I, Fischer A et al. Description of an adenovirus A31 outbreak in a paediatric haematology unit. *Bone Marrow Transplantation*. 2006; **38**(1): 23–8.
262. Venard V, Carret A, Corsaro D, Bordigoni P, Le Faou A. Genotyping of adenoviruses isolated in an outbreak in a bone marrow transplant unit shows that diverse strains are involved. *The Journal of Hospital Infection*. 2000; **44**(1): 71–4.
263. Yamada T, Hara K, Kadowaki T. Association of adenovirus 36 infection with obesity and metabolic markers in humans: A meta-analysis of observational studies. *PloS One*. 2012; **7**(7): e42031.
264. Esposito S, Preti V, Consolo S, Nazzari E, Principi N. Adenovirus 36 infection and obesity. *Journal of Clinical Virology: The Official Publication of the Pan American Society for Clinical Virology*. 2012; **55**(2): 95–100.
265. Almgren M, Atkinson R, He J, Hilding A, Hagman E, Wolk A et al. Adenovirus-36 is associated with obesity in children and adults in Sweden as determined by rapid ELISA. *PloS One*. 2012; **7**(7): e41652.
266. Dey SK, Hoq I, Okitsu S, Hayakawa S, Ushijima H. Prevalence, seasonality, and peak age of infection of enteric adenoviruses in Japan, 1995–2009. *Epidemiology and Infection*. 2013; **141**: 958–60.
267. Slatter MA, Read S, Taylor CE, Crooks BN, Abinun M, Flood TJ et al. Adenovirus type F subtype 41 causing disseminated disease following bone marrow transplantation for immunodeficiency. *Journal of Clinical Microbiology*. 2005; **43**(3): 1462–4.
268. Jeulin H, Salmon A, Bordigoni P, Venard V. Diagnostic value of quantitative PCR for adenovirus detection in stool samples as compared with antigen detection and cell culture in haematopoietic stem cell transplant recipients. *Clinical Microbiology and Infection: The Official Publication of the European Society of Clinical Microbiology and Infectious Diseases*. 2011; **17**(11): 1674–80.
269. Echavarria MS, Ray SC, Ambinder R, Dumler JS, Charache P. PCR detection of adenovirus in a bone marrow transplant recipient: Hemorrhagic cystitis as a presenting manifestation of disseminated disease. *Journal of Clinical Microbiology*. 1999; **37**(3): 686–9.
270. Ganzenmueller T, Heim A. Adenoviral load diagnostics by quantitative polymerase chain reaction: Techniques and application. *Reviews in Medical Virology*. 2012; **22**(3): 194–208.
271. Erard V, Huang ML, Ferrenberg J, Nguy L, Stevens-Ayers TL, Hackman RC et al. Quantitative real-time polymerase chain reaction for detection of adenovirus after T cell-replete hematopoietic cell transplantation: Viral load as a marker for invasive disease. *Clinical Infectious Diseases: An Official Publication of the Infectious Diseases Society of America*. 2007; **45**(8): 958–65.
272. Lankester AC, Heemskerk B, Claas EC, Schilham MW, Beersma MF, Bredius RG et al. Effect of ribavirin on the plasma viral DNA load in patients with disseminating adenovirus infection. *Clinical Infectious Diseases: An Official Publication of the Infectious Diseases Society of America*. 2004; **38**(11): 1521–5.
273. Morfin F, Dupuis-Girod S, Mundweiler S, Falcon D, Carrington D, Sedlacek P et al. *In vitro* susceptibility of adenovirus to antiviral drugs is species-dependent. *Antiviral Therapy*. 2005; **10**(2): 225–9.
274. Hoffman JA, Shah AJ, Ross LA, Kapoor N. Adenoviral infections and a prospective trial of cidofovir in pediatric hematopoietic stem cell transplantation. *Biology of Blood and Marrow Transplantation: Journal of the American Society for Blood and Marrow Transplantation*. 2001; **7**(7): 388–94.
275. Doan ML, Mallory GB, Kaplan SL, Dishop MK, Schecter MG, McKenzie ED et al. Treatment of adenovirus pneumonia with cidofovir in pediatric lung transplant recipients. *Journal of Heart Lung Transplant*. 2007; **26**(9): 883–9.
276. Wallot MA, Dohna-Schwake C, Auth M, Nadalin S, Fiedler M, Malago M et al. Disseminated adenovirus infection with respiratory failure in pediatric liver transplant recipients: Impact of intravenous cidofovir and inhaled nitric oxide. *Pediatric Transplant*. 2006; **10**(1): 121–7.
277. Ljungman P, Ribaud P, Eyrich M, Matthes-Martin S, Einsele H, Bleakley M et al. Cidofovir for adenovirus infections after allogeneic hematopoietic stem cell transplantation: A survey by the Infectious Diseases Working Party of the European Group for Blood and Marrow Transplantation. *Bone Marrow Transplantation*. 2003; **31**(6): 481–6.
278. Legrand F, Berrebi D, Houhou N, Freymuth F, Faye A, Duval M et al. Early diagnosis of adenovirus infection and treatment with cidofovir after bone marrow transplantation in children. *Bone Marrow Transplantation*. 2001; **27**(6): 621–6.
279. Nagafuji K, Aoki K, Henzan H, Kato K, Miyamoto T, Eto T et al. Cidofovir for treating adenoviral hemorrhagic cystitis in hematopoietic stem cell transplant recipients. *Bone Marrow Transplantation*. 2004; **34**(10): 909–14.

280. Paolino K, Sande J, Perez E, Loechelt B, Jantausch B, Painter W et al. Eradication of disseminated adenovirus infection in a pediatric hematopoietic stem cell transplantation recipient using the novel antiviral agent CMX001. *Journal of Clinical Virology: The Official Publication of the Pan American Society for Clinical Virology*. 2011; **50**(2): 167–70.
281. Chakrabarti S, Mautner V, Osman H, Collingham KE, Fegan CD, Klapper PE et al. Adenovirus infections following allogeneic stem cell transplantation: Incidence and outcome in relation to graft manipulation, immunosuppression, and immune recovery. *Blood*. 2002; **100**(5): 1619–27.
282. Heemskerk B, Lankester AC, van Vreeswijk T, Beersma MF, Claas EC, Veltrop-Duits LA et al. Immune reconstitution and clearance of human adenovirus viremia in pediatric stem-cell recipients. *The Journal of Infectious Diseases*. 2005; **191**(4): 520–30.
283. van Tol MJ, Claas EC, Heemskerk B, Veltrop-Duits LA, de Brouwer CS, van Vreeswijk T et al. Adenovirus infection in children after allogeneic stem cell transplantation: Diagnosis, treatment and immunity. *Bone Marrow Transplantation*. 2005; **35** (Suppl 1): S73–6.
284. Pagliara D, Savoldo B. Cytotoxic T lymphocytes for the treatment of viral infections and posttransplant lymphoproliferative disorders in transplant recipients. *Current Opinion in Infectious Diseases*. 2012; **25**(4): 431–7.
285. Binn LN, Sanchez JL, Gaydos JC. Emergence of adenovirus type 14 in US military recruits—A new challenge. *The Journal of Infectious Diseases*. 2007; **196**(10): 1436–7.

20 Human Rhinovirus Infections

Stephen B. Greenberg

CONTENTS

20.1 INTRODUCTION

More than 50% of all common colds are caused by rhinoviruses (HRVs).[1–3] Clinically, the common cold includes rhinitis and pharyngitis, as well as sneezing, hoarseness, and nonproductive cough.[4,5] Although self-limited in healthy people, the illness is associated with complications in individuals who suffer from heart or lung disease, or who are immunosuppressed.[6–11] In infants and young children, HRVs are associated with many cases of acute otitis media and sinusitis.[12,13] Since it was first identified by Price as a cause of respiratory illness over 50 years ago, several diagnostic tests have been developed for the detection of HRV.[14] Over the past 10 years, diagnostic tests employing polymerase chain reaction (PCR) technologies have increased the percentage of respiratory illnesses attributable to these viruses.[15]

20.2 VIROLOGY

HRVs are members of the *Picornaviridae* family and positive-sense, single-stranded ribonucleic acid (RNA) viruses with icosahedral symmetry. The capsid is composed of four proteins; VP1, VP2, VP3, and VP4 (Figure 20.1). Proteins VP1, VP2, and VP3 are responsible for antigenic diversity and the host immune response following infection.[3,16] VP4 is on the inside of the virus and

TABLE 20.1
Epidemiology of HRV Infections

"Common cold" illnesses	50%
Worldwide distribution	+
Acquisition in childhood	+
Incubation period	12–72 h
Prevalence	Peaks in early fall and spring
Multiple strains co-circulating	+
Spread	Direct contact, hand-to-hand contact, or by aersol

in early childhood and into adulthood. As a frequent cause of the common cold, these viruses are responsible for millions of lost work days, school absenteeism, and physician visits. Most HRV infections are symptomatic, but asymptomatic virus shedding has been reported. URIs caused by respiratory viruses such as HRVs are a frequent reason for inappropriate antibiotic use.[45]

The home is the principal location for transmission of HRV.[46] School-aged children are frequently the introducer of the infection. Secondary attack rates range from 25% to 70%. Daycare centers and schools are important locations for the spread of HRV. Transmission of HRVs can occur by close contact, autoinoculation, fomites, or aerosols.

Lee et al. presented data showing a new clade of HRV strains called HRV-C.[20] Other investigators have confirmed these findings.[25,47–49] No significant clinical differences have been reported in patients with HRV-Cs detected in specimens with other viruses, especially RSV (respiratory syncytial virus).

Clinical outcomes appear to be similar between the HRV species. HRV-C infections can have symptoms of the common cold, pharyngitis, croup, acute otitis media, bronchiolitis, and/or pneumonia.[19,50–52] These infections have been reported in healthy children and adults as well as in those with asthma, immunocompromised conditions, CF, or multiple sclerosis.[53–56]

HRV-Cs, more than HRV-As and -Bs, are major causes of febrile wheezes in infants and of asthma exacerbations in older children.[54] Of all viruses detected from middle ear fluids in children with otitis media, HRV-Cs accounted for half the documented infections.[57] Although reported infections have come mainly from respiratory tract specimens, HRV-Cs have been reported in blood and pericardium.[53,58,59]

With more sensitive PCR methods for HRV detection, reports of long periods (>2–3 weeks) of HRV positivity have increased.[60,61] Where strain typing has been used, however, HRV shedding normally stops within 11–21 days (Figure 20.5).[62–64] Therefore, persistence may represent serial or overlapping infections by multiple untyped strains.[65] In immunocompromised children, HRV-C strains were detected threefold longer (53 days vs. 16) than in immunocompetent children.[66]

Recent studies have documented HRV species in all months of the year in tropical, subtropical, and semi-arid regions.[67–69] Many HRV-C strains have been found to circulate during a single year and may be detected in subsequent years.[70,71]

Potential risk factors for HRV infection and illness include chronic stress, inflammation, and telomere length.[72–74] An increased susceptibility to developing a common cold among subjects experimentally infected with HRV, who had increased stress, has been reported in several studies. Volunteers who had exposure to long-term stressful experiences had glucocorticoid receptor resistance and were found to have a higher risk of developing a cold following experimental HRV infection. Greater glucocorticoid receptor resistance predicted increased production of local inflammatory cytokines. There were no effects of cortisol levels on illness risk, glucocorticoid receptor resistance, and inflammation. In a challenge model of HRV in healthy adults, shorter CD8 CD28-T cell telomere length was associated with greater odds of infection.[73]

Cigarette smoke extract alters the production of epithelial cytokines in response to HRV infections and suppresses HRV-induced expression of several epithelial genes that directly lost antiviral

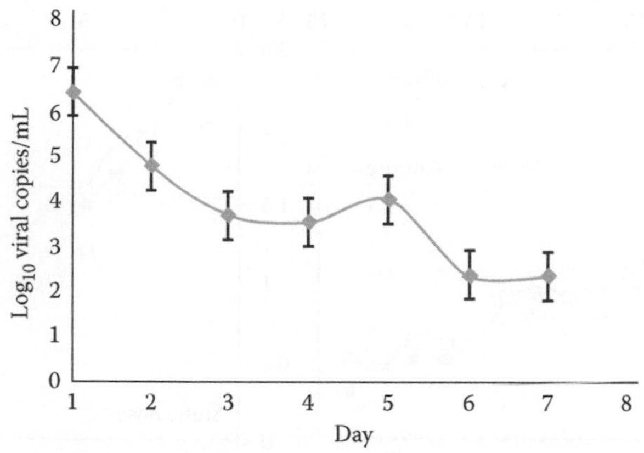

FIGURE 20.5 Longitudinal surveillance of HRV viral loads in university students. Self-collected mid-turbinate nasal swabs ($n = 98$) were serially submitted over a 7-day period by undergraduate students ($n = 14$) following the onset of URI. Fourteen nasal swabs were tested per time point. Data are plotted as mean viral loads ($\log_{10}$ viral copies/mL) and SEM for various days following onset of symptoms ($P < 0.001$). (Reprinted from *Diagnostic Microbiology and Infectious Disease*, Vol. 74, Granados A et al., Use of an improved quantitative polymerase chain reaction assay to determine differences in human rhinovirus viral loads in different populations, pp. 384–387, Copyright 2012, with permission from Elsevier.)

defenses and contribute to antiviral immunity. This could explain a basis for more severe clinical outcomes observed in smokers.[75,76]

20.5 DIAGNOSIS

Standard tissue culture methods for isolation are useful for detecting HRV. HRVs can be differentiated from other picornaviruses, such as EVs because of their acid lability.

With the development of PCR techniques, the ability to detect respiratory viruses has increased significantly. Detection of HRVs in respiratory specimens was enhanced by reverse transcription PCR (RT-PCR), involving the use of hybridization probes or double-stranded DNA binding dye. Several other studies have found increased sensitivity of RT-PCR compared with viral culture techniques.[77–84]

Antibody assays are reported for HRVs but are not readily available or helpful clinically. Since there is no common antigen for HRVs, serotype-specific neutralizing antibody assays are necessary to detect rises in serum antibodies following acute infections, and the large number of HRV serotypes makes this approach impractical.

20.6 CLINICAL FEATURES

20.6.1 Common Cold in Immunocompetent Adults

The incubation period for the common cold is 12–72 h. Rhinorrhea and sneezing plus nasal congestion are usually the initial symptoms. Sore throat is common and may be an early symptom. Fever is unusual but reported. Headache and malaise are often mild. Resolution of symptoms occurs in almost all cases within 4–9 days without complications (Figure 20.6).[85,86]

With the use of PCR techniques, HRVs have been reported commonly in asymptomatic children.[3] This may be a result of prolonged shedding from a previous respiratory illness, a mild illness that went unrecognized, or a virus during the incubation period. Asymptomatic HRV shedding is not as common in adults as it appears to be in children. In addition, coinfections with other respiratory viruses during respiratory illnesses is well described.[1]

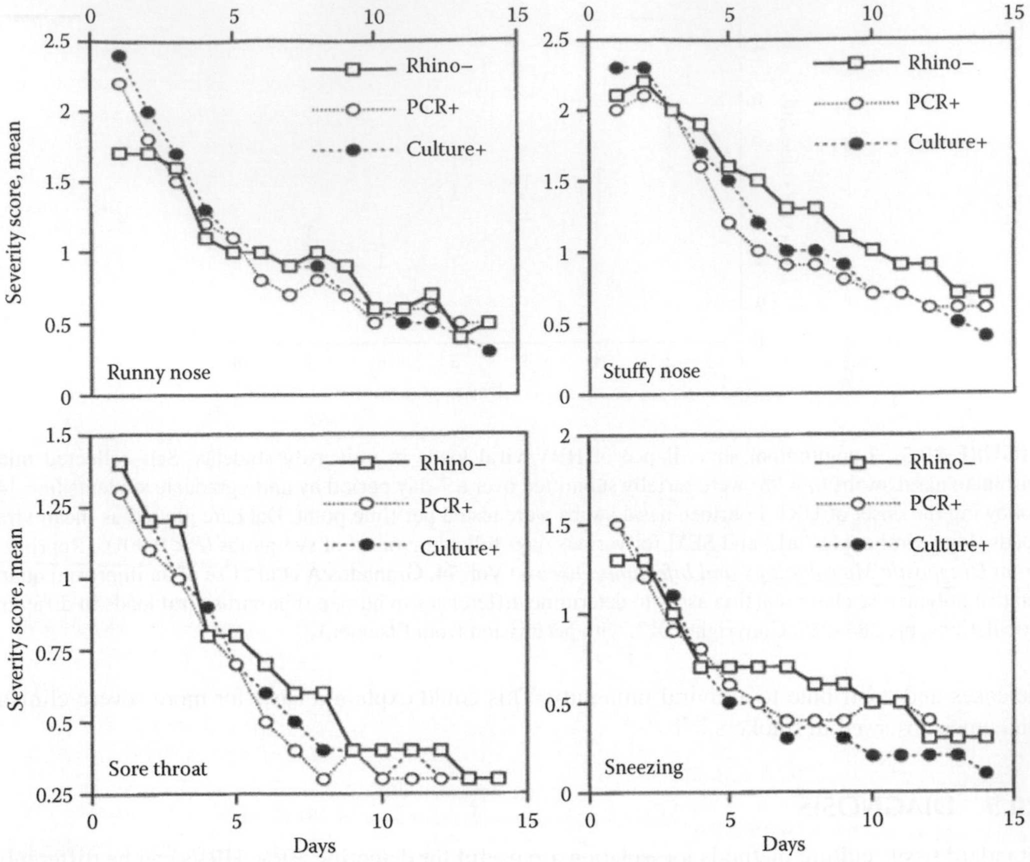

FIGURE 20.6 Mean severity of runny or stuffy nose, sore throat, and sneezing in adults with self-diagnosed common colds positive for HRV. Mean severity of runny or stuffy nose, sore throat, and sneezing in adults with self-diagnosed common colds positive for HRV by cell culture (filled circles), RT-PCR (empty circles), or negative for HRV (squares). Symptom severity was highest upon presentation and declined over the study period. Symptoms were scored twice daily on a scale ranging from 0 (absence of the symptom) to 4 (very severe). (Reprinted from *J Clin Microbiol* 1997; 35: 2864–2868, Arruda E et al., Frequency and natural history of rhinovirus infections in adults during autumn, with permission from American Society for Microbiology.)

20.6.2 HRV Infection in Influenza-Like Illnesses during H1N1 Pandemic

With the global spread of influenza A (H1N1) in 2009, a series of surveillance protocols were activated to monitor and characterize the pandemic. Many countries have reported on their findings in patients with influenza-like illnesses (ILI) who had respiratory specimens tested for a wide range of respiratory viruses. Most of the reports used PCR techniques in children or adults (Table 20.2).[87–95] The percentage of specimens that were positive with HRV ranged from 6.3% to 29.8%. In all the studies, the authors comment that they could not distinguish influenza illnesses from HRV-related illnesses by clinical characteristics, although influenza illnesses were more likely to have fever. Thus, during influenza outbreaks, other respiratory viruses, and especially HRV, continue to cause significant cases of URIs and lower respiratory infections (LRIs).

20.6.3 HRV Infections in Asthma Patients

Asthma exacerbations in children and adults are frequently associated with respiratory virus infections, especially HRVs.[10,54,56,96–98] Naturally occurring HRV infections lead to more severe and

TABLE 20.2
Human Rhinovirus Isolates from Patients with Influenza-Like Illness during the Influenza A (H1N1) 2009 Pandemic[a]

Reference	Location	Specimen[a]	Age Group	% Positive for HRV
Hombrouck[87]	Belgium	NP	Children	13
Schnepf[88]	France	NS	Children and adults	20
Memish[89]	Saudi Arabia	NP/TS	Adults (health care workers)	21
Pascalis[90]	Reunion Island	NS	Children and adults	13.4
Chang[91]	Texas, USA	NP	Children	29.8
Thiberville[92]	Vietnam	NS	Children and adults	20.3
Yang[93]	China	NP/TS	Adults	6.3
Nisii[94]	Italy	NP	Adults	10
Kraft[95]	USA/CDC	?	Immunocompromised adults	12.6

[a] NP = nasopharyngeal swab; NS = nasal swab; TS = throat swab.

longer lasting lower respiratory tract symptoms and changes in peak flow rate in asthmatic versus normal subjects.[99]

Experimental HRV-16 infections in volunteers with mild atopic asthma resulted in significantly reduced forced expiratory volume in 1 s (FEV_1) in home recordings.[99] In allergic subjects, HRV-16 infection resulted in increased airway inflammation after bronchoprovocation.[100] During other experimental HRV infections, significant increases in submucosal CD3+ lymphocytes and eosinophils were detected in bronchial mucosal biopsies.[101]

Lower airway dysfunction following HRV infection may result from direct infection of the lower airway or by stimulating inflammatory, immunologic, or neurogenic mechanisms in the upper airway, thereby impacting the lower airways. Papadopoulos et al. detected HRV in the columnar and basal cell layers of the lower airways.[102] Using *in situ* hybridization, the replicative strand of HRV in the lower airways has been detected.[103]

Experimental HRV infections in asthmatic subjects have demonstrated (1) airway narrowing; (2) markers of eosinophil activation, IL-8, and neutrophils; (3) bronchial infiltration with eosinophils, CD4 cells, and CD8 cells; (4) activation of prostaglandin and leukotriene pathways; and (5) induction of nitric oxide (NO).[104–107] Recently, innate immune responses were found to be defective in bronchial epithelial cells obtained from asthmatic subjects.[107] There is also evidence of impaired acquired immune responses in asthmatic patients. Impaired Th1 responses to HRV were found in peripheral blood mononuclear cells as reflected by significantly lower levels of IFN-α and IL-12, and higher levels of IL-10 from asthmatic patients compared to normal healthy volunteers (Figure 20.5).[108]

Several studies have found deficient induction of interferon-λ by HRV in bronchial epithelial cells from asthmatic patients.[109,110,111] Contoli et al. found that IFN-λs are induced by HRV infection of human bronchial epithelial cells, monocytes, and macrophages.[112] Induction of IFN-λ1 and IFN-λ2/3 mRNAs was significantly reduced in asthmatic compared with nonasthmatic subjects. Bronchoalveolar cells in asthma patients were deficient in IFN-λ after HRV was added. These studies support the view that innate immune responses in asthmatic subjects have deficiencies in two IFN families, in several lung cell types, and in response to HRV infection.

HRV infections are a major cause of wheezing episodes in infants and children.[113–118] Wheezing episodes in infancy that are virus-induced are often associated with asthma development in children. HRV infections that resulted in hospitalization during infancy were recently implicated as early predictors of subsequent development of asthma.[119] Almost 90% of wheezing children in year

TABLE 20.3
Human Rhinovirus Isolates in Childhood Community-Acquired Pneumonia and/or Bronchiolitis

Reference	Country	Design	Clinical	Specimen	Of All ⊕ %± HRV
Choi[156]	Korea	Retrospective	Pn	BAL	23.8
Launes[155]	Spain	Prospective	Pn	NPA	52
García-García[157]	Spain	Prospective	Pn	NPA	19
Miller[158]	Argentina	Prospective	Br	NS	40
Esposito[159]	Italy	Prospective	Pn	NS	29
Homaira[160]	Bangladesh	Prospective	Pn	NW	12
Guerrier[161]	Cambodia	Prospective	Pn/Br	NPS	34
Cho[162]	Korea	Prospective	Pn	NS	18.5
Suzuki[163]	Philippines	Prospective	Pn	NPS	30.5
Uršič[164]	Slovenia	Prospective	Pn/Br	NPS/TS	33.1
Pretorius[165]	South Africa	Prospective	SARI	NPS	25
Lu[154]	China	Prospective	Pn	NPA	30.9
Chidlow[166]	New Guinea	Prospective	Pn	NS	63
Ghani[167]	South Africa	Retrospective	Pn/Br	NPS/TS/BAL	39
Chen[168]	Taiwan	Prospective	Br	NPS	12.4
Antunest[169]	Portugal	Prospective	Br	?	0
Mansbach[170]	USA	Prospective	Br	NPA	25.6

Note: BAL = bronchoalveolar lavage; Br = bronchiolitis; NPA = nasopharyngeal aspirate; NS = nasal swab; NW = nasal wash; Pn = pneumonia; TS = throat swab.

20.6.8 HRV Infections in CF Patients

A few studies have examined the role of respiratory viral infections in CF patients. Collinson et al. detected picornavirus in over 40% of URIs in children with underlying CF.[181] There was no difference in pulmonary function in those children with proven HRV infection versus other respiratory viruses. Smyth et al. followed 108 patients with CF for one year, and detected HRV in 16% of exacerbations.[182] Those patients with proven HRV infection did not show deterioration in clinical activity but did receive more days of intravenous antibiotics.

Olesen et al. obtained sputum cultures in 75 children with CF and 45 were virus positive.[183] HRV infection did not appear to affect lung function. Having respiratory or "viral" symptoms had low positive predictive value, sensitivity, and specificity. Another study assayed for HRV in 71 patients with 165 episodes of URI. Forty percent were virus positive who had symptoms. URI symptoms correlated with positive virus detection independent of bacterial culture result.[184] de Almeida has reported infections by HRV-C in CF patients.[185]

20.6.9 HRV Infections in Immunocompromised Hosts

Respiratory virus infections are common causes of acute respiratory illness in patients after solid organ transplantation or following bone marrow transplantation.[186–191] In these immunocompromised patients, HRV was the number one detected respiratory virus by PCR assays. Ison et al. found an 83% (5/6) fatality rate in HSCT (hematopoietic stem cell transplantation) patients with bronchoalveolar lavage (BAL)-positive samples for HRV.[187] In a study of 215 patients with underlying HCT, 30% had infections at 100 days post-transplant.[191] The incidence for HRV was 22.3%. Median duration of virus shedding was 3 weeks. HRV infection was associated with URI symptoms. Two patients with HRV before 100 days developed an LRI and one patient with HRV.

In a prospective study of patients with malignancies and therapy-induced neutropenia, a virus was detected in 35% of patients.[192] HRVs were the number one virus detected by quantitative PCR in nasopharyngeal aspirates and associated with upper respiratory symptoms. In a prospective, multicenter study in children with cancer and fever and neutropenia, 57% had a virus detected by PCR-DNA. A third of the patients had mixed HRV bacterial infections.[193] HRVs were the second most frequently detected virus; RSV was most frequently identified.

20.6.10 HRV Infections in Health Care Facilities

Hospital outbreaks of HRV infections have been reported in neonatal intensive care units (ICUs) and long-term care facilities.[194–202] In one study, neonates acquired HRV infection during their hospital stay.[196] In long-term care facilities where HRV outbreaks have occurred, there were potential deaths associated with the infection. Recent guidelines for hospital isolation recommend droplet precautions for patients with known HRV infection.[203]

20.7 TREATMENT

Because there are currently no approved antiviral medications for HRV respiratory tract infections, symptomatic treatment should be considered.[204] Anticholinergic medications could be used for the commonly reported symptom, rhinorrhea. Anticholinergic nasal sprays have been reported to reduce rhinorrhea by approximately 30%. Nasal congestion can be alleviated by nasal and systemic decongestants. Several studies have suggested that heated, humidified steam may reduce nasal congestion in common colds, but the data are not conclusive.[205] Cough is a common accompanying problem in respiratory viral infections and can be suppressed with nonprescription cough suppressants. Other symptoms such as sore throat, myalgia, fever, or headache can be controlled with nonsteroidal anti-inflammatory drugs. Antibiotics are inappropriate for treating viral infections, although they are frequently prescribed by physicians.

Using our understanding of the cellular changes following HRV infection and replication, several antiviral agents and treatment strategies have been tested.[206] Compounds targeting cell susceptibility, virus attachment, receptor blockage, virus uncoating, RNA replication, and viral protein synthesis have been evaluated. Although several agents have demonstrated both *in vitro* and *in vivo* success, none have received U.S. Food and Drug Administration approval due to poor bioavailability, poor side-effect profile, or limited potency.[206–209]

Viral capsid-binding compounds, such as pleconaril, block virus uncoating in vitro.[210,211] Clinical trials demonstrated significant reduction in duration of respiratory symptoms in individuals receiving pleconaril for naturally occurring colds, but the drug was not approved. Several low molecular weight compounds inhibit the 3C protease, which is essential for viral replication and assembly. In volunteer trials, a 3C-protease inhibitor, ruprintrivir, was found to reduce viral shedding, but was associated with blood-tinged mucus and irritation of the nasal passages.[212]

Alternative medications, such as *Echinacea angustifolia* or zinc lozenges, have been tested in several volunteer trials but are not currently thought to be clinically effective.[213–217] A recent study in children with "common cold" reported to show shorter mean duration of symptoms in those taking zinc sulfate compared with placebo.[218] All of these studies suffer from poor control groups or incomplete virology. However, most reports show few side effects from taking alternative therapies.

Recent studies using primary airway fibroblasts have shown that inhibition of NF-KB by specific inhibitors did not reduce HRV stimulated cytokine release.[219] Salmeterol increased HRV-induced IL-6 and IL-8. Dexamethasone and fluticasone had the opposite effect. These drugs did alter HRV replication.

In a recent Cochrane Review of corticosteroids for the common cold, only two trials that used randomized, double-blind, controlled designs were found.[220] These two trials compared intranasal corticosteroids to placebo. No benefit was found for duration or severity of symptoms, adverse events, or treatment for secondary infections. No trials have compared oral corticosteroids to placebo. Larger randomized placebo-controlled trials would be required to completely answer the question of corticosteroid efficacy in the common cold.

In a pilot study using patients with mild asthma, inoculation with HRV-16 did not lead to improved asthma control or cold symptoms in the group receiving montelukast, a leukotriene receptor antagonist, compared with control subjects.[221]

HRV infection increases the expression of cell adhesion molecules such as fibronectin and carcinoembryonic antigen-related cell adhesion molecules.[222] Levocetirizine is a drug that interferes with NF-KB activation. In a study of HRV-16 infection in human nasal epithelial cells, *S. aureus* and *H. influenzae* have significantly reduced adhesion levels in the levocetirizine-treated epithelial cells compared with untreated control cells.

Quercetin, a plant flavanol, was recently reported to decrease expression of noninflammatory cytokines and improve lung function in HRV-1B and HRV-39 infected mice.[223] Quercetin also decreases viral load *in vivo*, probably by suppressing transcription of the HRV genome. Additionally, quercetin decreases HRV-induced cleavage of eIF4GI and increases phosphorylation of eIF2α. Thus, this antioxidant and anti-inflammatory agent appears to have antirhinoviral activity and should be evaluated further as a potential antiviral therapy for HRV infections.

Quinolones have been used to treat exacerbation of COPD because of their broad antibacterial spectrum and anti-inflammatory properties. Levofloxacin has been found to inhibit HRV infection in primary cell cultures employing human tracheal epithelial cells.[224] Levofloxacin pretreatment decreased mRNA levels of ICAM-1. Macrolides have also been reported to reduce ICAM-1 expression and HRV-induced cytokines *in vitro* and *in vivo*.[225]

20.8 PREVENTION

Spread of HRV from the respiratory tract to susceptible individuals may occur by aerosol, and/or directly by contact spread or by fomite.[226] HRV can be recovered from the hands of approximately 40% of adults with colds. Hand-to-hand transmission of HRV has led to evaluation of disinfectants that will eliminate virus on human skin and that are thought to be clinically nontoxic. A study using 2% aqueous iodine decreased transmission in family members who were exposed to HRV-infected individuals. An evaluation of virucidal hand treatments confirmed the prevention of HRV infections by organic acids but not ethanol.[227] Hand washing with soap and water effectively cleans HRV-contaminated hands better than single treatment with ethanol hand rub.[228]

Vaccines have not been thought to be useful against HRVs because of the serotype-specific neutralizing antibodies produced following infection and because of the numerous serotypes (>100). However, recent studies in a mouse model have reported development of cross-serotype reactive antibodies to VP1, suggesting a basis for successful antibody-mediated vaccine development.[229] Future studies will need to confirm and expand these preliminary observations.

20.9 CONCLUSION

HRVs cause significant morbidity in immunocompetent people and in patients with underlying chronic or immunosuppressed medical conditions. Newer diagnostic tests have expanded our understanding of these respiratory viruses in clinical infections. These sensitive diagnostic tests have been used to detect new HRVs, such as HRV-C. Recent studies on the pathogenesis of HRVs and the host response to this group of viruses have provided insights into potential targets for therapeutic interventions. The epidemiology of these viruses has helped to expand our understanding of these infections in severe chronic diseases such as asthma and COPD.

REFERENCES

1. Greenberg SB. Update on rhinovirus and coronavirus infections. *Semin Respir Crit Care Med* 2011; 32: 433–446.
2. Kennedy JL, Turner RB, Braciale T, Heymann PW, Borish L. Pathogenesis of rhinovirus infection. *Curr Opin Virol* 2012; 2: 287–293.
3. Jacobs SE, Lamson DM, St George K, Walsh TJ. Human rhinoviruses. *Clin Microbiol Rev* 2013; 26: 135–162.
4. Gwaltney JM Jr, Phillips CD, Miller RD, Riker DK. Computed tomographic study of the common cold. *N Engl J Med* 1994; 330: 25–30.
5. Gwaltney JM Jr, Winther B, Patrie JT, Hendley JO. Combined antiviral–antimediator treatment for the common cold. *J Infect Dis 2002*; 186: 147–154.
6. Whimbey E, Champlin RE, Couch RB et al. Community respiratory virus infections among hospitalized adult bone marrow transplant recipients. *Clin Infect Dis* 1996; 22: 778–782.
7. Greenberg SB, Allen M, Wilson J, Atmar RL. Respiratory viral infections in adults with and without chronic obstructive pulmonary disease. *Am J Respir Crit Care Med* 2000; 162: 167–173.
8. El-Sahly HM, Atmar RL, Glezen WP, Greenberg SB. Spectrum of clinical illness in hospitalized patients with "common cold" virus infections. *Clin Infect Dis* 2000; 31: 96–100.
9. Wedzicha JA. Role of viruses in exacerbations of chronic obstructive pulmonary disease. *Proc Am Thorac Soc* 2004; 1: 115–120.
10. Johnston SL, Pattemore PK, Sanderson G et al. Community study of role of viral infections in exacerbations of asthma in 9–11 year old children. *BMJ* 1995; 310: 1225–1229.
11. Hiatt PW, Grace SC, Kozinetz CA et al. Effects of viral lower respiratory tract infection on lung function in infants with cystic fibrosis. *Pediatrics* 1999; 103: 619–626.
12. Chonmaitree T, Howie VM, Truant AL. Presence of respiratory viruses in middle ear fluids and nasal wash specimens from children with acute otitis media. *Pediatrics* 1986; 77: 698–702.
13. Pitkaranta A, Virolainen A, Jero J, Arruda E, Hayden FG. Detection of rhinovirus, respiratory syncytial virus, and coronavirus infections in acute otitis media by reverse transcriptase polymerase chain reaction. *Pediatrics* 1998; 102: 291–295.
14. Price WH. The isolation of a new virus associated with respiratory clinical disease in humans. *Proc Natl Acad Sci USA* 1956; 42: 892–896.
15. Arden KE, Mackay IM. Human rhinoviruses: Coming in from the cold. *Genome Med* 2009; 1: 44.
16. Hayden FG. Rhinovirus and the lower respiratory tract. *Rev Med Virol* 2004; 14: 17–31.
17. Palmenberg AC, Spiro D, Kuzmickas R et al. Sequencing and analyses of all known human rhinovirus genomes reveal structure and evolution. *Science* 2009; 324: 55–59.
18. ICTV HRV C proposal. http://talk.ictvonline.org/media/p/1201.aspx30August2009.
19. Blomqvist S, Savolainen C, Råman L, Roivainen M, Hovi T. Human rhinovirus 87 and enterovirus 68 represent a unique serotype with rhinovirus and enterovirus features. *J Clin Microbiol* 2002; 40: 4218–4223.
20. Lee W-M, Kiesner C, Pappas T et al. A diverse group of previously unrecognized human rhinoviruses are common causes of respiratory illness in infants. *PLoS One* 2007; 2: e966.
21. Bochkov YA, Gern JE. Clinical and molecular features of human rhinovirus C. *Microbes Infect* 2012; 14: 485–494.
22. Fuchs R, Blaas D. Productive entry pathways of human rhinoviruses. *Adv Virol* 2012; 2012: 826301.
23. Roy A, Post CB. Long-distance correlations of rhinovirus capsid dynamics contribute to uncoating and antiviral activity. *Proc Natl Acad Sci USA* 2012; 109: 5271–5276.
24. Rahamat-Langendoen J, Riezebos-Brilman A, Borger R et al. Up surge of human enterovirus 68 infections in patients with severe respiratory tract infections. *J Clin Virol* 2011; 52: 103–106.
25. Tapparel C, Junier T, Germann D et al. New respiratory enterovirus and recombinant rhinoviruses among circulating strains. *Emerg Infect Dis* 2009; 15: 719–726.
26. Hasegawa S, Hirano R, Okamoto-Nakagawa R, Ichiyama T, Shirabe K. Enterovirus 68 infection in children with asthma attacks: Virus-induced asthma in Japanese children. *Allergy* 2011; 66: 1618–1620.
27. Imamura T, Fuji N, Suzuki A et al. Enterovirus 68 among children with severe acute respiratory infection, the Philippines. *Emerg Infect Dis* 2011; 17: 1430–1435.
28. Jacques J, Moret H, Minette D et al. Epidemiological, molecular, and clinical features of enterovirus respiratory infections in French children between 1999 and 2005. *J Clin Microbiol* 2008; 46: 206–213.
29. Piralla A, Lilleri D, Sarasini A et al. Human rhinovirus and human respiratory enterovirus (EV68 and EV104) infections in hospitalized patients in Italy, 2008–2009. *Diagn Microbiol Infect Dis* 2012; 73: 162–167.

185. de Almeida MB, Zerbinati RM, Tateno AF et al. Rhinovirus C and respiratory exacerbations in children with cystic fibrosis. *Emerg Infect Dis* 2010; 16: 996–999.
186. Garbino J, Gerbase MW, Wunderli W et al. Respiratory viruses and severe lower respiratory tract complications in hospitalized patients. *Chest* 2004; 125: 1033–1039.
187. Ison MG, Hayden FG, Kaiser L, Corey L, Boeckh M. Rhinovirus infections in hematopoietic stem cell transplant recipients with pneumonia. *Clin Infect Dis* 2003; 36: 1139–1143.
188. Hassan IA, Chopra R, Swindell R, Mutton KJ. Respiratory viral infections after bone marrow/peripheral stem-cell transplantation: The Christie hospital experience. *Bone Marrow Transplant* 2003; 32: 73–77.
189. Ljungman P, Ward KN, Crooks BN et al. Respiratory virus infections after stem cell transplantation: A prospective study from the infectious diseases working party of the European Group for blood and marrow transplantation. *Bone Marrow Transplant* 2001; 28: 479–484.
190. Ghosh S, Champlin R, Couch R et al. Rhinovirus infections in myelosuppressed adult blood and marrow transplant recipients. *Clin Infect Dis* 1999; 29: 528–532.
191. Milano F, Campbell AP, Guthrie KA et al. Human rhinovirus and coronavirus detection among allogeneic hematopoietic stem cell transplantation recipients. *Blood* 2010; 115: 2088–2094.
192. Ohrmalm L, Wong M, Aust C et al. Viral findings in adult hematological patients with neutropenia. *PLoS One* 2012; 7: e36543.
193. Torres JP, Labraña Y, Ibañez C et al. Frequency and clinical outcome of respiratory viral infections and mixed viral–bacterial infections in children with cancer, fever and neutropenia. *Pediatr Infect Dis J* 2012; 31: 889–893.
194. Valenti WM, Clarke TA, Hall CB, Menegus MA, Shapiro DL. Concurrent out breaks of rhinovirus and respiratory syncytial virus in anintensive care nursery: Epidemiology and associated risk factors. *J Pediatr* 1982; 100: 722–776.
195. Reid AB, Anderson TL, Cooley L, Williamson J, Mcgregor AR An outbreak of human rhinovirus species C infections in a neonatal intensive care unit. *Pediatr Infect Dis J* 2011; 30(12): 1096–1098.
196. vanPiggelen RO, vanLoon AM, Krediet TG, Verboon-Maciolek MA. Human rhinovirus causes severe infection in preterm infants. *Pediatr Infect Dis J* 2010; 29: 364–365.
197. Longtin J, Marchand-Austin A, Winter AL et al. Rhinovirus outbreaks in long-term care facilities, Ontario, Canada. *Emerg Infect Dis* 2010; 16: 1463–1465.
198. Wald TG, Shult P, Krause P, Miller BA, Drinka P, Gravenstein S. A rhinovirus outbreak among residents of a long-term care facility. *Ann Intern Med* 1995; 123: 588–593.
199. Longtin J, Winter AL, Heng D et al. Severe human rhinovirus outbreak associated with fatalities in a long-term care facility in Ontario, Canada. *J Am Geriatr Soc* 2010; 58: 2036–2038.
200. Louie JK, Yagi S, Nelson FA et al. Rhinovirus outbreak in a long term care facility for elderly persons associated with unusually high mortality. *Clin Infect Dis* 2005; 41: 262–265.
202. Hicks LA, Shepard CW, Britz PH et al. Two outbreaks of severe respiratory disease in nursing homes associated with rhinovirus. *J Am Geriatr Soc* 2006; 54: 284–289.
203. Siegel JD, Rhinehart E, Jackson M, Chiarello L; Health Care Infection Control Practices Advisory Committee. 2007 Guideline for isolation precautions: Preventing transmission of infectious agents in health care settings. *Am J Infect Control* 2007; 35: S65–S164.
204. Eccles R. Efficacy and safety of over-the-counter analgesics in the treatment of common cold and flu. *J Clin Pharm Ther* 2006; 31: 309–319.
205. Singh M. Heated, humidified air for the common cold. *Cochrane Database Syst Rev* 2004; 2: CD001728.
206. Rotbart HA. Antiviral therapy for enteroviruses and rhinoviruses. *Antivir Chem Chemother* 2000; 11: 261–271.
207. Hayden FG, Gwaltney JM Jr. Intranasal interferon-alpha 2 treatment of experimental rhinoviral colds. *J Infect Dis* 1984; 150: 174–180.
208. Higgins PG, Phillpotts RJ, Scott GM, Wallace J, Bernhardt LL, Tyrrell DA. Intranasal interferon as protection against experimental respiratory coronavirus infection in volunteers. *Antimicrob Agents Chemother* 1983; 24: 713–715.
209. Sasaki T, Yamaya M, Yasuda H et al. The proton pump inhibitor lansoprazole inhibits rhinovirus infection in cultured human tracheal epithelial cells. *Eur J Pharmacol* 2005; 509: 201–210.
210. Hayden FG, Herrington DT, Coats TL et al.; Pleconaril Respiratory Infection Study Group. Efficacy and safety of oral pleconaril for treatment of colds due to picornaviruses in adults: Results of 2 double-blind, randomized, placebo-controlled trials. *Clin Infect Dis* 2003; 36: 1523–1532.
211. Patick AK, Brothers MA, Maldonado F et al. *In vitro* antiviral activity and single-dose pharmacokinetics in humans of a novel, orally bioavailable inhibitor of human rhinovirus 3C protease. *Antimicrob Agents Chemother* 2005; 49: 2267–2275.

212. Hayden FG, Turner RB, Gwaltney JM et al. Phase II, randomized, double-blind, placebo-controlled studies of ruprintrivir nasal spray 2-percent suspension for prevention and treatment of experimentally induced rhinovirus colds in healthy volunteers. *Antimicrob Agents Chemother* 2003; 47: 3907–3916.
213. Kang EJ, Kim SY, Hwang IH, Ji YJ. The effect of probiotics on prevention of common cold: A meta-analysis of randomized controlled trial studies. *Korean J Fam Med* 2013; 34: 2–10.
214. Hemilä H, Chalker E. Vitamin C for preventing and treating the common cold. .*Cochrane Database Syst Rev* 2013; 1: CD000980.
215. Schoop R, Klein P, Suter A, Johnston SL. Echinacea in the prevention of induced rhinovirus colds: A meta-analysis. *Clin Ther* 2006; 28: 174–183.
216. Sperber SJ, Shah LP, Gilbert RD, Ritchey TW, Monto AS. *Echinacea purpurea* for prevention of experimental rhinovirus colds. *Clin Infect Dis* 2004; 38:1367–1371.
217. Turner RB. Ineffectiveness of intranasal zinc gluconate for prevention of experimental rhinovirus colds. *Clin Infect Dis* 2001; 33: 1865–1870.
218. Kurugöl Z, Akilli M, Bayram N, Koturoglu G. The prophylactic and therapeutic effectiveness of zinc sulphate on common cold in children. *Acta Paediatr* 2006; 95: 1175–1181.
219. Van Ly D, King NJ, Moir LM, Burgess JK, Black JL, Oliver BG. Effects of β(2) Agonists, corticosteroids, and novel therapies on rhinovirus-induced cytokine release and rhinovirus replication in primary airway fibro blasts. *J Allergy (Cairo)* 2011: 457169.
220. Hayward G, Thompson MJ, Perera R, Del Mar CB, Glasziou PP, Heneghan CJ. Corticosteroids for the common cold. *Cochrane Database Syst Rev* 2012 Aug 15; 8: CD008116.
221. Kloepfer KM, DeMore JP, Vrtis RF et al. Effects of montelukast on patients with asthma after experimental inoculation with human rhinovirus 16. *Ann Allergy Asthma Immunol* 2011; 106: 252–257.
222. Min JY, Shin SH, Kwon HJ, Jang YJ. Levocetirizine inhibits rhinovirus-induced bacterial adhesion to nasal epithelial cells through down-regulation of cell adhesion molecules. *Ann Allergy Asthma Immunol* 2012; 108: 44–48.
223. Ganesan S, Faris AN, Comstock AT et al. Quercetin inhibits rhinovirus replication *in vitro* and in vivo. *Antiviral Res* 2012; 94: 258–271.
224. Yamaya M, Nishimura H, Hatachi Y et al. Levofloxacin inhibits rhinovirus infection in primary cultures of human tracheal epithelial cells. *Antimicrob Agents Chemother* 2012; 56: 4052–4061.
225. Min JY, Jang YJ. Macrolide therapy in respiratory viral infections. *Mediators Inflamm* 2012; 2012: 649570.
226. Turner RB, Hendley JO. Virucidal hand treatments for prevention of rhinovirus infection. *J Antimicrob Chemother* 2005; 56: 805–807.
227. Turner RB, Biedermann KA, Morgan JM, Keswick B, Ertel KD, Barker MF. Efficacy of organic acids in hand cleansers for prevention of rhinovirus infections. *Antimicrob Agents Chemother* 2004; 48: 2595–2598.
228. Savolainen-Kopra C, Korpela T, Simonen-Tikka ML et al. Single treatment with ethanol hand rub is ineffective against human rhinovirus—Hand washing with soap and water removes the virus efficiently. *J Med Virol* 2012; 84: 543–547.
229. McLean GR, Walton RP, Shetty S et al. Rhinovirus infections and immunisation induce cross-serotype reactive antibodies to VP1. *Antiviral Res* 2012; 95: 193–201.
230. Baines KJ, Hsu AC, Tooze M et al. Novel immune genes associated with excessive inflammatory and antiviral responses to rhinovirus in COPD. *Respiratory Research* 2013; 14: 15.
231. Granados A, Luinstra K, Chong S et al. Use of an improved quantitative polymerase chain reaction assay to determine differences in human rhinovirus viral loads in different populations. *Diagnostic Microbiology and Infectious Disease* 2012; 74(4): 384–387.
232. Gern JE. Rhinovirus and the initiation of asthma. *Curr Opin Allergy Clin Immunol* 2009; 9: 73–78.

21 Human Respiratory Syncytial Virus Infections

Marcello Lanari, Silvia Vandini, and Giacomo Faldella

CONTENTS

21.1 INTRODUCTION

Respiratory syncytial virus (RSV) is a member of the pneumovirus genus and paramyxoviridae family, discovered in 1956. It is an RNA virus with an enveloped, nonsegmented, negative-sense, single-stranded genome with 10 genes encoded for 11 proteins.

The envelope is composed of four proteins in a lipid bilayer: the matrix (M) protein, the small hydrophobic (SH) protein, and the two glycosylated surface (G) and fusion (F) proteins. The G protein plays a key role in the infection process: the G protein determines adhesion of the virus to the respiratory epithelial cells, while the F protein mediates the entry of the virus into the cells and induces the insertion of viral RNA into the cell, leading to the formation of syncytia (Chanock et al., 1957). The surface proteins also mediate the production of neutralizing antibodies by the infected host.

The circulating RSV exists in two different subtypes, A and B; the two subtypes coexist during each RSV season, and subtype A seems to be associated with a more severe infection (Martinello et al., 2002; Gilca et al., 2006). Variations in G proteins determine antigenic differences between and within A and B subtypes, with a 35% homology of G glycoprotein between A and B (Johnson et al., 2004). Neutralizing antibodies versus G protein are subtype-specific, while antibodies against F protein neutralize both subtypes and could be more useful for active and passive immunization.

21.2 EPIDEMIOLOGY

RSV is a worldwide infection with a large diffusion, since specific antibodies can be detected in 87% of infants younger than 18 months (Simoes, 1999) and in virtually all 3-year-old infants.

RSV is the most important cause of acute lower respiratory tract infections (LRTIs) in infants and it is associated with hospitalization and mortality during the first years of life (Boyce et al., 2000; Leader and Kohlhase, 2003).

The widespread diffusion of RSV determines epidemics in infants younger than 5 years with an important economic impact related to an increase in pediatric visits, emergency room accesses, and hospital admissions. In the United States in 2000, there were approximately 86,000 hospitalizations,

402,000 emergency room visits, 1.7 million office visits, and 236,000 hospital outpatient visits, with a total cost estimated at $258 million (Paramore et al., 2004).

RSV is also an important cause of death in young infants. In infants younger than 1 year of age, RSV-associated mortality is ninefold higher than influenza-associated mortality (Thompson et al., 2003).

It was estimated (Nair et al., 2011) that, during 2005, over 33 million episodes of RSV-related LRTIs occurred worldwide in children younger than 5 years of age. During the same year, the estimated hospitalization rate for severe acute LRTI in young children was 3.4 (2.8–4.3) million (16.9 per 1000 infants aged 0–5 months and, 5.1 per 1000 infants aged 6–11 months). The mortality rate was 66,000–199,000/year for children younger than 5 years; 99% of deaths were observed in the developing countries (Hall et al., 2009). The mortality rate in the developing countries is up to 7%—much higher than the mortality rate observed in the developed countries (0.5%–2%), where severe RSV infections are observed in a well-defined high-risk population (Simoes, 1999).

In the developing countries, RSV-related mortality is an outstanding problem, since RSV is responsible for 70% of all cases of LRTI; risk factors for severe diseases are crowding, indoor smoke pollution, and malnutrition.

The rate of hospitalization for RSV bronchiolitis in the United States increased from 22.2% in 1980 to 47% in 1996 in infants younger than 1 year of age, and from 5.4% to 16.4% among total hospitalizations (Shay et al., 1999). The estimated rate of hospitalization during the first year of life is 388/1000 infants with bronchopulmonary dysplasia, 92/1000 infants with congenital heart disease (CHD), 70/1000 infants ≤28 weeks' gestation, 66/1000 infants born at 29–32 weeks' gestation, 57/1000 infants born at 33–36 weeks' gestation, and 30/1000 healthy infants born at term.

RSV is also an important cause of severe acute respiratory infections in elderly people (≥65 years old) and high-risk adults (those with chronic heart or lung disease; Falsey, 2005).

RSV infections are observed worldwide with some differences related to environmental factors that determine difference in epidemic trends: RSV activity peaks during winter season in temperate climates and is nearly continuous in cold climates, probably because of different meteorological factors conditioning virus activity and transmission.

Many authors registered a correlation between RSV epidemics and meteorological factors as relative humidity and minimum temperature (Meerhoff et al., 2009; Noyola and Mandeville, 2008; Vandini et al., 2013). Minimum temperature, 2–6°C, and relative humidity, 45–65%, are associated with greater stability of RSV in respiratory secretions; moreover, cold climate induces people to spend more time indoors, facilitating transmission of respiratory tract infections.

Some authors (Karr et al., 2009) observed a modest increased risk for RSV hospitalization (OR 1.14; 95% CI, 0.88–1.46) correlated to exposure to a higher concentration of fine particulate matter ($PM_{2,5}$) related to traffic-derived air pollution.

RSV disease is particularly severe in some groups of high-risk infants, in whom the infection often leads to severe respiratory failure, cardiac complications, and death.

Infants at high risk of RSV morbidity and mortality include preterm infants, especially those with chronic lung disease (CLD), infants with CHD, neuromuscular diseases, cystic fibrosis (CF), or immunodeficiency (Welliver, 2003; Resch et al., 2009).

Prematurity is one of the major risk factors for severe RSV infections in young infants for several reasons; the two most important mechanisms that predispose preterm infants to severe infections are inadequate antibody production and incomplete development of the lungs and the airways.

Broughton et al. (2006) observed that abnormal airway function (higher airway resistance) at 36 weeks postmenstrual age predisposes prematurely born infants to severe RSV LRTIs.

Several multicenter studies examined RSV epidemiology in large cohorts of term and preterm infants and reported a higher risk for RSV infections among preterm infants, including late preterm infants (33–35 weeks GA); these studies also evaluated risk factors for infection and hospitalization in this unique population (Wang et al., 1995, Weigl et al., 2003, Lanari et al., 2003 and 2011, Liese et al., 2003, Sampalis, 2003, Simoes, 2003, Figueras-Aloy et al., 2004, Simões et al., 2011).

A study performed in Italy (Lanari et al., 2002) reported a higher prevalence of RSV infections in infants with a GA ≤35 weeks than in infants born at term.

Infants born at 33–35 weeks GA are at risk for severe RSV infections, which may require hospitalization due to impaired lung development, relative immaturity of the immune system, and discharge at earlier age from the neonatal unit than infants born before 32 weeks GA (Carbonell-Estrany et al., 2004, Lanari et al., 2002).

Late preterm infants also have a higher risk of severe RSV infections than infants born at an earlier GA, with a higher rate of intubation and a higher ICU stay and length of hospital stay (Horn and Smout, 2003).

Risk factors for severe RSV infections in infants born at 33–35 weeks GA were analyzed in the Pediatric Investigators Collaborative Network on Infections in Canada (PICNIC) study by Wang et al. (1995) and in the FLIP study (Figueras-Aloy et al., 2004).

The PICNIC study was a prospective, multicenter, cohort study that enrolled 1,516 infants born at 33–35 weeks GA during 2 RSV seasons; hospitalization rate for RSV infections in the entire cohort was 3.6%; the mean length of hospital stay was 8.6–11.8 days in infants with pre-existing morbidity and 4.6–6.7 in healthy infants.

The FLIP study was a prospective case-control study evaluating risk factors for RSV-related respiratory infections in 186 infants born at 33–35 weeks GA in Spain during one epidemic season and hospitalized for a proven RSV infection, compared to 371 controls.

Since November 2009, infants born at GA ≥33 weeks were recruited into a multicenter cohort Italian study in order to examine the incidence of LRTIs during the first year of life: preliminary data showed that infants of the lower GA group (33 weeks + 0 days – 34 weeks + 6 days) were at a slightly higher risk of hospitalization for LRTI. In this study a protective effect of exclusive breast-feeding was also observed (Lanari et al., 2011).

Risk factors for RSV hospitalization in the three studies above were birth in the first part of RSV season (November, December, and January), age ≤10 weeks at the beginning of the RSV epidemic season, male gender, birth weight <10th percentile for sex and GA, preschool-age siblings, daycare attendance, number of inhabitants in household, exposure to tobacco smoke, and family history of wheezing.

CLD is a chronic pulmonary disease of premature infants defined as the need for oxygen supplementation after 28 days of age; CLD is related to high morbidity and high risk of hospitalization during the first years of life (Baraldi and Filippone, 2007). CLD is caused by prenatal (chorioamnionitis and intrauterine growth restriction) and postnatal (ventilator-induced lung injury, oxidative stress, infections, steroids, pulmonary fluids overload, and nutritional deficits) injuries, which damage the immature lung of the preterm newborn.

RSV infection is one of the most important causes of rehospitalization and respiratory deterioration in preterm infants with CLD.

The RSV-related hospitalization rate in infants with CLD is 56.2/100 children-years during the first 6 months of life (Boyce et al., 2000). The severity of RSV infections in infants with CLD can be explained by the reduction of lung volume and the airways hyperreactivity, deformation, and inflammation. These conditions predispose the immature and impaired lung to a severe obstructive airway disease during an acute respiratory infection.

Infants with CHD are also at high risk for severe acute respiratory disease following RSV infections. RSV-related rate of hospitalization is 12.1/100 children-years from birth to 6 months of age and 6.3/100 children-years from 6 to 12 months of age (Boyce et al., 2000); in a cohort of 1091 patients evaluated in Texas during four consecutive winter seasons from 1994 to 1998 and hospitalized with an RSV infection, 6% had CHD and more than a half of them were awaiting surgical repair. RSV infections in infants with CHD are often more severe, since they require more days of hospitalization and ICU and have a higher incidence of death and respiratory failure. In a Canadian study (Navas et al., 1992), 1/3 of infants with CHD hospitalized for an RSV infection required admission to the ICU, 20% required mechanical ventilation, and 9.4% died.

In our experience (Lanari et al., 2004), infants with CHD before surgical correction are at high risk of nosocomial RSV infections (9.8%), with high risk of subsequent respiratory failure and mortality.

Children with cyanotic CHD or pulmonary hypertension have impaired blood oxygenation, which is worsened by acute RSV infection.

Other congenital malformations are related to increased risk for hospitalization due to RSV-LRTI: in a birth cohort study performed in Colorado from 1997 to 2004, the risk for RSV-related hospitalization during the first 2 years of life was higher in infants with spina bifida, agenesis, hypoplasia or dysplasia of the lung, cleft palate alone, and biliary atresia (Zachariah et al., 2012).

Infants with congenital or acquired conditions related to immunodeficiency with deficits of cell-mediated immunity are at risk of severe RSV infections.

Luján-Zilbermann et al. (2001) reported that the risk of a severe respiratory virus infection increased after hematopoietic stem cells transplantation; 14% of infection detected in this pediatric population was caused by RSV.

Neuromuscular diseases also increase the severity of RSV infections, especially those requiring technology dependence and respiratory support (Panitch, 2004): in a prospective multicenter study performed in Germany during six consecutive RSV seasons (1999–2005), 4.7% of infants with infection had a clinically relevant neuromuscular disease: these patients were at higher risk for seizures (15.1% vs. 1.6%), need for mechanical ventilation (9.6% vs. 1.9%), and death (5.5% vs. 0.2%; Wilkesmann et al., 2007). As reviewed by Resch et al. (2009), RSV infections are frequently severe in infants with neuromuscular diseases because of low basal functional residual capacity, coexisting gastro-oesophageal reflux, and muscle weakness, which may lead to impaired cough mechanism and immobilization.

The severity of viral LRTI in infants with muscular weakness is probably due to impaired ability to clear respiratory secretions from the airways (deficits in cough mechanism and compromised swallowing coordination); these conditions lead to an increased risk of aspiration and atelectasis, and a respiratory infection determines an acute respiratory deterioration.

Limited data are available about RSV infection in children with CF; a longitudinal observational study published by Armstrong et al. in 1998 reported only seven cases of severe RSV infections among children with CF, and the PICNIC study did not identify CF patients as especially vulnerable to severe RSV LRTI.

21.3 CLINICAL FEATURES

Clinical manifestations of the RSV infection include both upper respiratory tract infections (URTIs) and LRTIs.

The most common clinical manifestation of RSV infection is a URTI characterized by rhinitis, cough, and sometimes fever. Signs of upper respiratory tract involvement commonly precede those of the lower respiratory tract by a few days. This clinical manifestation is more common in children older than 2 years of age and adults, while in younger infants RSV often determines an LRTI.

RSV infection typically causes an LRTI in infants 4–6 days from contact with the virus: symptoms include fever (75%), nasal congestion, cough (98%), tachypnea, breathing difficulty with retractions (73%), wheezing (65%), rales, prolonged respiratory phase, crackles, and cyanosis (Hall et al., 2009; Simoes, 1999); in very young infants, RSV can determine apneic episodes or a "sepsis-like presentation" with lethargy, irritability, poor feeding, and dehydration.

Food intake during the previous day was observed to be a reliable marker of hypoxia in infants with bronchiolitis (Corrard et al., 2013), since food intake <50% is predictive of mean SpO2 <90% (odds ratio 13.8, specificity 90%, and sensitivity 60%). This parameter might be extremely useful in the management of bronchiolitis in outpatients, since it is easy to monitor and can be registered daily by parents.

RSV can also cause pneumonia, with fine crackles and a radiographic pattern of alveolar, segmental, or lobar consolidation. The difference in clinical presentation (pneumonia or bronchiolitis) is subsequent to genetic, environmental, viral, and geographic factors.

Bacterial superinfection is common only in the developing countries and is related to a higher mortality rate.

Severity of the RSV infection is variable, from mild symptoms to severe respiratory failure; pediatric intensive care unit (PICU) admission and the subsequent need for mechanical ventilation occur in 7%–21% of infants with an acute RSV LRTI (Prodhan et al., 2009). Risk factors for PICU admission and the need for mechanical ventilation in healthy infants at initial presentation of the LRTI are the presence of lethargy (odds ratio (OR) 12.2; $P = 0.005$), a $PaCO_2$ of 65 mm Hg or greater (OR 9.3; $P = 0.01$), and grunting (OR 11.8; $P = 0.013$).

Infants with one or more risk factors for severe RSV LRTI (prematurity, bronchopulmonary dysplasia, and CHD) have a higher rate of hospitalization, respiratory failure, and mortality subsequent to RSV infections (Boyce et al., 2000; Leader and Kohlhase, 2003).

In a large hospital-based cohort, risk factors for severe LRTI were examined in hospitalized infants younger than 2 years: RSV detection, male gender, prematurity, CHD, CLD, and congenital syndromes increased the severity of bronchiolitis in the study cohort, since these conditions were related to longer hospitalization and higher rates of oxygen requirement, PICU admission, and mechanical ventilation (García et al., 2010).

Otitis media is often associated with RSV infections in young infants. Both viral and bacterial otitis media were found in 30%–40% infants with RSV LRTI, with a mean duration of symptoms of five days (Patel et al., 2007; Pettigrew et al., 2011; Kristjánsson et al., 2010). A complex interaction among virus and bacteria was hypothesized: viral infection probably promotes the replication of bacteria and increases the inflammation in the nasopharynx and in the eustachian tubes (Bakaletz, 2010).

Infants with RSV infection associated with acute otitis media (AOM) have a higher incidence of fever than infants without AOM (96% vs. 76%, OR 2.26, 95% confidence interval 1.53–30.01, $p = 0.0005$) at 6–35 months of age (Tomochika et al., 2009).

Cardiac complications may also occur in healthy infants without CHD hospitalized for severe RSV LRTI: sinoatrial block, tachyarrythmias, atrioventricular block, pericarditis, myocarditis, complete heart block, and reduced right ventricular function. Moreover, in infants with CHD, RSV bronchiolitis determines severe complications, including severe hypoxia, pulmonary edema, pulmonary hypertension, and heart failure (Geskey and Cyran, 2012)

A rare complication of RSV infections, especially in infants younger than 2 years with severe muscle weakness, is encephalopathy with seizures. Nakamura et al. (2012) reported the case of a 23-month-old Japanese child with a severe congenital myopathy who presented consciousness disturbances and seizures, followed by severe brain damage subsequent to an acute RSV infection.

RSV is also related to long-term respiratory sequelae through interactions with genetic, pulmonary, immunological, and cardiovascular functions (Bont and Ramilo, 2011). RSV infection in preterm infants with altered lung development subsequent to preterm birth and CLD is related to long-term abnormal lung function.

Respiratory morbidity of preterm infants increases after an episode of RSV LRTI, with an increase of respiratory symptoms, daycare attendance, hospitalization for respiratory disease, and use of drugs as inhaled bronchodilators (Greenough and Broughton, 2005).

A cohort study comparing preterm infants born before 32 weeks GA with and without RSV LRTI demonstrated that RSV bronchiolitis is associated with higher airway resistance, higher incidence of wheezing, and a greater use of bronchodilators (Broughton et al., 2007).

Long-term follow-up studies demonstrated a strong correlation between RSV bronchiolitis and atopy and allergy (Stein et al., 1999; Korppi et al., 2004; Sigurs et al., 2005; Henderson et al., 2005; Broughton et al., 2006).

In a cohort of 7-year-old children, RSV bronchiolitis was associated with an increased risk of recurrent wheezing at 30–42 months (28.1% vs. 13.1%) and 69–81 months (22.6% vs. 9.6%).

In another cohort, 13-year-old children hospitalized for RSV infections during the first year of life presented a higher rate of asthma (28% vs. 3.3%), recurrent wheezing (15% vs. 4.3%), and allergic rhinoconjunctivitis (39% vs. 15%) with mild airway obstruction both at rest and after bronchodilator inhalation, and slightly higher bronchial reactivity (Sigurs et al., 2005).

Lung function abnormalities in flow-volume spirometry (one or more abnormal results in spirometry and a decrease in forced expiratory volume (FEV) % and mid-expiratory flow (MEF_{50})) were found in young adults hospitalized in infancy for an RSV infection (Korppi et al., 2004).

21.4 PATHOGENESIS AND IMMUNITY

RSV infection can have different clinical features according to the virus, the host (age, coexisting respiratory disorders, and immunological factors), and the environment.

RSV causes upper respiratory symptoms in healthy adults, but it determines severe respiratory infections in immunosuppressed individuals, the elderly, and infants younger than 2 years.

Similar to other respiratory viruses, RSV can re-infect the host after the first contact (Le Nouën et al., 2011), but the severity of disease is usually reduced during the reinfection. The antibodies developed by the host after the first infection contribute poorly to protection; a possible explanation for this phenomenon could be the low immunogenicity of the viral protein domain and the large production of other viral proteins, such as that secreted form of the G glycoprotein. For these reasons the immune response against RSV is mainly mediated by IFN-γ secreting CD4+ and CD8+ T cells that promote virus clearance (González et al., 2012).

The immune response and the subsequent respiratory symptoms are determined by two different mechanisms: the necrosis of epithelial cells directly damaged by the virus and the immune response of the host (Bont and Kimpen, 2002).

The pathogenesis (van Drunen Littel-van den Hurk and Watkiss, 2012) of RSV infection is immune-mediated, and this was demonstrated by some authors through the failure of the vaccine that led to severe, nonprotective, Th2-biased immunopathology and through the association with other Th2-related conditions such as asthma and atopy.

The severity of the infection is related to environmental and social factors: age <3–6 months at onset of the RSV season, passive smoking, daycare attendance, presence of young siblings in the household, stay in a nursing home or hospital, and exposure to traffic-derived air pollution increase the risk of a severe RSV bronchiolitis (American Academy of Pediatrics, 2009; Karr et al., 2009).

RSV infects type I alveolar cells, nonbasilar airway epithelial cells, and alveolar macrophages (Johnson et al., 2007), and determines the impairment of the ciliary action, sloughing of infected epithelial cells, mononuclear cells infiltration, submucosal edema, mucus secretion, and sometimes syncytia formation. Even if RSV is not a highly cytopathic virus, the level of viral replication is related to the disease severity (DeVincenzo et al., 2010; El Saleeby et al., 2011).

Considering the viral factors related to the pathogenesis of the disease, subgroup A strain 19 was recently shown to increase mucus secretion, airway hypersensitivity, and IL-13 production. The RSV subgroup A2001/2-20 is related to greater disease severity since it determines higher IL-13 secretion, airway mucine expression, and higher lung gob-5 levels (Moore et al., 2009; Stokes et al., 2011). The severity of the disease is mediated by histopathological changes (epithelial desquamation, bronchiolitis, and airway hyper-responsiveness) correlated to RSV 2–20 higher replication.

After infection, the host response is modulated by several RSV proteins (NS1, NS2, and G protein) that interact with the immune response of the host.

The NS1 and NS2 proteins block IFN regulatory factor 3 activation and block the IFNα/β production and improve virus survival in the infected cells through activation of the phosphoinositide-3-kinase pathway, which reduces the apoptosis of the infected cells.

The G protein is a highly glycosylated and highly variable protein (with 53% amino acid identity and 1%–7% antigenic variability) protein, which impedes immune recognition, is responsible for the immune evasion of RSV, and reduces the influx of CXCR1 leucocytes such as natural killer cells and CD4+ or CD8+ T cells. Moreover, a truncated form (sG) is secreted during infection: it downregulates the TLR-mediated inflammatory response and binds RSV-specific antibodies, reducing their effect in virus neutralization (Bukreyev et al., 2008; Tripp et al., 2001; Polack, 2005).

RSV can also interfere with immune response through infection of immune cells as macrophages and dendritic cells and impairment of their antigen presenting activity (Lukacs et al., 2008; LeNouen et al., 2011).

Finally, RSV infects bone marrow stromal cells determining altered chemokine/cytokine expression and decreases the ability to stimulate B cell maturation: this condition contributes both to acute disease and long-term sequelae (Rezaee et al., 2011).

The host factors related to the pathogenesis of RSV infection include the conditions related to incomplete lung development or airways damage, immunodeficiency, or immunosuppression (premature birth, CLD, CHD, and T cell immunodeficiency).

Some authors (Miyairi and DeVincenzo, 2008) hypothesized the existence of genetic factors related to the host response to RSV infection and involved in the determination of the severity of the disease. Several polymorphisms were identified in genes involved in the innate defense, surfactant protein genes, host cell receptor genes, Th1/Th2 response genes, gene effectors of neutrophil response, and adaptive immunity.

Epithelial cells and macrophages also play an important role in the innate immune response to RSV, producing many cytokines and chemokines (IL-8/CXCL8, IP-10/CXCL10, MCP-1/CCL2, MIP-1α/CCL3, MIP-1β/CCL4, RANTES/CCL5, IL-6, TNF-α, IL-1αβ, and IFN-α/β) that were found in high concentrations in the respiratory secretions of infants hospitalized for RSV infections (McNamara et al., 2005). IL-8 concentration is correlated to the severity of the infection and it determines recruitments of neutrophils; the subsequent increase in the number of neutrophils leads to the secretion of further cytokines and degranulation products involved in the RSV-induced immunopathogenesis (McNamara et al., 2003).

The concentration of IL-8 in the amniotic fluid was found to have a protective effect against wheezing and severe bronchiolitis, probably through the positive effect on maturation of the fetal lung (van Bleek et al., 2011).

Moreover, regulatory T cells (T-regs) were found to be involved in the innate and adaptive response to the virus during the latest phases of the disease, since a depletion of T-regs causes a delay in virus elimination and an increase in the severity of disease (Fulton, 2010).

Other cytokines (IL-17, IL-6, and IL-23) are probably involved in the pathogenesis of the disease (Mukherjee et al., 2011).

The pathogenesis of RSV disease was studied through autopsy studies performed in an infant who died of an acute trauma after an acute episode of RSV infection (Johnson et al., 2007) and in 11 infants who died of a severe RSV infection (Welliver et al., 2008). These two studies allowed for the analysis of the histological features of two different patterns of RSV disease: in the first study the infection was self-limiting, while in the second study the infection was extremely severe and led to death the 11 infected infants.

In the severe cases, RSV antigen was found in exfoliated alveolar cells to be associated with high levels of neutrophils and monocytes and a low number of T cells, while in the nonfatal case the antigen was found only in the bronchial epithelial cells and the infiltrate was made predominantly of CD8+ T cells and B cells. These differences could explain the different clinical feature of the infection, with an acute and uncontrolled inflammatory response leading to a lethal disease (Rosenberg and Domachowske, 2012).

RSV may also alter T cell activation through interference with the synapses between dendritic cells and CD4+ T cells (González et al., 2012); in this way the virus impairs the T-cell activation mediated by the antigen presentation.

Moreover, RSV determines an interference with T cell polarization through an increase of Th1 polarized RSV-specific T cells and alters T cell migration in the lungs through the interaction between the viral G glycoprotein and a chemokine domain that activates T cells migration.

Since the antibody serum concentration decreases after cardiac bypass, patients undergoing cardiopulmonary bypass should receive a dose of palivizumab as soon as possible after the procedure.

The monthly dose of 15 mg/kg should be administered by aseptic technique in the anterolateral region of the thigh, avoiding the gluteal area because of the risk of damage to the sciatic nerve. Volumes over 1 mL should be injected in divided doses.

The efficacy and safety of palivizumab was determined through two randomized, double-blind, placebo-controlled trials: the impact-RSV trial (Null et al., 2005) and another study conducted in children with hemodinamically significant CHD (Feltes et al., 2003).

The IMpact trial was conducted during one RSV season in 1998 in a cohort of 1,502 infants younger than 2 years with CLD, or infants born before 36 weeks GA younger than 6 months: 1,002 randomized children received monthly 15 mg/kg palivizumab and 500 received placebo during the RSV season; all children were followed up for 150 days after randomization. Hospital admission for a respiratory illness with a positive test for RSV or a positive RSV test with a moderate respiratory disease during a previous hospital stay were evaluated as primary endpoints: the incidence of RSV-related hospitalization significantly decreased by 55% in the overall palivizumab group, with a reduction of the length of hospitalization; the duration of mechanical ventilation, days of hospitalization for nonrespiratory illness, and the incidence of otitis media were not lower in the palivizumab group. This reduction was greater in preterm infants (78%; 95% CI, 66%–90%) than in infants with CLD (39%; 95% CI, 20%–58%), who often required hospitalization for mild respiratory acute diseases. The incidence of adverse events did not differ in the two groups; the reported adverse events included injection side reactions (2.7% in the palivizumab group vs. 1.8% in the placebo group), fever (2.8% vs. 3%), rash (0.9% vs. 0.2%), and nervousness (2.6% vs. 2.5%). The incidence of death was 0.4% in the palivizumab group and 1% in the placebo group; none of the deaths were related to palivizumab.

Mortality due to RSV infection reported by some studies was 6.7%, including deaths for causes not related to the infection (Wang et al., 1995; Sampalis, 2003).

The efficacy and safety of palivizumab in two seasons were evaluated in 88 infants enrolled in the impact study (Null et al., 2005). The prevalence of antipalivizumab antibodies (titer >1/40) was observed in one subject and was not related to serious adverse events.

A randomized, double-blind, placebo-controlled multicenter study was conducted in 1,287 children aged ≤2 years with hemodinamically significant CHD (Feltes et al., 2003) who received monthly palivizumab 15 mg/kg for 5 doses. This trial demonstrated that palivizumab reduced the incidence of hospitalization (5.3% vs. 9.7%), the number of days of hospitalization for RSV infection, and total hospital days with increased supplemental oxygen. The study cohort included cyanotic CHD and noncyanotic CHD: the reduction of hospitalization was 29% in the cyanotic group and 58% in the noncyanotic group.

The reported adverse events (injection site reactions, fever, conjunctivitis, and cyanosis) were not different in the palivizumab group and in the placebo group, and never required drug discontinuation. Mortality did not differ in the two groups and was not related to palivizumab; moreover, the drug did not influence the management of cardiac disease.

A recent review (Resch and Michel-Behnke, 2013) confirmed that immunoprophylaxis with palivizumab is the most useful tool to prevent hospitalization for RSV bronchiolitis in infants with CHD, since an effective vaccine is not in use. Authors also reviewed pharmacoeconomic studies that confirmed the cost-effectiveness of palivizumab prophylaxis in pediatric patients with CHD.

Prophylaxis with palivizumab was also demonstrated to decrease by 80% the risk of recurrent wheezing in premature infants aged 2–5 years, with a 68% decrease in infants with no family history of asthma and 80% in infants with no atopic background, while the effect was not observed in infants with an atopic family history (Simões et al., 2010). This result suggests that RSV-induced recurrent wheezing is not mediated by an atopic mechanism.

A prospective Italian study comparing 154 palivizumab-recipients to 71 palivizumab-nonrecipients (Faldella et al., 2010) reported a reduction in hospitalization after palivizumab administration in infants younger than 6 months during their first RSV season.

Another monoclonal antibody (motavizumab, Medi-524 MedImmune) was subsequently introduced: it is a molecule derived from palivizumab, differing in 13 amino acid residuals; both antibodies target a highly conserved antigenic side A of F protein of RSV, but the neutralizing capacity measured in a murine model is higher in motavizumab (Mejías et al., 2005).

Motavizumab had higher neutralization activity than palivizumab *in vitro* and in animal models (Wu et al., 2005, 2007).

Clinical trials investigated safety and efficacy of motavizumab for the prophylaxis of RSV infection. A double-blind, randomized, phase 2 study (Fernández et al., 2010) compared properties of palivizumab and motavizumab administered sequentially during the same seasons to 260 high-risk infants ≤2 years who received five 15 mg/kg doses of palivizumab or motavizumab IM every 30 days. The incidence of adverse events was equal in the three study groups; deaths were not related to drug administration. Mean drug serum concentration was comparable in the study groups.

A multicenter phase 3 trial including over 300 locations (Simoes et al., 2007) investigated the safety and efficacy of motavizumab in 6,635 preterm infants <6 months or <24 months with CLD. The infants received five 15 mg/kg doses of palivizumab or motavizumab monthly and were followed for 5 months. Motavizumab was not inferior to palivizumab in the reduction of RSV hospitalization or RSV LRTI in outpatients; the incidence of adverse events was comparable for the two antibodies.

The safety, immunogenicity, and pharmacokinetics of motavizumab were investigated in a randomized, open-label, phase I–II trial run on 217 high-risk children: motavizumab properties were comparable to palivizumab (Abarca et al., 2009).

In January 2008, Medimmune submitted to the Food and Drug Administration a biological license application for motavizumab, but the Advisory Committee declined to endorse the request to approve the use of motavizumab because it has the same safety and efficacy of palivizumab, which has been in use since the 1990s.

Besides the use of mAbs for prophylaxis, the use of a vaccine against RSV was recently hypothesized.

The development of RSV vaccines is studied with different techniques (live-attenuated viruses, protein subunit-based, and vector-based). The vaccine should be started at birth to prevent the infection in the first months of life, but the immune system is still immature, RSV proteins G and F are weakly immunogenic, and the presence of maternal antibodies could interfere with the vaccine. Moreover, repeated booster doses could be necessary because of incomplete and short-lived immunity. Finally, the use of formalin-inactivated RSV may enhance the disease severity, inducing the release of cytokines related to lung inflammatory response (Chang, 2011).

The cost-effectiveness of a potential vaccination against RSV was analyzed in a decision-analysis model developed in The Netherlands (Meijboom et al., 2012), which hypothesized that the introduction of the vaccine might be cost-effective since it might lead to higher costs associated with a significant reduction of hospitalization and deaths (Sàez-Llorens et al., 2004).

Since palivizumab is a safe, effective, but expensive drug, the development of prophylaxis guidelines should be related to studies of pharmacoeconomics.

The extension of prophylaxis to late preterm infants has been a matter of concern for many years (Carbonell-Estrany et al., 2008; Lanari et al., 2010), since this population is susceptible to respiratory infections because of the immaturity of the lungs and the immune system, even though the AAP recommends the prophylaxis for late preterms only in the first 3 months of life (Rossi et al., 2010). The prophylaxis might be useful, especially in late preterm infants with >1 risk factors for RSV-LRTI, including chronological age, birth weight, presence and age of siblings, and daycare attendance (Lanari et al., 2009).

A prospective, multicenter Italian study (Lanari et al., 2002) enrolling 1,232 infants <2 years confirmed these risk factors and also observed an increase in risk for severe RSV LRTI determined by tobacco smoke exposure.

Clinical studies aiming to determine the cost-effectiveness of prophylaxis in this population and to optimize the national guidelines for prophylaxis schedule according to epidemiological data are ongoing.

A cost-utility analysis was conducted in four subgroups of preterm infants (Weiner et al., 2012): palivizumab was observed to save costs and improve QALY (quality-adjusted-life-year) in preterm infants <32 weeks. Moreover, it proved to be cost-effective in infants 32–34 weeks GA with the risk factors stated by the AAP in 2009 and in infants 32–35 weeks GA with >1 of the 2006 AAP risk factors.

The positive impact of prophylaxis with palivizumab on health care costs was confirmed by retrospective analysis performed in Austria (Resch et al., 2012) and in Spain (Nuijten and Wittenberg, 2010).

A pharmacoeconomic analysis could also be applied to the guidelines in use for the prophylaxis with palivizumab in different groups of high-risk children (Manzoni et al., 2012).

RSV prophylaxis is recommended in children with neuromuscular diseases or congenital diaphragmatic hernia for the documented cost-effectiveness, while it is still controversial in infants with Down syndrome, CF, and immunodeficiency.

REFERENCES

Abarca K, Jung E, Fernández P, Zhao L, Harris B, Connor EM, Losonsky GA, Motavizumab study group. Safety, tolerability, pharmacokinetics, and immunogenicity of motavizumab, a humanized, enhanced-potency monoclonal antibody for the prevention of respiratory syncytial virus infection in at-risk children. *Pediatr Infect Dis J*. 2009;28(4):267–272.

Abbott Laboratories. *Data on File*. Abbott Laboratories; International Division; Abbott Park; IL; 2000.

Abman SH, Griebel JL, Parker DK, Schmidt JM, Swanton D, Kinsella JP. Acute effects of inhaled nitric oxide in children with severe hypoxemic respiratory failure. *J Pediatr*. 1994;124(6):881–888.

Aldous WK, Gerber K, Taggart EW, Thomas J, Tidwell D, Daly JA. A comparison of Binax NOW to viral culture and direct fluorescent assay testing for respiratory syncytial virus. *Diagn Microbiol Infect Dis*. 2004;49(4):265–268.

American Academy of Pediatrics Subcommittee on Diagnosis and Management of Bronchiolitis. Diagnosis and management of bronchiolitis. *Pediatrics*. 2006;118(4):1774–1793.

American Academy of Pediatrics. Committee on Infectious Disease. Policy statement—modified recommendations for use of palivizumab for prevention of respiratory syncytial virus infections. *Pediatrics*. 2009;124(6):1694–1701.

Antonis AF, de Jong MC, van der Poel WH, van der Most RG, Stockhofe-Zurwieden N, Kimman T, Schrijver RS. Age-dependent differences in the pathogenesis of bovine respiratory syncytial virus infections related to the development of natural immunocompetence. *J Gen Virol*. 2010;91(Pt 10):2497–2506.

Arbiza J, Taylor G, López JA, Furze J, Wyld S, Whyte P, Stott EJ, Wertz G, Sullender W, Trudel M. Characterization of two antigenic sites recognized by neutralizing monoclonal antibodies directed against the fusion glycoprotein of human respiratory syncytial virus. *J Gen Virol*. 1992;73(Pt 9):2225–2234.

Bakaletz LO. Immunopathogenesis of polymicrobial otitis media. *J Leukoc Biol*2010;87(2):213–222.

Bar A, Srugo I, Amirav I, Tzverling C, Naftali G, Kugelman A. Inhaled furosemide in hospitalized infants with viral bronchiolitis: A randomized, double-blind, placebo-controlled pilot study. *Pediatr Pulmonol*. 2008;43(3):261–267.

Baraldi E, Filippone M. Chronic lung disease after premature birth. *N Engl J Med*. 2007;357(19):1946–1955.

Beeler JA, van Wyke Coelingh K. Neutralization epitopes of the F glycoprotein of respiratory syncytial virus: Effect of mutation upon fusion function. *J Virol*. 1989;63(7):2941–2950.

Bentley DL, Rabbits TH. Human immunoglobulin variable region genes—DNA sequences of two V kappa genes and a pseudogene. *Nature*. 1980;288(5792):730–733.

Berner ME, Hanquinet S, Rimensberger PC. High frequency oscillatory ventilation for respiratory failure due to RSV bronchiolitis. *Intensive Care Med*. 2008;34(9):1698–1702.

Bont L, Kimpen JL. Immunological mechanisms of severe respiratory syncytial virus bronchiolitis. *Intensive Care Med.* 2002;28(5):616–621.

Bont L, Ramilo O. The relationship between RSV bronchiolitis and recurrent wheeze: The chicken and the egg. *Early Hum Dev.* 2011;87 Suppl 1:S51–S54.

Boogaard R, Hulsmann AR, van Veen L, Vaessen-Verberne AA, Yap YN, Sprij AJ, Brinkhorst G et al. Recombinant human deoxyribonuclease in infants with respiratory syncytial virus bronchiolitis. *Chest.* 2007;131(3):788–795.

Boyce TG, Mellen BG, Mitchel EF Jr, Wright PF, Griffin MR. Rates of hospitalization for respiratory syncytial virus infection among children in medicaid. *J Pediatr.* 2000;137(6):865–870.

Brandenburg AH, Groen J, van Steensel-Moll HA, Claas EC, Rothbarth PH, Neijens HJ, Osterhaus AD. Respiratory syncytial virus specific serum antibodies in infants under six months of age: Limited serological response upon infection. *J Med Virol.* 1997;52(1):97–104.

Broughton S, Bhat R, Roberts A, Zuckerman M, Rafferty G, Greenough A. Diminished lung function, RSV infection, and respiratory morbidity in prematurely born infants. *Arch Dis Child.* 2006;91(1):26–30.

Broughton S, Sylvester KP, Fox G, Zuckerman M, Smith M, Milner AD, Rafferty GF, Greenough A. Lung function in prematurely born infants after viral lower respiratory tract infections. *Pediatr Infect Dis J.* 2007;26(11):1019–1024.

Brown KL, Walker G, Grant DJ, Tanner K, Ridout DA, Shekerdemian LS, Smith JH, Davis C, Firmin RK, Goldman AP. Predicting outcome in ex-premature infants supported with extracorporeal membrane oxygenation for acute hypoxic respiratory failure. *Arch Dis Child Fetal Neonatal Ed.* 2004;89(5):F423–F427.

Bukreyev A, Yang L, Fricke J, Cheng L, Ward JM, Murphy BR, Collins PL. The secreted form of respiratory syncytial virus G glycoprotein helps the virus evade antibody-mediated restriction of replication by acting as an antigen decoy and through effects on Fc receptor-bearing leukocytes. *J Virol.* 2008;82(24):12191–12204.

Carbonell-Estrany X, Figueras-Aloy J. Law BJ. Infección Respiratoria Infantil por Virus Respiratorio Sincitial Study Group, Pediatric Investigators Collaborative Network on Infections in Canada Study Group. Identifying risk factors for severe respiratory syncytial virus among infants born after 33 through 35 completed weeks of gestation: different methodologies yield consistent findings. *Pediatr Infect Dis J.* 2004;23(11 Suppl):S193–S201.

Carbonell-Estrany X, Bont L, Doering G, Gouyon JB, Lanari M. Clinical relevance of prevention of respiratory syncytial virus lower respiratory tract infection in preterm infants born between 33 and 35 weeks gestational age. *Eur J Clin Microbiol Infect Dis.* 2008;27(10):891–899.

Carbonell-Estrany X, Simões EA, Dagan R, Hall CB, Harris B, Hultquist M, Connor EM, Losonsky GA. Motavizumab Study Group. Motavizumab for prophylaxis of respiratory syncytial virus in high-risk children: A noninferiority trial. *Pediatrics.* 2010;125(1):e35–e51.

Chang J. Current progress on development of respiratory syncytial virus vaccine. *BMB Rep.* 2011;44(4):232–237.

Chanock, R., Roizman, B., Myers, R. Recovery from infants with respiratory illness of a virus related to chimpanzee coryza agent. Part 1: Isolation; properties and characterization. *Am. J. Hyg.*, 1957;66(3):281–290.

Cormier SA, You D, Honnegowda S. The use of a neonatal mouse model to study respiratory syncytial virus infections. *Expert Rev Anti Infect Ther.* 2010;8(12):1371–1380.

Corneli HM, Zorc JJ, Mahajan P, Shaw KN, Holubkov R, Reeves SD, Ruddy RM et al. Bronchiolitis Study Group of the Pediatric Emergency Care Applied Research Network (PECARN). A multicenter, randomized, controlled trial of dexamethasone for bronchiolitis. *N Engl J Med.* 2007;357(4):331–339.

Corrard F, de La Rocque F, Martin E, Wollner C, Elbez A, Koskas M, Wollner A, Boucherat M, Cohen R. Food intake during the previous 24 h as a percentage of usual intake: A marker of hypoxia in infants with bronchiolitis: An observational, prospective, multicenter study. *BMC Pediatr.* 2013;13:6.

DeVincenzo JP, Hall CB, Kimberlin DW, Sánchez PJ, Rodriguez WJ, Jantausch BA, Corey L et al. Surveillance of clinical isolates of respiratory syncytial virus for palivizumab (Synagis)-resistant mutants. *J Infect Dis.* 2004;190(5):975–978.

DeVincenzo JP, Wilkinson T, Vaishnaw A, Cehelsky J, Meyers R, Nochur S, Harrison L et al. Viral load drives disease in humans experimentally infected with respiratory syncytial virus. *Am J Respir Crit Care Med.* 2010;182(10):1305–13014.

Di Nardo M, Perrotta D, Stoppa F, Cecchetti C, Marano M, Pirozzi N. Independent lung ventilation in a newborn with asymmetric acute lung injury due to respiratory syncytial virus: A case report. *J Med Case Rep.* 2008;2:212.

Dowell SF, Anderson LJ, Gary HE Jr, Erdman DD, Plouffe JF, File TM Jr, Marston BJ, Breiman RF. Respiratory syncytial virus is an important cause of community-acquired lower respiratory infection among hospitalized adults. *J Infect Dis*. 1996;174(3):456–462.

Eiland LS. Respiratory syncytial virus: Diagnosis, treatment and prevention. *J Pediatr Pharmacol Ther*. 2009;14(2):75–85.

El Saleeby CM, Bush AJ, Harrison LM, Aitken JA, Devincenzo JP. Respiratory syncytial virus load, viral dynamics, and disease severity in previously healthy naturally infected children. *J Infect Dis*. 2011;204(7):996–1002.

Faldella G, Alessandroni R, Aquilano G, Vandini S, Lanari M, Silvestri M, Pistorio A, Rossi GA. Hospitalization for lower respiratory tract disease in preterm infants: Effects of prophylaxis with palivizumab. *J Chemother*. 2010;22(1):30–35.

Falsey AR. Respiratory syncytial virus infection in elderly and high-risk adults. *Exp Lung Res*. 2005;31 Suppl 1:77.

Feltes TF, Cabalka AK, Meissner HC, Piazza FM, Carlin DA, Top FH Jr, Connor EM, Sondheimer HM, Cardiac Synagis Study Group. Palivizumab prophylaxis reduces hospitalization due to respiratory syncytial virus in young children with hemodynamically significant congenital heart disease. *J Pediatr*. 2003;143(4):532–540.

Fernández P, Trenholme A, Abarca K, Griffin MP, Hultquist M, Harris B, Losonsky GA, Motavizumab Study Group. A phase 2, randomized, double-blind safety and pharmacokinetic assessment of respiratory syncytial virus (RSV) prophylaxis with motavizumab and palivizumab administered in the same season. *BMC Pediatr*. 2010;10:38.

Figueras-Aloy J, Carbonell-Estrany X, Quero J, IRIS Study Group. Case-control study of the risk factors linked to respiratory syncytial virus infection requiring hospitalization in premature infants born at a gestational age of 33–35 weeks in Spain. *Pediatr Infect Dis J*. 2004;23(9):815–820.

Fiore AE, Fry A, Shay D, Gubareva L, Bresee JS, Uyeki TM, Centers for Disease Control and Prevention (CDC). Antiviral agents for the treatment and chemoprophylaxis of influenza—recommendations of the Advisory Committee on Immunization Practices (ACIP). *MMWR Recomm Rep*. 2011;60(1):1–24.

Fulton RB, Meyerholz DK, Varga SM. Foxp3+ CD4 regulatory T cells limit pulmonary immunopathology by modulating the CD8 T cell response during respiratory syncytial virus infection. *J Immunol*. 2010;185(4):2382–2392.

Gadomski AM, Brower M. Bronchodilators for bronchiolitis. *Cochrane Database Syst Rev*. 2010 Dec 8;(12):CD001266.

García CG, Bhore R, Soriano-Fallas A, Trost M, Chason R, Ramilo O, Mejias A. Risk factors in children hospitalized with RSV bronchiolitis versus non-RSV bronchiolitis. *Pediatrics*. 2010;126(6):e1453–e1460. PubMed PMID: 21098154.

Garcia-Barreno B, Palomo C, Peñas C, Delgado T, Perez-Breña P, Melero JA. Marked differences in the antigenic structure of human respiratory syncytial virus F and G glycoproteins. *J Virol*. 1989;63(2):925–932.

Geevarghese B, Simões EA. Antibodies for prevention and treatment of respiratory syncytial virus infections in children. *Antivir Ther*. 2012;17(1 Pt B):201–211.

Gershwin LJ. Immunology of bovine respiratory syncytial virus infection of cattle. *Comp Immunol Microbiol Infect Dis*. 2012;35(3):253–257.

Geskey JM, Cyran SE. Managing the morbidity associated with respiratory viral infections in children with congenital heart disease. *Int J Pediatr*. 2012;2012:646–780.

Gilca R, De Serres G, Tremblay M, Vachon ML, Leblanc E, Bergeron MG, Dery P, Boivin G. Distribution and clinical impact of human respiratory syncytial virus genotypes in hospitalized children over 2 winter seasons. *J Infect Dis*. 2006;193(1):54–58.

González PA, Bueno SM, Carreño LJ, Riedel CA, Kalergis AM. Respiratory syncytial virus infection and immunity. *Rev Med Virol*. 2012;22(4):230–244.

Greenough A, Broughton S. Chronic manifestations of respiratory syncytial virus infection in premature infants. *Pediatr Infect Dis J*. 2005;24(11 Suppl):S184–S187, discussion S187–S188.

Greenough A. Role of ventilation in RSV disease: CPAP, ventilation, HFO, ECMO. *Paediatr Respir Rev*. 2009;10 Suppl 1:26–28.

Groothuis JR, Hoopes JM, Hemming VG. Prevention of serious respiratory syncytial virus-related illness II: Immunoprophylaxis. *Adv Ther*. 2011a;28(2):110–125.

Groothuis JR, Hoopes JM, Jessie VG. Prevention of serious respiratory syncytial virus-related illness I: Disease pathogenesis and early attempts at prevention. *Adv Ther*. 2011b;28(2):91–109.

Groothuis JR, Levin MJ, Rodriguez W, Hall CB, Long CE, Kim HW, Lauer BA, Hemming VG. Use of intravenous gamma globulin to passively immunize high-risk children against respiratory syncytial virus: Safety and pharmacokinetics The RSVIG Study Group. *Antimicrob Agents Chemother.* 1991;35(7):1469–1473.

Groothuis JR, Nishida H. Prevention of respiratory syncytial virus infections in high-risk infants by monoclonal antibody (palivizumab). *Pediatr Int.* 2002;44(3):235–241.

Groothuis JR, Simoes EA. Immunoprophylaxis and immunotherapy: Role in the prevention and treatment of repiratory syncytial virus. *Int J Antimicrob Agents.* 1993;2(2):97–103.

Groothuis JR, Simoes EA, Levin MJ, Hall CB, Long CE, Rodriguez WJ, Arrobio J, Meissner HC, Fulton DR, Welliver RC. Prophylactic administration of respiratory syncytial virus immune globulin to high-risk infants and young children. The Respiratory Syncytial Virus Immune Globulin Study Group. *N Engl J Med.* 1993;329(21):1524–1530.

Guglielmo BJ, Brooks GF. Antimicrobial therapy Cost-benefit considerations. *Drugs.* 1989;38(4):473–480.

Hacimustafaoglu M, Celebi S, Aynaci E, Sinirtas M, Koksal N, Kucukerdogan A, Ercan I, Goral G, Ildirim I. The progression of maternal RSV antibodies in the offspring. *Arch Dis Child.* 2004;89(1):52–53.

Hall CB, Weinberg GA, Iwane MK, Blumkin AK, Edwards KM, Staat MA, Auinger P et al. The burden of respiratory syncytial virus infection in young children. *N Engl J Med.* 2009;360(6):588–598.

Han J, Jia Y, Takeda K, Shiraishi Y, Okamoto M, Dakhama A, Gelfand EW. Montelukast during primary infection prevents airway hyperresponsiveness and inflammation after reinfection with respiratory syncytial virus. *Am J Respir Crit Care Med.* 2010;182(4):455–463.

Hartling L, Bialy LM, Vandermeer B, Tjosvold L, Johnson DW, Plint AC, Klassen TP, Patel H, Fernandes RM. Epinephrine for bronchiolitis. *Cochrane Database Syst Rev.* 2011 Jun 15;(6):CD003123.

Henderson J, Hilliard TN, Sherriff A, Stalker D, Al Shammari N, Thomas HM. Hospitalization for RSV bronchiolitis before 12 months of age and subsequent asthma, atopy and wheeze: A longitudinal birth cohort study. *Pediatr Allergy Immunol.* 2005;16(5):386–392.

Henrickson KJ. Advances in the laboratory diagnosis of viral respiratory disease. *Pediatr Infect Dis J.* 2004;23(1 Suppl):S6–S10.

Henrickson KJ. Cost-effective use of rapid diagnostic techniques in the treatment and prevention of viral respiratory infections. *Pediatr Ann.* 2005;34(1):24–31.

Henrickson KJ, Hall CB. Diagnostic assays for respiratory syncytial virus disease. *Pediatr Infect Dis J.* 2007;26(11 Suppl):S36–S40.

Hilliard TN, Archer N, Laura H, Heraghty J, Cottis H, Mills K, Ball S, Davis P. Pilot study of vapotherm oxygen delivery in moderately severe bronchiolitis. *Arch Dis Child.* 2012;97(2):182–183.

Horn SD, Smout RJ. Effect of prematurity on respiratory syncytial virus hospital resource use and outcomes. *J Pediatr.* 2003;143(5 Suppl):S133–S141.

Huang K, Incognito L, Cheng X, Ulbrandt ND, Wu H. Respiratory syncytial virus-neutralizing monoclonal antibodies motavizumab and palivizumab inhibit fusion. *J Virol.* 2010;84(16):8132–8140.

Jat KR, Chawla D. Surfactant therapy for bronchiolitis in critically ill infants. *Cochrane Database Syst Rev.* 2012 Sep 12;9:CD009194.

Johnson TR, Varga SM, Braciale TJ, Graham BS. Vbeta14(+) T cells mediate the vaccine-enhanced disease induced by immunization with respiratory syncytial virus (RSV) G glycoprotein but not with formalin-inactivated RSV. *J Virol.* 2004;78(16):8753–8760.

Johnson JE, Gonzales RA, Olson SJ, Wright PF, Graham BS. The histopathology of fatal untreated human respiratory syncytial virus infection. *Mod Pathol.* 2007;20(1):108–119.

Johnson S, Oliver C, Prince GA, Hemming VG, Pfarr DS, Wang SC, Dormitzer M, O'Grady J, Koenig S, Tamura JK, Woods R, Bansal G, Couchenour D, Tsao E, Hall WC, Young JF. Development of a humanized monoclonal antibody (MEDI-493) with potent *in vitro* and *in vivo* activity against respiratory syncytial virus. *J Infect Dis.* 1997;176(5):1215–1224.

Johnson TR, Rao S, Seder RA, Chen M, Graham BS. TLR9 agonist, but not TLR7/8, functions as an adjuvant to diminish FI-RSV vaccine-enhanced disease, while either agonist used as therapy during primary RSV infection increases disease severity. *Vaccine.* 2009;27(23):3045–3052.

Jorgensen J, Wei JL, Sykes KJ, Klem SA, Weatherly RA, Bruegger DE, Latz AD, Nicklaus PJ. Incidence of and risk factors for airway complications following endotracheal intubation for bronchiolitis. *Otolaryngol Head Neck Surg.* 2007;137(3):394–399.

Kapikian AZ, Mitchell RH, Chanock RM, Shvedoff RA, Stewart CE. An epidemiologic study of altered clinical reactivity to respiratory syncytial (RS) virus infection in children previously vaccinated with an inactivated RS virus vaccine. *Am J Epidemiol.* 1969;89(4):405–421.

Karr CJ, Rudra CB, Miller KA, Gould TR, Larson T, Sathyanarayana S, Koenig JQ. Infant exposure to fine particulate matter and traffic and risk of hospitalization for RSV bronchiolitis in a region with lower ambient air pollution. *Environ Res*. 2009;109(3):321–327.

Korppi M, Piippo-Savolainen E, Korhonen K, Remes S. Respiratory morbidity 20 years after RSV infection in infancy. *Pediatr Pulmonol*. 2004;38(2):155–160.

Kristjánsson S, Skúladóttir HE, Sturludóttir M, Wennergren G. Increased prevalence of otitis media following respiratory syncytial virus infection. *Acta Paediatr*. 2010;99(6):867–870.

Kuzik BA, Al-Qadhi SA, Kent S, Flavin MP, Hopman W, Hotte S, Gander S. Nebulized hypertonic saline in the treatment of viral bronchiolitis in infants. *J Pediatr*. 2007;151(3):266–270, 270.e1.

Lanari M, Adorni F, Silvestri M, Coscia A, Musicco M. Italian Study Group on Risk Factors for RSV-related Hospitalization. The multicenter Italian birth cohort study on incidence and determinants of lower respiratory tract infection hospitalization in infants at 33 weeks GA or more: preliminary results. *Early Hum Dev*. 2011;87 Suppl 1:S43–S46.

Lanari M, Giovannini M, Giuffré L, Marini A, Rondini G, Rossi GA, Merolla R, Zuccotti GV, Salvioli GP. Investigators R.A.DA.R. Study Group. Prevalence of respiratory syncytial virus infection in Italian infants hospitalized for acute lower respiratory tract infections, and association between respiratory syncytial virus infection risk factors and disease severity. *Pediatr Pulmonol*. 2002;33(6):458–465.

Lanari M, Rossi GA, Merolla R, di Luzio Paparatti U. High risk of nosocomial-acquired RSV infection in children with congenital heart disease. *J Pediatr*. 2004;145(1):140.

Lanari M, Silvestri M, Rossi GA. Respiratory syncytial virus risk factors in late preterm infants. *J Matern Fetal Neonatal Med*. 2009;22 Suppl 3:102–107.

Lanari M, Silvestri M, Rossi GA. Palivizumab prophylaxis in "late preterm" newborns. *J Matern Fetal Neonatal Med*. 2010;23 Suppl 3:53–55.

Lanari M, Silvestri M, Rossi GA. Clinical and pharmacological aspects of immunoprophylaxis for respiratory syncytial virus infection in high-risk infants. *Curr Drug Metab*. 2013;14(2):216–225.

Law BJ, Wang EE, MacDonald N, McDonald J, Dobson S, Boucher F, Langley J, Robinson J, Mitchell I, Stephens D. Does ribavirin impact on the hospital course of children with respiratory syncytial virus (RSV) infection? An analysis using the pediatric investigators collaborative network on infections in Canada (PICNIC) RSV database. *Pediatrics*. 1997;99(3):E7.

Leader S, Kohlhase K. Recent trends in severe respiratory syncytial virus (RSV) among US infants, 1997 to 2000. *J Pediatr*. 2003;143(5 Suppl):S127–S132.

Le Nouën C, Hillyer P, Munir S, Winter CC, McCarty T, Bukreyev A, Collins PL, Rabin RL, Buchholz UJ. Effects of human respiratory syncytial virus, metapneumovirus, parainfluenza virus 3 and influenza virus on CD4+ T cell activation by dendritic cells. *PLoS One*. 2010;5(11):e15017.

Leclerc F, Scalfaro P, Noizet O, Thumerelle C, Dorkenoo A, Fourier C. Mechanical ventilatory support in infants with respiratory syncytial virus infection. *Pediatr Crit Care Med*. 2001;2(3):197–204.

Liese JG, Grill E, Fischer B, Roeckl-Wiedmann I, Carr D, Belohradsky BH, Munich RSV Study Group. Incidence and risk factors of respiratory syncytial virus-related hospitalizations in premature infants in Germany. *Eur J Pediatr*. 2003;162(4):230–236.

Liet JM, Millotte B, Tucci M, Laflammme S, Hutchison J, Creery D, Ducruet T, Lacroix J, Canadian Critical Care Trials Group. Noninvasive therapy with helium-oxygen for severe bronchiolitis. *J Pediatr*. 2005;147(6):812–817.

Luján-Zilbermann J, Benaim E, Tong X, Srivastava DK, Patrick CC, DeVincenzo JP. Respiratory virus infections in pediatric hematopoietic stem cell transplantation. *Clin Infect Dis*. 2001;33(7):962–968.

Lukacs NW, Smit JJ, Schaller MA, Lindell DM. Regulation of immunity to respiratory syncytial virus by dendritic cells, toll-like receptors, and notch. *Viral Immunol*. 2008;21(2):115–122.

Malley R, DeVincenzo J, Ramilo O, Dennehy PH, Meissner HC, Gruber WC, Sanchez PJ et al. Reduction of respiratory syncytial virus (RSV) in tracheal aspirates in intubated infants by use of humanized monoclonal antibody to RSV F protein. *J Infect Dis*. 1998;178(6):1555–1561.

Manzoni P, Paes B, Resch B, Carbonell-Estrany X, Bont L. High risk for RSV bronchiolitis in late preterms and selected infants affected by rare disorders: A dilemma of specific prevention. *Early Hum Dev*. 2012;88 Suppl 2:S34–S41.

Martinello RA, Chen MD, Weibel C, Kahn JS. Correlation between respiratory syncytial virus genotype and severity of illness. *J Infect Dis*. 2002;186(6):839–842.

Martinón-Torres F, Rodríguez-Núñez A, Martinón-Sánchez JM. Nasal continuous positive airway pressure with heliox versus air oxygen in infants with acute bronchiolitis: A crossover study. *Pediatrics*. 2008;121(5):e1190–e1195.

McNamara PS, Flanagan BF, Hart CA, Smyth RL. Production of chemokines in the lungs of infants with severe respiratory syncytial virus bronchiolitis. *J Infect Dis*. 2005;191(8):1225–1232.

McNamara PS, Ritson P, Selby A, Hart CA, Smyth RL. Bronchoalveolar lavage cellularity in infants with severe respiratory syncytial virus bronchiolitis. *Arch Dis Child*. 2003;88(10):922–926.

Meerhoff TJ, Paget JW, Kimpen JL, Schellevis F. Variation of respiratory syncytial virus and the relation with meteorological factors in different winter seasons. *Pediatr Infect Dis J*. 2009;28(10):860–866.

Meijboom MJ, Rozenbaum MH, Benedictus A, Luytjes W, Kneyber MC, Wilschut JC, Hak E, Postma MJ. Cost-effectiveness of potential infant vaccination against respiratory syncytial virus infection in The Netherlands. *Vaccine*. 2012;30(31):4691–4700.

Meissner HC, Groothuis JR, Rodriguez WJ¸ Welliver RC, Hogg G, Gray PH, Loh R et al. Safety and pharmacokinetics of an intramuscular monoclonal antibody to RSV (SB 209763) in infants and young children at risk for severe RSV disease. *Antimicrob. Agents Chemother.* 1999;43(5):1183–1188.

Meissner HC, Fulton DR, Groothuis JR, Geggel RL, Marx GR, Hemming VG, Hougen T, Snydman DR. Controlled trial to evaluate protection of high-risk infants against respiratory syncytial virus disease by using standard intravenous immune globulin. *Antimicrob Agents Chemother*. 1993;37(8): 1655–1658.

Mejías A, Chávez-Bueno S, Ríos AM, Aten MF, Raynor B, Peromingo E, Soni P, Olsen KD, Kiener PA, Gómez AM, Jafri HS, Ramilo O. Comparative effects of two neutralizing anti-respiratory syncytial virus (RSV) monoclonal antibodies in the RSV murine model: Time versus potency. *Antimicrob Agents Chemother*. 2005;49(11):4700–4707.

Miernyk K, Bulkow L, DeByle C, Chikoyak L, Hummel KB, Hennessy T, Singleton R. Performance of a rapid antigen test (Binax NOW® RSV) for diagnosis of respiratory syncytial virus compared with real-time polymerase chain reaction in a pediatric population. *J Clin Virol*. 2011;50(3):240–243.

Mitchell I. Treatment of RSV bronchiolitis: Drugs, antibiotics. *Paediatr Respir Rev*. 2009;10 Suppl 1:14–15.

Miyairi I, DeVincenzo JP. Human genetic factors and respiratory syncytial virus disease severity. *Clin Microbiol Rev*. 2008;21(4):686–703.

Moore ML, Newcomb DC, Parekh VV, Van Kaer L, Collins RD, Zhou W, Goleniewska K et al. STAT1 negatively regulates lung basophil IL-4 expression induced by respiratory syncytial virus infection. *J Immunol*. 2009;183(3):2016–2026.

Mukherjee S, Allen RM, Lukacs NW, Kunkel SL, Carson WF 4th. STAT3-mediated IL-17 production by post-septic T cells exacerbates viral immunopathology of the lung. *Shock*. 2012;38(5):515–523.

Nair H, Verma VR, Theodoratou E, Zgaga L, Huda T, Simões EA, Wright PF, Rudan I, Campbell H. An evaluation of the emerging interventions against Respiratory Syncytial Virus (RSV)-associated acute lower respiratory infections in children. *BMC Public Health*. 2011;11 Suppl 3:S30.

Nakamura K, Kato M, Sasaki A, Shiihara T, Hayasaka K. Respiratory syncytial virus-associated encephalopathy complicated by congenital myopathy. *Pediatr Int*. 2012;54(5):709–711.

Navas L, Wang E, de Carvalho V, Robinson J. Improved outcome of respiratory syncytial virus infection in a high-risk hospitalized population of Canadian children Pediatric Investigators Collaborative Network on Infections in Canada. *J Pediatr*. 1992;121(3):348–354.

Noyola DE, Mandeville PB. Effect of climatological factors on respiratory syncytial virus epidemics. *Epidemiol Infect*. 2008;136(10):1328–1332.

Nuijten MJ, Wittenberg W. Cost effectiveness of palivizumab in Spain: An analysis using observational data. *Eur J Health Econ*. 2010;11(1):105–115.

Null D Jr, Pollara B, Dennehy PH, Steichen J, Sánchez PJ, Givner LB, Carlin D, Landry B, Top FH Jr, Connor E. Safety and immunogenicity of palivizumab (Synagis) administered for two seasons. *Pediatr Infect Dis J*. 2005;24(11):1021–1023.

Okoko JB, Wesumperuma HL, Hart CA. The influence of prematurity and low birthweight on transplacental antibody transfer in a rural West African population. *Trop Med Int Health*. 2001;6(7):529–534.

Oravax. Oravax Company Press Release; 19 March 1997.

Panitch HB. Bronchiolitis in infants. *Curr Opin Pediatr*. 2001;13(3):256–260.

Paramore LC, Ciuryla V, Ciesla G, Liu L. Economic impact of respiratory syncytial virus-related illness in the US: An analysis of national databases. *Pharmacoeconomics*. 2004;22(5):275–284.

Patel JA, Nguyen DT, Revai K, Chonmaitree T. Role of respiratory syncytial virus in acute otitis media: Implications for vaccine development. *Vaccine*. 2007;25(9):1683–1689.

Pavia AT. Viral infections of the lower respiratory tract: Old viruses, new viruses, and the role of diagnosis. *Clin Infect Dis*. 2011;52 Suppl 4:S284–S289.

Pediatrics. Palivizumab; a humanized respiratory syncytial virus monoclonal antibody reduces hospitalization from respiratory syncytial virus infection in high-risk infants. *Pediatrics*. 1998;102(3 Pt 1):531–537.

Pérez-Ruiz M, Pedrosa-Corral I, Sanbonmatsu-Gámez S, Navarro-Marí M. Laboratory detection of respiratory viruses by automated techniques. *Open Virol J*. 2012;6:151–159.
Perrotta C, Ortiz Z, Roque M. Chest physiotherapy for acute bronchiolitis in paediatric patients between 0 and 24 months old. *Cochrane Database Syst Rev*. 2007 Jan 24;(1):CD004873.
Pettigrew MM, Gent JF, Pyles RB, Miller AL, Nokso-Koivisto J, Chonmaitree T. Viral-bacterial interactions and risk of acute otitis media complicating upper respiratory tract infection. *J Clin Microbiol*. 2011;49(11):3750–3755.
Plint AC, Johnson DW, Patel H, Wiebe N, Correll R, Brant R, Mitton C et al. Pediatric Emergency Research Canada (PERC). Epinephrine and dexamethasone in children with bronchiolitis. *N Engl J Med*. 2009;360(20):2079–2089.
Polack FP, Irusta PM, Hoffman SJ, Schiatti MP, Melendi GA, Delgado MF, Laham FR et al. The cysteine-rich region of respiratory syncytial virus attachment protein inhibits innate immunity elicited by the virus and endotoxin. *Proc Natl Acad Sci U S A*. 2005;102(25):8996–9001.
Press EM, Hogg NM. The amino acid sequences of the Fd fragments of two human gamma-1 heavy chains. *Biochem J*. 1970;117(4):641–660.
Prince GA, Hemming VG, Horswood RL, Chanock RM. Immunoprophylaxis and immunotherapy of respiratory syncytial virus infection in the cotton rat. *Virus Res*. 1985;3(3):193–206.
Prodhan P, Westra SJ, Lin J, Karni-Sharoor S, Regan S, Noviski N. Chest radiological patterns predict the duration of mechanical ventilation in children with RSV infection. *Pediatr Radiol*. 2009;39(2):117–123.
Reduction of respiratory syncytial virus hospitalization among premature infants and infants with bronchopulmonary dysplasia using respiratory syncytial virus immune globulin prophylaxis The PREVENT Study Group. *Pediatrics*. 1997;99(1):93–99.
Resch B, Manzoni P, Lanari M. Severe respiratory syncytial virus (RSV) infection in infants with neuromuscular diseases and immune deficiency syndromes. *Paediatr Respir Rev*. 2009;10(3):148–153.
Resch B, Michel-Behnke I. Respiratory syncytial virus infections in infants and children with congenital heart disease: update on the evidence of prevention with palivizumab. *Curr Opin Cardiol*. 2013; 28(2):85–91.
Resch B, Sommer C, Nuijten MJ, Seidinger S, Walter E, Schoellbauer V, Mueller WD. Cost-effectiveness of palivizumab for respiratory syncytial virus infection in high-risk children, based on long-term epidemiologic data from Austria. *Pediatr Infect Dis J*. 2012;31(1):e1–e8.
Rezaee F, Gibson LF, Piktel D, Othumpangat S, Piedimonte G. Respiratory syncytial virus infection in human bone marrow stromal cells. *Am J Respir Cell Mol Biol*. 2011;45(2):277–286.
Rochelet M, Solanas S, Grossiord C, Maréchal P, Résa C, Vienney F, Barranger C, Joannes M. A thin layer-based amperometric enzyme immunoassay for the rapid and sensitive diagnosis of respiratory syncytial virus infections. *Talanta*. 2012;100:139–144.
Rodriguez WJ, Bui RH, Connor JD, Kim HW, Brandt CD, Parrott RH, Burch B, Mace J. Environmental exposure of primary care personnel to ribavirin aerosol when supervising treatment of infants with respiratory syncytial virus infections. *Antimicrob Agents Chemother*. 1987;31(7):1143–1146.
Rosenberg HF, Domachowske JB. Inflammatory responses to respiratory syncytial virus (RSV) infection and the development of immunomodulatory pharmacotherapeutics. *Curr Med Chem*. 2012;19(10): 1424–1431.
Rossi GA, Silvestri M, Lanari M. Should the American Academy of Pediatrics respiratory syncytial virus guidelines be modified?. *Pediatrics*. 2010;125(4):e1021; author reply e1022.
Sáez-Llorens X, Moreno MT, Ramilo O, Sánchez PJ, Top FH Jr, Connor EM, MEDI-493 Study Group. Safety and pharmacokinetics of palivizumab therapy in children hospitalized with respiratory syncytial virus infection. *Pediatr Infect Dis J*. 2004;23(8):707–712.
Sáez-Llorens X, Castaño E, Null D, Steichen J, Sánchez PJ, Ramilo O, Top FH Jr, Connor E. Safety and pharmacokinetics of an intramuscular humanized monoclonal antibody to respiratory syncytial virus in premature infants and infants with bronchopulmonary dysplasia The MEDI-493 Study Group. *Pediatr Infect Dis J*. 1998;17(9):787–791.
Sampalis JS. Morbidity and mortality after RSV-associated hospitalizations among premature Canadian infants. *J Pediatr*. 2003;143(5 Suppl):S150–S156.
Schindler M. Do bronchodilators have an effect on bronchiolitis?. *Crit Care*. 2002;6(2):111–112.
Shay DK, Holman RC, Newman RD, Liu LL, Stout JW, Anderson LJ. Bronchiolitis-associated hospitalizations among US children, 1980–1996. *JAMA*. 1999;282(15):1440–1446.
Siber GR, Leombruno D, Leszczynski J, McIver J, Bodkin D, Gonin R, Thompson CM, Walsh EE, Piedra PA, Hemming VG. Comparison of antibody concentrations and protective activity of respiratory syncytial virus immune globulin and conventional immune globulin. *J Infect Dis*. 1994;169(6):1368–1373.

Sigurs N, Gustafsson PM, Bjarnason R, Lundberg F, Schmidt S, Sigurbergsson F, Kjellman B. Severe respiratory syncytial virus bronchiolitis in infancy and asthma and allergy at age 13. *Am J Respir Crit Care Med.* 2005;171(2):137–141.

Simoes EA. Respiratory syncytial virus infection. *Lancet*, 1999;354(9181):847–852.

Simoes EA. Environmental and demographic risk factors for respiratory syncytial virus lower respiratory tract disease. *J Pediatr.* 2003;143(5 Suppl):S118–S126. PubMed PMID: 14615710.

Simoes EA, Sondheimer HM, Top FH Jr, Meissner HC, Welliver RC, Kramer AA, Groothuis JR. Respiratory syncytial virus immune globulin for prophylaxis against respiratory syncytial virus disease in infants and children with congenital heart disease The Cardiac Study Group. *J Pediatr.* 1998;133(4):492–499.

Simoes, EA, Carbonell-Estrany X, Losonsky G, Hultquist M, Harris B, Connor E. Phase III trial of motavizumab; an enhanced potency respiratory syncytial virus (RSV)-specific monoclonal antibody for the prevention of serious RSV disease in high risk infants. *Acta Paediatrica*, 2007;96(s456):232–233.

Simões EA, Carbonell-Estrany X, Fullarton JR, Rossi GA, Barberi I, Lanari M, European RSV Risk Factor Study Group. European risk factors' model to predict hospitalization of premature infants born 33–35 weeks' gestational age with respiratory syncytial virus: Validation with Italian data. *J Matern Fetal Neonatal Med.* 2011;24(1):152–157.

Simões EA, Carbonell-Estrany X, Rieger CH, Mitchell I, Fredrick L, Groothuis JR, Palivizumab Long-Term Respiratory Outcomes Study Group. The effect of respiratory syncytial virus on subsequent recurrent wheezing in atopic and nonatopic children. *J Allergy Clin Immunol.* 2010;126(2):256–262.

Sow FB, Gallup JM, Olivier A, Krishnan S, Patera AC, Suzich J, Ackermann MR. Respiratory syncytial virus is associated with an inflammatory response in lungs and architectural remodeling of lung-draining lymph nodes of newborn lambs. *Am J Physiol Lung Cell Mol Physiol.* 2011;300(1):L12–L24.

Spurling GK, Doust J, Del Mar CB, Eriksson L. Antibiotics for bronchiolitis in children. *Cochrane Database Syst Rev.* 2011 Jun 15;(6):CD005189.

Stein RT, Sherrill D, Morgan WJ, Holberg CJ, Halonen M, Taussig LM, Wright AL, Martinez FD. Respiratory syncytial virus in early life and risk of wheeze and allergy by age 13 years. *Lancet.* 1999;354(9178):541–545.

Stokes KL, Chi MH, Sakamoto K, Newcomb DC, Currier MG, Huckabee MM, Lee S et al. Differential pathogenesis of respiratory syncytial virus clinical isolates in BALB/c mice. *J Virol.* 2011;85(12):5782–5793.

Subramanian KN, Weisman LE, Rhodes T, Ariagno R, Sánchez PJ, Steichen J, Givner LB et al. Safety, tolerance and pharmacokinetics of a humanized monoclonal antibody to respiratory syncytial virus in premature infants and infants with bronchopulmonary dysplasia MEDI-493 Study Group. *Pediatr Infect Dis J.* 1998;17(2):110–115.

Takahashi N, Noma T, Honjo T. Rearranged immunoglobulin heavy chain variable region (VH) pseudogene that deletes the second complementarity-determining region. *Proc Natl Acad Sci USA.* 1984;81(16):5194–5198.

Tal G, Cesar K, Oron A, Houri S, Ballin A, Mandelberg A. Hypertonic saline/epinephrine treatment in hospitalized infants with viral bronchiolitis reduces hospitalization stay: 2 years experience. *Isr Med Assoc J.* 2006;8(3):169–173.

Teeratakulpisarn J, Limwattananon C, Tanupattarachai S, Limwattananon S, Teeratakulpisarn S, Kosalaraksa P. Efficacy of dexamethasone injection for acute bronchiolitis in hospitalized children: A randomized, double-blind, placebo-controlled trial. *Pediatr Pulmonol.* 2007;42(5):433–439.

Thompson WW, Shay DK, Weintraub E, Brammer L, Cox N, Anderson LJ, Fukuda K. Mortality associated with influenza and respiratory syncytial virus in the United States. *JAMA.* 2003;289(2):179–186.

Tomochika K, Ichiyama T, Shimogori H, Sugahara K, Yamashita H, Furukawa S. Clinical characteristics of respiratory syncytial virus infection-associated acute otitis media. *Pediatr Int.* 2009;51(4):484–487.

Tripp RA, Jones LP, Haynes LM, Zheng H, Murphy PM, Anderson LJ. CX3C chemokine mimicry by respiratory syncytial virus G glycoprotein. *Nat Immunol.* 2001;2(8):732–738.

van Bleek GM, Osterhaus AD, de Swart RL. RSV 2010: Recent advances in research on respiratory syncytial virus and other pneumoviruses. *Vaccine.* 2011;29(43):7285–7291.

van Drunen Littel-van den Hurk S, Watkiss ER. Pathogenesis of respiratory syncytial virus. *Curr Opin Virol.* 2012;2(3):300–305.

Vandini S, Corvaglia L, Alessandroni R, Aquilano G, Marsico C, Spinelli M, Lanari M, Faldella G. Respiratory syncytial virus infection in infants and correlation with meteorological factors and air pollutants. *Ital J Pediatr.* 2013;39(1):1.

Ventre K, Randolph A. WITHDRAWN: Ribavirin for respiratory syncytial virus infection of the lower respiratory tract in infants and young children. *Cochrane Database Syst Rev.* 2010 May 12;(5):CD000181.

Villenave R, Thavagnanam S, Sarlang S, Parker J, Douglas I, Skibinski G, Heaney LG, McKaigue JP, Coyle PV, Shields MD, Power UF. *in vitro* modeling of respiratory syncytial virus infection of

pediatric bronchial epithelium, the primary target of infection in vivo. *Proc Natl Acad Sci U S A*. 2012;109(13):5040–5045.
Wang EE, Law BJ, Stephens D. Pediatric Investigators Collaborative Network on Infections in Canada (PICNIC) prospective study of risk factors and outcomes in patients hospitalized with respiratory syncytial viral lower respiratory tract infection. *J Pediatr*. 1995;126(2):212–219.
Weigl JA, Puppe W, Schmitt HJ. Can respiratory syncytial virus etiology be diagnosed clinically? A hospital-based case-control study in children under two years of age. *Eur J Epidemiol*. 2003;18(5):431–439.
Weiner LB, Masaquel AS, Polak MJ, Mahadevia PJ. Cost-effectiveness analysis of palivizumab among preterm infant populations covered by Medicaid in the United States. *J Med Econ*. 2012;15(5):997–1018.
Welliver RC. Review of epidemiology and clinical risk factors for severe respiratory syncytial virus (RSV) infection. *J Pediatr*. 2003;143(5 Suppl):S112–S117.
Welliver TP, Reed JL, Welliver RC Sr. Respiratory syncytial virus and influenza virus infections: Observations from tissues of fatal infant cases. *Pediatr Infect Dis J*. 2008;27(10 Suppl):S92–S96.
Wilkesmann A, Ammann RA, Schildgen O, Eis-Hübinger AM, Müller A, Seidenberg J, Stephan V et al. DSM RSV Ped Study Group. Hospitalized children with respiratory syncytial virus infection and neuromuscular impairment face an increased risk of a complicated course. *Pediatr Infect Dis J*. 2007;26(6):485–491.
Wu H, Pfarr DS, Tang Y, An LL, Patel NK, Watkins JD, Huse WD, Kiener PA, Young JF. Ultra-potent antibodies against respiratory syncytial virus: Effects of binding kinetics and binding valence on viral neutralization. *J Mol Biol*. 2005;350(1):126–144.
Wu H, Pfarr DS, Johnson S, Brewah YA, Woods RM, Patel NK, White WI, Young JF, Kiener PA. Development of motavizumab, an ultra-potent antibody for the prevention of respiratory syncytial virus infection in the upper and lower respiratory tract. *J Mol Biol*. 2007;368(3):652–665.
Wu SY, Bonaparte J, Pyati S. Palivizumab use in very premature infants in the neonatal intensive care unit. *Pediatrics*. 2004;114(5):e554–e556.
Young J. Development of a potent respiratory syncytial virus-specific monoclonal antibody for the prevention of serious lower respiratory tract disease in infants. *Respir Med*. 2002;96 Suppl B:S31–S35.
Zachariah P, Ruttenber M, Simões EA. Down syndrome and hospitalizations due to respiratory syncytial virus: A population-based study. *J Pediatr*. 2012;160(5):827–831.e1.
Zhang L, Mendoza-Sassi RA, Wainwright C, Klassen TP. Nebulized hypertonic saline solution for acute bronchiolitis in infants. *Cochrane Database Syst Rev*. 2008 Oct 8;(4):CD006458.
Zhu Q, McAuliffe JM, Patel NK, Palmer-Hill FJ, Yang CF, Liang B, Su L et al. Analysis of respiratory syncytial virus preclinical and clinical variants resistant to neutralization by monoclonal antibodies palivizumab and/or motavizumab. *J Infect Dis*. 2011;203(5):674–682.

22 Human Influenza Virus Infections

Judith M. Fontana, Daniel P. Eiras, and Mirella Salvatore

CONTENTS

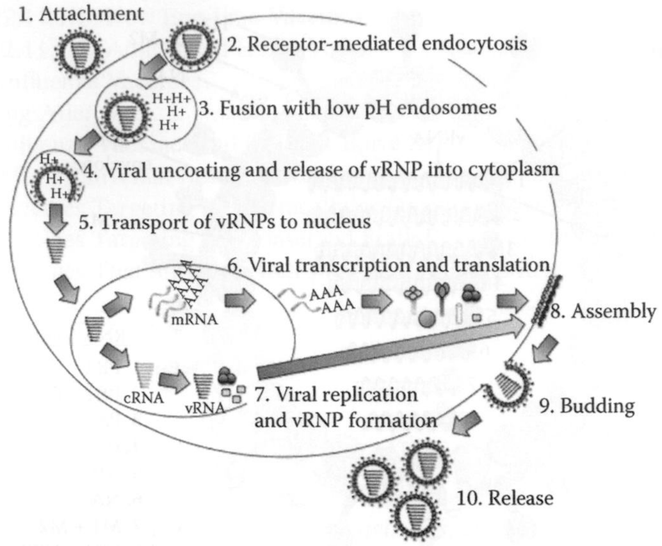

FIGURE 22.2 Schematic overview of the influenza virus replication cycle.

endosomal membranes (Figure 22.2).[17] The low pH environment within the endosome also triggers the acidification of the virion interior through the action of the M2 protein, a tetrameric ion channel that resides within the viral membrane and allows a flow of protons into the virion. This acidification weakens the interactions between the viral RNA-dependent RNA polymerase complex (vRNP) and M1 protein, which lines the interior of the viral envelope and provides structure and support for the virion, allowing the vRNP to be released into the host cell cytoplasm (Figure 22.2).[1,18] Because of its crucial role in viral entry, the M2 protein is an attractive target for the development of vaccines and antiviral drugs against influenza virus.

The vRNP complex of influenza virus comprises the eight viral RNA (vRNA) segments; NP; and three polymerase proteins, PB1, PB2, and PA. Influenza NP is known to homo-oligomerize with other NP molecules and bind with strong affinity and low specificity to vRNA at a stoichiometry of approximately 1 NP for every 24 nucleotides.[19,20] These interactions are believed to maintain the structure of the vRNP. Additionally, NP possesses two nuclear localization sequences that are recognized by host cellular nuclear import machinery, and function to bring the vRNP into the nucleus.[21] In addition to the vRNA, NP also binds to the PB1 and PB2 subunits of the viral polymerase, and may therefore function to facilitate the interaction between the viral genome and the polymerase.[20,22] Once in the nucleus, the heterotrimeric polymerase of influenza virus catalyzes vRNA transcription (Figure 22.2).[1] In a process called "cap snatching," the PB2 subunit of the polymerase binds to the 5′-7-methylguanosine cap region of cellular messenger RNA (mRNA), and the PA subunit uses its endonuclease activity to cleave the mRNA 10–15 nucleotides downstream of binding.[23] This short region of mRNA is used to prime the synthesis of polyadenylated viral mRNA, which is catalyzed by the polymerase activity of the PB1 subunit.[24] Following transcription, the viral mRNAs are exported from the nucleus into the cytoplasm, where they are translated by cellular machinery into viral proteins. Through its interaction with the viral polymerase,[25] cellular elongation initiation factor 4F,[26] and the 5′ untranslated region of viral mRNAs,[27] the NS1 protein selectively enhances viral translation over cellular translation.

In addition to its role in transcribing viral mRNAs, the influenza virus polymerase also produces exact positive-sense RNA copies (cRNA) of the viral genome, which are neither capped nor polyadenylated, and are used as templates to generate more negative-sense vRNA for packaging into nascent virions (Figure 22.2).[1,28] Although the exact mechanism behind this switch from transcription to replication is not fully elucidated, there is evidence to support the necessity of certain stabilizing forces, such as the presence of threshold amounts of NP and polymerase proteins, for this process to commence.[29] Additionally, the NEP, which is produced from a spliced form of the same vRNA segment that codes for NS1, is thought to regulate the accumulation of vRNA species, possibly contributing to the switch from transcription to replication.[30,31] Central to the evolutionary strategy of influenza virus, the viral polymerase does not possess any proofreading capabilities, producing an average of one error per replicated genome.[32] This unfaithful genomic replication leads to continual changes in viral proteins, called antigenic drift, which allow for evasion of the host immune response and escape from currently available antiviral drugs and seasonal vaccines.[1] Additionally, the PB1 component of the viral polymerase has been shown to play a role in the virulence of influenza virus and, depending on its origin, may confer increased transcription and replication efficiency.[33,34]

Influenza viral assembly is believed to occur at the site of specialized lipid domains, or rafts, on the apical plasma membrane in polarized epithelial cells (Figure 22.2).[35] These lipid rafts are enriched in cholesterol, sphingolipids, and phospholipids containing fatty acids, and have been shown to play a role in the entry, assembly, and budding of many viruses.[36] In influenza virus, the M1 protein orchestrates viral assembly at lipid rafts.[35] Although not a membrane-spanning protein, M1 may attach to the plasma membrane through the cooperative action of several binding sites, and is a determinant for virion morphology because of its interactions with all other viral proteins.[35,37] The HA and NA surface proteins bind weakly to the M1 protein and are intrinsically recruited to lipid rafts, where interactions with other M1 proteins increase the strength of these interactions.[38–40] The M2 protein is excluded from lipid rafts,[39] but may be incorporated into the virion through direct interactions with the M1 protein.[41,42] Following replication of the viral genome, the newly formed vRNA assembles with the NP, PB1, PB2, and PA proteins, which accumulate in the nucleus after their translation, to form the vRNP.[43,44] With the assistance of NEP, the vRNP is subsequently exported from the nucleus to the cytoplasm,[45] and though the mechanism for vRNP transport to the site of viral assembly is unknown, the M1 protein may be involved through its interaction with NP.[46,47] The M1 protein may also interact with NEP, resulting in its incorporation in small amounts into the virion.[48,49] The final virion includes a complete set of eight distinct vRNPs that are arranged as seven segments of varying lengths surrounding one central segment.[50]

Once all components of the virion are assembled, pleiomorphic spherical and filamentous virus particles bud and are released from the surface of the infected cell (Figure 22.2). This process is characterized by the induction of membrane curvature, and formation of an Ω-shaped bud.[51] Budding is thought to be initiated by the HA protein, and may be further supported by the helical structure of the M1 protein, which may possess an intrinsic ability to alter membrane structure.[52–54] The M2 protein also plays an important role in the budding process by inducing a specific curvature to the membrane that stabilizes the site long enough for filament formation, and mediates membrane scission in a cholesterol-dependent manner.[55,56] Following the completion of membrane scission, the NA protein allows for the release of progeny virions by enzymatically cleaving sialic acid moieties that tether the viral particle to the host cell surface.[1] Finally, NEP facilitates the efficient egress of budding virions through recruitment of a cellular ATPase.[57]

In addition to the nine structural proteins, influenza virus expresses two nonstructural proteins in the context of infected cells. The NS1 protein is a multifunctional accessory protein that plays a primary role in the virulence of influenza virus by antagonizing the host interferon (IFN) response to viral infection.[1] NS1, which likely exists as a homodimer, has two major domain regions, the N-terminal RNA-binding domain and the C-terminal effector domain.[58] In some influenza viruses, the NS1 protein may contain either a deletion in the linker region between the N- and C-terminal domains, or a truncation of the C-terminal domain.[59] Both of these changes have been associated with varying levels of virulence in mammals[60,61] and birds.[62,63] The PB1-F2 protein is expressed in most influenza viruses from an alternate open reading frame of the PB1 gene.[64,65] In virus-infected cells, PB1-F2 localizes to the mitochondria, where it disrupts the mitochondrial membrane potential and induces apoptosis.[66–68] In addition, the PB1-F2 protein has been implicated in the antagonism of the host IFN response.[69,70] The expression of PB1-F2 is also associated with the virulence of influenza virus in a strain-specific manner.[71,72]

with influenza virus, but cannot rule it out. In the case of a negative result, a second diagnostic test should always be used.[203]

22.7.3 Molecular Assays

Molecular assays for influenza, such as RT-PCR, use conserved gene targets to accurately identify the presence of vRNA in respiratory secretions. These assays can also be multiplexed to simultaneously detect several respiratory viruses in the same specimen, or can be used in real time to give quantitative information on virus present in the sample. There are several Food and Drug Administration (FDA)-approved commercially available kits that can discriminate between influenza A and B viruses, or that can also distinguish between HA gene sequences, allowing for the determination of some influenza A virus subtypes. Sometimes these tests identify the strain as influenza A virus, but they cannot identify the subtype. These strains that are "unsubtypable" may represent new influenza strains that need to be isolated and characterized by sequencing.[204,205]

The main advantage of molecular assays is that they are highly sensitive and specific, and can rapidly produce results in 3–6 h. These tests can only be performed in specialized laboratories, however, and therefore may not be widely available. Molecular testing is not indicated for all patients with suspected influenza, or to confirm the diagnosis of influenza when the disease is known to be circulating. Instead, it should be performed when an influenza diagnosis would change clinical management of the patient, or when it is necessary to identify influenza virus as the cause of respiratory outbreaks in nursing homes, hospitals, or other institutions.[204,205]

Although molecular assays are highly sensitive, several factors may cause false-negative results. These include low influenza virus load in the specimen from delayed sample collection, absence of influenza viral replication in the upper respiratory tract because of lower respiratory influenza disease, or general errors in the collection or handling of the specimen. Therefore, a negative result may not always exclude a diagnosis of influenza. Conversely, the detection of influenza RNA in respiratory secretions confirms the diagnosis of influenza virus infection, but is not necessarily an indication that viable virus is still present. Therefore, this technique is not useful for monitoring response to therapy.

22.7.4 Serologic Tests

Serologic tests, such as hemagglutination inhibition performed on paired specimens of acute and convalescent sera, have no diagnostic utility. They can be used to retrospectively establish a diagnosis of influenza infection or to evaluate the response to vaccination in clinical trials.

22.8 TREATMENT OF INFLUENZA

The development of antiviral therapies for influenza has been very slow, and the therapeutic armamentarium against this virus is still very limited. The adamantanes, developed in the 1960s, were the first approved class of antiviral agents against influenza. The second class of influenza antivirals, the NA inhibitors, was developed 30 years later. Since then, no new antiviral drugs active against influenza have been added to the market. Although a few new molecules are currently under development, only four drugs are currently approved for the treatment and prevention of influenza. The ever-present threat of emerging drug resistance and of new circulating influenza virus strains is a constant reminder of the substantial limitations in treating individuals affected by severe disease.

22.8.1 M2 Inhibitors: Adamantanes

This class of drugs, which includes amantadine and rimantadine, inhibits the ion channel activity of the M2 protein, thus preventing viral uncoating and entry. Since influenza B viruses lack the M2 protein, these drugs are only active against influenza A viruses. Amantadine and rimantadine share the same mechanism of action and spectrum of activity; however, they have different pharmacological properties. Amantadine is not metabolized in the body and is excreted unchanged in the urine, whereas rimantadine undergoes extensive metabolism. Therefore, the dosage of amantadine needs to be adjusted in patients with renal failure and in older adults. Amantadine use may be associated with minor, reversible CNS side effects, such as insomnia and dizziness. It may also cause seizures in individuals with preexisting seizure disorder.[206] These effects have not been described with rimantadine use.[207]

Amantadine and rimantadine have been shown to be effective in the treatment of influenza and to lead to a faster resolution of symptoms.[208] Cross-resistance to the adamantanes frequently emerges during treatment, and is frequently caused by a single-point mutation (S31N) in the M2 gene.[209] Surveillance studies have shown that, since 2005, approximately 98% of the circulating H3N2 influenza virus strains have developed resistance to these drugs.[210] Also, the circulating A(H1N1)pdm09 isolates and most H5N1 isolates are resistant to adamantanes.[211] Therefore, this class of drug is not recommended for treatment or prophylaxis of currently circulating influenza A virus strains.[212]

22.8.2 Neuraminidase Inhibitors

Neuraminidase inhibitors (NAIs) inhibit the ability of the influenza virus NA protein to cleave sialic acid groups from host glycoproteins, thus preventing the release and spread of nascent influenza virus particles from the cell surface. Oseltamivir (Tamiflu) and zanamivir (Relenza), the two FDA-approved NAIs, were rationally designed based on the crystal structure of the NA protein, and they are active against both influenza A and B viruses.[170] These two drugs differ in their pharmacologic characteristics, administration routes, and safety profiles. Oseltamivir is administered orally, either in capsules (30, 45, and 75 mg) or as a liquid suspension, whereas zanamivir is not orally bioavailable and must be delivered as an orally inhaled dry powder using the diskhaler device included in the medication package. Oseltamivir is rapidly absorbed and converted by the liver into its active metabolite, oseltamivir carboxylate, which is excreted unchanged in the urine. Therefore, the dosage of this drug must be adjusted in the case of decreased renal function. Oseltamivir is well tolerated, and its only major side effects are nausea and gastrointestinal upset. Zanamivir has been associated with bronchoconstriction in patients with asthma or chronic obstructive pulmonary disease.[170]

The recommended dosages of oseltamivir and zanamivir for influenza prophylaxis and treatment are indicated in Table 22.1. Oseltamivir was successfully used in infants during the 2009

TABLE 22.1
Recommended Dosage of Approved NAI for Treatment and Prophylaxis of Influenza

	Treatment		Prophylaxis	
	Children	Adults	Children	Adults
Oseltamivir	≥1 year of age Dose varies by child's weight: ≤15 kg: 30 mg twice a day >15 kg to 23 kg: 45 mg twice a day >23 kg to 40 kg: 60 mg twice a day >40 kg: adult dose	75 mg twice daily[a]	≥1 year of age Dose varies by child's weight: ≤15 kg: 30 mg once a day >15 kg to 23 kg: 45 mg once a day >23 kg to 40 kg: 60 mg once a day >40 kg: adult dose	75 mg once daily[a]
Zanamivir	≥7 years of age 10 mg (two inhalations) twice daily	10 mg (two inhalations) twice daily	≥5 years of age 10 mg (two inhalations) once daily	10 mg (two inhalations) once daily

[a] For patients with creatinine clearance of 10–30 mL per minute, a reduction of the treatment dosage of oseltamivir to 75 mg once daily, and in the chemoprophylaxis dosage to 75 mg every other day is recommended.

22.12.2 Influenza Vaccines and Guillain-Barré Syndrome

Guillain-Barré Syndrome (GBS) is an acute, inflammatory, demyelinating polyradiculoneuropathy that has been described after influenza virus infection[293,294] or vaccination.[295] The mechanism behind development of GBS is likely autoimmune, and possibly due to molecular mimicry. Following the isolation of a swine-origin influenza A (H1N1) virus that caused a small outbreak in humans in 1976, the United States began a mass vaccination program out of fear that a new pandemic was imminent because of similarities between this strain and the one that caused the 1918 pandemic. This vaccination campaign was discontinued, however, because of an unusually elevated number of individuals who developed GBS (an estimated risk of 1 per 100,000 vaccines).[296] Following this episode, there has been careful surveillance to identify whether an association between influenza vaccination and GBS exists. Much of this monitoring took place before and after the introduction of the vaccine for A(H1N1)pdm09. All of the studies have found either no association, or a risk of only about 1 case per million doses of vaccine.[297] Since GBS is recurrent in a small percentage of cases, it is currently recommended for subjects who have previously developed GBS within 6 weeks of influenza vaccination to avoid subsequent immunization with influenza vaccine. Patients with a history of GBS that was not temporally associated with receipt of the influenza vaccine can likely receive the vaccine without recurrence.

22.13 THE QUEST FOR A UNIVERSAL INFLUENZA VACCINE

Current influenza vaccines target the HA protein, which is the major antigenic determinant on the surface of the influenza virion. Because this protein is subject to variability driven by antigenic drift and shift, it is essential to reformulate the vaccine annually. Therefore, a current strategy for the development of a universal influenza vaccine is to target antigens that are critical for the viral life cycle, and that are both stable and conserved among influenza virus strains. Although this approach has not yet resulted in a commercial vaccine, the research in this area is extremely active. Here, we will briefly review the most promising strategies that are in preclinical development or clinical studies in humans.

22.13.1 Vaccines Targeting the Extracellular Domain of the M2 Protein

M2 is an integral transmembrane protein that is essential for acidification and uncoating of the influenza virion. The 24 amino acid N-terminal M2 extracellular domain, called M2e, is highly conserved among human influenza viruses,[298] and therefore it has been considered to be a good target for human vaccines. The M2e peptide is not very immunogenic, necessitating its attachment to a larger protein carrier, and/or the addition of an adjuvant in order to increase its immunogenicity and potential utility in the context of a vaccine.[299] To date, phase I trial studies in humans have demonstrated the safety and immunogenicity of several M2e fusion vaccine candidates with or without adjuvant[300]; however, there are currently no data supporting their efficacy in protecting against influenza. A recent study also showed that adding one of these M2e-based vaccines to TIV increased antibody responses to H1 and H3, but not to influenza B, by approximately 50%,[301] suggesting that M2 could be added to conventional vaccines to increase vaccine response.

22.13.2 Vaccines Targeting the Conserved Stalk Region of HA

Influenza HA is expressed on the surface of the virion, and mediates viral attachment and entry. Structurally, HA consists of a globular head and a stalk. The globular head is highly variable, and contains the epitopes against which the host antibody response is directed. Recent studies have shown that the stalk is highly conserved among influenza species.[302,303] In humans immunized for influenza, low frequencies of antibodies directed against nonimmunodominant epitopes in the HA stalk have also been identified. Some of these antibodies are broadly neutralizing and can confer protection against multiple influenza strains in the animal models.[304] This discovery has sparked new research aimed at identifying specific epitopes of the HA stalk that elicit broadly neutralizing antibodies, and that can be used for the development of a universal influenza vaccine. A comprehensive description of these strategies goes beyond the scope of this chapter, but has been thoroughly reviewed by Pica and Palese.[139]

22.13.3 Vaccines That Stimulate Cell-Mediated Immune Responses

Natural influenza virus infection stimulates both antibody and cell-mediated responses. Since influenza virus has the propensity to mutate its external antigenic composition to escape host immune defenses, antibody responses tend to be strain-specific, whereas T cell responses against internal, conserved proteins are cross-reactive. CTLs contribute significantly to viral clearance and clinical recovery from influenza, and can also help to protect against an otherwise lethal influenza virus challenge.[305] A major target for the host CTL response to influenza virus is NP, which is >90% conserved among influenza virus strains,[306,307] and cell-mediated responses against this protein are protective against heterologous challenge in mice.[308,309] These responses are essentially absent in humans who have been vaccinated with TIV. Therefore, several attempts have been made at developing an influenza vaccine that could elicit cross-reactive cell-mediated responses to NP. In humans, vector-based vaccines expressing the NP and M1 proteins have been shown to be safe and to induce CTL responses.[310] Following an influenza virus challenge in one study, vaccinated individuals had a decreased duration of viral shedding, though it is difficult to draw conclusions on vaccine efficacy due to the small number of subjects enrolled.[311]

REFERENCES

1. Palese PS, ML. Orthomyxoviridae: The viruses and their replication. In: Knipe DMH, Peter M., eds. *Fields Virology*, 5th ed. Philadelphia: Lippincott Williams & Wilkins; 2007. p. 1648–1689.
2. Wright P, Neumann, G., Kawaoka, Y. Orthomyxoviruses. In: Knipe DMH, Peter M., eds. *Fields Virology*, 5th ed. Philadelphia: Lippincott Williams & Wilkins; 2007. p. 1693–1740.
3. Presti RM, Zhao G, Beatty WL, Mihindukulasuriya KA, da Rosa AP, Popov VL et al. Quaranfil, Johnston Atoll, and Lake Chad viruses are novel members of the family Orthomyxoviridae. *J Virol*. 2009; 83(22): 11599–11606.
4. Shaw MW, Xu X, Li Y, Normand S, Ueki RT, Kunimoto GY et al. Reappearance and global spread of variants of influenza B/Victoria/2/87 lineage viruses in the 2000–2001 and 2001–2002 seasons. *Virology*. 2002; 303(1): 1–8.
5. Yamashita M, Krystal M, Fitch WM, Palese P. Influenza B virus evolution: Co-circulating lineages and comparison of evolutionary pattern with those of influenza A and C viruses. *Virology*. 1988; 163(1): 112–122.
6. Matsuzaki Y, Katsushima N, Nagai Y, Shoji M, Itagaki T, Sakamoto M et al. Clinical features of influenza C virus infection in children. *J Infect Dis*. 2006; 193(9): 1229–1235.
7. World Health Organization. A revision of the system of nomenclature for influenza viruses: A WHO memorandum. *Bull World Health Organ*. 1980; 58(4): 585–591.
8. Standardization of terminology of the pandemic A(H1N1) 2009 virus. *Wkly Epidemiol Rec*. 2011; 86(43): 480.
9. Palese P, Schulman JL. Mapping of the influenza virus genome: Identification of the hemagglutinin and the neuraminidase genes. *Proc Natl Acad Sci USA*. 1976; 73(6): 2142–2146.
10. Ritchey MB, Palese P, Kilbourne ED. RNAs of influenza A, B, and C viruses. *J Virol*. 1976; 18(2): 738–744.
11. Ghedin E, Sengamalay NA, Shumway M, Zaborsky J, Feldblyum T, Subbu V et al. Large-scale sequencing of human influenza reveals the dynamic nature of viral genome evolution. *Nature*. 2005; 437(7062): 1162–1126.
12. Bouvier NM, Palese P. The biology of influenza viruses. *Vaccine*. 2008; 26 Suppl 4: D49–D53.
13. Klenk HD, Garten W. Host cell proteases controlling virus pathogenicity. *Trends Microbiol*. 1994; 2(2): 39–43.

66. Chen W, Calvo PA, Malide D, Gibbs J, Schubert U, Bacik I et al. A novel influenza A virus mitochondrial protein that induces cell death. *Nat Med*. 2001; 7(12): 1306–1312.
67. Gibbs JS, Malide D, Hornung F, Bennink JR, Yewdell JW. The influenza A virus PB1-F2 protein targets the inner mitochondrial membrane via a predicted basic amphipathic helix that disrupts mitochondrial function. *J Virol*. 2003; 77(13): 7214–7224.
68. Yamada H, Chounan R, Higashi Y, Kurihara N, Kido H. Mitochondrial targeting sequence of the influenza A virus PB1-F2 protein and its function in mitochondria. *FEBS Lett*. 2004; 578(3): 331–336.
69. Varga ZT, Grant A, Manicassamy B, Palese P. Influenza virus protein PB1-F2 inhibits the induction of type I interferon by binding to MAVS and decreasing mitochondrial membrane potential. *J Virol*. 2012; 86(16): 8359–8366.
70. Varga ZT, Ramos I, Hai R, Schmolke M, Garcia-Sastre A, Fernandez-Sesma A et al. The influenza virus protein PB1-F2 inhibits the induction of type I interferon at the level of the MAVS adaptor protein. *PLoS Pathog*. 2011; 7(6): e1002067.
71. McAuley JL, Zhang K, McCullers JA. The effects of influenza A virus PB1-F2 protein on polymerase activity are strain specific and do not impact pathogenesis. *J Virol*. 2010; 84(1): 558–564.
72. Hai R, Schmolke M, Varga ZT, Manicassamy B, Wang TT, Belser JA et al. PB1-F2 expression by the 2009 pandemic H1N1 influenza virus has minimal impact on virulence in animal models. *J Virol*. 2010; 84(9): 4442–4450.
73. Swayne DE. Avian influenza vaccines and therapies for poultry. *Comp Immunol Microbiol Infect Dis*. 2009; 32(4): 351–363.
74. Tong S, Li Y, Rivailler P, Conrardy C, Castillo DA, Chen LM et al. A distinct lineage of influenza A virus from bats. *Proc Natl Acad Sci USA*. 2012; 109(11): 4269–4274.
75. Webster RG, Bean WJ, Gorman OT, Chambers TM, Kawaoka Y. Evolution and ecology of influenza A viruses. *Microbiol Rev*. 1992; 56(1): 152–179.
76. Alexander DJ. A review of avian influenza in different bird species. *Vet Microbiol*. 2000; 74(1–2): 3–13.
77. Suarez DL. Avian influenza: Our current understanding. *Anim Health Res Rev*. 2010; 11(1): 19–33.
78. Hoye BJ, Munster VJ, Nishiura H, Klaassen M, Fouchier RA. Surveillance of wild birds for avian influenza virus. *Emerg Infect Dis*. 2010; 16(12): 1827–1834.
79. Bankowski RA. *Proceedings of the First International Symposium on Avian Influenza*. In: Bankowski RA, ed. *Symposium on Avian Influenza*; 1981 April 22–24, 1981; Beltsville, MD; 1981.
80. World Organization for Animal Health (OIE). In: *Manual of Standards for Diagnostic Tests and Vaccines for Terrestrial Animals*. World Trade Organization, editor; 2012.
81. Alexander DJ. An overview of the epidemiology of avian influenza. *Vaccine*. 2007; 25(30): 5637–5644.
82. Harder TC, Werner, O. Avian Influenza; 2006.
83. Kalthoff D, Globig A, Beer M. (Highly pathogenic) avian influenza as a zoonotic agent. *Vet Microbiol*. 2010; 140(3–4): 237–245.
84. Medina RA, Garcia-Sastre A. Influenza A viruses: New research developments. *Nat Rev Microbiol*. 2011; 9(8): 590–603.
85. Ito T, Couceiro JN, Kelm S, Baum LG, Krauss S, Castrucci MR et al. Molecular basis for the generation in pigs of influenza A viruses with pandemic potential. *J Virol*. 1998; 72(9): 7367–7373.
86. Ito T. Interspecies transmission and receptor recognition of influenza A viruses. *Microbiol Immunol*. 2000; 44(6): 423–430.
87. Shinya K, Ebina M, Yamada S, Ono M, Kasai N, Kawaoka Y. Avian flu: Influenza virus receptors in the human airway. *Nature*. 2006; 440(7083): 435–436.
88. Garcia-Sastre A. Induction and evasion of type I interferon responses by influenza viruses. *Virus Res*. 2011; 162(1–2): 12–18.
89. Guillot L, Le Goffic R, Bloch S, Escriou N, Akira S, Chignard M et al. Involvement of toll-like receptor 3 in the immune response of lung epithelial cells to double-stranded RNA and influenza A virus. *J Biol Chem*. 2005; 280(7): 5571–5580.
90. Le Goffic R, Balloy V, Lagranderie M, Alexopoulou L, Escriou N, Flavell R et al. Detrimental contribution of the Toll-like receptor (TLR)3 to influenza A virus-induced acute pneumonia. *PLoS Pathog*. 2006; 2(6): e53.
91. Le Goffic R, Pothlichet J, Vitour D, Fujita T, Meurs E, Chignard M et al. Cutting Edge: Influenza A virus activates TLR3-dependent inflammatory and RIG-I-dependent antiviral responses in human lung epithelial cells. *J Immunol*. 2007; 178(6): 3368–3372.
92. Jeisy-Scott V, Kim JH, Davis WG, Cao W, Katz JM, Sambhara S. TLR7 recognition is dispensable for influenza virus A infection but important for the induction of hemagglutinin-specific antibodies in response to the 2009 pandemic split vaccine in mice. *J Virol*. 2012; 86(20): 10988–10998.

93. Garcia MA, Gil J, Ventoso I, Guerra S, Domingo E, Rivas C et al. Impact of protein kinase PKR in cell biology: From antiviral to antiproliferative action. *Microbiol Mol Biol Rev*. 2006; 70(4): 1032–1060.
94. Silverman RH. Viral encounters with 2',5'-oligoadenylate synthetase and RNase L during the interferon antiviral response. *J Virol*. 2007; 81(23): 12720–12729.
95. Haller O, Kochs G, Weber F. The interferon response circuit: Induction and suppression by pathogenic viruses. *Virology*. 2006; 344(1): 119–130.
96. Randall RE, Goodbourn S. Interferons and viruses: An interplay between induction, signalling, antiviral responses and virus countermeasures. *J Gen Virol*. 2008; 89(Pt 1): 1–47.
97. Hatada E, Takizawa T, Fukuda R. Specific binding of influenza A virus NS1 protein to the virus minus-sense RNA in vitro. *J Gen Virol*. 1992; 73 (Pt 1): 17–25.
98. Hatada E, Fukuda R. Binding of influenza A virus NS1 protein to dsRNA in vitro. *J Gen Virol*. 1992; 73 (Pt 12): 3325–3329.
99. Guo Z, Chen LM, Zeng H, Gomez JA, Plowden J, Fujita T et al. NS1 protein of influenza A virus inhibits the function of intracytoplasmic pathogen sensor, RIG-I. *Am J Respir Cell Mol Biol*. 2007; 36(3): 263–269.
100. Lu Y, Wambach M, Katze MG, Krug RM. Binding of the influenza virus NS1 protein to double-stranded RNA inhibits the activation of the protein kinase that phosphorylates the elF-2 translation initiation factor. *Virology*. 1995; 214(1): 222–228.
101. Min JY, Li S, Sen GC, Krug RM. A site on the influenza A virus NS1 protein mediates both inhibition of PKR activation and temporal regulation of viral RNA synthesis. *Virology*. 2007; 363(1): 236–243.
102. Min JY, Krug RM. The primary function of RNA binding by the influenza A virus NS1 protein in infected cells: Inhibiting the 2'-5' oligo (A) synthetase/RNase L pathway. *Proc Natl Acad Sci USA*. 2006; 103(18): 7100–7105.
103. Munir M, Zohari S, Berg M. Non-structural protein 1 of avian influenza A viruses differentially inhibit NF-kappaB promoter activation. *Virol J*. 2011; 8: 383.
104. Talon J, Horvath CM, Polley R, Basler CF, Muster T, Palese P et al. Activation of interferon regulatory factor 3 is inhibited by the influenza A virus NS1 protein. *J Virol*. 2000; 74(17): 7989–7996.
105. Hale BG, Randall RE, Ortin J, Jackson D. The multifunctional NS1 protein of influenza A viruses. *J Gen Virol*. 2008; 89(Pt 10): 2359–2376.
106. Jia D, Rahbar R, Chan RW, Lee SM, Chan MC, Wang BX et al. Influenza virus non-structural protein 1 (NS1) disrupts interferon signaling. *PLoS One*. 2010; 5(11): e13927.
107. Nemeroff ME, Barabino SM, Li Y, Keller W, Krug RM. Influenza virus NS1 protein interacts with the cellular 30 kDa subunit of CPSF and inhibits 3'end formation of cellular pre-mRNAs. *Mol Cell*. 1998; 1(7): 991–1000.
108. Kochs G, Garcia-Sastre A, Martinez-Sobrido L. Multiple anti-interferon actions of the influenza A virus NS1 protein. *J Virol*. 2007; 81(13): 7011–7021.
109. Conenello GM, Tisoncik JR, Rosenzweig E, Varga ZT, Palese P, Katze MG. A single N66S mutation in the PB1-F2 protein of influenza A virus increases virulence by inhibiting the early interferon response in vivo. *J Virol*. 2011; 85(2): 652–662.
110. Pang IK, Iwasaki A. Inflammasomes as mediators of immunity against influenza virus. *Trends Immunol*. 2011; 32(1): 34–41.
111. Ichinohe T, Lee HK, Ogura Y, Flavell R, Iwasaki A. Inflammasome recognition of influenza virus is essential for adaptive immune responses. *J Exp Med*. 2009; 206(1): 79–87.
112. Allen IC, Scull MA, Moore CB, Holl EK, McElvania-TeKippe E, Taxman DJ et al. The NLRP3 inflammasome mediates *in vivo* innate immunity to influenza A virus through recognition of viral RNA. *Immunity*. 2009; 30(4): 556–565.
113. Mandell GL, Bennett, J.E., Dolin, R. *Principles and Practice of Infectious Diseases*. 7th ed. Philadelphia: Elsevier Inc.; 2010.
114. de Jong JC, Palache AM, Beyer WE, Rimmelzwaan GF, Boon AC, Osterhaus AD. Haemagglutination-inhibiting antibody to influenza virus. *Dev Biol (Basel)*. 2003; 115: 63–73.
115. Wiley DC, Wilson IA, Skehel JJ. Structural identification of the antibody-binding sites of Hong Kong influenza haemagglutinin and their involvement in antigenic variation. *Nature*. 1981; 289(5796): 373–378.
116. Caton AJ, Brownlee GG, Yewdell JW, Gerhard W. The antigenic structure of the influenza virus A/PR/8/34 hemagglutinin (H1 subtype). *Cell*. 1982; 31(2 Pt 1): 417–427.
117. Marcelin G, Sandbulte MR, Webby RJ. Contribution of antibody production against neuraminidase to the protection afforded by influenza vaccines. *Rev Med Virol*. 2012; 22(4): 267–279.
118. Ekiert DC, Wilson IA. Broadly neutralizing antibodies against influenza virus and prospects for universal therapies. *Curr Opin Virol*. 2012; 2(2): 134–141.

172. Rothberg MB, Haessler SD. Complications of seasonal and pandemic influenza. *Crit Care Med.* 2010; 38(4 Suppl): e91–e97.
173. Hajjar LA, Mauad T, Galas FR, Kumar A, da Silva LF, Dolhnikoff M et al. Severe novel influenza A (H1N1) infection in cancer patients. *Ann Oncol.* 2010; 21(12): 2333–2341.
174. Memoli MJ, Harvey H, Morens DM, Taubenberger JK. Influenza in pregnancy. *Influenza Other Respi Viruses.* 2012.
175. Louria DB, Blumenfeld HL, Ellis JT, Kilbourne ED, Rogers DE. Studies on influenza in the pandemic of 1957–1958. II. Pulmonary complications of influenza. *J Clin Invest.* 1959; 38(1 Part 2): 213–265.
176. Centers for Disease Control and Prevention. Bacterial coinfections in lung tissue specimens from fatal cases of 2009 pandemic influenza A (H1N1)—United States, May–August 2009. *MMWR Morb Mortal Wkly Rep.* 2009; 58(38): 1071–1074.
177. Warren-Gash C, Smeeth L, Hayward AC. Influenza as a trigger for acute myocardial infarction or death from cardiovascular disease: A systematic review. *Lancet Infect Dis.* 2009; 9(10): 601–610.
178. Mamas MA, Fraser D, Neyses L. Cardiovascular manifestations associated with influenza virus infection. *Int J Cardiol.* 2008; 130(3): 304–309.
179. Paddock CD, Liu L, Denison AM, Bartlett JH, Holman RC, Deleon-Carnes M et al. Myocardial injury and bacterial pneumonia contribute to the pathogenesis of fatal influenza B virus infection. *J Infect Dis.* 2012; 205(6): 895–905.
180. Davis LE. Neurologic and muscular complications of the 2009 influenza A (H1N1) pandemic. *Curr Neurol Neurosci Rep.* 2010; 10(6): 476–483.
181. Ekstrand JJ. Neurologic complications of influenza. *Semin Pediatr Neurol.* 2012; 19(3): 96–100.
182. Maheady DC. Reye's syndrome: Review and update. *J Pediatr Health Care.* 1989; 3(5): 246–250.
183. Claas EC, Osterhaus AD, van Beek R, De Jong JC, Rimmelzwaan GF, Senne DA et al. Human influenza A H5N1 virus related to a highly pathogenic avian influenza virus. *Lancet.* 1998; 351(9101): 472–477.
184. Gambotto A, Barratt-Boyes SM, de Jong MD, Neumann G, Kawaoka Y. Human infection with highly pathogenic H5N1 influenza virus. *Lancet.* 2008; 371(9622): 1464–1475.
185. Beigel JH, Farrar J, Han AM, Hayden FG, Hyer R, de Jong MD et al. Avian influenza A (H5N1) infection in humans. *N Engl J Med.* 2005; 353(13): 1374–1385.
186. Matrosovich M, Zhou N, Kawaoka Y, Webster R. The surface glycoproteins of H5 influenza viruses isolated from humans, chickens, and wild aquatic birds have distinguishable properties. *J Virol.* 1999; 73(2): 1146–1155.
187. Herfst S, Schrauwen EJ, Linster M, Chutinimitkul S, de Wit E, Munster VJ et al. Airborne transmission of influenza A/H5N1 virus between ferrets. *Science.* 2012; 336(6088): 1534–1541.
188. Imai M, Watanabe T, Hatta M, Das SC, Ozawa M, Shinya K et al. Experimental adaptation of an influenza H5 HA confers respiratory droplet transmission to a reassortant H5 HA/H1N1 virus in ferrets. *Nature.* 2012; 486(7403): 420–428.
189. Gao R, Cao B, Hu Y, Feng Z, Wang D, Hu W et al. Human infection with a novel avian-origin influenza A (H7N9) virus. *N Engl J Med.* 2013; 368(20): 1888–1897.
190. Zhu H, Wang D, Kelvin DJ, Li L, Zheng Z, Yoon SW et al. Infectivity, transmission and pathology of human H7N9 influenza in ferrets and pigs. 2013; 341(6142): 183–186.
191. Yu H, Cowling BJ, Feng L, Lau EH, Liao Q, Tsang TK et al. Human infection with avian influenza A H7N9 virus: An assessment of clinical severity. *The Lancet.* 2013; 382(9887): 138–145.
192. Weber TP, Stilianakis NI. Inactivation of influenza A viruses in the environment and modes of transmission: A critical review. *J Infect.* 2008; 57(5): 361–373.
193. Tellier R. Review of aerosol transmission of influenza A virus. *Emerg Infect Dis.* 2006; 12(11): 1657–1662.
194. Tellier R. Aerosol transmission of influenza A virus: A review of new studies. *J R Soc Interface.* 2009; 6 Suppl 6: S783–S790.
195. Fabian P, McDevitt JJ, DeHaan WH, Fung RO, Cowling BJ, Chan KH et al. Influenza virus in human exhaled breath: An observational study. *PLoS One.* 2008; 3(7): e2691.
196. Noti JD, Lindsley WG, Blachere FM, Cao G, Kashon ML, Thewlis RE et al. Detection of infectious influenza virus in cough aerosols generated in a simulated patient examination room. *Clin Infect Dis.* 2012; 54(11): 1569–1577.
197. Greatorex JS, Digard P, Curran MD, Moynihan R, Wensley H, Wreghitt T et al. Survival of influenza A(H1N1) on materials found in households: Implications for infection control. *PLoS One.* 2011; 6(11): e27932.

198. Greatorex JS, Page RF, Curran MD, Digard P, Enstone JE, Wreghitt T et al. Effectiveness of common household cleaning agents in reducing the viability of human influenza A/H1N1. *PLoS One*. 2010; 5(2): e8987.
199. Webster RG, Yakhno M, Hinshaw VS, Bean WJ, Murti KG. Intestinal influenza: Replication and characterization of influenza viruses in ducks. *Virology*. 1978; 84(2): 268–278.
200. Webster RG. Influenza: An emerging disease. *Emerg Infect Dis*. 1998; 4(3): 436–441.
201. de Jong MD, Bach VC, Phan TQ, Vo MH, Tran TT, Nguyen BH et al. Fatal avian influenza A (H5N1) in a child presenting with diarrhea followed by coma. *N Engl J Med*. 2005; 352(7): 686–691.
202. Kumar S, Henrickson KJ. Update on influenza diagnostics: Lessons from the novel H1N1 influenza A pandemic. *Clin Microbiol Rev*. 2012; 25(2): 344–361.
203. Chartrand C, Leeflang MM, Minion J, Brewer T, Pai M. Accuracy of rapid influenza diagnostic tests: A meta-analysis. *Ann Intern Med*. 2012; 156(7): 500–511.
204. Mahony JB. Nucleic acid amplification-based diagnosis of respiratory virus infections. *Expert Rev Anti Infect Ther*. 2010; 8(11): 1273–1292.
205. Centers for Disease Control and Prevention. Guidance for clinicians on the user of RT-PCR and other molecular assays for diagnosis of influenza virus infection. 2012 [cited Accessed 04/09/13]; Available from: http://www.cdc.gov/flu/professionals/diagnosis/molecular-assays.htm
206. Atkinson WL, Arden NH, Patriarca PA, Leslie N, Lui KJ, Gohd R. Amantadine prophylaxis during an institutional outbreak of type A (H1N1) influenza. *Arch Intern Med*. 1986; 146(9): 1751–1756.
207. Dolin R, Reichman RC, Madore HP, Maynard R, Linton PN, Webber-Jones J. A controlled trial of amantadine and rimantadine in the prophylaxis of influenza A infection. *N Engl J Med*. 1982; 307(10): 580–584.
208. Togo Y, Hornick RB, Felitti VJ, Kaufman ML, Dawkins AT, Jr., Kilpe VE et al. Evaluation of therapeutic efficacy of amantadine in patients with naturally occurring A2 influenza. *JAMA*. 1970; 211(7): 1149–1156.
209. Hay AJ, Wolstenholme AJ, Skehel JJ, Smith MH. The molecular basis of the specific anti-influenza action of amantadine. *EMBO J*. 1985; 4(11): 3021–3024.
210. Bright RA, Shay DK, Shu B, Cox NJ, Klimov AI. Adamantane resistance among influenza A viruses isolated early during the 2005–2006 influenza season in the United States. *JAMA*. 2006; 295(8): 891–894.
211. Hayden FG. Antiviral resistance in influenza viruses—Implications for management and pandemic response. *N Engl J Med*. 2006; 354(8): 785–788.
212. Fiore AE, Uyeki TM, Broder K, Finelli L, Euler GL, Singleton JA et al. Prevention and control of influenza with vaccines: Recommendations of the Advisory Committee on Immunization Practices (ACIP), 2010. *MMWR Recomm Rep*. 2010; 59(RR-8): 1–62.
213. Roche Laboratories Inc. Tamiflu (oseltamivir phosphate) capsules and oral suspension [package insert]. Nutley, NJ: Roche laboratories, Inc.; 2009.
214. Monto AS, Robinson DP, Herlocher ML, Hinson JM, Jr., Elliott MJ, Crisp A. Zanamivir in the prevention of influenza among healthy adults: A randomized controlled trial. *JAMA*. 1999; 282(1): 31–35.
215. Nicholson KG, Aoki FY, Osterhaus AD, Trottier S, Carewicz O, Mercier CH et al. Efficacy and safety of oseltamivir in treatment of acute influenza: A randomised controlled trial. Neuraminidase Inhibitor Flu Treatment Investigator Group. *Lancet*. 2000; 355(9218): 1845–1850.
216. Whitley RJ, Hayden FG, Reisinger KS, Young N, Dutkowski R, Ipe D et al. Oral oseltamivir treatment of influenza in children. *Pediatr Infect Dis J*. 2001; 20(2): 127–133.
217. Heinonen S, Silvennoinen H, Lehtinen P, Vainionpaa R, Vahlberg T, Ziegler T et al. Early oseltamivir treatment of influenza in children 1–3 years of age: A randomized controlled trial. *Clin Infect Dis*. 2010; 51(8): 887–894.
218. Johnston SL, Ferrero F, Garcia ML, Dutkowski R. Oral oseltamivir improves pulmonary function and reduces exacerbation frequency for influenza-infected children with asthma. *Pediatr Infect Dis J*. 2005; 24(3): 225–232.
219. Lee N, Chan PK, Choi KW, Lui G, Wong B, Cockram CS et al. Factors associated with early hospital discharge of adult influenza patients. *Antivir Ther*. 2007; 12(4): 501–508.
220. Lee N, Cockram CS, Chan PK, Hui DS, Choi KW, Sung JJ. Antiviral treatment for patients hospitalized with severe influenza infection may affect clinical outcomes. *Clin Infect Dis*. 2008; 46(8): 1323–1324.
221. Louie JK, Acosta M, Winter K, Jean C, Gavali S, Schechter R et al. Factors associated with death or hospitalization due to pandemic 2009 influenza A(H1N1) infection in California. *JAMA*. 2009; 302(17): 1896–1902.
222. Louie JK, Acosta M, Jamieson DJ, Honein MA. Severe 2009 H1N1 influenza in pregnant and postpartum women in California. *N Engl J Med*. 2010; 362(1): 27–35.

223. Ariano RE, Sitar DS, Zelenitsky SA, Zarychanski R, Pisipati A, Ahern S et al. Enteric absorption and pharmacokinetics of oseltamivir in critically ill patients with pandemic (H1N1) influenza. *CMAJ*. 2010; 182(4): 357–363.
224. Armitage JM, Williams SJ. Inhaler technique in the elderly. *Age Ageing*. 1988; 17(4): 275–278.
225. Kiatboonsri S, Kiatboonsri C, Theerawit P. Fatal respiratory events caused by zanamivir nebulization. *Clin Infect Dis*. 2010; 50(4): 620.
226. Smith JR, Ariano RE, Toovey S. The use of antiviral agents for the management of severe influenza. *Crit Care Med*. 2010; 38(4 Suppl): e43–e51.
227. Medeiros R, Rameix-Welti MA, Lorin V, Ribaud P, Manuguerra JC, Socie G et al. Failure of zanamivir therapy for pneumonia in a bone-marrow transplant recipient infected by a zanamivir-sensitive influenza A (H1N1) virus. *Antivir Ther*. 2007; 12(4): 571–576.
228. Hayden FG. Newer influenza antivirals, biotherapeutics and combinations. *Influenza Other Respi Viruses*. 2013; 7 Suppl 1: 63–75.
229. Gaur AH, Bagga B, Barman S, Hayden R, Lamptey A, Hoffman JM et al. Intravenous zanamivir for oseltamivir-resistant 2009 H1N1 influenza. *N Engl J Med*. 2010; 362(1): 88–89.
230. Dulek DE, Williams JV, Creech CB, Schulert AK, Frangoul HA, Domm J et al. Use of intravenous zanamivir after development of oseltamivir resistance in a critically Ill immunosuppressed child infected with 2009 pandemic influenza A (H1N1) virus. *Clin Infect Dis*. 2010; 50(11): 1493–1496.
231. Gubareva LV, Robinson MJ, Bethell RC, Webster RG. Catalytic and framework mutations in the neuraminidase active site of influenza viruses that are resistant to 4-guanidino-Neu5Ac2en. *J Virol*. 1997; 71(5): 3385–3390.
232. Moscona A. Neuraminidase inhibitors for influenza. *N Engl J Med*. 2005; 353(13): 1363–1373.
233. Moscona A. Oseltamivir resistance—Disabling our influenza defenses. *N Engl J Med*. 2005; 353(25): 2633–2636.
234. Baranovich T, Webster RG, Govorkova EA. Fitness of neuraminidase inhibitor-resistant influenza A viruses. *Curr Opin Virol*. 2011; 1(6): 574–581.
235. Hurt AC, Holien JK, Parker MW, Barr IG. Oseltamivir resistance and the H274Y neuraminidase mutation in seasonal, pandemic and highly pathogenic influenza viruses. *Drugs*. 2009; 69(18): 2523–2531.
236. Meijer A, Lackenby A, Hungnes O, Lina B, van-der-Werf S, Schweiger B et al. Oseltamivir-resistant influenza virus A (H1N1), Europe, 2007–08 season. *Emerg Infect Dis*. 2009; 15(4): 552–560.
237. Centers for Disease Control and Prevention. Update: Influenza activity—United States and worldwide, May 20–September 22, 2012. *MMWR Morb Mortal Wkly Rep*. 2012; 61(39): 785–789.
238. Okomo-Adhiambo M, Sleeman K, Lysen C, Nguyen HT, Xu X, Li Y et al. Neuraminidase inhibitor susceptibility surveillance of influenza viruses circulating worldwide during the 2011 Southern Hemisphere season. *Influenza Other Respi Viruses*. 2013; 7(5): 645–658.
239. Centers for Disease Control and Prevention. Licensure of a high-dose inactivated influenza vaccine for persons aged > or = 65 years (Fluzone High-Dose) and guidance for use—United States, 2010. *MMWR Morb Mortal Wkly Rep*. 2010; 59(16): 485–486.
240. Murphy BR, Coelingh K. Principles underlying the development and use of live attenuated cold-adapted influenza A and B virus vaccines. *Viral Immunol*. 2002; 15(2): 295–323.
241. Ison MG, Gubareva LV, Atmar RL, Treanor J, Hayden FG. Recovery of drug-resistant influenza virus from immunocompromised patients: A case series. *J Infect Dis*. 2006; 193(6): 760–764.
242. Nguyen HT, Fry AM, Loveless PA, Klimov AI, Gubareva LV. Recovery of a multidrug-resistant strain of pandemic influenza A 2009 (H1N1) virus carrying a dual H275Y/I223R mutation from a child after prolonged treatment with oseltamivir. *Clin Infect Dis*. 2010; 51(8): 983–984.
243. Hurt AC, Holien JK, Parker M, Kelso A, Barr IG. Zanamivir-resistant influenza viruses with a novel neuraminidase mutation. *J Virol*. 2009; 83(20): 10366–10373.
244. Hernandez JE, Adiga R, Armstrong R, Bazan J, Bonilla H, Bradley J et al. Clinical experience in adults and children treated with intravenous peramivir for 2009 influenza A (H1N1) under an Emergency IND program in the United States. *Clin Infect Dis*. 2011; 52(6): 695–706.
245. Kohno S, Yen MY, Cheong HJ, Hirotsu N, Ishida T, Kadota J et al. Phase III randomized, double-blind study comparing single-dose intravenous peramivir with oral oseltamivir in patients with seasonal influenza virus infection. *Antimicrob Agents Chemother*. 2011; 55(11): 5267–5276.
246. Kohno S, Kida H, Mizuguchi M, Hirotsu N, Ishida T, Kadota J et al. Intravenous peramivir for treatment of influenza A and B virus infection in high-risk patients. *Antimicrob Agents Chemother*. 2011; 55(6): 2803–2812.
247. Ikematsu H, Kawai N. Laninamivir octanoate: A new long-acting neuraminidase inhibitor for the treatment of influenza. *Expert Rev Anti Infect Ther*. 2011; 9(10): 851–857.

248. Chamni S, De-Eknamkul W. Recent progress and challenges in the discovery of new neuraminidase inhibitors. *Expert Opin Ther Pat.* 2013; 23(4): 409–423.
249. Kiso M, Kubo S, Ozawa M, Le QM, Nidom CA, Yamashita M et al. Efficacy of the new neuraminidase inhibitor CS-8958 against H5N1 influenza viruses. *PLoS Pathog.* 2010; 6(2): e1000786.
250. Watanabe A, Chang SC, Kim MJ, Chu DW, Ohashi Y. Long-acting neuraminidase inhibitor laninamivir octanoate versus oseltamivir for treatment of influenza: A double-blind, randomized, noninferiority clinical trial. *Clin Infect Dis.* 2010; 51(10): 1167–1175.
251. Sugaya N, Ohashi Y. Long-acting neuraminidase inhibitor laninamivir octanoate (CS-8958) versus oseltamivir as treatment for children with influenza virus infection. *Antimicrob Agents Chemother.* 2010; 54(6): 2575–2582.
252. Furuta Y, Takahashi K, Shiraki K, Sakamoto K, Smee DF, Barnard DL et al. T-705 (favipiravir) and related compounds: Novel broad-spectrum inhibitors of RNA viral infections. *Antiviral Res.* 2009; 82(3): 95–102.
253. Furuta Y, Takahashi K, Fukuda Y, Kuno M, Kamiyama T, Kozaki K et al. *in vitro* and *in vivo* activities of anti-influenza virus compound T-705. *Antimicrob Agents Chemother.* 2002; 46(4): 977–981.
254. Furuta Y, Takahashi K, Kuno-Maekawa M, Sangawa H, Uehara S, Kozaki K et al. Mechanism of action of T-705 against influenza virus. *Antimicrob Agents Chemother.* 2005; 49(3): 981–986.
255. Malakhov MP, Aschenbrenner LM, Smee DF, Wandersee MK, Sidwell RW, Gubareva LV et al. Sialidase fusion protein as a novel broad-spectrum inhibitor of influenza virus infection. *Antimicrob Agents Chemother.* 2006; 50(4): 1470–1479.
256. Darwish I, Mubareka S, Liles WC. Immunomodulatory therapy for severe influenza. *Expert Rev Anti Infect Ther.* 2011; 9(7): 807–822.
257. Barik S. New treatments for influenza. *BMC Med.* 2012; 10: 104.
258. Centers for Disease Control and Prevention. Prevention and control of influenza with vaccines: Recommendations of the Advisory Committee on Immunization Practices (ACIP), 2011. *MMWR Morb Mortal Wkly Rep.* 2011; 60(33): 1128–1132.
259. World Health Organization. WHO recommendations on the composition of the 2013/14 influenza virus vaccines in the northern hemisphere. *Euro Surveill.* 2013; 18(9):pii=20411. Available online: http://www.eurosurveillance.org/ViewArticle.aspx?ArticleId=20411.
260. Belshe RB, Coelingh K, Ambrose CS, Woo JC, Wu X. Efficacy of live attenuated influenza vaccine in children against influenza B viruses by lineage and antigenic similarity. *Vaccine.* 2010; 28(9): 2149–2156.
261. Centers for Disease Control and Prevention. FluView: A Weekly Influenza Surveillance Report Prepared by the Influenza Division. 2012–2013 Influenza Season Week 14 ending April 6, 2013. 2013 [cited Accessed 04/16/13]; Available from: http://www.cdc.gov/flu/weekly
262. Frenck RW, Jr., Belshe R, Brady RC, Winokur PL, Campbell JD, Treanor J et al. Comparison of the immunogenicity and safety of a split-virion, inactivated, trivalent influenza vaccine (Fluzone(R)) administered by intradermal and intramuscular route in healthy adults. *Vaccine.* 2011; 29(34): 5666–5674.
263. Lerman SJ, Wright PF, Patil KD. Antibody decline in children following A/New Jersey/76 influenza virus immunization. *J Pediatr.* 1980; 96(2): 271–274.
264. Danke NA, Kwok WW. HLA class II-restricted CD4+ T cell responses directed against influenza viral antigens postinfluenza vaccination. *J Immunol.* 2003; 171(6): 3163–3169.
265. Edwards KM, Dupont WD, Westrich MK, Plummer WD, Jr., Palmer PS, Wright PF. A randomized controlled trial of cold-adapted and inactivated vaccines for the prevention of influenza A disease. *J Infect Dis.* 1994; 169(1): 68–76.
266. Tasker SA, Treanor JJ, Paxton WB, Wallace MR. Efficacy of influenza vaccination in HIV-infected persons. A randomized, double-blind, placebo-controlled trial. *Ann Intern Med.* 1999; 131(6): 430–433.
267. Frasca D, Diaz A, Romero M, Landin AM, Phillips M, Lechner SC et al. Intrinsic defects in B cell response to seasonal influenza vaccination in elderly humans. *Vaccine.* 2010; 28(51): 8077–8084.
268. Agarwal N, Ollington K, Kaneshiro M, Frenck R, Melmed GY. Are immunosuppressive medications associated with decreased responses to routine immunizations? A systematic review. *Vaccine.* 2012; 30(8): 1413–1424.
269. Ansaldi F, de Florentiis D, Durando P, Icardi G. Fluzone((R)) Intradermal vaccine: A promising new chance to increase the acceptability of influenza vaccination in adults. *Expert Rev Vaccines.* 2012; 11(1): 17–25.
270. Sullivan SJ, Jacobson R, Poland GA. Advances in the vaccination of the elderly against influenza: Role of a high-dose vaccine. *Expert Rev Vaccines.* 2010; 9(10): 1127–1133.
271. Couch RB, Winokur P, Brady R, Belshe R, Chen WH, Cate TR et al. Safety and immunogenicity of a high dosage trivalent influenza vaccine among elderly subjects. *Vaccine.* 2007; 25(44): 7656–7663.

While HPIVs themselves primarily cause asymptomatic infection outside their natural hosts, several closely related *Paramyxovirinae* viruses have been associated with respiratory infections in nonhuman mammals. For example, the Sendai virus shares many antigenic and genetic properties with HPIV-1 and is capable of causing respiratory disease in mice, hamsters, and pigs.[79] Simian viruses 5 and 41 are similar to HPIV-2 and can infect primates, while canine parainfluenza virus, also closely related to HPIV-2, can cause croup and lower respiratory disease in dogs.[81,117–120] Finally, bovine PIV-3 is antigenically related to HPIV-3 and has been associated with "shipping fever" in cattle and can also infect horses, sheep, goats, water buffaloes, deer, dogs, cats, monkeys, guinea pigs, rats, and pigs.[79,113,121–123] These models may be used to further understand the manifestations of HPIV disease in humans.

23.2.7 Viral Antigens

Antibodies to most of the HPIV viral proteins can be detected in the sera of both humans and animals following infection; however, only the HN and F proteins are capable of producing neutralizing antibodies.[5] Administration of polyclonal or monoclonal antibodies, vaccinia virus recombinants expressing HN or F glycoproteins, or purified HN and F glycoproteins have been shown to induce a high-level, long-lasting, protective immunological response.[119,124–131] While antibodies to proteins other than the HN and F proteins can be induced following infection, these antibodies elicit a weaker immune response and are only found in the serum for a short time following infection.[132]

There are a wide variety of HPIV-derived reagents designed to help scientists and clinicians better detect, identify, study, prevent, and further understand HPIVs. Preparations of HPIV proteins are among the easiest of these reagents to produce and can consist of purified HPIV virions (propagated *in vitro*), as well as purified HPIV virions that have been chemically and physically disrupted. These protein preparations can be used for several important functions. Whole virus preparations can be used in SDS-PAGE and Western blot analysis for detection of HPIV antibodies (or for differentiating which HPIV proteins specific antibodies react to). HPIV preparations can also be separated into the membrane-bound proteins (the HN, F, and M proteins) and the nucleocapsid (containing HPIV N, L, and P proteins in addition to genomic RNA) by disrupting the viral envelope with detergent followed by ultracentrifugation. This process is relatively straightforward and can be used to create HPIV protein preparations for antibody detection, antibody production, and vaccination.

A second useful type of HPIV viral reagents is monoclonal or polyclonal antibodies. These antibodies are often made by inoculating animals with virus preparations or purified viral antigens and are most commonly used in detection and differentiation of HPIV types. MAbs and PAbs can be used for viral detection with enzyme-linked immunosorbent assays (ELISAs), immunofluorescence assays (IFAs), hemagglutination inhibition assays (HIs), and Western blotting.

The third class of commonly used HPIV reagents is recombinant viral proteins. Recombinant viral proteins are prepared when viral proteins are cloned into bacterial or viral expression vectors, which in turn create a large amount of viral protein. Recombinant viral proteins have several advantages over whole virus or virus subunit preparations. For example, recombinant proteins can eliminate the presence of unwanted additional viral antigens from a protein preparation. These proteins are frequently used in the detection of viral antibodies from serum to indicate whether infection has occurred, or may also be used as subunit vaccines.

Finally, HPIV is one of the few negative-sense RNA viruses for which a reverse genetics system has been developed. Reverse genetics systems are a way of making infectious viruses starting with only nucleic acid. These systems are frequently used as research tools, allowing researchers to introduce specific mutations into the virus to determine their effect on virulence, replication, and so on. Reverse genetic systems are often used to introduce mutations that are known to attenuate viruses in an effort to create immunogenic, viable viruses with little or no ill effects on those individuals infected. These properties are the hallmark of a good vaccine and HPIV reverse genetic systems are already being widely used in that pursuit. These systems require transfection of cell cultures with either a plasmid encoding the complete genome or antigenomic RNA in addition to plasmids encoding the NP, P, and L proteins. The plasmids contain a T7 RNA polymerase promoter and RNA is expressed via T7 polymerase, which is supplied by a recombinant vaccinia virus or is constitutively expressed in the cell line. The viral components are expressed and translated forming a viral nucleocapsid, which then goes on to produce a true infection. This process is very inefficient, but it can produce enough infectious virus particles to infect a new culture in the same manner as a wild-type virus and create a significant amount of HPIV containing the desired mutations for use in future studies or downstream applications.[16,133–135]

23.3 EPIDEMIOLOGY

23.3.1 Geographic and Age Distribution

HPIV-1 to -4 have a wide geographic distribution and have been identified in virtually all areas where tissue culture, HAd, and RT-PCR have been used to study respiratory disease in children. These viruses are common community-acquired respiratory pathogens. Taken together, they are responsible for a significant amount of serious lower respiratory viral disease in children and adults. They are less frequent causes of upper respiratory tract infection (URI). One study of 4755 patients with "respiratory tract infections" indicates the following prevalence for HPIVs: HPIV-3 (2.1%), HPIV-1 (1.2%), HPIV-2 (0.4%), and HPIV-4 (0.2%).[136] Unlike some viruses, HPIV is not specifically associated with certain ethnic, economic, gender, or geographic characteristics, though HPIV infection is more likely in individuals who are malnourished, living in overcrowded environments, vitamin A deficient, or subjected to environmental smoke or toxins.[137–141] Upper respiratory tract infections with HPIVs are commonly found in people of all ages, from infants to the elderly, while lower respiratory tract infections with HPIV are most commonly associated with infants, young children, the elderly, and the immunocompromised.[79,142–148] In children under 5 years of age living in the United States, there are greater than 5 million cases of lower respiratory illness each year, with HPIV-1, -2, and -3 being the causative agent in as many as one-third of these cases; second only to respiratory syncytial virus (RSV).[11,144,147,149] Recent studies have indicated that approximately 500,000 children are hospitalized each year with acute respiratory infection or with lower respiratory illness, and that 23,000 and 65,000 of these cases, respectively, are caused by HPIV-1, -2, or -3.[149,150] HPIV-4 has been isolated more infrequently than HPIVs 1 through 3, likely owing to the fact that it is more difficult to recover.[5] However, serological studies indicate that most children between the ages of 6 and 10 have evidence of past infection, indicating that despite being recovered far less frequently, HPIV-4 is quite prevalent in the community.[151] Immunity to HPIVs is incomplete and reinfection with the same type of HPIV (particularly with HPIV-1 and -3) is not uncommon. One study showed that three outbreaks of HPIV-3 occurred in the same nursery over a 9-month time period and that 17% of the children infected in one outbreak were also infected during one of the subsequent outbreaks.[152]

23.3.1.1 HPIV-1

HPIV-1 commonly occurs in the fall and winter and is frequently defined by biennial epidemics.[138,147,153,154] During these epidemics, estimates indicate that 18,000–35,000 children under age 5 are hospitalized in the United States alone.[11,144,153,155–158] Many of these children are admitted with croup, and while all HPIVs are capable of causing croup, HPIV-1 is the most frequent cause, with estimates indicating that HPIV-1 may be the causative agent of >50% of all croup cases in the United States.[11,153,156] In addition to croup, HPIV-1 can also cause bronchiolitis, tracheobronchitis, pneumonia, and febrile and afebrile wheezing. The majority of HPIV-1 infections occur in children aged 7–36 months of age, with peak incidence occurring between 24 and 36 months of age (Table 23.1). HPIV-1 can also lead to hospitalization of normally healthy adults and has been linked to cases of bacterial pneumonia and deaths of nursing home citizens.

of HPIV infection can be measured in terms of lives lost, whereas in developed countries like the United States, fatal HPIV infection is very rare and the economic burden is more in terms of medical bills and loss of wages. One study in the early 1990s indicated that HPIV-1 and -2 could be collectively responsible for as many as 250,000 emergency room visits and 70,000 hospitalizations, at a cost of $50 million and $140 million, respectively.[180]

23.11 PATHOGENESIS AND IMMUNITY

23.11.1 Pathogenesis

The pathogenesis of HPIV still needs further clarification; however, there has been significant progress in the past decade, owing primarily to the development of the HAE culture model. As discussed earlier, the HAE model involves the use of cultured airway epithelium cells that are propagated at a liquid/air interface and mimic epithelial cells of the human airway. The epithelium of the respiratory tract is the primary site of HPIV infection, which begins with the binding of HN protein to the appropriate cellular receptors. HPIVs bind and enter superficial ciliated cells on the apical (lumenal) face and do not spread to the underlying basal cells or the goblet cells.[233–235] The release of progeny also occurs at the apical interface, which is consistent with the lack of viremia found in otherwise healthy individuals and also serves to limit viral exposure to blood-borne components of the host immune system.[236]

HPIV infection in nonpolarized cell lines *in vitro* often shows CPE characterized by significant cell-to-cell fusion/syncytium formation. However, examination of postmortem lung tissue from otherwise healthy individuals who died due to HPIV infection frequently shows very little evidence of syncytia formation, suggesting that this phenomenon may be relatively uncommon (though it has been observed in immunocompromised patients).[197,201,237–239] Unlike standard tissue culture models, HAE models of HPIV infection show very little sign of syncytia formation and may more closely mimic what happens *in vivo* during an HPIV infection. HPIV-infected HAE cultures do not show overt cytopathology; however, they do have accelerated rates of epithelial cell shedding and replacement, increased numbers of mucin-containing cells, and decreased ciliary function.[233,236] One recent study suggests that HPIV infection, possibly during the attachment phase of replication, leads to an increase in chloride ion secretion and decrease in sodium ion absorption across tracheal endothelium, which in turn leads to a buildup of fluid in the respiratory tract.[240] Collectively, these phenomena would increase the amount of fluid and mucus in the respiratory tract, while limiting the patient's ability to clear this excess buildup of fluid, mucus, and sloughed cells, which explains many of the clinical manifestations of HPIV infection.[236] The use of HAE cultures is a recent and powerful development in the study of HPIV infection and ongoing studies using this model will continue to reveal additional details of HPIV pathogenesis.

23.11.2 Immunology

Host defenses against HPIV infection are primarily mediated by humoral immunity to the major surface antigens (HN and F proteins).[131,241] Most children are born with neutralizing antibodies to all four HPIV serotypes; however, like most antibodies present at birth, the titer falls dramatically during the first 6 months of life. By age 5, most children have regained detectable levels of antibody to the surface antigens of at least one serotype of HPIV.[242] Shortly after infection, most children develop IgM responses, followed later by the presence of IgG, most often consisting of the IgG1 class.[243]

Primary infections with HPIV-3 frequently induce a much stronger response to the HN protein than the F protein, and subsequent infections with the same HPIV serotype are often required before a strong response is made to the F protein.[112,144] Early studies with SV5 indicated that neutralizing antibodies to the F protein appear to be more effective at preventing reinfection than those antibodies to the HN protein due to their ability to neutralize infectious virus and prevent cell-to-cell spread (HN antibodies have a lesser ability to disrupt cell-to-cell spread of HPIV).[244,245] These observations were initially described as the rationale for why reinfection with the same HPIV serotype is not uncommon, especially in children. However, subsequent studies have demonstrated that HPIVs require the HN and F proteins to function synergistically and that antibodies to the HN protein will significantly decrease the function of the F protein as well.[246,247] In addition, studies with recombinant HPIV-3 glycoproteins indicate that, in the cotton rat, recombinant HN protein provides a more effective immune response than does the F protein.[131,248] Therefore, a preferential immune response toward the HN protein is not necessarily the reason that infants and children are susceptible to reinfections with the same HPIV serotype. An alternative hypothesis for this phenomenon is that while children and adults both produce secretory IgA following HPIV infection, only older children and adults produce IgA that is capable of preventing and/or ameliorating clinical disease manifestations.[170,249–252] Children have decreased levels of HN antibody compared to adults, which may also contribute to the frequency of HPIV reinfection in infants and young children.[5,253]

In addition to neutralizing antibodies, studies have shown that cytotoxic lymphocytes (CTLs) also seem to play an important role in clearing HPIV from the lower respiratory tract.[114,254,255] Immunization of mice with a peptide containing a major epitope for CD+ CTLs induces a high level of resistance to Sendai virus, while mice that lack a specific CD8+ CTL response still managed to clear the infection, but succumb to a significantly lower lethal dose.[256] For mice lacking all classes of T cells but still producing natural killer cells, the lethal dose of Sendai virus was 300-fold lower than for wild-type mice. In addition, the survival time of Sendai virus-infected nude mice could be increased by nearly 32% or 79% following treatment with Sendai virus-specific CD8+ or CD4+ T cells, respectively. Furthermore, treatment with both CD4+ and CD8+ T cells could increase survival time by greater than 500%.[256] Meanwhile, treatment with interleukin 2 (IL-2) had no effect on the survival time in Sendai infected mice.[256] In nonlethal infection of mice with HPIV, removal of CD8+ T-cells resulted in a delayed viral clearance and a 20% mortality rate. Meanwhile, antibody-mediated depletion of CD4+ T cells inhibited antibody production and delayed viral clearance by 20%, but did not cause any mortality. Removal of these cells did not have any effect on the mouse's ability to mount a CD8+ CTL response, but removal of both CD4+ and CD8+ cell types led to failure to clear the HPIV infection and was 100% lethal.[255] Infections of infants and children with profound T-cell deficiencies can lead to fatal pneumonia, as CD8+ T cells play an important role in killing infected cells, while CD4+ T cells help antibody production in B cells.[197,255,256] Consistent with the observations seen in mice with Sendai virus, studies have shown that immunocompromised children and adults more commonly develop severe forms of disease and are capable of shedding virus for a much greater timeframe.[197,198,214,257] HPIV-induced pneumonia in patients recovering from bone marrow transplant carries a 30% mortality rate.[194]

Cytokines also likely play a role in protecting and clearing HPIV from the host. Gamma interferon, tumor necrosis factor, IL-2, IL-6, and IL-10 were all detected in the lungs of Sendai virus-infected mice.[258] Human peripheral leukocytes stimulated by Sendai virus produce macrophage inflammatory protein 1 alpha, monocyte chemotactic protein 1, tumor necrosis factor alpha, IL-6, and IL-8, all of which play an important role in clearing viral infection.[259]

23.12 DIAGNOSIS

Rapid and accurate diagnosis of HPIVs, and respiratory viruses in general, can play an important role in the treatment of hospitalized patients. Viruses are thought to be the causative agent of a majority of lower respiratory tract infections in children and at least 12% in hospitalized adults, and yet a disproportionate amount of patients are given antibiotics prior to determining the offending pathogen. Rapid and sensitive diagnostics can limit the number of unnecessary antibiotics given to hospitalized patients, decrease the number of unnecessary medical procedures and diagnostic tests

Following centrifugation, cells are placed onto a microscope slide via Pasteur pipet. Alternatively, in samples with low cellular content, cells may be added to the slide via cytocentrifugation. Once adhered to the slide, they are fixed in acetone, stained with the appropriate fluorescent antibodies, and visualized with a fluorescent microscope. The presence of fluorescence on the slide is indicative of the presence of HPIV antigen. If the viral load in the sample is low, detection rates may increase by first using the clinical sample to infect a tissue culture and then using the DFA stain on the cultured cells to determine if the offending virus is HPIV. The primary method of HPIV detection was (and may still be in some laboratories) to look for the presence of HPIV via DFA directly from the specimen and inoculate any negative samples into tissue culture for additional testing. However, with the advent of molecular diagnostics, commercial DFA reagents are harder to find, as are those laboratories with the appropriate equipment and technical expertise to perform these assays. For HPIV detection, the sensitivity of DFA from clinical specimens compared to detection by tissue culture is approximately 50–60%, though the specificity is generally considered to be excellent.[79]

23.12.8 Molecular Detection

The most common method of HPIV detection in the United States is via molecular detection of viral nucleic acid directly from the patient specimen. There are a large number of commercially available molecular diagnostics for the detection of HPIVs using several different approaches. All of these techniques begin via extraction of nucleic acid from the patient specimen, which may be performed via phenol/chloroform extraction, with commercial spin column extraction kits, or automated extraction machines. The extracted nucleic acid is then used in the appropriate molecular assay, the most common of which is real-time reverse transcriptase polymerase chain reaction (rRT-PCR), where a small, conserved portion of the HPIV genome is amplified and detected using HPIV-specific detection reagents. At present, the number of commercially available molecular diagnostics designed solely for the detection of HPIVs is limited. However, there are quite a few molecular diagnostic assays commercially available for use in simultaneously detecting several respiratory viruses, including HPIVs. Most of these assays are designed to differentiate HPIV-1, -2, and -3, but do not detect the presence of HPIV-4. As scientists/clinicians discover that HPIV-4 is an important cause of respiratory illness, it too is being incorporated into new molecular diagnostic assays. Studies have shown that molecular diagnostics can detect double or triple the number of HPIV-positive clinical specimens and can often do it in a fraction of the time associated with the classical HPIV detection methods.[276–278] The increased turnaround time is nearly as important as the increased detection rate. Standard detection methods can take days, while molecular tests can be completed in hours. This shorter turnaround time allows physicians to more effectively utilize the test results in patient treatment and can decrease the number of antibiotics prescribed, the number of additional diagnostic tests ordered, and even decrease the duration of stay in hospitalized patients.[260] One drawback of molecular diagnostics is the limited amount of genetic data available for HPIVs, which makes it more difficult to select appropriate target regions for each assay. Recent studies, including one that sequenced the complete genome of about 40 HPIV-1 strains, continue to add to our knowledge of HPIV genetics and demonstrate that there are numerous highly conserved regions of the genome that can be used as targets for new molecular diagnostics.[85] Similar studies are being performed with HPIV-3 and to a lesser extent HPIV-2 and -4.

23.13 PREVENTION AND CONTROL

As described earlier, estimates of HPIV infection in infants and young children indicate that HPIVs cause as at least as many episodes of acute respiratory infection and hospitalization as influenza viruses.[149,150] Influenza vaccination of this age group is universally recommended; however, there are currently no vaccines available for HPIV. The lack of a safe, efficacious HPIV vaccine is not for lack of trying, and development is hampered by two primary hurdles, including (1) most natural infections with HPIV occur in children at a very young age, and (2) the first natural HPIV infection often fails to confer sufficient immunity to prevent asymptomatic or even symptomatic reinfection.[279] These facts mean that a safe, efficacious vaccine would likely need to be administered at a very young age and would have to lead to a more robust immune response than is even seen during natural infection with HPIV. These are particularly difficult constraints given the fact that infants and young children have a less diverse B-cell repertoire, less efficient antibody affinity maturation, and the presence of maternal antibodies can decrease the immunogenicity of parenterally administered nonlive vaccines and mucosally administered live vaccines. These attributes all make the feasibility of creating a safe and efficacious vaccine to be administered to infants and young children a daunting task, yet progress is being made and several vaccine candidates are currently in clinical trials.[279]

Initial efforts toward an HPIV vaccine began in the 1960s, with clinical trials using formalin-killed HPIV-1, -2, and -3. These vaccines elicited antibodies to all three serotypes; however, the levels were not as high as those seen during natural infection and these vaccines were not effective in preventing children from subsequent severe HPIV infections.[280,281] In addition to inducing lower levels of antibody, the inactivated virus vaccines frequently lead to the production of nonneutralizing antibodies (at least nonneutralizing toward native viruses) and failed to induce the production of mucosal antibodies.[282]

Subsequent vaccines were prepared using naturally occurring attenuated HPIV strains. One of these vaccines made use of bovine HPIV-3. Human and bovine HPIV-3 viruses are similar antigenically and the bovine PIV-3 virus (bPIV-3) is capable of inducing strong immune responses to HPIV-3 in rats and primates. This vaccine exhibited similar results in children, but did not elicit a strong response in seropositive adults.[283–285] Similar efforts to make an HPIV-1 vaccine have been performed utilizing Sendai virus, which is the murine equivalent to HPIV-1.[279] A second type of live attenuated vaccine was developed by cold adaption. Cold-adapted vaccines are produced by passaging wild-type HPIVs in cell culture at a suboptimal temperature (in this case, 20°C or 22°C). After 45 passages, an isolate with good infectivity, immunogenicity, and stability was identified; however, this virus was still not an effective vaccine.[286,287] A final method for the production of a live-attenuated HPIV vaccine was to create "protease-activation" mutants, which are resistant to trypsin cleavage, but not to other proteases. These viruses can lead to an attenuated infection in humans; however, they have not been successfully developed into HPIV vaccines.[6,288,289]

Subunit vaccines for HPIV-3 have also been developed with little success. These vaccines generally consist of HPIV-3 HN and F glycoproteins that have been isolated from purified virus preparations or that have been produced using baculovirus expression systems.[130,248,290–292] The baculovirus-derived glycoproteins appeared very similar to native antigens, induced an acceptable amount of neutralizing HN and F protein antibodies, induced an IgA response, and elicited a neutralizing immune response in cotton rats against intranasal HPIV-3 infection.[129] However, these proteins, which were highly immunogenic in small mammals, proved to be much less immunogenic in chimpanzees or humans.[293] In addition, studies have shown that subunit vaccines can be less immunogenic to completely naïve hosts and that the presence of passively acquired antibodies can also further suppress the immune response induced by subunit vaccines. This makes the utility of such vaccines questionable in the group that needs them the most; infants and young children who are at the highest risk for severe HPIV infection are the least capable of benefitting from subunit vaccines.[294]

Current approaches to HPIV vaccines make use of recombinant viruses. These are also live attenuated viruses; however, the difference between these viruses and the ones previously described are that the attenuating mutations are engineered into the genome by scientists. Reverse genetics systems for HPIV are among the first such systems to be ever used and have been around for quite some time. Scientists have tried to engineer several different recombinant vaccines in recent years. The first approach has been to replace the HN and F genes from a bovine HPIV-3 virus with those from a human HPIV-3.[295–297] A second approach has been to swap the HN and F genes of the previously described cold-passaged HPIV-1 with wild-type HPIV-1 HN and F genes.[298,299] Third, site-directed mutagenesis has been used to alter specific nucleotides corresponding with attenuating mutations in other *Paramyxoviruses*. This strategy has been implemented for HPIV-1 and -2 and incorporates specific attenuating mutations into the P/C and L genes of wild-type viruses.[300–302] Finally, two different vaccines have been made in which the previously described recombinant virus containing the HPIV-3 HN and F genes in the bovine HPIV-3 backbone were further altered to also include either the RSV G and F genes or the F gene alone. These vaccines are an effort to create a bivalent vaccine for RSV and HPIV-3, and the vaccine containing the RSV F gene alone has shown success in clinical trials.[303–306] Recombinant viruses currently appear to be the most promising approach to creating a safe, efficacious HPIV (and RSV) vaccine, and several candidates remain in development and clinical trials.[279]

23.14 TREATMENT

In addition to vaccination for disease prevention, scientists are also working on the development of antiviral compounds that can be used to effectively treat HPIV infection. To date there is no currently licensed antiviral compound for treatment of HPIV, but several treatments have shown anecdotal success in controlling/treating HPIV infection in humans.

Possible treatment options currently available for HPIV infection include high-titer pooled immunoglobulins (immunotherapy), steroids, and ribavirin (inhaled and/or IV) administered alone or in some combination. These therapies have been shown to decrease pulmonary virus titer and inflammation in cotton rats.[307–311] In addition, oral and systemic steroids have shown possible benefit in decreasing symptoms of croup in as little as 6 h posttreatment.[312] Meanwhile, combination therapy with ribavirin and methylprednisolone have demonstrated some success in treating immunocompromised patients with pneumonia, and immunotherapy combined with intravenous ribavirin has been used to treat HPIV-2 viremia and myocarditis.[313–315]

Several additional therapies have been tried in the treatment of HPIV infection. One study showed that in a patient with severe HPIV-3 pneumonia, a combination of the anti-influenza medication peramivir and intravenous erythromycin may have rapidly improved the patient's lung function (the erythromycin served more as an immune system modulator rather than having a direct antiviral effect).[316] Another study indicated that the novel sialidase fusion protein DAS181 may be successfully used in the treatment of HPIV-3 infections in immunocompromised hosts.[317]

Finally, several compounds have been recently identified as having anti-HPIV activity *in vitro*. These compounds include novel small molecules, small interfering RNAs, neuraminidase inhibitors (zanamivir), protein synthesis inhibitors (puromycin), nucleic acid synthesis inhibitors, benzithiazole derivatives, carbocyclic-3-deezaadenosine, α-glucosidase inhibitors, α-mannosidase inhibitors, ascorbic acid, calcium elenolate, extracts of *Sanicula europaea* leaves, and legume lectins (including concanavalin A).[318–335] Despite having some *in vitro* activity, none of these compounds has yet been used in a clinical setting.

REFERENCES

1. Chanock RM, Parrott RH, Bell JA, Rowe WP, Huebner RJ. New viruses observed in children with respiratory diseases. *Public Health Rep* 1958; 73: 193–195.
2. Chanock RM, Parrott RH, Cook K, Andrews BE, Bell JA, Reichelderfer T et al. Newly recognized myxoviruses from children with respiratory disease. *N Engl J Med* 1958; 258: 207–213.
3. Chanock RM. Association of a new type of cytopathogenic myxovirus with infantile croup. *J Exp Med* 1956; 104: 555–576.
4. Howe C, Morgan C, de Vaux St Cyr C, Hsu KC, Rose HM. Morphogenesis of type 2 parainfluenza virus examined by light and electron microscopy. *J Virol* 1967; 1: 215–237.
5. Chanock RM, Murphy BR, Collins PL. Parainfluenza Viruses. In: Knipe DM, Howley PM, eds. *Fields Virology*. 4th ed. Philadelphia , PA: Lippincott, Williams and Wilkins; 2001. 1341–1379.

6. Tashiro M, Homma M. Protection of mice from wild-type Sendai virus infection by a trypsin-resistant mutant, TR-2. *J Virol* 1985; 53: 228–234.
7. Sánchez A, Banerjee AK. Studies on human parainfluenza virus 3: Characterization of the structural proteins and *in vitro* synthesized proteins coded by mRNAs isolated from infected cells. *Virology* 1985; 143: 45–54.
8. Cowley JA, Barry RD. Characterization of human parainfluenza viruses. I. The structural proteins of parainfluenza virus 2 and their synthesis in infected cells. *J Gen Virol* 1983; 64: 2117–2125.
9. Storey DG, Dimock K, Kang CY. Structural characterization of virion proteins and genomic RNA of human parainfluenza virus 3. *J Virol* 1984; 52: 761–766.
10. Wechsler SL, Lambert DM, Galinski MS, Heineke BE, Pons MW. Human parainfluenza virus 3: Purification and characterization of subviral components, viral proteins and viral RNA. *Virus Res* 1985; 3: 339–351.
11. Denny FW, Clyde WA. Acute lower respiratory tract infections in nonhospitalized children. *J Pediatr* 1986; 108: 635–646.
12. Spriggs MK, Collins PL. Human parainfluenza virus type 3: Messenger RNAs, polypeptide coding assignments, intergenic sequences, and genetic map. *J Virol* 1986; 59: 646–654.
13. Komada H, Tsurudome M, Bando H, Nishio M, Ueda M, Tsumura H et al. Immunological response of monkeys infected intranasally with human parainfluenza virus type 4. *J Gen Virol* 1989; 70: 3487–3492.
14. Kolakofsky D, Pelet T, Garcin D, Hausmann S, Curran J, Roux L. Paramyxovirus RNA synthesis and the requirement for hexamer genome length: The rule of six revisited. *J Virol* 1998; 72: 891–899.
15. Durbin AP, Siew JW, Murphy BR, Collins PL. Minimum protein requirements for transcription and RNA replication of a minigenome of human parainfluenza virus type 3 and evaluation of the rule of six. *Virology* 1997; 234: 74–83.
16. Hoffman MA, Banerjee AK. An infectious clone of human parainfluenza virus type 3. *J Virol* 1997; 71: 4272–4277.
17. Horikami SM, Curran J, Kolakofsky D, Moyer SA. Complexes of Sendai virus NP-P and P-L proteins are required for defective interfering particle genome replication in vitro. *J Virol* 1992; 66: 4901–4908.
18. Buchholz CJ, Spehner D, Drillien R, Neubert WJ, Homann HE. The conserved N-terminal region of Sendai virus nucleocapsid protein NP is required for nucleocapsid assembly. *J Virol* 1993; 67: 5803–5812.
19. Curran J, Homann H, Buchholz C, Rochat S, Neubert W, Kolakofsky D. The hypervariable C-terminal tail of the Sendai paramyxovirus nucleocapsid protein is required for template function but not for RNA encapsidation. *J Virol* 1993; 67: 4358–4364.
20. Buchholz CJ, Retzler C, Homann HE, Neubert WJ. The carboxy-terminal domain of Sendai virus nucleocapsid protein is involved in complex formation between phosphoprotein and nucleocapsid-like particles. *Virology* 1994; 204: 770–776.
21. Byrappa S, Gupta KC. Human parainfluenza virus type 1 phosphoprotein is constitutively phosphorylated at Ser-120 and Ser-184. *J Gen Virol* 1999; 80: 1199–1209.
22. Byrappa S, Hendricks DD, Pan YB, Seyer JM, Gupta KC. Intracellular phosphorylation of the Sendai virus P protein. *Virology* 1995; 208: 408–413.
23. Byrappa S, Pan YB, Gupta KC. Sendai virus P protein is constitutively phosphorylated at serine249: high phosphorylation potential of the P protein. *Virology* 1996; 216: 228–234.
24. Bowman MC, Smallwood S, Moyer SA. Dissection of individual functions of the Sendai virus phosphoprotein in transcription. *J Virol* 1999; 73: 6474–6483.
25. Komada H, Tsurudome M, Ueda M, Nishio M, Bando H, Ito Y. Isolation and characterization of monoclonal antibodies to human parainfluenza virus type 4 and their use in revealing antigenic relation between subtypes 4A and 4B. *Virology* 1989; 171: 28–37.
26. Curran J, Boeck R, Kolakofsky D. The Sendai virus P gene expresses both an essential protein and an inhibitor of RNA synthesis by shuffling modules via mRNA editing. *EMBO J* 1991; 10: 3079–3085.
27. Spriggs MK, Collins PL. Sequence analysis of the P and C protein genes of human parainfluenza virus type 3: Patterns of amino acid sequence homology among paramyxovirus proteins. *J Gen Virol* 1986; 67: 2705–2719.
28. Curran J. A role for the Sendai virus P protein trimer in RNA synthesis. *J Virol* 1998; 72: 4274–4280.
29. Curran J. Reexamination of the Sendai virus P protein domains required for RNA synthesis: A possible supplemental role for the P protein. *Virology* 1996; 221: 130–140.
30. Ryan KW, Portner A. Separate domains of Sendai virus P protein are required for binding to viral nucleocapsids. *Virology* 1990; 174: 515–521.
31. Coronel EC, Murti KG, Takimoto T, Portner A. Human parainfluenza virus type 1 matrix and nucleoprotein genes transiently expressed in mammalian cells induce the release of virus-like particles containing nucleocapsid-like structures. *J Virol* 1999; 73: 7035–7038.

131. Spriggs MK, Murphy BR, Prince GA, Olmsted RA, Collins PL. Expression of the F and HN glycoproteins of human parainfluenza virus type 3 by recombinant vaccinia viruses: Contributions of the individual proteins to host immunity. *J Virol* 1987; 61: 3416–3423.
132. Tao T, Davoodi F, Cho CJ, Skiadopoulos MH, Durbin AP, Collins PL et al. A live attenuated recombinant chimeric parainfluenza virus (PIV) candidate vaccine containing the hemagglutinin-neuraminidase and fusion glycoproteins of PIV1 and the remaining proteins from PIV3 induces resistance to PIV1 even in animals immune to PIV3. *Vaccine* 2000; 18: 1359–1366.
133. He B, Paterson RG, Ward CD, Lamb RA. Recovery of infectious SV5 from cloned DNA and expression of a foreign gene. *Virology* 1997; 237: 249–260.
134. Durbin AP, Hall SL, Siew JW, Whitehead SS, Collins PL, Murphy BR. Recovery of infectious human parainfluenza virus type 3 from cDNA. *Virology* 1997; 235: 323–332.
135. Garcin D, Pelet T, Calain P, Roux L, Curran J, Kolakofsky D. A highly recombinogenic system for the recovery of infectious Sendai paramyxovirus from cDNA: Generation of a novel copy-back nondefective interfering virus. *EMBO J* 1995; 14: 6087–6094.
136. Liu WK, Liu Q, Chen DH, Liang HX, Chen XK, Huang WB et al. Epidemiology and clinical presentation of the four human parainfluenza virus types. *BMC Infect Dis* 2013; 13: 28.
137. Berman S. Epidemiology of acute respiratory infections in children of developing countries. *Rev Infect Dis* 1991; 13: S454–S462.
138. Carballal G, Videla CM, Espinosa MA, Savy V, Uez O, Sequeira MD et al. Multicentered study of viral acute lower respiratory infections in children from four cities of Argentina, 1993–1994. *J Med Virol* 2001; 64: 167–174.
139. Kim MR, Lee HR, Lee GM. Epidemiology of acute viral respiratory tract infections in Korean children. *J Infect* 2000; 41: 152–158.
140. McIntosh K. Pathogenesis of severe acute respiratory infections in the developing world: Respiratory syncytial virus and parainfluenza viruses. *Rev Infect Dis* 1991; 13: S492–S500.
141. Tsai HP, Kuo PH, Liu CC, Wang JR. Respiratory viral infections among pediatric inpatients and outpatients in Taiwan from 1997 to 1999. *J Clin Microbiol* 2001; 39: 111–118.
142. Falsey AR. Noninfluenza respiratory virus infection in long-term care facilities. *Infect Control Hosp Epidemiol* 1991; 12: 602–608.
143. Falsey AR, Cunningham CK, Barker WH, Kouides RW, Yuen JB, Menegus M et al. Respiratory syncytial virus and influenza A infections in the hospitalized elderly. *J Infect Dis* 1995; 172: 389–394.
144. Glezen WP, Frank AL, Taber LH, Kasel JA. Parainfluenza virus type 3: Seasonality and risk of infection and reinfection in young children. *J Infect Dis* 1984; 150: 851–857.
145. Glezen WP, Greenberg SB, Atmar RL, Piedra PA, Couch RB. Impact of respiratory virus infections on persons with chronic underlying conditions. *JAMA* 2000; 283: 499–505.
146. Lamy ME, Pouthier-Simon F, Debacker-Willame E. Respiratory viral infections in hospital patients with chronic bronchitis. Observations during periods of exacerbation and quiescence. *Chest* 1973; 63: 336–341.
147. Murphy B, Phelan PD, Jack I, Uren E. Seasonal pattern in childhood viral lower respiratory tract infections in Melbourne. *Med J Aust* 1980; 1: 22–24.
148. Whimbey E, Champlin RE, Couch RB, Englund JA, Goodrich JM, Raad I et al. Community respiratory virus infections among hospitalized adult bone marrow transplant recipients. *Clin Infect Dis* 1996; 22: 778–782.
149. Weinberg GA, Hall CB, Iwane MK, Poehling KA, Edwards KM, Griffin MR et al. Parainfluenza virus infection of young children: Estimates of the population-based burden of hospitalization. *J Pediatr* 2009; 154: 694–699.
150. Henrickson KJ, Hoover S, Kehl KS, Hua W. National disease burden of respiratory viruses detected in children by polymerase chain reaction. *Pediatr Infect Dis J* 2004; 23: S11–S18.
151. Gardner SD. The isolation of parainfluenza 4 subtypes A and B in England and serological studies of their prevalence. *J Hyg (Lond)* 1969; 67: 545–550.
152. Chanock RM, Parrott RH, Johnson KM, Kapikian AZ, Bell JA. Myxoviruses: Parainfluenza. *Am Rev Respir Dis* 1963; 88: S152–S166.
153. Marx A, Török TJ, Holman RC, Clarke MJ, Anderson LJ. Pediatric hospitalizations for croup (laryngotracheobronchitis): biennial increases associated with human parainfluenza virus 1 epidemics. *J Infect Dis* 1997; 176: 1423–1427.
154. Fry AM, Curns AT, Harbour K, Hutwagner L, Holman RC, Anderson LJ. Seasonal trends of human parainfluenza viral infections: United States, 1990–2004. *Clin Infect Dis* 2006; 43: 1016–1022.
155. Belshe RB, Van Voris LP, Mufson MA. Impact of viral respiratory diseases on infants and young children in a rural and urban area of southern West Virginia. *Am J Epidemiol* 1983; 117: 467–474.

156. Denny FW, Murphy TF, Clyde WA, Collier AM, Henderson FW. Croup: An 11-year study in a pediatric practice. *Pediatrics* 1983; 71: 871–876.
157. Henrickson KJ, Kuhn SM, Savatski LL, Sedmak J. Recovery of human parainfluenza virus types one and two. *J Virol Methods* 1994; 46: 189–205.
158. Skolnik NS. Treatment of croup. A critical review. *Am J Dis Child* 1989; 143: 1045–1049.
159. Downham MA, McQuillin J, Gardner PS. Diagnosis and clinical significance of parainfluenza virus infections in children. *Arch Dis Child* 1974; 49: 8–15.
160. Washburne JF, Bocchini JA, Jamison RM. Summertime respiratory syncytial virus infection: Epidemiology and clinical manifestations. *South Med J* 1992; 85: 579–583.
161. de Silva LM, Cloonan MJ. Brief report: Parainfluenza virus type 3 infections: Findings in Sydney and some observations on variations in seasonality world-wide. *J Med Virol* 1991; 35: 19–21.
162. Mufson MA, Mocega HE, Krause HE. Acquisition of parainfluenza 3 virus infection by hospitalized children. I. Frequencies, rates, and temporal data. *J Infect Dis* 1973; 128: 141–147.
163. Singh-Naz N, Willy M, Riggs N. Outbreak of parainfluenza virus type 3 in a neonatal nursery. *Pediatr Infect Dis J* 1990; 9: 31–33.
164. Karron RA, O'Brien KL, Froehlich JL, Brown VA. Molecular epidemiology of a parainfluenza type 3 virus outbreak on a pediatric ward. *J Infect Dis* 1993; 167: 1441–1445.
165. Chanock RM, Parrott RH. Acute respiratory disease in infancy and childhood: Present understanding and prospects for prevention. *Pediatrics* 1965; 36: 21–39.
166. Killgore GE, Dowdle WR. Antigenic characterization of parainfluenza 4A and 4B by the hemagglutination-inhibition test and distribution of HI antibody in human sera. *Am J Epidemiol* 1970; 91: 308–316.
167. Lindquist SW, Darnule A, Istas A, Demmler GJ. Parainfluenza virus type 4 infections in pediatric patients. *Pediatr Infect Dis J* 1997; 16: 34–38.
168. Lau SK, Li KS, Chau KY, So LY, Lee RA, Lau YL et al. Clinical and molecular epidemiology of human parainfluenza virus 4 infections in hong kong: Subtype 4B as common as subtype 4A. *J Clin Microbiol* 2009; 47: 1549–1552.
169. McLean DM, Bannatyne RM, Givan KF. Myxovirus dissemination by air. *Can Med Assoc J* 1967; 96: 1449–1453.
170. Smith CB, Purcell RH, Bellanti JA, Chanock RM. Protective effect of antibody to parainfluenza type 1 virus. *N Engl J Med* 1966; 275: 1145–1152.
171. Kapikian AZ, Bell JA, Mastrota FM, Huebner RJ, Wong DC, Chanock RM. An outbreak of parainfluenza 2 (croup-associated) virus infection. Association with acute undifferentiated febrile illness in children. *JAMA* 1963; 183: 324–330.
172. Tyrrell DA, Bynoe ML, Petersen KB, Sutton RN, Pereira MS. Inoculation of human volunteers with parainfluenza viruses types 1 and 3 (HA 2 and HA 1). *Br Med J* 1959; 2: 909–911.
173. Tyrrell DA, Bynoe ML. Studies on parainfluenza type 2 and 4 viruses obtained from patients with common colds. *Br Med J* 1969; 1: 471–474.
174. Murphy BR, Richman DD, Chalhub EG, Uhlendorf CP, Baron S, Chanock RM. Failure of attenuated temperature-sensitive influenza A (H3N2) virus to induce heterologous interference in humans to parainfluenza type 1 virus. *Infect Immun* 1975; 12: 62–68.
175. Kapikian AZ, Chanock RM, Reichelderfer TE, Ward TG, Huebner RJ, Bell JA. Inoculation of human volunteers with parainfluenza virus type 3. *JAMA* 1961; 178: 537–541.
176. Lessler J, Reich NG, Brookmeyer R, Perl TM, Nelson KE, Cummings DA. Incubation periods of acute respiratory viral infections: A systematic review. *Lancet Infect Dis* 2009; 9: 291–300.
177. Frank AL, Taber LH, Wells CR, Wells JM, Glezen WP, Paredes A. Patterns of shedding of myxoviruses and paramyxoviruses in children. *J Infect Dis* 1981; 144: 433–441.
178. Gross PA, Green RH, Curnen MG. Persistent infection with parainfluenza type 3 virus in man. *Am Rev Respir Dis* 1973; 108: 894–898.
179. Ruuskanen O, Arola M, Heikkinen T, Ziegler T. Viruses in acute otitis media: Increasing evidence for clinical significance. *Pediatr Infect Dis J* 1991; 10: 425–427.
180. Henrickson KJ, Kuhn SM, Savatski LL. Epidemiology and cost of infection with human parainfluenza virus types 1 and 2 in young children. *Clin Infect Dis* 1994; 18: 770–779.
181. Woo PC, Young K, Tsang KW, Ooi CG, Peiris M, Yuen K. Adult croup: A rare but more severe condition. *Respiration* 2000; 67: 684–688.
182. van der Hoek L, Sure K, Ihorst G, Stang A, Pyrc K, Jebbink MF et al. Croup is associated with the novel coronavirus NL63. *PLoS Med* 2005; 2: e240.
183. van der Hoek L, Sure K, Ihorst G, Stang A, Pyrc K, Jebbink MF et al. Human coronavirus NL63 infection is associated with croup. *Adv Exp Med Biol* 2006; 581: 485–491.

184. Sung JY, Lee HJ, Eun BW, Kim SH, Lee SY, Lee JY et al. Role of human coronavirus NL63 in hospitalized children with croup. *Pediatr Infect Dis J* 2010; 29: 822–826.
185. Kellner G, Popow-Kraupp T, Kundi M, Binder C, Wallner H, Kunz C. Contribution of rhinoviruses to respiratory viral infections in childhood: A prospective study in a mainly hospitalized infant population. *J Med Virol* 1988; 25: 455–469.
186. Jennings LC, Dawson KP, Abbott GD, Allan J. Acute respiratory tract infections of children in hospital: A viral and Mycoplasma pneumoniae profile. *N Z Med J* 1985; 98: 582–585.
187. Dowell SF, Anderson LJ, Gary HE, Erdman DD, Plouffe JF, File TM et al. Respiratory syncytial virus is an important cause of community-acquired lower respiratory infection among hospitalized adults. *J Infect Dis* 1996; 174: 456–462.
188. Drews AL, Atmar RL, Glezen WP, Baxter BD, Piedra PA, Greenberg SB. Dual respiratory virus infections. *Clin Infect Dis* 1997; 25: 1421–1429.
189. Greenberg SB. Viral pneumonia. *Infect Dis Clin North Am* 1991; 5: 603–621.
190. Korppi M, Halonen P, Kleemola M, Launiala K. Viral findings in children under the age of two years with expiratory difficulties. *Acta Paediatr Scand* 1986; 75: 457–464.
191. Marx A, Gary HE, Marston BJ, Erdman DD, Breiman RF, Török TJ et al. Parainfluenza virus infection among adults hospitalized for lower respiratory tract infection. *Clin Infect Dis* 1999; 29: 134–140.
192. Fiore AE, Iverson C, Messmer T, Erdman D, Lett SM, Talkington DF et al. Outbreak of pneumonia in a long-term care facility: Antecedent human parainfluenza virus 1 infection may predispose to bacterial pneumonia. *J Am Geriatr Soc* 1998; 46: 1112–1117.
193. Srinivasan A, Wang C, Yang J, Inaba H, Shenep JL, Leung WH et al. Parainfluenza virus infections in children with hematologic malignancies. *Pediatr Infect Dis J* 2011; 30: 855–859.
194. Wendt CH, Weisdorf DJ, Jordan MC, Balfour HH, Hertz MI. Parainfluenza virus respiratory infection after bone marrow transplantation. *N Engl J Med* 1992; 326: 921–926.
195. Karp D, Willis J, Wilfert CM. Parainfluenza virus II and the immunocompromised host. *Am J Dis Child* 1974; 127: 592–593.
196. Henry RL, Hodges IG, Milner AD, Stokes GM. Respiratory problems 2 years after acute bronchiolitis in infancy. *Arch Dis Child* 1983; 58: 713–716.
197. Delage G, Brochu P, Pelletier M, Jasmin G, Lapointe N. Giant-cell pneumonia caused by parainfluenza virus. *J Pediatr* 1979; 94: 426–429.
198. Frank JA, Warren RW, Tucker JA, Zeller J, Wilfert CM. Disseminated parainfluenza infection in a child with severe combined immunodeficiency. *Am J Dis Child* 1983; 137: 1172–1174.
199. Little BW, Tihen WS, Dickerman JD, Craighead JE. Giant cell pneumonia associated with parainfluenza virus type 3 infection. *Hum Pathol* 1981; 12: 478–481.
200. McIntosh K, Kurachek SC, Cairns LM, Burns JC, Goodspeed B. Treatment of respiratory viral infection in an immunodeficient infant with ribavirin aerosol. *Am J Dis Child* 1984; 138: 305–308.
201. Weintrub PS, Sullender WM, Lombard C, Link MP, Arvin A. Giant cell pneumonia caused by parainfluenza type 3 in a patient with acute myelomonocytic leukemia. *Arch Pathol Lab Med* 1987; 111: 569–570.
202. King JC, Burke AR, Clemens JD, Nair P, Farley JJ, Vink PE et al. Respiratory syncytial virus illnesses in human immunodeficiency virus- and noninfected children. *Pediatr Infect Dis J* 1993; 12: 733–739.
203. King JC. Community respiratory viruses in individuals with human immunodeficiency virus infection. *Am J Med* 1997; 102: 19–24; discussion 5–6.
204. Beard LJ, Robertson EF, Thong YH. Para-influenza pneumonia in DiGeorge syndrome two years after thymic epithelial transplantation. *Acta Paediatr Scand* 1980; 69: 403–406.
205. Josephs S, Kim HW, Brandt CD, Parrott RH. Parainfluenza 3 virus and other common respiratory pathogens in children with human immunodeficiency virus infection. *Pediatr Infect Dis J* 1988; 7: 207–209.
206. Apalsch AM, Green M, Ledesma-Medina J, Nour B, Wald ER. Parainfluenza and influenza virus infections in pediatric organ transplant recipients. *Clin Infect Dis* 1995; 20: 394–399.
207. Lewis VA, Champlin R, Englund J, Couch R, Goodrich JM, Rolston K et al. Respiratory disease due to parainfluenza virus in adult bone marrow transplant recipients. *Clin Infect Dis* 1996; 23: 1033–1037.
208. Ljungman P, Gleaves CA, Meyers JD. Respiratory virus infection in immunocompromised patients. *Bone Marrow Transplant* 1989; 4: 35–40.
209. Waner JL, Whitehurst NJ, Downs T, Graves DG. Production of monoclonal antibodies against parainfluenza 3 virus and their use in diagnosis by immunofluorescence. *J Clin Microbiol* 1985; 22: 535–538.
210. Nichols WG, Corey L, Gooley T, Davis C, Boeckh M. Parainfluenza virus infections after hematopoietic stem cell transplantation: Risk factors, response to antiviral therapy, and effect on transplant outcome. *Blood* 2001; 98: 573–578.

211. Luján-Zilbermann J, Benaim E, Tong X, Srivastava DK, Patrick CC, DeVincenzo JP. Respiratory virus infections in pediatric hematopoietic stem cell transplantation. *Clin Infect Dis* 2001; 33: 962–968.
212. Arola M, Ruuskanen O, Ziegler T, Salmi TT. Respiratory virus infections during anticancer treatment in children. *Pediatr Infect Dis J* 1995; 14: 690–694.
213. Zambon M, Bull T, Sadler CJ, Goldman JM, Ward KN. Molecular epidemiology of two consecutive outbreaks of parainfluenza 3 in a bone marrow transplant unit. *J Clin Microbiol* 1998; 36: 2289–2293.
214. Fishaut M, Tubergen D, McIntosh K. Cellular response to respiratory viruses with particular reference to children with disorders of cell-mediated immunity. *J Pediatr* 1980; 96: 179–186.
215. Bitnun A, Ford-Jones EL, Petric M, MacGregor D, Heurter H, Nelson S et al. Acute childhood encephalitis and Mycoplasma pneumoniae. *Clin Infect Dis* 2001; 32: 1674–1684.
216. Vreede RW, Schellekens H, Zuijderwijk M. Isolation of parainfluenza virus type 3 from cerebrospinal fluid. *J Infect Dis* 1992; 165: 1166.
217. Lewandowski LJ, Lief FS, Verini MA, Pienkowski MM, ter Meulen V, Koprowski H. Analysis of a viral agent isolated from multiple sclerosis brain tissue: Characterization as a parainfluenzavirus type 1. *J Virol* 1974; 13: 1037–1045.
218. ter Meulen V, Koprowski H, Iwasaki Y, Käckell YM, Müller D. Fusion of cultured multiple-sclerosis brain cells with indicator cells: Presence of nucleocapsids and virions and isolation of parainfluenza-type virus. *Lancet* 1972; 2: 1–5.
219. Román G, Phillips CA, Poser CM. Parainfluenza virus type 3: Isolation from CSF of a patient with Guillain-Barré syndrome. *JAMA* 1978; 240: 1613–1615.
220. Arguedas A, Stutman HR, Blanding JG. Parainfluenza type 3 meningitis. Report of two cases and review of the literature. *Clin Pediatr (Phila)* 1990; 29: 175–178.
221. McCarthy VP, Carlile JR, Reichelderfer PS, Clark JS. Parainfluenza type 3 in newborns. *Pediatr Infect Dis J* 1987; 6: 217–218.
222. Meissner HC, Murray SA, Kiernan MA, Snydman DR, McIntosh K. A simultaneous outbreak of respiratory syncytial virus and parainfluenza virus type 3 in a newborn nursery. *J Pediatr* 1984; 104: 680–684.
223. Seidman DS, Nass D, Mendelson E, Shehtman I, Mashiach S, Achiron R. Prenatal ultrasonographic diagnosis of fetal hydrocephalus due to infection with parainfluenza virus type 3. *Ultrasound Obstet Gynecol* 1996; 7: 52–54.
224. Kashiwagi Y, Kawashima H, Kanetaka Y, Ioi H, Takekuma K, Hoshika A et al. Sudden infant death syndrome due to parainfluenza virus 2 associated with hemophagocytic syndrome. *J Infect* 2004; 49: 329–332.
225. Hotez PJ, Goldstein B, Ziegler J, Doveikis SA, Pasternack MS. Adult respiratory distress syndrome associated with parainfluenza virus type 1 in children. *Pediatr Infect Dis J* 1990; 9: 750–752.
226. Grattan-Smith T, Forer M, Kilham H, Gillis J. Viral supraglottitis. *J Pediatr* 1987; 110: 434–435.
227. Perämäki E, Salmi I, Kava T, Romppanen T, Hakkarainen T. Unilateral bronchiolitis obliterans organizing pneumonia and bronchoalveolar lavage neutrophilia in a patient with parainfluenza 3 virus infection. *Respir Med* 1991; 85: 159–161.
228. Phillips MJ, Blendis LM, Poucell S, offterson J, Petric M, Roberts E et al. Syncytial giant-cell hepatitis. Sporadic hepatitis with distinctive pathological features, a severe clinical course, and paramyxoviral features. *N Engl J Med* 1991; 324: 455–460.
229. Abenhaim Halpern L, Agyeman P, Steinlin M, El-Koussy M, Grunt S. Mild encephalopathy with splenial lesion and parainfluenza virus infection. *Pediatr Neurol* 2013; 48: 252–254.
230. Mastroyianni SD, Voudris KA, Katsarou E, Gionnis D, Mavromatis P, Vagiakou EA et al. Acute necrotizing encephalopathy associated with parainfluenza virus in a Caucasian child. *J Child Neurol* 2003; 18: 570–572.
231. Phillips PE, Christian CL. Myxovirus antibody increases in human connective tissue disease. *Science* 1970; 168: 982–984.
232. Wilks D, Burns SM. Myopericarditis associated with parainfluenza virus type 3 infection. *Eur J Clin Microbiol Infect Dis* 1998; 17: 363–365.
233. Zhang L, Bukreyev A, Thompson CI, Watson B, Peeples ME, Collins PL et al. Infection of ciliated cells by human parainfluenza virus type 3 in an *in vitro* model of human airway epithelium. *J Virol* 2005; 79: 1113–1124.
234. Bartlett EJ, Hennessey M, Skiadopoulos MH, Schmidt AC, Collins PL, Murphy BR et al. Role of interferon in the replication of human parainfluenza virus type 1 wild type and mutant viruses in human ciliated airway epithelium. *J Virol* 2008; 82: 8059–8070.

235. Schaap-Nutt A, Scull MA, Schmidt AC, Murphy BR, Pickles RJ. Growth restriction of an experimental live attenuated human parainfluenza virus type 2 vaccine in human ciliated airway epithelium *in vitro* parallels attenuation in African green monkeys. *Vaccine* 2010; 28: 2788–2798.
236. Schomacker H, Schaap-Nutt A, Collins PL, Schmidt AC. Pathogenesis of acute respiratory illness caused by human parainfluenza viruses. *Curr Opin Virol* 2012; 2: 294–299.
237. Downham MA, Gardner PS, McQuillin J, Ferris JA. Role of respiratory viruses in childhood mortality. *Br Med J* 1975; 1: 235–239.
238. Aherne W, Bird T, Court SD, Gardner PS, McQuillin J. Pathological changes in virus infections of the lower respiratory tract in children. *J Clin Pathol* 1970; 23: 7–18.
239. Jarvis WR, Middleton PJ, Gelfand EW. Parainfluenza pneumonia in severe combined immunodeficiency disease. *J Pediatr* 1979; 94: 423–425.
240. Kunzelmann K, König J, Sun J, Markovich D, King NJ, Karupiah G et al. Acute effects of parainfluenza virus on epithelial electrolyte transport. *J Biol Chem* 2004; 279: 48760–48766.
241. Kasel JA, Frank AL, Keitel WA, Taber LH, Glezen WP. Acquisition of serum antibodies to specific viral glycoproteins of parainfluenza virus 3 in children. *J Virol* 1984; 52: 828–832.
242. Morgan OW, Chittaganpitch M, Clague B, Chantra S, Sanasuttipun W, Prapasiri P et al. Hospitalization due to human parainfluenza virus-associated lower respiratory tract illness in rural Thailand. *Influenza Other Respi Viruses* 2013; 7: 280–285.
243. Julkunen I, Hovi T, Seppälä I, Mäkelä O. Immunoglobulin G subclass antibody responses in influenza A and parainfluenza type 1 virus infections. *Clin Exp Immunol* 1985; 60: 130–138.
244. Merz DC, Scheid A, Choppin PW. Importance of antibodies to the fusion glycoprotein of paramyxoviruses in the prevention of spread of infection. *J Exp Med* 1980; 151: 275–288.
245. Merz DC, Scheid A, Choppin PW. Immunological studies of the functions of paramyxovirus glycoproteins. *Virology* 1981; 109: 94–105.
246. Portner A, Scroggs RA, Metzger DW. Distinct functions of antigenic sites of the HN glycoprotein of Sendai virus. *Virology* 1987; 158: 61–68.
247. Iorio RM, Glickman RL, Sheehan JP. Inhibition of fusion by neutralizing monoclonal antibodies to the haemagglutinin-neuraminidase glycoprotein of Newcastle disease virus. *J Gen Virol* 1992; 73: 1167–1176.
248. Brideau RJ, Oien NL, Lehman DJ, Homa FL, Wathen MW. Protection of cotton rats against human parainfluenza virus type 3 by vaccination with a chimeric FHN subunit glycoprotein. *J Gen Virol* 1993; 74: 471–477.
249. Hrusková J, Fedová D, Syrůcek L, Penningerová S, Holanová L, Berkovicová V. Haemagglutination inhibition antibodies in nasal secretions of persons after natural parainfluenza virus infection. *Acta Virol* 1978; 22: 203–208.
250. Tremonti LP, Lin JS, Jackson GG. Neutralizing activity in nasal secretions and serum in resistance of volunteers to parainfluenza virus type 2. *J Immunol* 1968; 101: 572–577.
251. Welliver R, Wong DT, Choi TS, Ogra PL. Natural history of parainfluenza virus infection in childhood. *J Pediatr* 1982; 101: 180–187.
252. Yanagihara R, McIntosh K. Secretory immunological response in infants and children to parainfluenza virus types 1 and 2. *Infect Immun* 1980; 30: 23–28.
253. Belshe RB, Karron RA, Newman FK, Anderson EL, Nugent SL, Steinhoff M et al. Evaluation of a live attenuated, cold-adapted parainfluenza virus type 3 vaccine in children. *J Clin Microbiol* 1992; 30: 2064–2070.
254. Henderson FW. Pulmonary cell-mediated cytotoxicity in hamsters with parainfluenza virus type 3 pneumonia. *Am Rev Respir Dis* 1979; 120: 41–47.
255. Hou S, Doherty PC, Zijlstra M, Jaenisch R, Katz JM. Delayed clearance of Sendai virus in mice lacking class I MHC-restricted CD8+ T cells. *J Immunol* 1992; 149: 1319–1325.
256. Kast WM, Bronkhorst AM, de Waal LP, Melief CJ. Cooperation between cytotoxic and helper T lymphocytes in protection against lethal Sendai virus infection. Protection by T cells is MHC-restricted and MHC-regulated; a model for MHC-disease associations. *J Exp Med* 1986; 164: 723–738.
257. Rabella N, Rodriguez P, Labeaga R, Otegui M, Mercader M, Gurguí M et al. Conventional respiratory viruses recovered from immunocompromised patients: Clinical considerations. *Clin Infect Dis* 1999; 28: 1043–1048.
258. Mo XY, Sarawar SR, Doherty PC. Induction of cytokines in mice with parainfluenza pneumonia. *J Virol* 1995; 69: 1288–1291.
259. Hua J, Liao MJ, Rashidbaigi A. Cytokines induced by Sendai virus in human peripheral blood leukocytes. *J Leukoc Biol* 1996; 60: 125–128.

260. Henrickson KJ. Cost-effective use of rapid diagnostic techniques in the treatment and prevention of viral respiratory infections. *Pediatr Ann* 2005; 34: 24–31.
261. Pavia AT. Viral infections of the lower respiratory tract: Old viruses, new viruses, and the role of diagnosis. *Clin Infect Dis* 2011; 52: S284–S289.
262. Mandell LA, Wunderink RG, Anzueto A, Bartlett JG, Campbell GD, Dean NC et al. Infectious Diseases Society of America/American Thoracic Society consensus guidelines on the management of community-acquired pneumonia in adults. *Clin Infect Dis* 2007; 44: S27–S72.
263. Kim JK, Jeon JS, Kim JW, Rheem I. Epidemiology of respiratory viral infection using multiplex rt-PCR in cheonan, Korea (2006–2010). *J Microbiol Biotechnol* 2013; 23: 267–273.
264. Pretorius MA, Madhi SA, Cohen C, Naidoo D, Groome M, Moyes J et al. Respiratory viral coinfections identified by a 10-plex real-time reverse-transcription polymerase chain reaction assay in patients hospitalized with severe acute respiratory illness—South Africa, 2009–2010. *J Infect Dis* 2012; 206: S159–S165.
265. Franková V, Holubová J, Grubhoffer L, Kasová V. Contribution to laboratory diagnosis of mumps and parainfluenza. *Acta Virol* 1988; 32: 503–514.
266. Julkunen I. Serological diagnosis of parainfluenza virus infections by enzyme immunoassay with special emphasis on purity of viral antigens. *J Med Virol* 1984; 14: 177–187.
267. Lennette EH, Jensen FW, Guenther RW, Magoffin RL. Serologic responses to para-influenza viruses in patients with mumps virus injection. *J Lab Clin Med* 1963; 61: 780–788.
268. Vuorinen T, Meurman O. Enzyme immunoassays for detection of IgG and IgM antibodies to parainfluenza types 1, 2, and 3. *J Virol Methods* 1989; 23: 63–70.
269. Herrmann EC, Hable KA. Experiences in laboratory diagnosis of parainfluenza viruses in routine medical practice. *Mayo Clin Proc* 1970; 45: 177–188.
270. Gardner PS, McQuillin J, McGuckin R, Ditchburn RK. Observations on clinical and immunofluorescent diagnosis of parainfluenza virus infections. *Br Med J* 1971; 2: 7–12.
271. Stout C, Murphy MD, Lawrence S, Julian S. Evaluation of a monoclonal antibody pool for rapid diagnosis of respiratory viral infections. *J Clin Microbiol* 1989; 27: 448–452.
272. Doane FW, Anderson N, Zbitnew A, Rhodes AJ. Application of electron microscopy to the diagnosis of virus infections. *Can Med Assoc J* 1969; 100: 1043–1049.
273. Hierholzer JC, Bingham PG, Coombs RA, Johansson KH, Anderson LJ, Halonen PE. Comparison of monoclonal antibody time-resolved fluoroimmunoassay with monoclonal antibody capture-biotinylated detector enzyme immunoassay for respiratory syncytial virus and parainfluenza virus antigen detection. *J Clin Microbiol* 1989; 27: 1243–1249.
274. Hietala J, Uhari M, Tuokko H. Antigen detection in the diagnosis of viral infections. *Scand J Infect Dis* 1988; 20: 595–599.
275. Sarkkinen HK, Halonen PE, Salmi AA. Type-specific detection of parainfluenza viruses by enzyme-immunoassay and radioimmunoassay in nasopharyngeal specimens of patients with acute respiratory disease. *J Gen Virol* 1981; 56: 49–57.
276. Kuypers J, Wright N, Ferrenberg J, Huang ML, Cent A, Corey L et al. Comparison of real-time PCR assays with fluorescent-antibody assays for diagnosis of respiratory virus infections in children. *J Clin Microbiol* 2006; 44: 2382–2388.
277. Lee BE, Robinson JL, Khurana V, Pang XL, Preiksaitis JK, Fox JD. Enhanced identification of viral and atypical bacterial pathogens in lower respiratory tract samples with nucleic acid amplification tests. *J Med Virol* 2006; 78: 702–710.
278. Freymuth F, Vabret A, Cuvillon-Nimal D, Simon S, Dina J, Legrand L et al. Comparison of multiplex PCR assays and conventional techniques for the diagnostic of respiratory virus infections in children admitted to hospital with an acute respiratory illness. *J Med Virol* 2006; 78: 1498–1504.
279. Schmidt AC, Schaap-Nutt A, Bartlett EJ, Schomacker H, Boonyaratanakornkit J, Karron RA et al. Progress in the development of human parainfluenza virus vaccines. *Expert Rev Respir Med* 2011; 5: 515–526.
280. Chin J, Magoffin RL, Shearer LA, Schieble JH, Lennette EH. Field evaluation of a respiratory syncytial virus vaccine and a trivalent parainfluenza virus vaccine in a pediatric population. *Am J Epidemiol* 1969; 89: 449–463.
281. Fulginiti VA, Eller JJ, Sieber OF, Joyner JW, Minamitani M, Meiklejohn G. Respiratory virus immunization. I. A field trial of two inactivated respiratory virus vaccines; an aqueous trivalent parainfluenza virus vaccine and an alum-precipitated respiratory syncytial virus vaccine. *Am J Epidemiol* 1969; 89: 435–448.
282. Murphy BR, Graham BS, Prince GA, Walsh EE, Chanock RM, Karzon DT et al. Serum and nasal-wash immunoglobulin G and A antibody response of infants and children to respiratory syncytial virus F and G glycoproteins following primary infection. *J Clin Microbiol* 1986; 23: 1009–1014.

325. Saladino R, Crestini C, Palamara AT, Danti MC, Manetti F, Corelli F et al. Synthesis, biological evaluation, and pharmacophore generation of uracil, 4(3H)-pyrimidinone, and uridine derivatives as potent and selective inhibitors of parainfluenza 1 (Sendai) virus. *J Med Chem* 2001; 44: 4554–4562.
326. Soret MG. Antiviral activity of calcium elenolate on parainfluenza infection of hamsters. *Antimicrob Agents Chemother (Bethesda)* 1969; 9: 160–166.
327. White LA, Freeman CY, Forrester BD, Chappell WA. *In vitro* effect of ascorbic acid on infectivity of herpesviruses and paramyxoviruses. *J Clin Microbiol* 1986; 24: 527–531.
328. Wyde PR, Ambrose MW, Meyer HL, Gilbert BE. Toxicity and antiviral activity of LY253963 against respiratory syncytial and parainfluenza type 3 viruses in tissue culture and in cotton rats. *Antiviral Res* 1990; 14: 237–247.
329. Wyde PR, Ambrose MW, Meyer HL, Zolinski CL, Gilbert BE. Evaluation of the toxicity and antiviral activity of carbocyclic 3-deazaadenosine against respiratory syncytial and parainfluenza type 3 viruses in tissue culture and in cotton rats. *Antiviral Res* 1990; 14: 215–225.
330. Wyde PR, Moore DK, Pimentel DM, Blough HA. Evaluation of the antiviral activity of N-(phosphonoacetyl)-L-aspartate against paramyxoviruses in tissue culture and against respiratory syncytial virus in cotton rats. *Antiviral Res* 1995; 27: 59–69.
331. Mao H, Thakur CS, Chattopadhyay S, Silverman RH, Gudkov A, Banerjee AK. Inhibition of human parainfluenza virus type 3 infection by novel small molecules. *Antiviral Res* 2008; 77: 83–94.
332. Bitko V, Musiyenko A, Shulyayeva O, Barik S. Inhibition of respiratory viruses by nasally administered siRNA. *Nat Med* 2005; 11: 50–55.
333. Uematsu J, Koyama A, Takano S, Ura Y, Tanemura M, Kihira S et al. Legume lectins inhibit human parainfluenza virus type 2 infection by interfering with the entry. *Viruses* 2012; 4: 1104–1115.
334. Tanaka Y, Kato J, Kohara M, Galinski MS. Antiviral effects of glycosylation and glucose trimming inhibitors on human parainfluenza virus type 3. *Antiviral Res* 2006; 72: 1–9.
335. Bumcrot D, Manoharan M, Koteliansky V, Sah DW. RNAi therapeutics: A potential new class of pharmaceutical drugs. *Nat Chem Biol* 2006; 2: 711–719.

24 Emergence and Pathogenesis of Avian Influenza in Humans

Jennifer R. Plourde and Kevin S. Harrod

CONTENTS

24.1 INTRODUCTION

Influenza viruses cause global epidemics annually and occasional pandemics, such as the 1918 "Spanish influenza" and the more recent 2009 H1N1 "Swine flu" pandemic.[1] Three to five million humans are infected with influenza viruses worldwide each year, with an estimated 250,000–500,000 deaths.[2] The virus typically causes a mild or severe respiratory illness that commonly presents as a sudden onset of fever, myalgia, dry cough, headache, sore throat, runny nose, anorexia, and generally feeling unwell.[2,3] This highly contagious virus is easily transmissible among humans, and an incubation time of approximately 1–5 days assists in the widespread transmission of the disease.[2,3] Vaccines are available for the expected circulating strains of seasonal influenza at the beginning of the influenza season each year, and vaccination has been estimated to prevent approximately 60% of influenza infections but varies each season.[4] Despite a global immunization effort, influenza epidemics continue with new strains arising with resistance to immunization. Unfortunately, immunized individuals can still be infected, and only about 40% of Americans were vaccinated each season over the past four influenza seasons (2009–2010, 2010–2011, 2011–2012, and 2012–present), leaving the majority of the population vulnerable to disease.[5]

Highly pathogenic avian influenza (HPAI) circulates among wild waterfowl and can infect humans through zoonotic transmission. HPAI, subtype H5N1, emerged in humans in 1997 without any reassortment with a human influenza strain.[6–19] Vaccines are being developed but are not readily available, and early vaccines were shown to be ineffective without the addition of an adjuvant.[20–22] Between 2003 and 2013, the World Health Organization (WHO) confirmed cases of H5N1 infection been identified, 13 of these have been considered inactive and have not been detected since 2008.[39] The eradication of the 13 strains could have been the result of limited or reduced fitness, or high mortality exhibited in the host that prohibited efficient transmission.

24.3 H5N1 VIRUS REPLICATION

Replication of influenza viruses begins with the attachment to host epithelial cells of the respiratory tract expressing specific host receptors. It has been shown that the surface glycoproteins (such as HA) bind to neuraminic acids (e.g., sialic acids) on the cell's surface to initiate infection and replication. Generally, human influenza viruses preferentially bind to an *N*-acetylneuraminic acid that is attached to the ending galactose sugar by an α2,6 linkage (SAα2,6Gal) commonly found in the upper respiratory tract, while avian influenza viruses preferentially attach to sialic acids with an α2,3 linkage, which are found in the lower respiratory tract of humans.[42] While human influenza virus receptors are prominent in the respiratory tract and lungs, receptors for avian influenza (SAα2,3Gal) have been found on type II pneumocytes, bronchi, bronchioli, trachea, a few epithelial cells in the upper respiratory tract, cells outside the respiratory tract, Kupffer cells, glomerular cells, splenic T lymphocytes, and neurons in the brain and intestine.[43] The absence of avian influenza receptors in the upper airway could explain the lack of efficient human-to-human transmission of H5N1. Importantly, some avian H7 viruses of North American lineages and H9N2 viruses that have infected humans possess increased binding of α2,6Gal similar to that of human influenza A viruses, which have significant implications for the transmissibility of these emerging viruses.[44–46] While there are species-specific receptor preferences, controversial research has shown that as few as four mutations in the HA segment can confer increased transmission of H5N1 in a ferret model of experimental infection.[47,48] Importantly, these findings suggest that H5N1 strains may only require a few mutations before acquiring significantly increased transmissibility in humans.

After attachment to the host cell, influenza viruses are internalized into endocytic compartments via clathrin-mediated endocytosis[49] or nonclathrin, noncaveoliae-mediated endocytosis.[50] The viral HA undergoes a structural change after the HA0 precursor is cleaved into HA1 and HA2. It has been suggested that the cleavage of human influenza virus HA proteins is completed by type II transmembrane serine proteases and human airway trypsin-like protease. HPAI viruses of the H5 and H7 subtype, however, do not require these specific proteases and the HA protein can be cleaved by ubiquitously expressed subtilisin-like and furin-like proteases.[51–54] Several cleaved HA molecules undergoing conformational changes in the acidic environment of the endosome results in uncoating and releasing contents of the virion into the cytoplasm.[55] The first few steps of the viral replication cycle occur quickly, with the majority of virus particles entering the cytoplasm from the endosome about 25 min after internalization and RNP complexes reaching the nucleus only 10 min later.[56]

Subsequent to fusion of the virus to the host cell, the ion channel activity of matrix 2 (M2), an integral membrane protein, induces the virus to dissociate the RNP complex from the virus. Additional roles of the M2 protein include assembly, budding, and the ratio of filamentous and spherical particles.[57–59] This protein is highly conserved and is believed to be a good target for developing a universal influenza vaccine.[60] The antiviral medicines amantadine and rimantadine target the influenza A M2 protein to inhibit viral uncoating or disassembly of the virion during endocytosis. New antiviral treatments need to be developed in light of many influenza A viruses that have now acquired resistance to amantadine through mutations in the M2 segment.[61,62]

The viral RNP (vRNP) consists of viral RNA, which is coated by NP, and has the PB1, PB2, and PA proteins bound to the partially complementary ends of the viral RNA. The vRNP enters the nucleus where viral RNA synthesis occurs. The vRNPs are too large for passive diffusion and use active nuclear import mechanisms of the cell to reach the nucleus. While all proteins in the vRNP have nuclear localization signals, it has been shown that the signals on the NP are both sufficient and necessary for viral RNA import into the nucleus.[32]

Once the negative-sense viral RNA is imported into the nucleus, replication occurs following a two-step process. A full-length positive-sense copy, termed complementary RNA (cRNA), of the viral RNA is made from the negative-sense strand. The cRNA is used as a template to generate more viral genomic RNA. Additionally, the negative-sense viral RNA is also transcribed into viral messenger RNA (mRNA) by a primer-dependent mechanism. The mRNA are not full copies of the viral RNA and are capped and polyadenylated. The reaction of viral RNA to mRNA, viral RNA to cRNA, and cRNA to viral RNA are all catalyzed by the same RNA-dependent RNA polymerase (RdRp) complex composed of the influenza PB1, PB2, and PA proteins and is packaged within the virion.[32]

Influenza RdRp replicates the viral genome and transcribes viral mRNA encoding proteins. Through a process known as "cap-snatching," a 5′ capped primer is taken from host pre-mRNA transcripts and used to initiate mRNA synthesis.[63,64] The same polymerase used for transcription is used for polyadenylation of the mRNA transcripts. A stretch of five to seven uracil residues and an adjacent double-stranded region of the viral RNA promoter are required for polyadenylation.[65–67] In addition to translation of eight influenza proteins from the eight mRNAs generated through transcription, the translation of M and NS mRNA can result in two proteins due to splicing (such as M1 and M2, and NS1 and NEP/NS2, respectively).[32]

In addition to acting as a template for mRNA synthesis, viral RNA is also used as a template for cRNA, which is full length and is not capped or polyadenylated. The RdRp used for mRNA synthesis in a primer-dependent manner is also used to generate cRNA independent of a primer.[32,64,68] Soon after the virion contents are released and imported to the nucleus, the RNPs are only capable of transcription.[32] If the process is interrupted at this step, there will be an accumulation of mRNA in the cell. The switch from mRNA synthesis to cRNA synthesis is not fully understood and several hypotheses have been suggested.[32,64,68] One hypothesis is that an accumulation of NP is required to produce full-length cRNA, which only occurs after translation.[32] An alternate model is that a switch does not occur, but NP and the polymerase have a stabilization role and both mRNA and cRNA are made early during infection but cRNA is degraded until enough NP exists to encapsidate the cRNA.[68] More recently, it has been shown that the concentrations of capped cellular mRNA, the 5′-end of the viral RNA, and the RdRp regulate the switch between transcription and replication.[64]

Once viral RNA has been synthesized from cRNA, it must be exported from the nucleus. However, before being exported to the cytoplasm, the newly generated viral RNA must be encapsidated by NP and form an RNP complex with PB1, PB2, and PA. These complexes are then exported through the functions of M1 and NEP/NS2. The M1 protein has been shown to associate with the lipid membrane and interact with vRNP and NEP/NS2. Following export to the cytoplasm, influenza viruses are packaged and assembled at the apical plasma membrane of polarized cells, where they can bud out of the host cell. Budding will not occur in the absence of M1. Additionally, once the virus particle buds from the cell, its envelope remains attached to the cell membrane and NA is required to remove the sialic acid from the carbohydrate to complete the budding process. Without NA, the particle cannot be released from the cell.[32]

24.4 EPIDEMIOLOGY

Wild aquatic birds are the natural reservoir for influenza A viruses, with only three known subtypes having emerged in humans as pandemic strains: H1N1 (1918 and 2009), H2N2 (1957), and H3N2 (1968).[69] Generally, influenza viruses are species-specific and interspecies transmission is not common. Recently, some avian influenza viruses have shown zoonotic transmission to other mammals such as horses,[70] pigs,[71] and whales[72] without reassortment. In fact, the influenza strains that caused the 1957 and 1968 human pandemics were reassortant strains of both human and avian viruses believed to have originated in pigs. Reassortant strains can arise when a host, such as a pig, acquires two or more influenza strains concurrently. Following replication of multiple strains, progeny virions can contain segments from one or more strains of influenza and continue to spread among new hosts.[28]

hospitalization.[10] Supplemental oxygen should be provided in the event of hypoxemia, and oxygen saturation should be monitored at presentation and routinely during care.[177] Broad-spectrum antibiotics are commonly used as an initial treatment along with antiviral agents, alone or with corticosteroids. Early intervention with antiviral agents may be beneficial, though no decrease in mortality has been observed when treatment is started late in infection.[78,106,177]

Currently, oseltamivir (trade name Tamiflu®), an oral antiviral agent, is the primary treatment recommended for H5N1 infection in humans, especially when administered in the early stages of the disease.[177,178] It has also been suggested that late treatment with oseltamivir may also be beneficial since H5N1 continues to replicate late in infection.[162] As soon as H5N1 infection is suspected, patients should be started on a standard 5-day course of therapy.[177] On a case-by-case basis, oseltamivir can be delivered at a twofold higher dosage, for longer periods of time, or in combination with amantadine or rimantadine. These combination therapies are thought to be especially useful in patients with pneumonia or progressive disease.[177] Despite early administration of standard doses of oseltamivir, H5N1 disease can still progress to a fatal outcome. The possibility of infection with an oseltamivir-resistant virus can also result in a poor outcome, despite treatment.[162] Zanamivir (trade name Relenza) is an inhaled NA inhibitor that can also be used to treat H5N1 infection and several others are under development: peramivir, pyrrolidine derivative A315675, and long-acting R-118958 and FLUNET compounds.[179] Currently, it is unknown whether other NA inhibitors will be beneficial in treating H5N1 infection.[177] When NA inhibitors are available, the WHO does not recommend monotherapy with amantadine or rimantadine.[177]

Adamantanes such as amantadine have been used in early treatment of H5N1 infections and have had clinical benefits.[105,177] In seasonal influenza infection, this drug has been associated with the emergence of resistant influenza strains, and the majority of H3N2 and H1N1 viruses are now resistant to adamantanes.[180–182] A combination of treatment with oseltamivir and adamantanes has been shown to have enhanced antiviral activity and a reduction in the emergence of resistant strains.[183] Therefore, combination therapy should be considered in areas where there are likely adamantane-susceptible strains of H5N1 and should not be used where virus isolates are known to be adamantane-resistant. When this combination is used, respiratory samples should be collected for serial virological monitoring to identify any emerging resistance.[177]

It is not advised to use corticosteroids routinely, but they can be used for septic shock with suspected adrenal insufficiency requiring vasopressors to cause vasoconstriction and maintain or increase blood pressure. Caution should be used when treating with corticosteroids for long periods or with high doses to reduce serious adverse events or opportunistic infection. Unless pneumonia is present, antibiotic chemoprophylaxis should not be used to treat H5N1 infection. However, antibiotics are appropriate for community-acquired pneumonia.[177]

24.11 PREVENTION AND CONTROL

Surveillance is critical for the identification of HPAI outbreaks as soon as possible in avian species and humans. It is especially important to conduct surveillance on poultry since most human infections are the result of contact with infected birds and because of the significant economic losses that result from infected poultry.[69] Humans most commonly acquire H5N1 influenza infection following contact with infected poultry, either through direct contact, plucking and preparing diseased birds, handling fighting cocks, playing with infected poultry, or consuming undercooked infected poultry.[77] The first step in identifying a potential outbreak in humans is to identify HPAI in poultry as soon as possible.[184] Currently, surveillance protocols are in place worldwide and include enhanced biosecurity, surveillance, culling of flocks, and restricting movement of poultry.[185]

Since human-to-human transmission of H5N1 influenza is inefficient and humans are most commonly infected through direct contact with infected poultry, the most efficient form of control is to avoid or limit contact with sick poultry or suspected cases of H5N1 infection, especially in geographic areas where H5N1 is known to circulate. When individuals must work with suspected or confirmed H5N1 patients or animals, full-barrier precautions should be implemented (e.g., washing hands; wearing gowns, gloves, face shields or goggles; using a particulate respirator such as an N95, EU FFP2, or equivalent; and negative-pressure isolation rooms).[69]

24.11.1 Vaccination in Poultry

Inactivated vaccines and some recombinant live virus vaccines were developed for use in poultry to prevent infection with H5N1 and have been successful in increasing resistance to infection and decreasing virus shedding, morbidity, mortality, transmissibility, and virus replication.[186,187] Despite the seeming success of existing vaccines in poultry, much discussion remains regarding whether or not they drive antigenic drift or conceal continued circulation of the virus among the poultry population.[179] Additional problems with vaccinating domestic poultry arise from the inability to control poultry smuggling, immunize domestic ducks, and maintain poultry vaccinations. These issues led to the re-emergence of H5N1 in Vietnam, after widespread vaccination of domestic poultry eliminated the incidence of infection in humans and domestic chickens between 2005 and 2007.[179] Additionally, vaccinations for all poultry imported to Hong Kong were successful for 7 years but are currently less effective due to the vaccine requiring an update.[179]

Several problems with the current vaccine strategy have been identified that reduce the efficiency of vaccinations to control H5N1 outbreaks in poultry.[188] The specificity to a single HA subtype is unlikely to be effective where multiple subtypes (e.g., H5, H7, and H9) are cocirculating. When birds are vaccinated, they develop antibodies against the specific subtype, which confounds routine serological surveillance and hinders the differentiation between previously infected birds and vaccinated birds. Another issue is that vaccination may prevent clinical signs of infection but not prevent infection, which may allow for "silent infection," the continued circulation of the virus, and incidental infection of humans. Vaccines can also induce immune pressure and increase the evolution rate and antigenic drift, resulting in viruses with better evasion of the host-immune response. The emergence of new variants can then render the vaccine inefficient or useless in the protection of birds until a new vaccine can be developed.[188]

24.11.2 Human Vaccines

The previous emergence of pandemic influenza strains and the subsequent development of vaccines demonstrated that prior immune priming is necessary to induce an effective antibody response. In the absence of priming, two doses are likely needed to confer protection in an individual.[69]

While new influenza vaccines are developed and produced for epidemic strains of human influenza each year, the methods used to test immunogenicity work poorly for H5N1 strains. Disagreement in procedures and the determination of protective titers have not been standardized and evaluation of new vaccines has been difficult. Additionally, the method used to generate seasonal vaccines does not work for H5N1 viruses, since highly pathogenic strains kill the embryonated eggs used in vaccine production before high viral antigen titers can develop. The use of nonattenuated H5N1 viruses also requires vaccine manufacturing plants with enhanced biosafety containment. Efforts have been made to overcome these obstacles, such as using low pathogenic avian influenza strains (e.g., H5N3) or reverse genetics to remove the multibasic amino acids at the HA cleavage site to reduce pathogenicity.[69] Additionally, using the HA and NA of the H5N1 candidate vaccine strain on the backbone of the laboratory strain A/PR8/34 results in a virus that can grow to high titers in eggs and enhance antigenic yield.[189]

Not knowing which H5N1 strain will become pandemic makes the development of an effective vaccine even more complicated. The high mutation rate of influenza viruses and antigenic drift constantly occurring warrant careful consideration when choosing a candidate vaccine strain. The WHO identified several strains from various clades as candidates for developing vaccines that will protect against currently circulating H5N1 viruses.[69]

Vaccines are under development, but early vaccines were shown to be ineffective without the addition of an adjuvant.[20–22] Vaccines generated using the plasmid-based reverse genetics system and one of the WHO recommended candidate viruses have been shown to be effective in healthy adults after two doses with 90 μg of HA. It is important to note that this amount of protein is much higher than what is found in seasonal influenza vaccines and complicates the production of such a vaccine on a large scale. Some studies have shown that H5N1 subunit vaccines adjuvanted with aluminum phosphate have modestly increased immunogenicity but not enough to justify large-scale production. The use of an alum-adjuvant in a whole virus H5N1 vaccine has been shown to result in reasonable immunogenicity at two doses of only 10 μg and may prove to be a better candidate for large-scale production.[190]

REFERENCES

1. Henry J, Smeyne RJ, Jang H, Miller B, Okun MS. Parkinsonism and neurological manifestations of influenza throughout the 20th and 21st centuries. *Parkinsonism Relat Disord* 2010; 16(9): 566–571.
2. WHO. Influenza (Seasonal) Fact Sheet. April 2009; Available at: http://www.who.int/mediacentre/factsheets/fs211/en/index.html. Accessed March 2013.
3. Studahl M. Influenza virus and CNS manifestations. *J Clin Virol* 2003; 28(3): 225–232.
4. Centers for Disease Control and Prevention. What you should know for the 2012–2013 influenza season. 2013; Available at: http://www.cdc.gov/flu/about/season/flu-season-2012-2013.htm. Accessed March 2013.
5. Centers for Disease Control and Prevention. National early season flu vaccination coverage, United States 2012–13 flu season. 2012; Available at: http://www.cdc.gov/flu/fluvaxview/nifs-estimates-nov2012.htm. Accessed March 2013.
6. World Health Organization. Summary of human infection with highly pathogenic avian influenza A (H5N1) virus reported to WHO, January 2003–March 2009: Cluster-associated cases. *Wkly Epidemiol Rec* 2010; 85(3): 13–20.
7. World Health Organization. Update on human cases of highly pathogenic avian influenza A (H5N1) infection: 2009. *Wkly Epidemiol Rec* 2010; 85(7): 49–51.
8. Influenza A virus subtype H5N1 infection in humans. *Commun Dis Rep CDR Wkly* 1997; 7(50): 441.
9. Centers for Disease Control and Prevention. Isolation of avian influenza A(H5N1) viruses from humans—Hong Kong, May–December 1997. *MMWR Morb Mortal Wkly Rep* 1997; 46(50): 1204–1207.
10. Beigel JH, Farrar J, Han AM et al. Avian influenza A (H5N1) infection in humans. *N Engl J Med* 2005; 353(13): 1374–1385.
11. De Martin S, Nicoll A. H5N1 avian influenza: Update on the global situation. *Euro Surveill* 2005; 10(12): E051215 1.
12. Ducatez MF, Olinger CM, Owoade AA et al. Avian flu: Multiple introductions of H5N1 in Nigeria. *Nature* 2006; 442(7098): 37.
13. Joseph T, Subbarao K. Human infections with avian influenza viruses. *Md Med* 2005; 6(1): 30–32.
14. Lye DC, Nguyen DH, Giriputro S, Anekthananon T, Eraksoy H, Tambyah PA. Practical management of avian influenza in humans. *Singapore Med J* 2006; 47(6): 471–475.
15. Malik Peiris JS. Avian influenza viruses in humans. *Rev Sci Tech* 2009; 28(1): 161–173.
16. Parry J. Mortality from avian flu is higher than in previous outbreak. *BMJ* 2004; 328(7436): 368.
17. Peiris JS, Yu WC, Leung CW et al. Re-emergence of fatal human influenza A subtype H5N1 disease. *Lancet* 2004; 363(9409): 617–619.
18. Subbarao K, Katz J. Avian influenza viruses infecting humans. *Cell Mol Life Sci* 2000; 57(12): 1770–1784.
19. Yu H, Shu Y, Hu S et al. The first confirmed human case of avian influenza A (H5N1) in Mainland China. *Lancet* 2006; 367(9504): 84.
20. Wu J, Liu SZ, Dong SS et al. Safety and immunogenicity of adjuvanted inactivated split-virion and whole-virion influenza A (H5N1) vaccines in children: A phase I-II randomized trial. *Vaccine* 2010; 28(38): 6221–6227.
21. Layton RC, Gigliotti A, Armijo P et al. Enhanced immunogenicity, mortality protection, and reduced viral brain invasion by alum adjuvant with an H5N1 split-virion vaccine in the ferret. *PLoS One* 2011; 6(6): e20641.
22. Layton RC, Petrovsky N, Gigliotti AP et al. Delta inulin polysaccharide adjuvant enhances the ability of split-virion H5N1 vaccine to protect against lethal challenge in ferrets. *Vaccine* 2011; 29(37): 6242–6251.

23. World Health Organization. Cumulative number of confirmed human cases of avian influenza A(H5N1) reported to WHO (2003–2013). 15 February 2013; Available at: http://www.who.int/influenza/human_animal_interface/EN_GIP_20130215CumulativeNumberH5N1cases.pdf. Accessed March 2013.
24. Gu J, Xie Z, Gao Z et al. H5N1 infection of the respiratory tract and beyond: A molecular pathology study. *Lancet* 2007; 370(9593): 1137–1145.
25. The Writing Committee of the Second World Health Organization Consultation on Clinical Aspects of Human Infection with Avian Influenza A (H5N1) Virus. Update on avian influenza A (H5N1) virus infection in humans. *N Engl J Med* 2008; 358(3): 261–273.
26. Ng WF, To KF. Pathology of human H5N1 infection: New findings. *Lancet* 2007; 370: 1106–1108.
27. Ashour MM, Khatab AM, El-Folly RF, Amer WA. Clinical features of avian influenza in Egyptian patients. *J Egypt Soc Parasitol* 2012; 42(2): 385–396.
28. Wang TT, Palese P. Unraveling the mystery of swine influenza virus. *Cell* 2009; 137: 983–985.
29. Centers for Disease Control and Prevention. Update: Isolation of avian influenza A(H5N1) viruses from humans—Hong Kong, 1997–1998. *MMWR Morb Mortal Wkly Rep* 1998; 46(52–53): 1245–1247.
30. From the Centers for Disease Control and Prevention. Update: Isolation of avian influenza A(H5N1) viruses from humans—Hong Kong, 1997–1998. *JAMA* 1998; 279(5): 347–348.
31. Avian strain of influenza A virus isolated from humans in Hong Kong. *Commun Dis Rep CDR Wkly* 1999; 9(15): 131–134.
32. Knipe DM, Howley PM, eds. *Fields Virology*, Volume 2. 5th ed. Philadelphia, PA: Lippincott, Wiliams, & Williams; 2007.
33. Hale BG, Randall RE, Ortin J, Jackson D. The multifunctional NS1 protein of influenza A viruses. *J Gen Virol* 2008; 89(Pt 10): 2359–2376.
34. Schneider J, Wolff T. Nuclear functions of the influenza A and B viruses NS1 proteins: Do they play a role in viral mRNA export? *Vaccine* 2009; 27(45): 6312–6316.
35. Zamarin D, Ortigoza MB, Palese P. Influenza A virus PB1-F2 protein contributes to viral pathogenesis in mice. *J Virol* 2006; 80(16): 7976–7983.
36. McAuley JL, Chipuk JE, Boyd KL, Van De Velde N, Green DR, McCullers JA. PB1-F2 proteins from H5N1 and 20 century pandemic influenza viruses cause immunopathology. *PLoS Pathog* 2010; 6(7): e1001014.
37. Lamb RA, Takeda M. Death by influenza virus protein. *Nat Med* 2001; 7(12): 1286–1288.
38. Chen W, Calvo PA, Malide D et al. A novel influenza A virus mitochondrial protein that induces cell death. *Nat Med* 2001; 7(12): 1306–1312.
39. Updated unified nomenclature system for the highly pathogenic H5N1 avian influenza viruses. 2011; Available at: http://www.who.int/influenza/gisrs_laboratory/h5n1_nomenclature/en/index.html. Accessed March 2013.
40. WHO/OIE/FAO H5N1 Evolution Working Group. Continuing progress towards a unified nomenclature for the highly pathogenic H5N1 avian influenza viruses: Divergence of clade 2 · 2 viruses. Influenza and Other Respiratory Viruses. *Influenza Other Resp Viruses* 2009; 3: 59–62.
41. WHO/OIE/FAO H5N1 Evolution Working Group. Continued evolution of highly pathogenic avian influenza A (H5N1): Updated nomenclature. *Influenza Other Resp Viruses* 2012; 6(1): 1–5.
42. Connor RJ, Kawaoka Y, Webster RG, Paulson JC. Receptor specificity in human, avian, and equine H2 and H3 influenza virus isolates. *Virology* 1994; 205(1): 17–23.
43. Yao L, Korteweg C, Hsueh W, Gu J. Avian influenza receptor expression in H5N1-infected and noninfected human tissues. *FASEB J* 2008; 22(3): 733–740.
44. Belser JA, Blixt O, Chen LM et al. Contemporary North American influenza H7 viruses possess human receptor specificity: Implications for virus transmissibility. *Proc Natl Acad Sci USA* 2008; 105(21): 7558–7563.
45. Matrosovich MN, Krauss S, Webster RG. H9N2 influenza A viruses from poultry in Asia have human virus-like receptor specificity. *Virology* 2001; 281(2): 156–162.
46. Butt KM, Smith GJ, Chen H et al. Human infection with an avian H9N2 influenza A virus in Hong Kong in 2003. *J Clin Microbiol* 2005; 43(11): 5760–5767.
47. Herfst S, Schrauwen EJ, Linster M et al. Airborne transmission of influenza A/H5N1 virus between ferrets. *Science* 2012; 336(6088): 1534–1541.
48. Imai M, Watanabe T, Hatta M et al. Experimental adaptation of an influenza H5 HA confers respiratory droplet transmission to a reassortant H5 HA/H1N1 virus in ferrets. *Nature* 2012; 486(7403): 420–428.
49. Matlin KS, Reggio H, Helenius A, Simons K. Infectious entry pathway of influenza virus in a canine kidney cell line. *J Cell Biol* 1981; 91(3 Pt 1): 601–613.
50. Sieczkarski SB, Whittaker GR. Influenza virus can enter and infect cells in the absence of clathrin-mediated endocytosis. *J Virol* 2002; 76(20): 10455–10464.

51. Bertram S, Glowacka I, Steffen I, Kuhl A, Pohlmann S. Novel insights into proteolytic cleavage of influenza virus hemagglutinin. *Rev Med Virol* 2010; 20(5): 298–310.
52. Bosch F, Garten W, Klenk H, Rott R. Proteolytic cleavage of influenza virus hemagglutinins: Primary structure of the connecting peptide between HA1 and HA2 determines proteolytic cleavability and pathogenicity of Avian influenza viruses. *Virology* 1981; 113(2): 725–735.
53. Steinhauer DA. Role of hemagglutinin cleavage for the pathogenicity of influenza virus. *Virology* 1999; 258(1): 1–20.
54. Walker J, Molloy S, Thomas G, Sakaguchi T, Yoshida T, Chambers T, Kawaoka Y. Sequence specificity of furin, a proprotein-processing endoprotease, for the hemagglutinin of a virulent avian influenza virus. *J Virol* 1994; 68(2): 1213–1218.
55. Stegmann T, Morselt HW, Scholma J, Wilschut J. Fusion of influenza virus in an intracellular acidic compartment measured by fluorescence dequenching. *Biochim Biophys Acta* 1987; 904(1): 165–170.
56. Martin K, Helenius A. Transport of incoming influenza virus nucleocapsids into the nucleus. *J Virol* 1991; 65(1): 232–244.
57. Roberts NA. Treatment of influenza with neuraminidase inhibitors: Virological implications. *Philos Trans Biol Sci* 2001; 356(1416): 1895–1897.
58. Hughey P, Roberts P, Holsinger L, Zebedee S, Lamb R, Compans R. Effects of antibody to the influenza A virus M2 protein on M2 surface expression and virus assembly. *Virology* 1995; 212(2): 411–421.
59. Schroeder C, Heider H, Möncke-Buchner E, Tse-I Lin. The influenza virus ion channel and maturation cofactor M2 is a cholesterol-binding protein. *Eur Biophys J* 2005; 34(1): 52–66.
60. Fiers W, De Filette M, Birkett A, Neirynck S, Min Jou W. A "universal" human influenza A vaccine. *Virus Res* 2004; 103(1–2): 173–176.
61. Pielak RM, Chou JJ. Flu channel drug resistance: A tale of two sites. *Protein Cell* 2010; 1(3): 246–258.
62. Ison MG. Antivirals and resistance: Influenza virus. *Curr Opin Virol* 2011; 1(6): 563–573.
63. Krug RM. Priming of influenza viral RNA transcription by capped heterologous RNAs. *Curr Top Microbiol Immunol* 1981; 93: 125–149.
64. Olson AC, Rosenblum E, Kuchta RD. Regulation of influenza RNA polymerase activity and the switch between replication and transcription by the concentrations of the vRNA 5' end, the cap source, and the polymerase. *Biochemistry* 2010; 49(47): 10208–10215.
65. Robertson JS, Schubert M, Lazzarini RA. Polyadenylation sites for influenza virus mRNA. *J Virol* 1981; 38(1): 157–163.
66. Li X, Palese P. Characterization of the polyadenylation signal of influenza virus RNA. *J Virol* 1994; 68(2): 1245–1249.
67. Luo GX, Luytjes W, Enami M, Palese P. The polyadenylation signal of influenza virus RNA involves a stretch of uridines followed by the RNA duplex of the panhandle structure. *J Virol* 1991; 65(6): 2861–2867.
68. Vreede FT, Jung TE, Brownlee GG. Model suggesting that replication of influenza virus is regulated by stabilization of replicative intermediates. *J Virol* 2004; 78(17): 9568–9572.
69. Peiris JS, de Jong MD, Guan Y. Avian influenza virus (H5N1): A threat to human health. *Clin Microbiol Rev* 2007; 20(2): 243–267.
70. Webster RG, Guo YJ. New influenza virus in horses. *Nature* 1991; 351: 527.
71. Kundin WD. Hong Kong A-2 influenza virus infection among swine during epidemic in Taiwan. *Nature* 1970; 228: 857.
72. Hinshaw VS, Bean WJ, Geraci J, Fiorelli P, Early G, Webster RG. Characterization of two influenza A viruses from a pilot whale. *J Virol* 1986; 58: 655–656.
73. Claas EC, Osterhaus AD, van Beek R et al. Human influenza A H5N1 virus related to a highly pathogenic avian influenza virus. *Lancet* 1998; 351(9101): 472–477.
74. Ku AS, Chan LT. The first case of H5N1 avian influenza infection in a human with complications of adult respiratory distress syndrome and Reye's syndrome. *J Paediatr Child Health* 1999; 35(2): 207–209.
75. Centers for Disease Control and Prevention. From the Centers for Disease Control and Prevention. Isolation of avian influenza A(H5N1) viruses from humans—Hong Kong, May–December 1997. *JAMA* 1998; 279(4): 263–264.
76. Mounts AW, Kwong H, Izurieta HS et al. Case-control study of risk factors for avian influenza A (H5N1) disease, Hong Kong, 1997. *J Infect Dis* 1999; 180(2): 505–508.
77. The Writing Committee of the World Health Organization (WHO) Consultation on Human Influenza A/H5. Avian influenza A (H5N1) infection in humans. *New Engl J Med* 2005; 353(13): 1374–1385.
78. Hien TT, Liem NT, Dung NT et al. Avian influenza A (H5N1) in 10 patients in Vietnam. *New Engl J Med* 2004; 350(12): 1179–1188.

79. Ungchusak K, Auewarakul P, Dowell SF et al. Probable person-to-person transmission of avian influenza A (H5N1). *New Engl J Med* 2005; 352(4): 333–340.
80. Bridges CB, Katz JM, Seto WH et al. Risk of influenza A (H5N1) infection among health care workers exposed to patients with influenza A (H5N1), Hong Kong. *J Infect Dis* 2000; 181(1): 344–348.
81. Tran TH, Nguyen TL, Nguyen TD et al. Avian influenza A (H5N1) in 10 patients in Vietnam. *N Engl J Med* 2004; 350(12): 1179–1188.
82. Parry J. WHO investigates possible human to human transmission of avian flu. *BMJ* 2004; 328(7435): 308.
83. Normile D, Enserink M. Infectious diseases. Avian influenza makes a comeback, reviving pandemic worries. *Science* 2004; 305(5682): 321.
84. Banks J, Speidel EC, McCauley JW, Alexander DJ. Phylogenetic analysis of H7 haemagglutinin subtype influenza A viruses. *Arch Virol* 2000; 145(5): 1047–1058.
85. Guan Y, Shortridge KF, Krauss S, Webster RG. Molecular characterization of H9N2 influenza viruses: Were they the donors of the "internal" genes of H5N1 viruses in Hong Kong? *Proc Natl Acad Sci USA* 1999; 96(16): 9363–9367.
86. Aamir UB, Wernery U, Ilyushina N, Webster RG. Characterization of avian H9N2 influenza viruses from United Arab Emirates 2000 to 2003. *Virology* 2007; 361(1): 45–55.
87. Jia N, de Vlas SJ, Liu YX et al. Serological reports of human infections of H7 and H9 avian influenza viruses in northern China. *J Clin Virol* 2009; 44(3): 225–229.
88. Peiris M, Yuen KY, Leung CW et al. Human infection with influenza H9N2. *Lancet* 1999; 354(9182): 916–917.
89. Peiris JS, Guan Y, Markwell D, Ghose P, Webster RG, Shortridge KF. Cocirculation of avian H9N2 and contemporary "human" H3N2 influenza A viruses in pigs in southeastern China: Potential for genetic reassortment? *J Virol* 2001; 75(20): 9679–9686.
90. Lin YP, Shaw M, Gregory V et al. Avian-to-human transmission of H9N2 subtype influenza A viruses: Relationship between H9N2 and H5N1 human isolates. *Proc Natl Acad Sci USA* 2000; 97(17): 9654–9658.
91. Webster RG, Geraci J, Petursson G, Skirnisson K. Conjunctivitis in human beings caused by influenza A virus of seals. *N Engl J Med* 1981; 304(15): 911.
92. Banks J, Speidel E, Alexander DJ. Characterisation of an avian influenza A virus isolated from a human—Is an intermediate host necessary for the emergence of pandemic influenza viruses? *Arch Virol* 1998; 143(4): 781–787.
93. Fouchier RA, Schneeberger PM, Rozendaal FW et al. Avian influenza A virus (H7N7) associated with human conjunctivitis and a fatal case of acute respiratory distress syndrome. *Proc Natl Acad Sci USA* 2004; 101(5): 1356–1361.
94. Koopmans M, Wilbrink B, Conyn M et al. Transmission of H7N7 avian influenza A virus to human beings during a large outbreak in commercial poultry farms in the Netherlands. *Lancet* 2004; 363(9409): 587–593.
95. Puzelli S, Di Trani L, Fabiani C et al. Serological analysis of serum samples from humans exposed to avian H7 influenza viruses in Italy between 1999 and 2003. *J Infect Dis* 2005; 192(8): 1318–1322.
96. Nguyen-Van-Tam JS, Nair P, Acheson P et al. Outbreak of low pathogenicity H7N3 avian influenza in UK, including associated case of human conjunctivitis. *Euro Surveill* 2006; 11(5): E060504.2.
97. Tweed SA, Skowronski DM, David ST et al. Human illness from avian influenza H7N3, British Columbia. *Emerg Infect Dis* 2004; 10(12): 2196–2199.
98. Hirst M, Astell CR, Griffith M et al. Novel avian influenza H7N3 strain outbreak, British Columbia. *Emerg Infect Dis* 2004; 10(12): 2192–2195.
99. Centers for Disease Control and Prevention (CDC). Update: Influenza activity—United States and worldwide, 2003–04 season, and composition of the 2004–05 influenza vaccine. *MMWR Morb Mortal Wkly Rep* 2004; 53(25): 547–552.
100. Centers for Disease Control and Prevention (CDC). Update: Influenza activity—United States, 2003–04 season. *MMWR Morb Mortal Wkly Rep* 2004; 53(13): 284–287.
101. Avian influenza A/(H7N2) outbreak in the United Kingdom. *Euro Surveill* 2007; 12(5): E070531.2.
102. Cheng VC, Chan JF, Wen X et al. Infection of immunocompromised patients by avian H9N2 influenza A virus. *J Infect* 2011; 62(5): 394–399.
103. Pawar SD, Tandale BV, Raut CG et al. Avian influenza H9N2 seroprevalence among poultry workers in Pune, India, 2010. *PLoS One* 2012; 7(5): e36374.
104. Cameron KR, Gregory V, Banks J, Brown IH, Alexander DJ, Hay AJ, Lin YP. H9N2 subtype influenza A viruses in poultry in Pakistan are closely related to the H9N2 viruses responsible for human infection in Hong Kong. *Virology* 2000; 278(1): 36–41.

105. Chan PKS. Outbreak of avian influenza A(H5N1) virus infection in Hong Kong in 1997. *Clin Infect Dis* 2002; 34(Supplement 2): S58–S64.
106. Chotpitayasunondh T, Ungchusak K, Hanshaoworakul W et al. Human disease from influenza A (H5N1), Thailand, 2004. *Emerg Infect Dis* 2005; 11(2): 201–209.
107. Tam JS. Influenza A (H5N1) in Hong Kong: An overview. *Vaccine* 2002; 20 Suppl 2: S77–S81.
108. de Jong MD, Bach VC, Phan TQ et al. Fatal avian influenza A (H5N1) in a child presenting with diarrhea followed by coma. *N Engl J Med* 2005; 352(7): 686–691.
109. Wang TT, Parides MK, Palese P. Seroevidence for H5N1 influenza infections in humans: Meta-analysis. *Science* 2012; 335(6075): 1463.
110. Mitchell H, Levin D, Forrest S et al. Higher level of replication efficiency of 2009 (H1N1) pandemic influenza virus than those of seasonal and avian strains: Kinetics from epithelial cell culture and computational modeling. *J Virol* 2011; 85(2): 1125–1135.
111. Skehel J, Wiley D. Receptor binding and membrane fusion in virus entry: The influenza hemagglutinin. *Annu Rev Biochem* 2000; 69: 531–569.
112. Hatta M, Gao P, Halfmann P, Kawaoka Y. Molecular basis for high virulence of Hong Kong H5N1 influenza A viruses. *Science* 2001; 293(5536): 1840–1842.
113. Belser J, Lu X, Maines T et al. Pathogenesis of avian influenza (H7) virus infection in mice and ferrets: Enhanced virulence of Eurasian H7N7 viruses isolated from humans. *J Virol* 2007; 81(20): 11139–11147.
114. Maines TR, Lu XH, Erb SM et al. Avian influenza (H5N1) viruses isolated from humans in Asia in 2004 exhibit increased virulence in mammals. *J Virol* 2005; 79(18): 11788–11800.
115. Tumpey TM, Lu X, Morken T, Zaki SR, Katz JM. Depletion of lymphocytes and diminished cytokine production in mice infected with a highly virulent influenza a (H5N1) virus isolated from humans. *J Virol* 2000; 74(13): 6105–6116.
116. Schrauwen EJA, Herfst S, Leijten LM et al. The multibasic cleavage site in H5N1 virus is critical for systemic spread along the olfactory and hematogenous routes in ferrets. *J Virol* 2012; 86(7): 3975–3984.
117. McNicholl IR, McNicholl JJ. Neuraminidase inhibitors: Zanamivir and oseltamivir. *Ann Pharmacother* 2001; 35(1): 57–70.
118. Wagner R, Matrosovich M, Klenk H. Functional balance between haemagglutinin and neuraminidase in influenza virus infections. *Rev Med Virol* 2002; 12(3): 159–166.
119. Wagner R, Wolff T, Herwig A, Pleschka S, Klenk H. Interdependence of hemagglutinin glycosylation and neuraminidase as regulators of influenza virus growth: A study by reverse genetics. *J Virol* 2000; 74(14): 6316–6323.
120. Baigent SJ, McCauley JW. Glycosylation of haemagglutinin and stalk-length of neuraminidase combine to regulate the growth of avian influenza viruses in tissue culture. *Virus Research* 2001; 79: 177–185.
121. Baigent SJ, Bethell RC, McCauley JW. Genetic analysis reveals that both haemagglutinin and neuraminidase determine the sensitivity of naturally occurring avian influenza viruses to Zanamivir in vitro. *Virology* 1999; 2(-2): 323–338.
122. Matsuoka Y, Swayne DE, Thomas C et al. Neuraminidase stalk length and additional glycosylation of the hemagglutinin influence the virulence of influenza H5N1 viruses for mice. *J Virol* 2009; 83: 4704–4708.
123. Maines TR, Chen L, Matsuoka Y et al. Lack of transmission of H5N1 avian-human reassortant influenza viruses in a ferret model. *Proc Natl Acad Sci USA* 2006; 103(32): 12121–12126.
124. Salomon R, Franks J, Govorkova EA et al. The polymerase complex genes contribute to the high virulence of the human H5N1 influenza virus isolate A/Vietnam/1203/04. *J Exp Med* 2006; 203(3): 689, 697; 689.
125. Brojer C, Agren EO, Uhlhorn H, Bernodt K, Jansson DS, Gavier-Widen D. Characterization of encephalitis in wild birds naturally infected by highly pathogenic avian influenza H5N1. *Avian Dis* 2012; 56(1): 144–152.
126. Cardona CJ, Xing Z, Sandrock CE, Davis CE. Avian influenza in birds and mammals. *Comp Immunol Microbiol Infect Dis* 2009; 32(4): 255–273.
127. Keawcharoen J, Oraveerakul K, Kuiken T et al. Avian influenza H5N1 in tigers and leopards. *Emerg Infect Dis* 2004; 10(12): 2189–2191.
128. Zhang Z, Zhang J, Huang K et al. Systemic infection of avian influenza A virus H5N1 subtype in humans. *Hum Pathol* 2009; 40(5): 735–739.
129. Korteweg C, Gu J. Pathology, molecular biology, and pathogenesis of avian influenza A (H5N1) infection in humans. *Am J Pathol* 2008; 172(5): 1155–1170.
130. Gao R, Dong L, Dong J et al. A systematic molecular pathology study of a laboratory confirmed H5N1 human case. *PLoS One* 2010; 5(10): e13315.

131. Kuiken T, van den Brand J, van Riel D, Pantin-Jackwood M, Swayne DE. Comparative pathology of select agent influenza a virus infections. *Vet Pathol* 2010; 47: 893–914.
132. Rowe T, Cho DS, Bright RA, Zitzow LA, Katz JM. Neurological manifestations of avian influenza viruses in mammals. *Avian Diseases* 2003; 47: 1122–1126.
133. Neurological complications of influenza. *Br Med J* 1970; 1(5691): 248–249.
134. Kapila CC, Kaul S, Kapur SC, Kalayanam TS, Banerjee D. Neurological and hepatic disorders associated with influenza. *Br Med J* 1958; 2(5108): 1311–1314.
135. Lu X, Tumpey TM, Morken T, Zaki SR, Cox NJ, Katz JM. A mouse model for the evaluation of pathogenesis and immunity to influenza A (H5N1) viruses isolated from humans. *J Virol* 1999; 73(7): 5903–5911.
136. Mori I, Nishiyama Y, Yokochi T, Kimura Y. Olfactory transmission of neurotropic viruses. *J Neurovirol* 2005; 11(2): 129–137.
137. Reinacher M, Bonin J, Narayan O, Scholtissek C. Pathogenesis of neurovirulent influenza A virus infection in mice. Route of entry of virus into brain determines infection of different populations of cells. *Lab Invest* 1983; 49(6): 686–692.
138. Tanaka H, Park C, Ninomiya A, Ozaki H, Takada A, Umemura T, Kida H. Neurotropism of the 1997 Hong Kong H5N1 influenza virus in mice. *Vet Microbiol* 2003; 95(1–2): 1–13.
139. Yoshikawa H, Yamazaki S, Watanabe T, Abe T. Study of influenza-associated encephalitis/encephalopathy in children during the 1997 to 2001 influenza seasons. *J Child Neurol* 2001; 16(12): 885–890.
140. Brahic M, Bureau JF, Michiels T. The genetics of the persistent infection and demyelinating disease caused by Theiler's virus. *Annu Rev Microbiol* 2005; 59: 279–298.
141. Katz J, Lu X, Frace A, Morken T, Zaki S, Tumpey T. Pathogenesis of and immunity to avian influenza A H5 viruses. *Biomed Pharmacother* 2000; 54(4): 178–187.
142. Lipatov AS, Krauss S, Guan Y, Peiris M, Rehg JE, Perez DR, Webster RG. Neurovirulence in mice of H5N1 influenza virus genotypes isolated from Hong Kong poultry in 2001. *J Virol* 2003; 77(6): 3816–3823.
143. Nishimura H, Itamura S, Iwasaki T, Kurata T, Tashiro M. Characterization of human influenza A (H5N1) virus infection in mice: Neuro-, pneumo- and adipotropic infection. *J Gen Virol* 2000; 81: 2503–2510.
144. Park CH, Ishinaka M, Takada A, Kida H, Kimura T, Ochiai K, Umemura T. The invasion routes of neurovirulent A/Hong Kong/483/97 (H5N1) influenza virus into the central nervous system after respiratory infection in mice. *Arch Virol* 2002; 147: 1425–1436.
145. Plourde JR, Pyles JA, Layton RC, Vaughan SE, Tipper JL, Harrod KS. Neurovirulence of H5N1 infection in ferrets is mediated by multifocal replication in distinct permissive neuronal cell regions. *PLoS One* 2012; 7(10): e46605.
146. Shinya K, Makino A, Hatta M et al. Subclinical brain injury caused by H5N1 influenza virus infection. *J Virol* 2010; 85(10): 5202–5207.
147. Shinya K, Shimada A, Ito T et al. Avian influenza virus intranasally inoculated infects the central nervous system of mice through the general visceral afferent nerve. *Arch Virol* 2000; 145(1): 187–195.
148. Zitzow LA, Rowe T, Morken T, Shieh W, Zaki S, Katz JM. Pathogenesis of avian influenza A (H5N1) viruses in ferrets. *J Virol* 2002; 76(9): 4420–4442.
149. Kreijtz JH, Bodewes R, van den Brand JM et al. Infection of mice with a human influenza A/H3N2 virus induces protective immunity against lethal infection with influenza A/H5N1 virus. *Vaccine* 2009; 27(36): 4983–4989.
150. Guillot L, Le Goffic R, Bloch S, Escriou N, Akira S, Chignard M, Si-Tahar M. Involvement of toll-like receptor 3 in the immune response of lung epithelial cells to double-stranded RNA and influenza a virus. *J Biol Chem* 2005; 280: 5571–5580.
151. Lund JM, Alexopoulou L, Sato A et al. Recognition of single-stranded RNA viruses by Toll-like receptor 7. *Proc Natl Acad Sci USA* 2004; 101(15): 5598–5603.
152. Garcia-Sastre A. Identification and characterization of viral antagonists of type I interferon in negative-strand RNA viruses. *Curr Top Microbiol Immunol* 2004; 283: 249–280.
153. Seo SH, Hoffmann E, Webster RG. The NS1 gene of H5N1 influenza viruses circumvents the host anti-viral cytokine responses. *Virus Res* 2004; 103(1–2): 107–113.
154. Jiao P, Tian G, Li Y et al. A single-amino-acid substitution in the NS1 protein changes the pathogenicity of H5N1 avian influenza viruses in mice. *J Virol* 2008; 82(3): 1146–1154.
155. Seo SH, Hoffmann E, Webster RG. Lethal H5N1 influenza viruses escape host anti-viral cytokine responses. *Nat Med* 2002; 8(9): 950–954.
156. Haye K, Burmakina S, Moran T, Garcia-Sastre A, Fernandez-Sesma A. The NS1 protein of a human influenza virus inhibits type I interferon production and the induction of antiviral responses in primary human dendritic and respiratory epithelial cells. *J Virol* 2009; 83: 6849–6862.

157. Gack MU, Albrecht RA, Urano T et al. Influenza A virus NS1 targets the ubiquitin ligase TRIM25 to evade recognition by the host viral RNA sensor RIG-I. *Cell Host Microbe* 2009; 5(5): 439–449.
158. Li S, Min JY, Krug RM, Sen GC. Binding of the influenza A virus NS1 protein to PKR mediates the inhibition of its activation by either PACT or double-stranded RNA. *Virology* 2006; 349(1): 13–21.
159. Ramos I, Fernandez-Sesma A. Innate immunity to H5N1 influenza viruses in humans. *Viruses* 2012; 4(12): 3363–3388.
160. Fukuyama S, Kawaoka Y. The pathogenesis of influenza virus infections: The contributions of virus and host factors. *Curr Opin Immunol* 2011; 23(4): 481–486.
161. Peiris JS, Cheung CY, Leung CY, Nicholls JM. Innate immune responses to influenza A H5N1: Friend or foe? *Trends Immunol* 2009; 30(12): 574–584.
162. de Jong MD, Simmons CP, Thanh TT et al. Fatal outcome of human influenza A (H5N1) is associated with high viral load and hypercytokinemia. *Nat Med* 2006; 12(10): 1203–1207.
163. Mok KP, Wong CH, Cheung CY et al. Viral genetic determinants of H5N1 influenza viruses that contribute to cytokine dysregulation. *J Infect Dis* 2009; 200(7): 1104–1112.
164. Potter CW, Oxford JS. Determinants of immunity to influenza infection in man. *Br Med Bull* 1979; 35(1): 69–75.
165. Treanor JJ, Tierney EL, Zebedee SL, Lamb RA, Murphy BR. Passively transferred monoclonal antibody to the M2 protein inhibits influenza A virus replication in mice. *J Virol* 1990; 64(3): 1375–1377.
166. Fiore AE, Bridges CB, Cox NJ. Seasonal influenza vaccines. *Curr Top Microbiol Immunol* 2009; 333: 43–82.
167. Plotkin JB, Dushoff J. Codon bias and frequency-dependent selection on the hemagglutinin epitopes of influenza A virus. *Proc Natl Acad Sci USA* 2003; 100(12): 7152–7157.
168. Bush RM, Bender CA, Subbarao K, Cox NJ, Fitch WM. Predicting the evolution of human influenza A. *Science* 1999; 286(5446): 1921–1925.
169. Liu W, Zou P, Ding J, Lu Y, Chen YH. Sequence comparison between the extracellular domain of M2 protein human and avian influenza A virus provides new information for bivalent influenza vaccine design. *Microbes Infect* 2005; 7(2): 171–177.
170. Kim MC, Song JM, O E, Kwon YM, Lee YJ, Compans RW, Kang SM. Virus-like particles containing multiple M2 extracellular domains confer improved cross-protection against various subtypes of influenza virus. *Mol Ther* 2013; 21(2): 485–492.
171. Kang SM, Kim MC, Compans RW. Virus-like particles as universal influenza vaccines. *Expert Rev Vaccines* 2012; 11(8): 995–1007.
172. Wang ML, Skehel JJ, Wiley DC. Comparative analyses of the specificities of anti-influenza hemagglutinin antibodies in human sera. *J Virol* 1986; 57(1): 124–128.
173. Doherty PC, Kelso A. Toward a broadly protective influenza vaccine. *J Clin Invest* 2008; 118(10): 3273–3275.
174. Roti M, Yang J, Berger D, Huston L, James EA, Kwok WW. Healthy human subjects have CD4+ T cells directed against H5N1 influenza virus. *J Immunol* 2008; 180(3): 1758–1768.
175. Lee LY, Ha do LA, Simmons C et al. Memory T cells established by seasonal human influenza A infection cross-react with avian influenza A (H5N1) in healthy individuals. *J Clin Invest* 2008; 118(10): 3478–3490.
176. Kreijtz JH, de Mutsert G, van Baalen CA, Fouchier RA, Osterhaus AD, Rimmelzwaan GF. Cross-recognition of avian H5N1 influenza virus by human cytotoxic T-lymphocyte populations directed to human influenza A virus. *J Virol* 2008; 82(11): 5161–5166.
177. World Health Organization. Clinical management of human infection with avian influenza A (H5N1) virus. 15 August 2007. Available at: http://www.who.int/influenza/resources/documents/ClinicalManagement07.pdf. Accessed March 2013.
178. Schunemann HJ, Hill SR, Kakad M et al. WHO Rapid Advice Guidelines for pharmacological management of sporadic human infection with avian influenza A (H5N1) virus. *Lancet Infect Dis* 2007; 7(1): 21–31.
179. Salomon R, Webster RG. The influenza virus enigma. *Cell* 2009; 136(3): 402–410.
180. Bright RA, Shay DK, Shu B, Cox NJ, Klimov AI. Adamantane resistance among influenza A viruses isolated early during the 2005–2006 influenza season in the United States. *JAMA* 2006; 295(8): 891–894.
181. Deyde VM, Xu X, Bright RA et al. Surveillance of resistance to adamantanes among influenza A(H3N2) and A(H1N1) viruses isolated worldwide. *J Infect Dis* 2007; 196(2): 249–257.
182. Deyde VM, Nguyen T, Bright RA et al. Detection of molecular markers of antiviral resistance in influenza A (H5N1) viruses using a pyrosequencing method. *Antimicrob Agents Chemother* 2009; 53(3): 1039–1047.

183. Ilyushina NA, Bovin NV, Webster RG, Govorkova EA. Combination chemotherapy, a potential strategy for reducing the emergence of drug-resistant influenza A variants. *Antiviral Res* 2006; 70(3): 121–131.
184. Mumford E, Bishop J, Hendrickx S, Embarek PB, Perdue M. Avian influenza H5N1: Risks at the human-animal interface. *Food Nutr Bull* 2007; 28(2 Suppl): S357–S363.
185. Yee KS, Carpenter TE, Cardona CJ. Epidemiology of H5N1 avian influenza. *Comp Immunol Microbiol Infect Dis* 2009; 32(4): 325–340.
186. van den Berg T, Lambrecht B, Marche S, Steensels M, Van Borm S, Bublot M. Influenza vaccines and vaccination strategies in birds. *Comp Immunol Microbiol Infect Dis* 2008; 31(2–3): 121–165.
187. Swayne DE, Perdue ML, Beck JR, Garcia M, Suarez DL. Vaccines protect chickens against H5 highly pathogenic avian influenza in the face of genetic changes in field viruses over multiple years. *Vet Microbiol* 2000; 74(1–2): 165–172.
188. Abdelwhab EM, Hafez HM. Insight into alternative approaches for control of avian influenza in poultry, with emphasis on highly pathogenic H5N1. *Viruses* 2012; 4(11): 3179–208.
189. Webby RJ, Perez DR, Coleman JS et al. Responsiveness to a pandemic alert: Use of reverse genetics for rapid development of influenza vaccines. *Lancet* 2004; 363(9415): 1099–1103.
190. Lin J, Zhang J, Dong X et al. Safety and immunogenicity of an inactivated adjuvanted whole-virion influenza A (H5N1) vaccine: A phase I randomised controlled trial. *Lancet* 2006; 368(9540): 991–997.

25 Emergence and Pathogenesis of Swine Influenza Viruses in Humans

Jennifer L. Smith, Frederick T. Koster, and Robert J. Hogan

CONTENTS

25.1 INTRODUCTION

Influenza A viruses belong to the Orthomyxoviridae family.[1] They are enveloped, single-stranded, negative-sense ribonucleic acid (RNA) viruses with a segmented genome.[2] The eight gene segments encode for 10, sometimes 11 viral proteins. The hemagglutinin (HA) and neuraminidase (NA) are the major surface glycoproteins of the virus as well as the major antigenic proteins, and thus the viruses are subtyped based on these proteins. Currently, there are 17 HA and 9 NA subtypes of influenza A.[3,4]

Animals play an important role in influenza epidemics through the introduction of novel viruses. There is a greater diversity of influenza A viruses in wild aquatic birds, and 16 HA and 9 NA subtypes have been found in these birds in almost every combination. Thus, wild aquatic birds, such as ducks and shorebirds, serve as the natural reservoir for influenza A viruses.[5] There are a limited number of influenza virus subtypes that have established permanent lineages in animal species other than birds. Avian viruses have sporadically transmitted to other hosts such as horses and pigs, in which they have adapted and formed stable lineages. It is unusual for wholly avian viruses to transmit to and become established in humans, and it is generally accepted that an intermediary host is required for novel influenza viruses to cross the species barrier.

Pigs have a unique position in the ecology of influenza. Because they can be infected with and support the replication of both avian and human influenza viruses, they play an important role in the generation of recombinant influenza viruses.[6] Owing to the segmented nature of the influenza genome, reassortment of gene segments can occur and produce variant viruses. The most common reassortments involve the genes for the surface glycoproteins, HA and NA, causing antigenic shift, a radical change of the antigenic properties of the surface proteins. Antigenic shift of influenza viruses results in the emergence of new subtypes of influenza A viruses, and these viruses can then be transmitted from pigs and cause outbreaks among humans.[7] Thus, pigs serve as a "mixing vessel" when they become infected by two distinct influenza strains.[6,8] This has been the generally accepted method by which new human pandemics arise.[9] This chapter discusses the role swine play in the appearance of influenza viruses in humans, the pathology of swine-origin influenza viruses (SOIV) in humans as well as measures to control and prevent the emergence of SOIVs.

25.2 HISTORY OF INFLUENZA IN NORTH AMERICAN SWINE

In the last century, three influenza A virus lineages had become established in North American swine populations; the "classical" swine H1N1 (cH1N1), human-like H3N2, and a reassortant H1N2.[10] The disease of pigs was first recognized in 1918 in the United States during the most notable pandemic of the twentieth century (Figure 25.1). Beginning in 1917 and continuing throughout 1918, an H1N1 influenza virus spread worldwide, causing roughly 20–40 million deaths.[11] During the 1918 pandemic, pigs suffered from an illness similar to humans, as noted by the close similarity of clinical disease signs. Influenza virus was first isolated in 1930 as the causative agent of swine influenza.[12] This H1N1 influenza virus was later shown to be similar to the influenza virus that caused the 1918 human pandemic.[13] Whether the virus originated in swine or was transmitted from humans into the swine population is unclear.

Since the time of initial isolation of influenza virus from pigs, cH1N1 became endemic in swine and continued to circulate for about 80 years with little to no change. This virus became the precursor for the generation of reassortants and establishment of other swine virus lineages. Prior to 1998, the isolation and detection of H3N2 influenza viruses from pigs was rare, with low seroprevelance of about 1%.[14,15] However, there was little to no surveillance occurring in swine herds, making it difficult to ascertain what viruses were cocirculating in pigs during this period. The

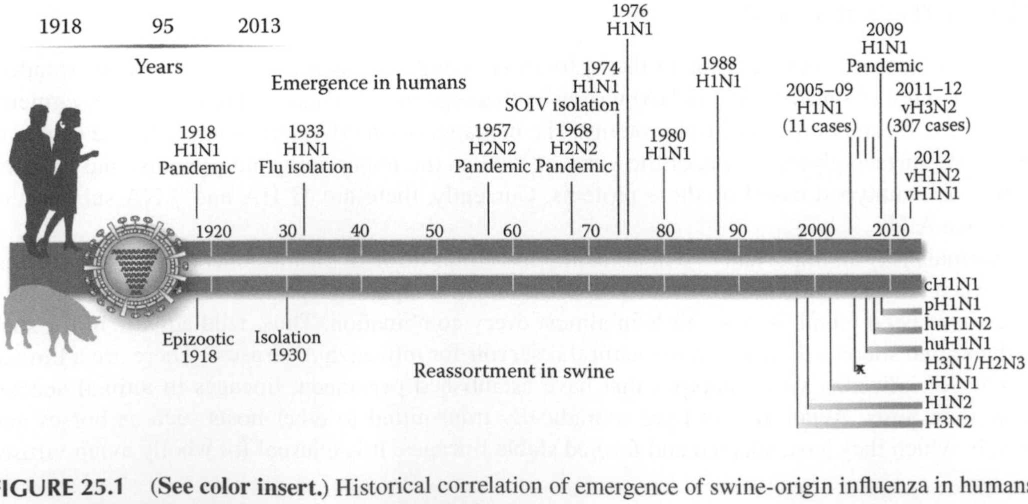

FIGURE 25.1 **(See color insert.)** Historical correlation of emergence of swine-origin influenza in humans. Dates in red indicate that fatal cases were reported.

epidemiology of influenza viruses in swine changed dramatically in 1997 when a human H3N2 virus was transmitted to pigs, thereby increasing the seroprevalence and isolation of H3N2 viruses from pigs (Figure 25.1).[10] The initial outbreak of influenza-like disease occurred in North Carolina and resulted in high morbidity among swine herds. Subsequent less severe outbreaks were reported in Texas, Minnesota, and Iowa. Genetic analysis showed that reassortment between the cH1N1 virus and the human H3N2 virus had generated three genotypes of H3N2 viruses, which included a wholly human, a double reassortant (classical swine and human H3N2), and triple reassortant (classical swine, human H3, and avian).[16] Published reports confirmed the spread of the triple reassortant H3N2 isolate throughout the Midwestern United States. This virus spread widely throughout the swine population accounting for up to 27% of swine influenza isolates during 2000 and into 2001.[10,17] Although the double and triple reassortant H3N2 viruses contained the same HA gene, the wholly human and double reassortant H3N2 viruses did not spread efficiently in pigs and have not been isolated again since their initial appearance. With the introduction of the human H3N2 into pigs, the diversity of swine viruses increased dramatically due to increased bidirectional transmission of viruses and subsequent reassortment between human and swine influenza viruses.

Influenza viruses continued to evolve and reassort in pigs with the appearance of an H1N2 isolate in Indiana in 1999 (Figure 25.1).[18] This virus was isolated when respiratory disease and abortion were noted on a farm over a 6-week period beginning in November 1999.[19] Genetic analysis showed that this virus was a triple reassortant H3N2 virus that had an H1 HA gene from the classical swine lineage.[18] In 2003, a human H1N2 transmitted to pigs in Canada, causing abortions in sows.[20] This caused the subsequent emergence of reassortant H1N2 viruses, some of which were shown to have several genes from a human H1N1 virus.[20] It was also reported that a unique H1N1 human/swine reassortant containing the PB1 from a human virus and the remaining genes from the classical swine H1N1 lineage was isolated. During this same time, H1N2 viruses were isolated from humans in many countries.[21] This provides more support for the idea that not only can pigs be infected with human influenza viruses, but that they can serve as a "mixing vessel" for the reassortment of influenza viruses that can then be transmitted to the human population.

In 2006, several other reassortant viruses were isolated from dead pigs in the United States, including viruses of the H3N1and H2N3 subtypes.[22,23] Phylogenetic analysis of the H3N1 isolates showed they were reassortant viruses that contained the HA gene closely related to a turkey H3N2 and an NA gene from a human H1N1; the remaining genes were obtained from circulating H3N2 and H1N2 swine viruses. However, because infection of turkeys with swine influenza viruses is common, the authors suggested the H3N2 turkey virus could have originated from swine.[24] Another novel virus was isolated from pigs with respiratory disease in Missouri and was later identified by sequence analysis as an H2N3 isolate. The HA gene was shown to be similar to that of a North American Mallard H2, while the NA was closely related to a blue-winged teal H4N3. Furthermore, the PA gene was homologous to an H6N5 mallard isolate and the rest of the internal genes were from a contemporary triple reassortant swine virus. Although these viruses have been detected, they have yet to become established in swine. Notably, this provided evidence that influenza viruses transmit from birds to pigs, and infection of pigs promotes reassortment of influenza viruses from different hosts.

The current picture of influenza in swine has become even more complex. With the continual introduction of genes from avian viruses, the swapping of genes between human seasonal influenza strains and swine lineages, the diversity of influenza viruses in pigs has increased dramatically. By 2008, all successful reassortants endemic in the swine population contained what has been referred to as the triple reassortant internal gene (TRIG) cassette.[25] The TRIG cassette includes the PA and PB2 genes from avian lineages; the NS, NP, and M genes from the classical swine lineage; and the human PB1 gene. Acquisition of the TRIG cassette by the H1 swine lineage has increased the rate of mutations among North American isolates, and reassortment with various HA and NA combinations has led to the generation of at least six lineages of influenza viruses circulating in swine; the cluster IV H3N2 and five H1 lineages (Figure 25.1).[25] One of the H1 lineages that had arisen from acquisition of the TRIG cassette included an H1N1 isolate that contained a human HA gene, the δ cluster.[26]

Two separate introductions of human seasonal HA genes caused the δ-cluster to be subdivided into distinct subclusters, δ1 (H1N2) and δ2 (H1N1). Between 2008 and 2010, outbreaks in swine were caused mainly by the H1 subtype (85%), with the δ-cluster accounting for about 40% of the total isolates by 2009.[27] The fact that swine maintained a virus containing an HA gene from a human isolate easily allowed these viruses to transmit back into the human population.

On June 11, 2009, a pandemic was declared by the World Health Organization (WHO) and it was shown to be caused by a novel swine-origin H1N1 isolate that crossed the species barrier and caused outbreaks in over 214 countries worldwide.[28] The human 2009 pandemic (pdmH1N1) strain was believed to have originated from a North American swine virus and contained a combination of genes not previously reported in humans or swine.[29] These genes were from Eurasian swine (NA and M), cH1N1 influenza (HA, NP, and NS), and the triple reassortant swine lineage (PB2, PB1, and PA).[29] Interestingly, the 2009 pdmH1N1 expressed an HA that was descendant from and antigenically similar to the 1918 virus. Several of the genes appear to have been originally acquired from avian influenza viruses (PB2, PA, NA, and M), whereas the PB1 gene appeared to have originated from the human H3N2 lineage, making this a quadruple reassortant virus. The 2009 pdmH1N1 formed a distinct lineage of H1 virus in pigs, and this has enhanced the potential for further change in the epidemiology of swine viruses due to reassortment of the novel 2009 pdmH1N1 with viruses of the other lineages of swine influenza viruses. The swine population now serves as a reservoir for influenza strains that have circulated in humans. With limitless reassortment potential comes the increased likelihood of the emergence of new variants in pigs with the ability to transmit to humans and perhaps cause future pandemics.

25.3 HISTORY OF INFLUENZA IN EURASIAN SWINE

The identification and evolution of swine influenza in Europe has been outlined in several excellent reviews, which will be discussed only briefly herein.[30,31] Influenza in swine was first reported in Great Britain between 1938 and 1940 and was most closely related to human H1N1 isolates. Classical swine H1N1 was first isolated in Europe from pigs imported from the United States to Italy. Then, in 1979, an avian H1N1 virus was transmitted from birds to pigs and established a stable lineage. This virus replaced the cH1N1 virus and became the endemic strain in Europe beginning in the early 1990s. In the early 1970s, a human H3N2 transmitted to pigs; this virus descended from the 1968 human pandemic H3N2 and circulated at a low level for about 10 years, causing sporadic cases. The H1N2 subtype was first isolated in France in 1987; this virus was a triple reassortant with an avian HA gene and NA gene from a human strain. This virus did not spread in the pig population and was later replaced with an H1N2 isolate, with a human HA gene and the remaining genes from a swine H3N2 isolate. This virus quickly spread throughout European swine herds. There are three lineages currently circulating in European swine; namely, the avian-like H1N1, human-like H3N2, and human-like H1N2. Therefore, swine influenza viruses from North American and Eurasian lineages are genetically and antigenically distinct. These three swine lineages continue to reassort with other circulating swine and human isolates.

The 2009 pdmH1N1 virus emerged in Europe shortly after its appearance in North America and has since introduced more variants into Eurasian swine herds. The major concern in Eurasia, however, is the existence of avian influenza viruses, especially the highly pathogenic H5 strains, in areas where swine are reared. Reassortment of swine viruses with avian virus could introduce additional genetic diversity to viruses already capable of transmitting to humans. The addition of genes from highly pathogenic avian influenza virus could have severe consequences for the human population, as such a reassortment could produce a virus that is highly transmissible and virulent.

25.4 INFECTION OF PIGS WITH AVIAN INFLUENZA VIRUSES

Pigs have receptors to support replication of both human and avian influenza viruses,[6] and though pigs have the necessary receptor type to support the replication of avian influenza viruses, the transmission of wholly avian viruses to pigs was thought to be a relatively rare event. A serological survey of pigs in China between 1977 and 1982 revealed evidence of avian H4 and H5 viruses, suggesting that pigs had been sporadically infected with avian viruses.[32] Pigs have been shown to support the replication of avian influenza viruses when high doses are experimentally inoculated intranasally.[33] Of the 38 avian viruses tested, influenza viruses of HA subtypes H2 through H13 replicated to similar levels as human influenza viruses for 4–7 days post-inoculation with little to no clinical disease signs. In addition, reassortant viruses were recovered after coinfection with a swine and an avian isolate that did not appear to replicate in pigs, contributing more evidence that reassortment can occur in pigs and generate novel influenza viruses.

Serology also provided evidence of antibodies to avian H9 influenza virus in pigs in China in 1998.[32] Interestingly, in 1999, an influenza A virus of the H9N2 subtype was isolated from two girls in Hong Kong.[34] Later, five more human cases of H9N2 influenza virus infection were reported from mainland China, and subsequent serological surveys suggested that there were other undetected cases of human infection.[35,36] In 2003, H9N2 viruses were isolated from swine suffering from respiratory disease in China.[37] Genetic analysis showed that these isolates were closely related to circulating chicken H9N2 viruses; however, they were distinct in that they were reassortants of H9 and H5 influenza viruses.

Then, in 1999, an outbreak of respiratory disease occurred on a swine farm in Ontario, Canada.[38] This outbreak was later shown to be caused by an H4N6 isolate genetically related to North American ducks. This was the first documented case of transmission of a wholly avian influenza virus to pigs and the first isolation of an influenza virus of the H4 subtype from naturally infected pigs. In October 2001, a wholly avian H3N3 influenza virus was isolated from pigs suffering from mild respiratory illness on the same Ontario farm where the H4N6 was previously isolated.[39] Three viruses were isolated and shown to be similar to North American avian influenza viruses. In May 2002, an H1N1 virus was isolated on a different pig farm in Canada.[39] This virus was also a wholly avian virus phylogenetically related to the North American avian lineage. None of these avian viruses become established in pigs.

In February 2003, avian H5N1 was directly transmitted to humans in Asia,[40] and transmission of avian H5N1 viruses continues to the present day. As of April 2013, 628 laboratory-confirmed cases of human infection were identified in several Asian countries as well as countries in the Middle East, with 374 reported fatalities[41] (http://www.who.int/influenza/human_animal_interface/EN_GIP_20130426CumulativeNumberH5N1cases.pdf), for a cumulative fatality rate of 59%. Introduction of highly pathogenic avian influenza viruses into the human population raised an alarm for a potential pandemic with severe consequences. Antibodies were detected in pigs in China, suggesting that pigs had been naturally infected with H5N1 isolates, though the incidence was low.[42] Two H5N1 influenza viruses were isolated from swine during routine surveillance in southern China in 2001 and 2003 and were shown to be closely related to H5N1 duck viruses.[43] It had been previously shown that H5N1 viruses isolated from humans and chickens during an outbreak in 1997 could replicate in the upper respiratory tract of pigs with no clinical disease signs after experimental inoculation.[44] Therefore, it was important to assess the ability of 2004 H5N1 viruses to replicate in pigs. Pigs intranasally inoculated with four 2004 H5N1 isolates supported replication. Virus could be isolated for at least 3 days from nasal swabs and disease signs were mild. Virus was also isolated from tissues of the respiratory tract 6 days post-inoculation. Further studies with H5N1 isolates showed that pigs could support their replication with no clinical signs or systemic spread.[45] During surveillance conducted between 2005 and 2009 in Indonesia, 52 H5N1 viruses were isolated, accounting for 7.4% of pigs sampled.[46] Viruses were isolated from apparently healthy pigs in regions where outbreaks of H5N1 had occurred and remained enzootic in poultry. Serological survey of pigs in China during 2004 and 2007 revealed no evidence of H5 infections,[47] while serological evidence of H5N1 in pigs was detected in Egypt during surveillance conducted in 2008.[48]

In early 2008, avian–swine H5N2 reassortants with internal genes (PB2, PA, NP, and M) from the 2006 Korean swine H3N1 lineage were isolated from pigs during routine surveillance.[49] Novel avian viruses have been isolated from pigs between 2008 and 2011 in China.[50,51,52,53] The H4N1,

H4N8, H6N6, and H10N5 isolates were the first of these subtypes to be isolated from pigs and they all were wholly avian viruses. Additionally, genetic analysis revealed the internal genes of the H10N5, the NP of the H4N8, and the PB2 of the H6N6 were most closely related to that of H5N1 avian isolates, suggesting that reassortment of H5 viruses with other avian viruses is already occurring. With continued introductions of H5N1 into swine, the potential for reassortment with human and other swine isolates increases, and so with it the potential for transmission of these novel viruses into the human population. In fact, reverse genetics was used recently to generate reassortants of an H5 avian virus with the 2009 pdmH1N1 strain. Some of these hybrid viruses were shown to be highly transmissible by respiratory droplets in guinea pigs.[54]

25.5 ROLE OF MODERNIZATION OF SWINE FARMING

One plausible explanation for the increased reassortment and introduction of SOIV into humans is industrialization of swine farming. Swine production in the United States has changed dramatically since the 1970s. Beginning in the early 1960s, the number of small-scale swine production facilities began to decrease (Figure 25.2). In the 1980s, the first concentrated animal feeding operations were built. Some facilities could house up to 300,000 hogs per year and about 25,000 heads at once (http://www.aphis.usda.gov/animal_health/emergingissues/downloads/1pigs.pdf). By 1995, farms with 2000 or more hogs accounted for about 43% of farms; this increased to 87% by 2010. Since 1993, the production from operations marketing less than 1000 hogs per year has decreased from 28% to 2.9%. Swine farming was industrialized over this time period, with fewer farms but more pigs per operation, reaching a peak in the average number of heads of swine per operation around 2005 (Figure 25.2). At the same time, the number of SOIV isolated from humans increased. The number of swine operations has remained unchanged since this time and the number of head per operation has also remained steady, with only modest changes, of about 1%, since 2009. Iowa and North Carolina contain 43.1% of the United States hog inventory, while Minnesota and Illinois are the third- and fourth-largest producers. It is interesting to note that North Carolina became the second-largest swine producing state in 1994, with the largest pork processing plant in the world built in 1995, and just a few years later an outbreak of H3N2 occurred there among pigs in 1998. This virus later became endemic in pigs. It appears that large-scale swine operations bring together more heads of swine in smaller indoor spaces and could have an impact on the generation and

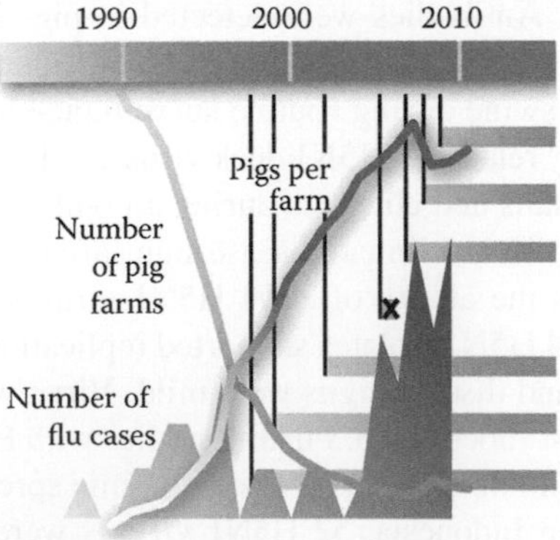

FIGURE 25.2 **(See color insert.)** Correlation between swine production and emergence of swine-origin influenza in humans. The red line indicates the total number of pig farms, the blue line indicates the average number of pigs per operation, and the green shaded area indicates the number of swine-origin influenza virus infections in humans by year up to but not including cases of 2009 pdmH1N1 infection. Scales are not included because the *y*-axis is variable for all three parameters. (Adapted from Figures 1 and 2 published in Krueger WS, Gray GC. Swine influenza virus infections in man. *Current Topics in Microbiology and Immunology* 2013; **370**: 201–225 and USDA Pork Industry data.)

maintenance of novel influenza viruses (Figure 25.2). It has also been noted that animals have fewer respiratory and disease problems in the open air. Therefore, indoor housing of large numbers of pigs aides in the spread and maintenance of respiratory infection.

Because swine workers can serve as a bridge for transmission of SOIV to the community, prospective surveillance among swine workers and pigs in Iowa was conducted during 2002–2004 to assess the risk factors associated with transmission of influenza viruses between pigs and humans.[55] Although there were 20 respiratory outbreaks among swine during the 2-year study, only one swine worker tested positive for influenza of the H3N2 subtype. While an outbreak of H3N2 in pigs was documented, the majority of isolates from swine outbreaks were triple reassortant H1N1 viruses (69%). Similar studies found that up to 23% of those occupationally exposed, such as swine farmers, swine veterinarians, and pork processing workers, were more likely to have elevated antibodies to cH1N1 and H1N2 viruses.[56]

25.6 HISTORY OF HUMAN INFECTION WITH SOIV

Transmission from pigs to humans is likely to occur via direct contact with pigs or indirectly through aerosols created by coughing and sneezing. Clinical signs cannot differentiate between SOIV and seasonal influenza in humans, so SOIV cases can go unrecognized or underreported due to the lack of surveillance. In addition, prior to the detection of SOIV for the first time in 1974, human cases were identified by serological evidence; however, it can be difficult to differentiate SOIV infection due to cross-reactivity of antibodies with annual influenza vaccine-induced antibodies.[57]

Although the first pandemic of the twentieth century occurred in 1918, the first isolation of influenza virus from humans did not occur until 1933, a few years after the isolation of influenza from pigs (Figure 25.1).[58] Case reports of SOIV infection in humans have been comprehensively reviewed for the period of 1958 up to 2009, so only a few important cases occurring during this time period will be highlighted herein.[59] Approximately 50 reported cases of human illness associated with swine influenza strains were identified worldwide between 1958 and 2005.[60] Thirty-seven of these cases were reported in the general population and 13 were military cases associated with the 1976 outbreak at Fort Dix in New Jersey.[61] The case fatality rate of 14% (7/50) was mainly associated with pneumonia. Six deaths (17%) from pneumonia were identified as being caused by an H1N1 virus, and four nonfatal cases were associated with the H3N2 subtype. Coinciding with the predominance in pigs, all human infections in the United States prior to 1998 were caused by cH1N1 virus. Of the 37 SOIV cases, most were young (median age 24.5 years), and there was an association with swine-rearing areas and exposure to pigs through county fairs and livestock shows. However, one fatal case was not associated with known exposure to pigs. Between 2005 and 2009, transmission of SOIV to humans was reported sporadically, with 11 human cases of triple reassortant H1 SOIV infection; 8 cases occurred after 2007.[62]

In April 2009, a novel swine-origin H1N1 influenza A virus was determined to be the cause of outbreaks of respiratory illness in Mexico.[63] Within weeks of discovery, this virus was transmitted across communities in North America and subsequently identified in many areas of the world by May 2009.[64,65] Worldwide transmission of pdmH1N1 continued in both the Northern and Southern hemispheres, until the pandemic was declared to be over in October 2010.[66] Although the number of cases was high worldwide, mortality remained low (about 1%).

Since the end of the 2009 pandemic, SOIVs have continued to be transmitted to humans mainly through exposure to pigs at county and state fairs. The continued circulation of the 2009 pdmH1N1 has led to the further change in the epidemiology of SOIV by further reassortment with viruses of the other swine lineages. During 2011, the first known human infection with variant H3N2 (vH3N2) SOIV containing the M gene from the pdmH1N1 influenza virus was reported after the patient attended a fair in Pennsylvania.[67] Investigation revealed 82 suspected and 3 confirmed cases of infection (Table 25.1). More cases were later identified, totaling 12 cases among people that had attended a county or state fair (Table 25.1). Subsequently, in the summer of 2012, vH3N2 was again of influenza virus pathogenesis and targeting of immunity toward highly conserved portions of the viral glycoproteins, may represent the best overall strategy for the prevention of the next influenza pandemic.

REFERENCES

1. Wright PF, Webster RG. Orthomyxoviruses. In: Knipe DM, Howley PM, Griffin DE et al., eds. *Fields Virology*. Philadelphia: Lippincott Williams and Wilkins; 2001: pp. 1533–1579.
2. Lamb RA, Krug RM. Orthomyxoviridae: The viruses and their replication. In: Knipe DM, Howley PM, Griffin DE et al., eds. *Fields Virology*. Philadelphia: Lippincott Williams and Wilkins; 2001: pp. 1487–1531.
3. Fouchier RA, Munster V, Wallensten A et al. Characterization of a novel influenza A virus hemagglutinin subtype (H16) obtained from black-headed gulls. *J Virol* 2005; 79(5): 2814–2822.
4. Sun X, Shi Y, Lu X et al. Bat-derived influenza hemagglutinin h17 does not bind canonical avian or human receptors and most likely uses a unique entry mechanism. *Cell Rep* 2013; 3(3): 769–778.
5. Webster RG, Yakhno M, Hinshaw VS, Bean WJ, Murti KG. Intestinal influenza: Replication and characterization of influenza viruses in ducks. *Virology* 1978; 84(2): 268–278.
6. Ito T, Couceiro JN, Kelm S et al. Molecular basis for the generation in pigs of influenza A viruses with pandemic potential. *J Virol* 1998; **72**(9): 7367–7373.
7. Scholtissek C. Pigs as "mixing vessels" for the creation of new pandemic influenza A viruses. *Med Princ Pract* 1990; **2**: 65–71.
8. Scholtissek C, Burger H, Kistner O, Shortridge KF. The nucleoprotein as a possible major factor in determining host specificity of influenza H3N2 viruses. *Virology* 1985; **147**(2): 287–294.
9. Hinshaw VS, Air GM, Gibbs AJ, Graves L, Prescott B, Karunakaran D. Antigenic and genetic characterization of a novel hemagglutinin subtype of influenza A viruses from gulls. *J Virol* 1982; **42**(3): 865–872.
10. Olsen CW. The emergence of novel swine influenza viruses in North America. *Virus Res* 2002; **85**(2): 199–210.
11. Barry JM. *The Great Influenza: The Epic Story of the Deadliest Plague in History*. New York: Penguin Group (USA) Inc.; 2004.
12. Shope R. Swine Influenza III. Filtration experiments and etiology. *J Exp Med* 1931; **54**: 373–380.
13. Taubenberger JK, Reid AH, Fanning TG. The 1918 influenza virus: A killer comes into view. *Virology* 2000; **274**(2): 241–245.
14. Hinshaw VS, Bean WJ, Jr., Webster RG, Easterday BC. The prevalence of influenza viruses in swine and the antigenic and genetic relatedness of influenza viruses from man and swine. *Virology* 1978; **84**(1): 51–62.
15. Chambers TM, Hinshaw VS, Kawaoka Y, Easterday BC, Webster RG. Influenza viral infection of swine in the United States 1988–1989. *Arch Virol* 1991; **116**(1–4): 261–265.
16. Zhou NN, Senne DA, Landgraf JS et al. Genetic reassortment of avian, swine, and human influenza A viruses in American pigs. *J Virol* 1999; **73**(10): 8851–8856.
17. Webby RJ, Swenson SL, Krauss SL, Gerrish PJ, Goyal SM, Webster RG. Evolution of swine H3N2 influenza viruses in the United States. *J Virol* 2000; **74**(18): 8243–8251.
18. Karasin AI, Olsen CW, Anderson GA. Genetic characterization of an H1N2 influenza virus isolated from a pig in Indiana. *J Clin Microbiol* 2000; **38**(6): 2453–2456.
19. Karasin AI, Landgraf J, Swenson S et al. Genetic characterization of H1N2 influenza A viruses isolated from pigs throughout the United States. *J Clin Microbiol* 2002; **40**(3): 1073–1079.
20. Karasin AI, Carman S, Olsen CW. Identification of human H1N2 and human-swine reassortant H1N2 and H1N1 influenza A viruses among pigs in Ontario, Canada (2003 to 2005). *J Clin Microbiol* 2006; **44**(3): 1123–1126.
21. Xu X, Smith CB, Mungall BA et al. Intercontinental circulation of human influenza A(H1N2) reassortant viruses during the 2001–2002 influenza season. *J Infect Dis* 2002; **186**(10): 1490–1493.
22. Lekcharoensuk P, Lager KM, Vemulapalli R, Woodruff M, Vincent AL, Richt JA. Novel swine influenza virus subtype H3N1, United States. *Emerg Infect Dis* 2006; **12**(5): 787–794.
23. Ma W, Vincent AL, Gramer MR et al. Identification of H2N3 influenza A viruses from swine in the United States. *Proc Natl Acad Sci U S A* 2007; **104**(52): 20949–20954.
24. Choi YK, Lee JH, Erickson G et al. H3N2 influenza virus transmission from swine to turkeys, United States. *Emerg Infect Dis* 2004; **10**(12): 2156–2160.
25. Vincent AL, Ma W, Lager KM, Janke BH, Richt JA. Swine influenza viruses a North American perspective. *Adv Virus Res* 2008; **72**: 127–154.

26. Ciacci Zanella JR, Vincent AL, Zanella EL et al. Comparison of human-like H1 (delta-Cluster) influenza a viruses in the swine host. *Influenza Res Treat* 2012; **2012**: 329029.
27. Lorusso A, Vincent AL, Gramer MR, Lager KM, Ciacci-Zanella JR. Contemporary epidemiology of North American lineage triple reassortant influenza a viruses in pigs. *Curr Top Microbiol Immunol* 2013; **370**: 113–132.
28. Peiris JS, Poon LL, Guan Y. Emergence of a novel swine-origin influenza A virus (S-OIV) H1N1 virus in humans. *J Clin Virol* 2009; **45**(3): 169–173.
29. Garten RJ, Davis CT, Russell CA et al. Antigenic and genetic characteristics of swine-origin 2009 A(H1N1) influenza viruses circulating in humans. *Science* 2009; **325**(5937): 197–201.
30. Kuntz-Simon G, Madec F. Genetic and antigenic evolution of swine influenza viruses in Europe and evaluation of their zoonotic potential. *Zoonoses Public Health* 2009; **56**(6–7): 310–325.
31. Vincent A, Awada L, Brown I et al. Review of influenza a virus in swine worldwide: A call for increased surveillance and research. *Zoonoses Public Health* 2013 Apr 5. doi: 10.1111/zph.12049. [Epub ahead of print].
32. Ninomiya A, Takada A, Okazaki K, Shortridge KF, Kida H. Seroepidemiological evidence of avian H4, H5, and H9 influenza A virus transmission to pigs in southeastern China. *Vet Microbiol* 2002; **88**(2): 107–114.
33. Kida H, Ito T, Yasuda J et al. Potential for transmission of avian influenza viruses to pigs. *J Gen Virol* 1994; **75(Pt 9)**: 2183–2188.
34. Peiris M, Yam WC, Chan KH, Ghose P, Shortridge KF. Influenza A H9N2: Aspects of laboratory diagnosis. *J Clin Microbiol* 1999; **37**(10): 3426–3427.
35. Peiris M, Yuen KY, Leung CW et al. Human infection with influenza H9N2. *Lancet* 1999; **354**(9182): 916–917.
36. Guo Y, Li J, Cheng X. Discovery of men infected by avian influenza A (H9N2) virus. *Zhonghua Shi Yan He Lin Chuang Bing Du Xue Za Zhi* 1999; **13**(2): 105–108.
37. Cong YL, Pu J, Liu QF et al. Antigenic and genetic characterization of H9N2 swine influenza viruses in China. *J Gen Virol* 2007; **88**(Pt 7): 2035–2041.
38. Karasin AI, Brown IH, Carman S, Olsen CW. Isolation and characterization of H4N6 avian influenza viruses from pigs with pneumonia in Canada. *J Virol* 2000; **74**(19): 9322–9327.
39. Karasin AI, West K, Carman S, Olsen CW. Characterization of avian H3N3 and H1N1 influenza A viruses isolated from pigs in Canada. *J Clin Microbiol* 2004; **42**(9): 4349–4354.
40. Peiris JS, Yu WC, Leung CW et al. Re-emergence of fatal human influenza A subtype H5N1 disease. *Lancet* 2004; **363**(9409): 617–619.
41. Tran TH, Nguyen TL, Nguyen TD et al. Avian influenza A (H5N1) in 10 patients in Vietnam. *N Engl J Med* 2004; **350**(12): 1179–1188.
42. Choi YK, Nguyen TD, Ozaki H et al. Studies of H5N1 influenza virus infection of pigs by using viruses isolated in Vietnam and Thailand in 2004. *J Virol* 2005; **79**(16): 10821–10825.
43. Zhu Q, Yang H, Chen W et al. A naturally occurring deletion in its NS gene contributes to the attenuation of an H5N1 swine influenza virus in chickens. *J Virol* 2008; **82**(1): 220–228.
44. Shortridge KF, Zhou NN, Guan Y et al. Characterization of avian H5N1 influenza viruses from poultry in Hong Kong. *Virology* 1998; **252**(2): 331–342.
45. Lipatov AS, Kwon YK, Sarmento LV et al. Domestic pigs have low susceptibility to H5N1 highly pathogenic avian influenza viruses. *PLoS Pathog* 2008; **4**(7): e1000102.
46. Nidom CA, Takano R, Yamada S et al. Influenza A (H5N1) viruses from pigs, Indonesia. *Emerg Infect Dis* 2010; **16**(10): 1515–1523.
47. Song XH, Xiao H, Huang Y et al. Serological surveillance of influenza A virus infection in swine populations in Fujian province, China: no evidence of naturally occurring H5N1 infection in pigs. *Zoonoses Public Health* 2010; **57**(4): 291–298.
48. El-Sayed A, Awad W, Fayed A, Hamann HP, Zschock M. Avian influenza prevalence in pigs, Egypt. *Emerg Infect Dis* 2010; **16**(4): 726–727.
49. Lee JH, Pascua PN, Song MS et al. Isolation and genetic characterization of H5N2 influenza viruses from pigs in Korea. *J Virol* 2009; **83**(9): 4205–4215.
50. Wang N, Zou W, Yang Y et al. Complete genome sequence of an H10N5 avian influenza virus isolated from pigs in central China. *J Virol* 2012; **86**(24): 13865–13866.
51. Hu Y, Liu X, Li S, Guo X, Yang Y, Jin M. Complete genome sequence of a novel H4N1 influenza virus isolated from a pig in central China. *J Virol* 2012; **86**(24): 13879.
52. Su S, Qi WB, Chen JD et al. Complete genome sequence of an avian-like H4N8 swine influenza virus discovered in southern China. *J Virol* 2012; **86**(17): 9542.

have challenged the historic concepts of measles pathogenesis. Here, we provide an overview of our current understanding of MV entry, dissemination, and transmission to the next host. Furthermore, we will discuss the main cause of measles-associated morbidity and mortality, the transient but profound immune suppression. Finally, this chapter includes a brief discussion on measles vaccination and eradication.

26.2 MOLECULAR BIOLOGY OF MV

MV belongs to the family *Paramyxoviridae*, genus *Morbillivirus*, and is the only virus within this genus that targets primates as its natural host. Virus particles are pleomorphic and average in size from 100 to 300 nm.[1] The viral genome consists of a single-stranded ribonucleic acid (RNA) molecule of negative polarity, typically 15,894 nucleotides (nt) in length, consisting of six genes that encode eight proteins (Figure 26.1a). The genome is contained in a helical nucleocapsid, which is surrounded by a lipid bilayer.[3] This envelope is derived from the membrane of the infected cell during budding.[4] Genes are transcribed by a start–stop mechanism from a single promoter at the 3′ end of the genome leading to a so-called transcription gradient, which means that mRNA transcribed from the genes closest to the 3′ end are present in greater abundance than those transcribed from the genes at the 5′ end.[5,6] This is due to the chance that between each open reading frame (ORF) the virus-associated RNA-dependent RNA-polymerase (RdRp) may dissociate from the genome, and thus has to re-initiate transcription at the 3′ end.

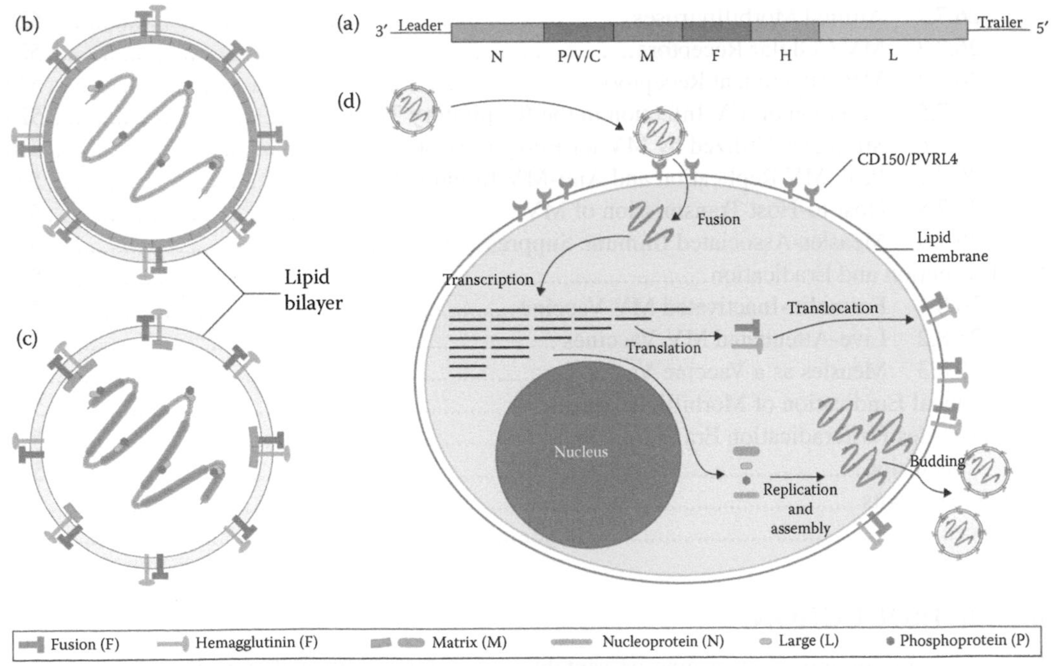

FIGURE 26.1 **(See color insert.)** (a) Schematic representation of the MV genome. The P gene also encodes the V and C protein. Gene lengths are not shown on scale. (b,c) Schematic representation of an MV virion. The enveloped virus contains six structural proteins: the transmembrane glycoproteins F and H, the N protein coating the genomic RNA, and the P and L proteins in a complex associated with the nucleoprotein. For the location of the M protein two models exist.[18] M is either present directly beneath the lipid bilayer (b) or directly interacts with the nucleoprotein (c). (d) Schematic representation of the MV replication cycle. MV enters via interaction between the H glycoprotein and a cellular receptor followed by fusion, replicates in the cytoplasm, and assembled virions are formed by budding at the plasma membrane.

The nucleoprotein (N) mRNA is produced first, since it is at the promoter-proximal position of the genome. The main function of the N protein is to encapsidate the genomic RNA. Since one N protein covers 6 nt, the genome lengths of morbilliviruses obey the "rule of six" (i.e., the genome length must be a multiple of six nt).[5]

The second gene in the morbillivirus genome is the phosphoprotein (P) gene, which encodes two different mRNAs and three proteins: P, V, and C. The P protein is a cofactor of the RdRp,[7] essential in transcription and replication. The C and V proteins are either translated from an overlapping reading frame or are cotranscriptionally edited products of the P mRNA.[8,9] The V protein is important in immune inhibition, potentially interfering with the type 1 interferon pathway by binding to DBB1, mda-5, STAT1, and STAT2.[10,11,226–229] The C protein has been suggested to modulate the viral polymerase activity and play a role in interference with the innate immune system.[12,13] An rMV defective for C proved to be growth-defective in peripheral blood mononuclear cells (PBMCs) and less virulent *in vivo*.[14,15]

The matrix (M) protein is assumed to associate with the inner leaflet of the virus envelope (Figure 26.1b).[16,17] However, a recent publication using electron cryotomography revealed that in MV particles the M protein coats the N-coated viral RNA, rather than localizing to the envelope (Figure 26.1c).[18] The M protein has an important role in the morphogenesis of viral particles,[19] and may be the driving force in viral budding. M is thought to interact with both the N protein[20] and the cytoplasmic tails of the viral envelope glycoproteins to ensure incorporation of the viral genome into nascent virions.[21,22]

The mRNAs encoding the two viral transmembrane glycoproteins, the fusion (F) and hemagglutinin (H) proteins are transcribed after M. The F glycoprotein mediates membrane fusion, either between the virus particle and a host cell (virus-to-cell fusion) or between two adjacent host cells (cell-to-cell fusion). The H glycoprotein mediates attachment of the viral particle to host cell receptors. The F glycoproteins form trimers, while H is present as a dimer of dimers, which interact to form the fusion complex.[23] Upon binding the cellular receptor, the H glycoprotein undergoes a conformational change and triggers the fusion activity of the F glycoprotein.[24,25] Therefore, the combination of the F and H glycoproteins is critical for viral entry and cell-to-cell spread.

The transcription unit encoding the large (L) protein mRNA is located at the 5′ end of the genome and accounts for more than 40% of the genome length. The L protein acts both as a transcriptase and as a replicase, in a complex with P.[7,26–28]

26.2.1 Virus Life Cycle

A schematic representation of the morbillivirus life cycle is shown in Figure 26.1d. To initiate infection of a target cell, the H glycoprotein interacts with an entry receptor present on the cell surface. After virus binding and fusion of the viral membrane with that of the host cell, the minimal unit of infectivity, the ribonucleoprotein (RNP) complex, is released into the cytoplasm. The RNP is comprised of the viral genome associated with the N, P, and L proteins. In the cytoplasm, the RdRp is responsible for primary transcription during the first 6 h postinfection (h.p.i.). In the second phase of infection (6–12 h.p.i.), newly synthesized RdRp leads to an exponential increase in mRNA synthesis. In the third phase of infection (12–24 h.p.i.), the emphasis shifts from transcription to genome replication: RdRp switches from functioning as a transcriptase to functioning as a replicase.

During the viral replication cycle, the F and H glycoproteins are modified in the Golgi apparatus and translocated to the cell membrane.[29] The presence of these glycoproteins at the cell membrane can generate syncytia or multinucleated giant cells, which can be seen in the lungs or lymphoid tissues of MV-infected hosts. Newly formed RNP associates with the M protein, which complex is recruited to the plasma membrane. Here, new viral particles are generated by budding from lipid rafts. The interaction between the M protein and the cytoplasmic tails of the transmembrane glycoproteins ensures that new viral particles have an envelope containing F and H glycoproteins on its surface. The M protein and the RNP are incorporated into the newly formed virus particles.

127. Kawamata N, Xu B, Nishijima H et al. Expression of endothelia and lymphocyte adhesion molecules in bronchus-associated lymphoid tissue (BALT) in adult human lung. *Respir Res* 2009; **10**: 97.
128. Geijtenbeek TBH, Torensma R, van Vliet SJ et al. Identification of DC-SIGN, a novel dendritic cell-specific ICAM-3 receptor that supports primary immune responses. *Cell* 2000; **100**: 575–85.
129. Turville SG, Santos JJ, Frank I et al. Immunodeficiency virus uptake, turnover, and 2-phase transfer in human dendritic cells. *Blood* 2004; **103**: 2170–9.
130. Avota E, Gassert E, Schneider-Schaulies S. Measles virus-induced immunosuppression: From effectors to mechanisms. *Med Microbiol Immunol* 2010; **199**: 227–37.
131. Lessler J, Reich NG, Brookmeyer R et al. Incubation periods of acute respiratory viral infections: A systematic review. *Lancet Infect Dis* 2009; **9**: 291–300.
132. Hall WC, Kovatch RM, Herman PH, Fox JG. Pathology of measles in rhesus monkeys. *Vet Pathol* 1971; **8**: 307–19.
133. Sakaguchi M, Yoshikawa Y, Yamanouchi K et al. Growth of measles virus in epithelial and lymphoid tissues of cynomolgus monkeys. *Microbiol Immunol* 1986; **30**: 1067–73.
134. Warthin AS. Occurrence of numerous large giant cells in the tonsils and pharyngeal mucosa in the prodromal stage of measles. *Arch Pathol* 1931; **11**: 864–74.
135. Finkeldey W. Über Riesenzellbefunde in den Gaumenmandeln, zugleich ein Beitrag zur Histopathologie der Mandelveränderungen im Maserninkubationsstadium. *Virchows Arch* 1931; **281**: 323–9.
136. Good RA, Zak SJ. Disturbances in gamma globulin synthesis as "experiments of nature". *Pediatrics* 1956; **18**: 109–49.
137. Nahmias A, Griffith D, Salsbury C, Yoshida K. Thymic aplasia with lymphopenia, plasma cells, and normal immunoglobulins. *JAMA* 1967; **201**: 103–8.
138. Burnet FM. Measles as an index of immunological function. *Lancet* 1968; **292**: 610–3.
139. Permar SR, Rao SS, Sun Y et al. Clinical measles after measles virus challenge in simian immunodeficiency virus-infected measles virus-vaccinated rhesus monkeys. *J Infect Dis* 2007; **196**: 1784–93.
140. Van Binnendijk RS, Poelen MCM, Kuijpers KC, Osterhaus ADME, UytdeHaag FGCM. The predominance of CD8+ T cells after infection with measles virus suggests a role for CD8+ class I MHC-restricted cytotoxic T lymphocytes (CTL) in recovery from measles. *J Immunol* 1990; **144**: 2394–9.
141. De Vries RD, Yüksel S, Osterhaus ADME, De Swart RL. Specific CD8+ T-lymphocytes control dissemination of measles virus. *Eur J Immunol* 2010; **40**: 388–95.
142. Van Binnendijk RS, Poelen MCM, De Vries P et al. Measles virus-specific human T cell clones. Characterization of specificity and function of CD4+ helper/cytotoxic and CD8+ cytotoxic T cell clones. *J Immunol* 1989; **142**: 2847–54.
143. Jaye A, Magnusen AF, Sadiq AD, Corrah T, Whittle HC. Ex vivo analysis of cytotoxic T lymphocytes to measles antigens during infection and after vaccination in Gambian children. *J Clin Invest* 1998; **102**: 1969–77.
144. Permar SR, Moss WJ, Ryon JJ et al. Increased thymic output during acute measles virus infection. *J Virol* 2003; **77**: 7872–9.
145. Permar SR, Klumpp SA, Mansfield KG et al. Limited contribution of humoral immunity to the clearance of measles viremia in rhesus monkeys. *J Infect Dis* 2004; **190**: 998–1005.
146. Pueschel K, Tietz A, Carsillo M, Steward M, Niewiesk S. Measles virus specific CD4 T cell activity does not correlate with protection against lung infection or viral clearance. *J Virol* 2007; **81**: 8571–8.
147. Frey S, Krempl CD, Schmitt-Graff A, Ehl S. Role of T cells in virus control and disease after infection with pneumonia virus of mice. *J Virol* 2008; **82**: 11619–27.
148. El Mubarak HS, Ibrahim SA, Vos HW et al. Measles virus protein-specific IgM, IgA, and IgG subclass responses during the acute and convalescent phase of infection. *J Med Virol* 2004; **72**: 290–8.
149. Chen RT, Markowitz LE, Albrecht P et al. Measles antibody: Reevaluation of protective titers. *J Infect Dis* 1990; **162**: 1036–42.
150. Samb B, Aaby P, Whittle HC et al. Serologic status and measles attack rates among vaccinated and unvaccinated children in rural Senegal. *Pediatr Infect Dis J* 1995; **14**: 203–9.
151. Black FL, YANNET H. Inapparent measles after gamma globulin administration. *JAMA* 1960; **173**: 1183–8.
152. Racaniello V. An exit strategy for measles virus. *Science* 2011; **334**: 1650–1.
153. Ludlow M, Lemon K, De Vries RD et al. Measles virus infection of epithelial cells in the macaque upper respiratory tract is mediated by sub-epithelial immune cells. *J Virol* 2013; **87**: 4033–42.
154. Ludlow M, Allen I, Schneider-Schaulies J. Systemic spread of measles virus: Overcoming the epithelial and endothelial barriers. *Thromb Haemost* 2009; **102**: 1050–6.
155. Griffin DE, Ward BJ, Jauregui E, Johnson RT, Vaisberg A. Immune activation in measles. *N Engl J Med* 1989; **320**: 1667–72.

156. Akramuzzaman SM, Cutts FT, Wheeler JG, Hossain MJ. Increased childhood morbidity after measles is short-term in urban Bangladesh. *Am J Epidemiol* 2000; **151**: 723–35.
157. Von Pirquet CE. Das Verhalten der kutanen Tuberkulin-reaktion während der Masern. *Dtsch Med Wochenschr* 1908; **34**: 1297–300.
158. Tamashiro VG, Perez HH, Griffin DE. Prospective study of the magnitude and duration of changes in tuberculin reactivity during uncomplicated and complicated measles. *Pediatr Infect Dis J* 1987; **6**: 451–4.
159. Lisse I, Samb B, Whittle H et al. Acute and long-term changes in T-lymphocyte subsets in response to clinical and subclinical measles. A community study from rural Senegal. *Scand J Infect Dis* 1998; **30**: 17–21.
160. Ryon JJ, Moss WJ, Monze M, Griffin DE. Functional and phenotypic changes in circulating lymphocytes from hospitalized Zambian children with measles. *Clin Diagn Lab Immunol* 2002; **9**: 994–1003.
161. Premenko-Lanier M, Rota PA, Rhodes GH, Bellini WJ, McChesney MB. Protection against challenge with measles virus (MV) in infant macaques by an MV DNA vaccine administered in the presence of neutralizing antibody. *J Infect Dis* 2004; **189**: 2064–71.
162. Bankamp B, Hodge G, McChesney MB, Bellini WJ, Rota PA. Genetic changes that affect the virulence of measles virus in a rhesus macaque model. *Virology* 2008; **373**: 39–50.
163. Hirsch RL, Griffin DE, Johnson RT et al. Cellular immune responses during complicated and uncomplicated measles virus infections of man. *Clin Immunol Immunopathol* 1984; **31**: 1–12.
164. Ward BJ, Johnson RT, Vaisberg A, Jauregui E, Griffin DE. Cytokine production *in vitro* and the lymphoproliferative defect of natural measles virus infection. *Clin Immunol Immunopathol* 1991; **61**: 236–48.
165. Avota E, Avots A, Niewiesk S et al. Disruption of Akt kinase activation is important for immunosuppression induced by measles virus. *Nat Med* 2001; **7**: 725–31.
166. Griffin DE, Ward BJ. Differential CD4 T cell activation in measles. *J Infect Dis* 1993; **168**: 275–81.
167. Ward BJ, Griffin DE. Changes in cytokine production after measles virus vaccination: predominant production of IL-4 suggests induction of a Th2 response. *Clin Immunol Immunopathol* 1993; **67**: 171–7.
168. Fugier-Vivier I, Servet-Delprat C, Rivailler P et al. Measles virus suppresses cell-mediated immunity by interfering with the survival and functions of dendritic and T cells. *J Exp Med* 1997; **186**: 813–23.
169. Grosjean I, Caux C, Bella C et al. Measles virus infects human dendritic cells and blocks their allostimulatory properties for CD4+ T cells. *J Exp Med* 1997; **186**: 801–12.
170. Schnorr J-J, Xanthakos S, Keikavoussi P et al. Induction of maturation of human blood dendritic cell precursors by measles virus is associated with immmunosuppression. *Proc Natl Acad Sci USA* 1997; **94**: 5326–31.
171. Condack C, Grivel J-C, Devaux P, Margolis L, Cattaneo R. Measles virus vaccine attenuation: suboptimal infection of lymphatic tissue and tropism alteration. *J Infect Dis* 2007; **196**: 541–9.
172. De Vries RD, McQuaid S, Van Amerongen G et al. Measles immune suppression: Lessons from the macaque model. *PLoS Pathog* 2012; **8**: e1002885.
173. Sallusto F, Lenig D, Forster R, Lipp M, Lanzavecchia A. Two subsets of memory T lymphocytes with distinct homing potentials and effector functions. *Nature* 1999; **401**: 708–12.
174. Mongkolsapaya J, Jaye A, Callan MFC et al. Antigen-specific expansion of cytotoxic T lymphocytes in acute measles virus infection. *J Virol* 1999; **73**: 67–71.
175. Beineke A, Puff C, Seehusen F, Baumgartner W. Pathogenesis and immunopathology of systemic and nervous canine distemper. *Vet Immunol Immunopathol* 2009; **127**: 1–18.
176. Kretschmer R, Janeway CA, Rosen FS. Immunologic amnesia. Study of an 11-year-old girl with recurrent severe infections associated with dysgammaglobulinemia, lymphopenia and lymphocytotoxic antibody, resulting in loss of immunologic memory. *Pediat Res* 1968; **2**: 7–16.
177. Enders JF, Peebles TC. Propagation in tissue cultures of cytophatic agents from patients with measles. *Proc Soc Exp Biol Med* 1954; **86**: 277–86.
178. Rauh LW, Schmidt R. Measles immunization with killed virus vaccine. *Am J Dis Child* 1965; **109**: 232–7.
179. Polack FP, Auwaerter PG, Lee SH et al. Production of atypical measles in rhesus macaques: Evidence for disease mediated by immune complex formation and eosinophils in the presence of fusion-inhibiting antibody. *Nat Med* 1999; **5**: 629–34.
180. Fulginiti VA, Eller JJ, Downte AW, Kempe CH. Altered reactivity to measles virus. Atypical measles in children previously immunized with inactivated measles virus vaccines. *JAMA* 1967; **202**: 1075–80.
181. Nader PR, Horwitz MS, Rousseau J. Atypical exanthem following exposure to natural measles: Eleven cases in children previously inoculated with killed vaccine. *J Pediatr* 1968; **72**: 22–8.
182. WHO. Measles vaccines. *Wkly Epidemiol Rec* 2004; **79**: 130–42.
183. Katz SL. Immunization with live attenuated measles virus vaccines: Five years' experience. *Arch Gesamte Virusforsch* 1965; **16**: 222–30.

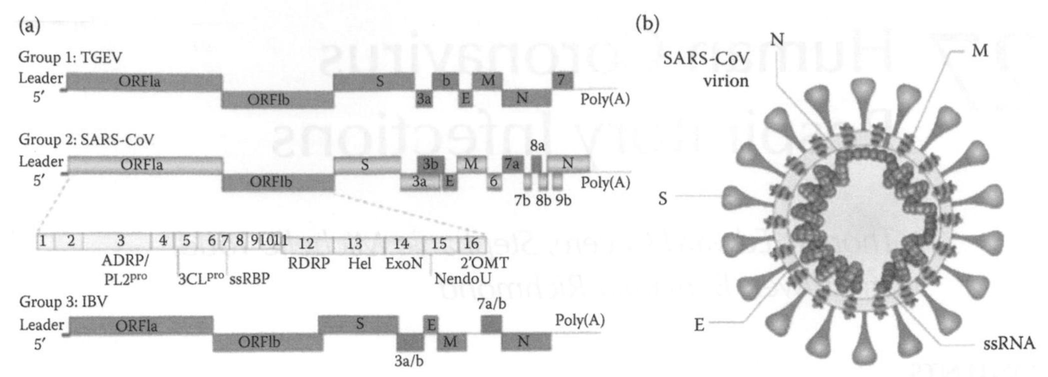

FIGURE 27.1 (**See color insert.**) (a) Schematic diagram of representative genomes from each of the coronavirus groups. Approximately the first two-thirds of the 26–32 kb, positive-sense RNA genome encodes a large polyprotein (ORF1a/b; green) that is proteolytically cleaved to generate 15 or 16 nonstructural proteins (nsps; nsps for severe acute respiratory syndrome coronavirus [SARS-CoV] are illustrated). The 3′-end third of the genome encodes four structural proteins—spike (S), membrane (M), envelope (E), and nucleocapsid (N) (all shown in blue)—along with a set of accessory proteins that are unique to each virus species (shown in red). Some group 2 coronaviruses express an additional structural protein, hemagglutinin esterase (not shown). (b) Schematic diagram of the coronavirus virion. 2′OMT, ribose-2′-*O*-methyltransferase; ExoN, 3′5′ exonuclease; Hel, helicase; IBV, infection bronchitis virus; NendoU, uridylate-specific endoribonuclease; RDRP, RNA-dependent RNA polymerase; ssRBP, single-stranded RNA binding protein; ssRNA, single-stranded RNA; TGEV, transmissible gastroenteritis virus. (Reproduced with permission from Perlman S, Netland J. *Nature Reviews Microbiology*. 2009; **7**(6): 439–50.)

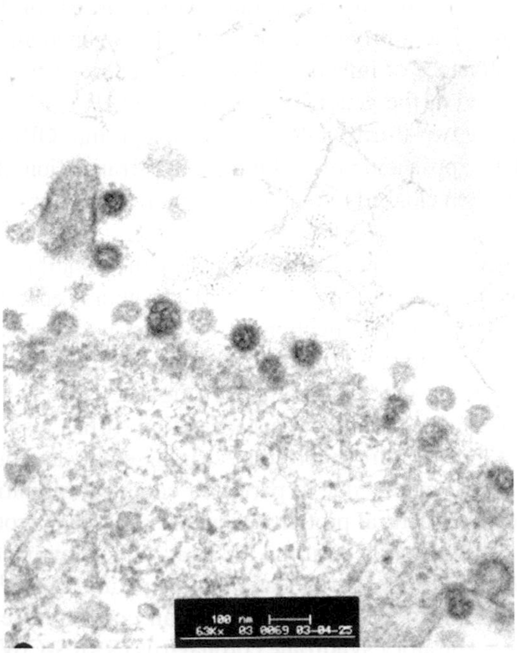

FIGURE 27.2 Thin-section electron micrograph of the surface of an infected FRhK4 cell showing SARS coronavirus with spikes. Bar = 100 nm. (Reproduced with permission from Poon LL et al. *The Lancet Infectious Diseases*. 2004; **4**(11): 663–71.)

1960s, whereas SARS-CoV was identified in 2003 and NL63 and HKU1 were identified in 2004 and 2005, respectively.[2,4,13] Four of these viruses (HCoV 229E, OC43, NL63, HKU1) are known to circulate continuously in the human population.[14]

There are three serogroups of coronaviruses, and within these serogroups, viruses are further subdivided based on their host range and genomic sequence.[4,14] Group 1 contains HCoVs 229E and NL63; group 2 contains HCoVs HKU1 and OC43 and SARS-CoV; and group 3 contains MERS-CoV.[14,15]

Although receptors for many coronaviruses are still unknown, several receptors have been identified. These include aminopeptidase N for multiple group 1 coronaviruses, 9-*O*-acetylated sialic acid for multiple group 2 coronaviruses, including HCoV-OC43, and angiotensin converting enzyme 2 (ACE2) for HCoV-NL63 and SARS-CoV.[3] Although both HCoV-NL63 and SARS-CoV bind to ACE2, these viruses bind to different portions of the receptor and with different affinity. This difference contributes, in part, to the different clinical outcomes: mild disease for HCoV-NL63 infection and severe respiratory disease for SARS-CoV.[16–19]

HCoV-NL63 was first isolated in the Netherlands from a 7-month-old child suffering from bronchiolitis, conjunctivitis, and fever. The virus was isolated using a virus-discovery-cDNA-amplified restriction fragment-length polymorphism technique (VIDISCA).[4] VIDISCA is a novel and rapid technique for amplification of unknown genomes based on the cDNA AFLP technique and it does not require prior knowledge of the genomic sequence.[4,14] Based on the genomic sequence, this virus is classified as a group 1 coronavirus and is most closely related to HCoV-229E. However, unlike HCoV-229E, which is fastidious and exhibits a narrow host range *in vitro*, HCoV-NL63 replicates efficiently in monkey kidney cells.[4] The HCoV-NL63 viral genome contains several notable features, including a unique N-terminal fragment within the S protein.[4]

27.2 EPIDEMIOLOGY

Infections of the respiratory tract rank as one of the top three causes of death in children under the age of 5 years worldwide, and while many of these infections are of unknown cause, HCoVs have been suggested as the etiological agent for up to 10% of all respiratory diseases.[14]

The first cases of severe acute respiratory syndrome (SARS) were reported in Foshan, in the Guangdong province of China in November 2002. Within months, the disease spread to 29 countries worldwide, ultimately affecting greater than 8000 patients and causing close to 800 fatalities. An important feature that contributed to the 2002–2003 SARS epidemic was the ability of SARS-CoV to cross species from animals to humans. The virus was isolated from Himalayan palm civets, raccoon dogs, and Chinese ferret badgers found in a live-animal market in Guangdon, China where transmission to animal handlers occurred.[20] However, subsequent screening suggested that these animals were not the primary reservoir for SARS-CoV. Rather, Chinese horseshoe bats have been suggested as an animal reservoir, and the virus may have spread from bats, to the mammals listed above, to humans (Figure 27.3)[11,21] One patient who acquired SARS in Guangdong traveled to Hong Kong, and served as the index case for greater than 50% of the total cases of SARS, highlighting the efficacy of modern global travel for spreading infectious disease.[22] SARS-CoV was spread primarily via airborne droplets and fomites.

HCoV-NL63 and HCoV-HKU1 are associated with acute respiratory disease in young children (less than 1 year of age) and immunocompromised adults. Based on RT-PCR screening, HCoV-NL63 virus was detected in 7% of patients suffering from respiratory disease at one hospital during January 2003, whereas no samples collected during the spring or summer of 2003 were positive.[4]

In June, 2012, a novel coronavirus was isolated from the sputum of a man in Jeddah, Saudi Arabia who presented with acute pneumonia and respiratory failure. This isolate was provisionally termed human coronavirus Erasmus Medical Center (HCoV-EMC), and later renamed Middle East respiratory syndrome coronavirus (MERS-CoV).[15,23,24] Since the index case in Saudi Arabia, 94 two enzymes $PL1^{pro}$ and $PL2^{pro}$ in other coronaviruses, for processing the N-terminal side of the replicative polyprotein at three specific sites. $PL2^{pro}$ of SARS-CoV also has unusually narrow substrate specificity, as compared to homologues of other coronaviruses.[12,30–38] The central portion and C-terminal end of the polyprotein are processed by a chymotrypsin-like protease $3CL^{pro}$ at 11 specific sites.[34,39,40] This protease is also known as the main protease, M^{pro}, as it releases the enzymes, RNA-dependent RNA polymerase (RdRp, nsp12) and helicase (nsp13), with both of these latter proteins being very important to viral replication. There are altogether 16 replicase gene products (nspl to nsp16). These nonstructural proteins range in size, from 13 to 1922 amino acid residues. Some of these proteins have novel predicted functions, including an ADP-ribose 1′-phosphatase activity (nsp3), 3′-to-5′ exonuclease activity (nsp14), uridylate-specific endoribonuclease (nsp15), and *S*-adenosylmethioine-dependent 2′-O-phosphatase (nsp16). As much as five of these nsp proteins have no known or predicted functions.[41–44]

28.2.4 Structural Proteins

There are four major structural proteins at the 3′ end, including nucleocapsid (N), envelope (E), membrane (M), and spike (S).[25,45–47] These known viral proteins confer the homologies necessary to initially classify the agents that caused the SARS syndrome to the group of coronavirus. In addition, eight unique accessory proteins are also encoded. These proteins showed no homology to any known viral or eukaryotic proteins. The functions of these accessory proteins are poorly understood. The open reading frames of these eight accessory proteins are inter-dispersing at the 3′ end of the viral genome between the ORFs of N and S. The subgenomic RNAs of these proteins are either monocistronic or bicistronic.

28.2.4.1 Spike Protein (S)

The Spike protein is a type I membrane protein that inserts into the viral envelope, conferring the crown-like appearance of the virus in electron microscopy. This protein interacts with the cellular receptor, angiotensin-converting enzyme 2 (ACE2),[48–50] mediating the entrance of the virus into the host cells. S protein induces membrane fusion between the viral envelope and the host plasma membrane. This protein is, thus, the major determining factor in the host range of SARS-CoV as well as tissue tropism of the virus.

Spike protein is synthesized as a 120 kDa protein and is immediately modified by glycosylation co-translationally.[48,51] Unlike the S protein of other coronaviruses that is cleaved into two domains and assembled into a trimer during virus packaging, the S protein of SARS-CoV is processed differently. During viral entry into the host cells, there might be multiple critical cleavage at the sites between the N-terminal S1 domain and C-terminal S2 domain, as well as within S2 domain.[51–54] Besides association with the receptor ACE2, a transmembrane protease/serine superfamily member 2 (TMPRSS2) might also be involved in mediating the entrance of the virus into the host cells.[55,56]

28.2.4.2 Envelope Protein (E)

Protein E is a transmembrane protein that is important in viral assembly. There was formation of viral-like particles with the expression of protein M and protein E only in culture models.[46,57–59] Overexpression experiments also suggested that protein E binded to Bcl-2 or Bcl-xL, subsequently inducing apoptosis.[60] Protein E also interacts with PALS1, the latter of which is essential for maintaining epithelial tight junctions.[61] This protein also has a cation-selective ion channel activity.[62] Hence, besides viral assembly, protein E might also have other roles in enhancing viral survival in the host.

28.2.4.3 Membrane Protein (M)

Protein M is a multiple transmembrane protein. It plays a crucial role during viral assembly and in the budding of virus from the host cells.[57,59,63–65] Protein M might also be able to induce interferon responses to infection.[66,67]

28.2.4.4 Nucleocapsid Protein (N)

Protein N is a basic RNA binding protein that complexes with the genomic RNA to form the viral capsid. Protein N interacts with protein M during viral assembly.[68–71] N also plays a role in subgenomic RNA synthesis. Protein N is associated with the replicase complex during subgenomic RNA synthesis.[72,73]

28.2.4.5 Accessory Proteins

The accessory proteins are dispensable for *in vivo* and *in vitro* growth of the coronavirus. Deletion of these accessory proteins in experimental models of coronavirus did not seem to affect viral replication, but there was attenuation in the natural host. These accessory proteins appear to contribute to various growth and immune advantages to the virus, thus allowing their sequences to prevail in the SARS-CoV genome, even if there should be strong selection pressure.[45,74–78] These proteins in the SARS-CoV genome are labeled according to their position in the genome from the 5′ end as: ORFs 3a, 3b, 6, 7a, 7b, 8a, 8b, and 9b.

28.2.4.5.1 ORF 3a

ORF 3a is 274 amino acid residues in size. It is found in the Golgi complex and rough endoplasmic reticulum. This protein might be secreted out of the cells or undergo endocytosis.[79,80] The expression of ORF 3a was confirmed in tissue specimens from SARS patients.[81] Circulating antibodies against ORF 3a were also detected.[82] In *in vitro* cell culture models, ORF 3a activates pro-inflammatory genes in host cells, through activation of JNK (c-Jun NH_2-terminal kinase)[83] and NK-κB.[83,84] There was upregulation of cytokines and chemokines, including IL-8 and RANTES (regulated on activation, normal T cell expressed and secreted).[83,85] Expression of ORF 3a induced apoptosis via caspase 8 and caspase 9 pathways.[86,87] The links with induction of apoptosis via Bax, p53 and p38 MAP kinase were uncertain.[86] ORF 3a might also play a role in viral replication and viral release.[88–90]

28.2.4.5.2 ORF 3b

ORF 3b is 154 amino acid residues in size. It is found in multiple subcellular locations, which might be related to different functions. In tissue culture models, ORF 3b was found accumulated in the nucleolus and subsequently translocated to the cytoplasm and inside the mitochondrion.[91–93] By modulating the activity of RUNX1b, there were upregulations of cytokines and chemokines.[94] Through activation of JNK and ERK (extracellular signal-regulated kinases) pathways, AP-1 activity was also induced.[95] Caspase-3 activity might be increased, resulting in apoptosis and necrosis.[96] Expression of ORF 3b, however, has not been confirmed in human tissue specimens. The presence of circulating serum antibodies has also not been ascertained.[81,97]

28.2.4.5.3 ORF 6

ORF 6 is 63 amino acid residues in size and is found in the membranes of the rough endoplasmic reticulum. Its expression in the target cells of patients' specimen has been detected.[81] ORF 6 is considered to be one of the important virulent factors for SARS-CoV. ORF 6 might act as an antagonist to IFN, suppressing IFN induction and the IFN signaling pathways.[98,99] ORF 6 binds to karyopherin α2 (KPNA2), inhibiting recruitment of KPNB1 (a component of classical nuclear import complex) and preventing translocation of ISGF3 (STAT1/STAT2/IRF-9) to the nuclei indirectly.[98] ORF 6 appears to play an important role in assisting SARS-CoV to evade the host innate immune responses. When ORF 6 was expressed in the host cells, double-membrane structures were formed, recapturing features observed during viral replications.[98,100] Together with the finding of colocalization of this protein with nonstructural protein nsp3, ORF 6 may also play a role in viral replication.[99,100]

28.2.4.5.4 ORF 7a

ORF 7a is 122 amino acid residues in size and is a type I membrane protein. ORF 7a is expressed in an *in vitro* culture model and in target cells in patients' specimens.[81] ORF 7a might be located in the rough endoplasmic reticulum, Golgi apparatus, inside mitochondria, or in the cytoplasm.[101,102] It interacts with structural proteins M and E, and can be found in the perinuclear region.[103] Overexpression of ORF 7a induces caspase-3-dependent apoptosis.[104,105] and activating the NF-κB and IL-8 promoter with subsequent production of pro-inflammatory chemokines, including IL-8 and RANTES.[83,106] ORF 7a might interact with members of Bcl-2 proteins, thus inducing apoptosis.[107] Overexpression of ORF 7a also inhibited cellular protein synthesis and activation of p38 mitogen-activated protein kinase.[108,109] Cell cycle arrest at G_0/G_1 was also observed.[110] ORF 7b was known to be expressed in infected cells, but there were little hints to its cellular function.

28.2.4.5.5 ORFs 8a and 8b

ORFs 8a and 8b were expressed as separate peptides of 39 and 84 amino acid residues in sizes, respectively, but it appeared to be expressed as a single peptide ORF 8ab in human specimens obtained during the early phase of the outbreak and in some animal models. This was a 29-nucleotide deletion, which divided the single ORF to two in the former cases. Overexpression of ORF 8a induced apoptosis using a mitochondrion-dependent pathway.[111] Overexpression of ORF 8b induced DNA synthesis. ORF 8a interacted with viral protein E, resulting in the downregulation of the latter protein.[112,113] The functions and cellular stabilities of ORF 8ab, ORF 8a, and ORF 8b appeared to be completely different. Their differential roles in the pathogenesis and replication of SARS-CoV remained unknown.

28.2.4.5.6 ORF 9b

ORF 9b is a 98 amino acid peptide synthesized from an alternative open reading frame within the N-gene, in the subgenomic mRNA 9. Anti-9b antibody and ORF 9b proteins have been detected in clinical specimens of SARS patients.[81,114] ORF 9b is present in the endoplasmic reticulum as well as being exported outside the host cell. This peptide might induce apoptosis, requiring export of this protein from the nucleus to endoplasmic reticulum.[115] ORF 9b also interacts with ORF 6, but the significance of this interaction is unknown.[116]

28.3 EPIDEMIOLOGY

Severe acute respiratory syndrome (SARS) is a novel infectious disease first recognized in late February 2003. The disease appeared earlier in Guangdong Province of southern China around November 2002. Rumors of a fatal infectious respiratory disease, mixed with rumor of preventive measures such as herbal medicine and acts of "fumigating with vinegar," had been spreading in the locality but were not enough to alert the world. This emerging disease only caught the attention of authorities when it spread to the neighborhood, the Hong Kong Special Administration Region (HKSAR). From this small, densely populated, busy city, the disease escalated to epidemic, via the rich international air-travel network of Hong Kong.

Hong Kong, Hanoi, Singapore, and Toronto were considered the initial SARS "hot zones." The disease spread rapidly among health care workers and their close contacts. This was partially due to the lack of awareness of this emerging disease and failure to implement timely measures of infectious control in the initial phase of the epidemic. In parallel, there was also rapid increase in the number of cases through secondary transmission to nonhealth care workers, in which the disease spread to the community. This virus, however, appeared to have low communicability, as outbreak only occurred in close contact, within family, and in high-density accommodation.

On March 15, 2003, the World Health Organization (WHO) issued emergency travel recommendations, marking a turning point in the outbreak. All countries with imported cases were able to prevent further transmission, and were able to keep the number of additional cases low. This is achieved through prompt detection of cases, isolation, and quarantine measures. There were, however, "atypical patients" with unusual clinical presentation or contact histories, or "superspreaders" with relatively mild or no symptoms, yet continuously shedding the virus. These patients served as reservoirs of the virus that easily evaded the preliminary surveillance system.[117]

At the beginning of July 2003, without an effective vaccine or well-proven therapeutic measures, SARS appeared to be under control. The WHO recorded 8000 patients with a total death toll of 774 (9.6%) in the period from November 2002 through July 31, 2003. The most affected regions included mainland China (5327 cases, 349 deaths), Hong Kong (1755 cases, 299 deaths), Taiwan (346 cases, 37 deaths), and Singapore (238 cases, 33 deaths).[118]

28.3.1 Starting Point at Hong Kong

Since November 2002, clusters of cases of severe, atypical pneumonia appeared among health care workers and their household members in the Guangdong Province of southern China. On February 21, 2003, an infected medical doctor spent a single night in the Room 911, 9th floor of a Hong Kong hotel (Hotel M). This doctor visited the Emergency Department on arrival to Hong Kong. He had a fever and respiratory symptoms for a few days before entering Hong Kong. He was discharged with remedies for symptomatic relief, unaware of the possible link to the mysterious illness just across the border. He became seriously ill the next day and was admitted to a loco-regional hospital. He died 10 days later. His brief stay in Hotel M was already enough to infect guests and visitors staying or briefly visiting the hotel's ninth floor. These visitors brought the virus home with them to other parts of Hong Kong, Vietnam, Singapore, and Toronto.[119]

The index patient from Hong Kong infected 12 other persons who had been staying or visiting the same hotel. Two of these patients were subsequently seeding further outbreaks in two other regional hospitals. One of these individuals appeared to be a "superspreader." Unaware of this new contagious disease, a nebulizer was used on this patient in the ward, simultaneously infecting nearby patients, health care workers, and a group of medical students doing their junior clerkship.[120] At the end of March 2003, an outbreak occurred in a single block of apartments in a private housing estate (Amoy Gardens). There were 320 SARS cases in less than 3 weeks. The probable index patient had chronic renal failure and was on continuous ambulatory peritoneal dialysis (CAPD). Used CAPD fluid, infected with virus, was discarded into the toilet, contaminating the sewage system and subsequently infecting the neighborhood. Quarantine measures were installed.[121,122]

Public health measures and improving personal hygiene measures appeared to impose control over the disease, and the rate of appearance of new cases dropped in April 2003. In the outbreaks in Hong Kong, there were 1755 cases of SARS. Among these patients, 295 of them died (16.8%). Around 30% of cases occurred in health care workers. Nurses were the top category of workers being affected. Among them, eight medical workers died.[123] Finally, the WHO removed Hong Kong from its list of areas with SARS on June 23, 2003, marking the end of the SARS outbreaks in this city.[124]

28.3.2 China

The Chinese authorities reported only 37 cases in Beijing by April 19, 2003, but escalated to 400 in the following days, when the epidemic was well underway in other countries.[125] By this time, SARS had spread to many provinces, including western Guangxi, northern Gansu, and Inner Mongolia.[126] On April 23, 2003, the WHO extended its SARS-related travel advice to Beijing and the Shanxi Province of China. Strict measures were imposed by the Chinese Authorities in the following 4 days, closing temporarily all recreational facilities, including theaters, Internet cafes, discos, and so on.[127] In this outbreak, there were 5327 cases of SARS, with a death toll of 349 patients. Beijing was removed from the list of SARS areas on June 24, 2003.[128]

28.3.3 Taiwan

Taiwan's epidemic was the third-worst in the world, after China and Hong Kong. The story began when a man with history of travel in the Guangdong Province and Hong Kong was diagnosed with

SARS, together with his wife, on March 14, 2003.[129] Twelve days later, an individual from the quarantined private estate of Hong Kong flew to Taiwan and took a train to Taichung to celebrate the traditional festival, Qing Ming. He infected his brother and a passenger on the train. At the end of April, the number of new cases increased steadily. A laundry worker with diabetes mellitus remained on duty in a hospital even though he was having fever and diarrhea since April 12, 2003. He had frequent contact with visitors and hospital staff. His symptoms worsened on April 16, 2003 and he was admitted to the hospital. Two days later, he developed bilateral lung infiltrates. Due to the huge number of potential contacts, the hospital was contained. Clusters of infected health care workers in eight other hospitals were linked to this outbreak.[130] Secondary transmission occurred throughout different regions of Taiwan. This outbreak in Taiwan was an example of extensive transmission from one single, unrecognized, atypical patient. The saga in Taiwan ended on July 5, 2003, when the WHO removed Taiwan from the list of SARS areas.[131]

28.3.4 Singapore

A previously healthy 23-year-old woman of Chinese ethnicity who had been staying on the 9th floor of Hotel M during a vacation to Hong Kong became the index case of SARS. She was admitted to a hospital due to worsening respiratory symptoms. Unaware of this new contagious diseases, strict infection control measures were not implemented and this index patient infected at least 20 other persons, including many health care workers.[132] This pattern of spread among health care workers of the same hospital and a different hospital was typical for outbreaks of SARS in Singapore. "Superspreaders" were also identified. In one study, 144 of Singapore's 206 probable cases were traced back to contact with only 5 patients. Another characteristic measure used was demonstrated in a prompt identification of cases clustering at a wholesale market on April 20, 2003. The market was immediately ordered to be closed for 15 days. About 400 persons were put under home quarantine. This measure successfully limited the total number of infected people to 15. In Singapore, 238 cases of SARS were diagnosed, with a death toll of 33.[133–136] The outbreaks ended on May 31, 2003 when Singapore was removed from the WHO list of SARS areas.[137]

28.3.5 Toronto

The index patient stayed with her husband on the 9th floor of Hotel M when the index patient of Hong Kong was there, from February 13, 2003 to February 23, 2003. Upon returning to Toronto, she developed symptoms 2 days later and passed away 9 days after onset. Five out of six family members living in the same household developed SARS in the first week of March. The outbreak seemed to be under control.[138] A second outbreak occurred when an undiagnosed case underwent surgery at a hospital and spread the disease to the health care workers and other patients. Another patient transferred from this hospital to another medical center carried SARS to the latter and resulted in another outbreak. The stories in Toronto were characterized by outbreaks occurring among health care workers despite full awareness of the disease and its specific mode of spread.[139] In Toronto, there were altogether 251 cases of SARS and 43 died.[140,141] On July 2, 2003, the WHO removed Toronto from the list of SARS areas.[142]

28.3.6 Vietnam

The index patient in Vietnam also got the disease from a brief visit to the 9th floor of Hotel M in Hong Kong. The outbreak followed the usual route of passing the disease to health care workers and their close contacts. Vietnam appeared very successful in containing the disease and was the first to be removed from the list of SARS areas on April 28, 2003.[143]

28.4 CLINICAL FEATURES

High fever, more than 38°C, was the most common symptom in SARS. It was also the main criterion in the WHO case definition to qualify at least a suspected or probable case. This fact had also been incorporated into public health measures, including screening for travelers in the major ports. Most of the so-called "atypical" cases were those patients that failed to launch a fever at presentation. They might be febrile at a later stage of the disease, but such window period was usually enough to create a high risk of secondary outbreaks.[119,122,139,144–146]

The other symptoms of SARS fit the common description for "atypical pneumonia" or other viral pneumonias. There might be chills, rigors, headache, malaise, and myalgia. There might not be a lot of upper respiratory tract symptoms. Sputum production was not prominent unless the clinical course of the patient was complicated by secondary infection. Diarrhea was only common in the cohort of the outbreak in Amoy Gardens in Hong Kong.[147–150]

It was suspected that some patients infected with SARS-CoV might only have mild symptoms or even be asymptomatic.[151] The existence of such patients would have strong implications to public health, as these patients would be able to evade the public health surveillance system. Unfortunately, convincing population-wise study data is not available.[123,146,152–154]

SARS patients did not have any specific biochemical disturbance. High serum lactate dehydrogenase was observed and had been linked to poor outcome. The enzyme might originate from the primary effect of viral infection causing lung injury. Alternatively, it might be the side effect of treatment such as the known hemolytic effect of ribavirin.[119,122,139,146]

Hematological changes seemed to be more consistent.[155] There were lymphopenia and thrombocytopenia. Both CD4 and CD8 counts were reduced in the early phase of the disease. Prothrombin time, activated partial-thromboplastin time, international normalized ratio, and the level of D-dimer may be deranged.[156,157]

28.4.1 Clinical Course

The incubation period of SARS was about 6 days. In the WHO guidelines, the estimated maximum incubation period was 10 days. SARS might then evolve with highly variable clinical courses, ranging from mild, trivial symptoms to severe, fatal diseases.

In the first week, the disease was characterized by fever, myalgia, and other systemic symptoms. All patients were managed with intravenous amoxicillin-clavulanate, oral azithromycin, intravenous ribavirin, and a tailing regimen of corticosteroids. In the second week, there might be recurrence of fever and oxygen desaturation. Some patients might develop diarrhea. From this second week onwards, some patients might start to have deteriorating courses. This was, paradoxically, associated with sero-conversion and a drop in viral load. Chest x-ray might show initial improvement but was subsequently followed by diffuse bilateral shadowing. This phase of disease might be related to indirect immune-mediated damage rather than due to direct viral infection in the first week.[119,122,139,144–146]

About 20% of patients progressed to the third phase of acute respiratory distress syndrome, requiring intensive care and ventilatory support. These patients might develop severe lymphopenia and might be complicated by secondary nosocomial infection. The WHO estimated that case fatality is in the range of 14–19%. There were loco-regional variations: 11–17% in Hong Kong, 13–15% in Singapore, 15–19% in Canada, and 5–13% in China. Old-age and comorbidities were shown to be independent predictors of poor outcome.[158–161]

For patients recovered from fever and respiratory symptoms, they were advised to practice isolation and cross-contamination precautions, and should refrain from social interactions, including work or school, for at least 10–14 days. The period of viral shedding was variable. In fact, some asymptomatic patients or patients recovered from SARS might continue to shed virus for variable periods of time. These latter "superspreaders" were important reservoirs for outbreaks.[162,163]

Arden, K.E., Chang, A.B., Lambert, S.B., Nissen, M.D., Sloots, T.P., Mackay, I.M., 2010. Newly identified respiratory viruses in children with asthma exacerbation not requiring admission to hospital. *J. Med. Virol.* 82, 1458–1461.

Arden, K.E., McErlean, P., Nissen, M.D., Sloots, T.P., Mackay, I.M., 2006. Frequent detection of human rhinoviruses, paramyxoviruses, coronaviruses, and bocavirus during acute respiratory tract infections. *J. Med. Virol.* 78, 1232–1240.

Arnott, A., Vong, S., Rith, S., Naughtin, M., Ly, S., Guillard, B., Deubel, V., Buchy, P., 2012. Human bocavirus amongst an all-ages population hospitalised with acute lower respiratory infections in Cambodia. *Influenza Other Respi. Viruses*. 7(2), 201–210.

Arthur, J.L., Higgins, G.D., Davidson, G.P., Givney, R.C., Ratcliff, R.M., 2009. A novel bocavirus associated with acute gastroenteritis in Australian children. *PLoS Pathog.* 5, e1000391.

Babady, N.E., Mead, P., Stiles, J., Brennan, C., Li, H., Shuptar, S., Stratton, C.W., Tang, Y.W., Kamboj, M., 2012. Comparison of the Luminex xTAG RVP Fast assay and the Idaho Technology FilmArray RP assay for detection of respiratory viruses in pediatric patients at a cancer hospital. *J. Clin. Microbiol.* 50, 2282–2288.

Babkin, I.V., Tumentsev, A.I., Tikunov, A.Y., Kurilschikov, A.M., Ryabchikova, E.I., Zhirakovskaya, E.V., Netesov, S.V., Tikunova, N.V., 2013. Evolutionary time-scale of primate bocaviruses. *Infect. Genet. Evol* 14, 265–274.

Balada-Llasat, J.M., LaRue, H., Kelly, C., Rigali, L., Pancholi, P., 2011a. Evaluation of commercial ResPlex II v2.0, MultiCode-PLx, and xTAG respiratory viral panels for the diagnosis of respiratory viral infections in adults. *J. Clin. Virol.* 50, 42–45.

Balada-Llasat, J.M., LaRue, H., Kelly, C., Rigali, L., Pancholi, P., 2011b. Evaluation of commercial ResPlex II v2.0, MultiCode-PLx, and xTAG respiratory viral panels for the diagnosis of respiratory viral infections in adults. *J. Clin. Virol.* 50, 42–45.

Bastien, N., Brandt, K., Dust, K., Ward, D., Li, Y., 2006. Human bocavirus infection, Canada. *Emerg. Infect. Dis.* 12, 848–850.

Bohmer, A., Schildgen, V., Lusebrink, J., Ziegler, S., Tillmann, R.L., Kleines, M., Schildgen, O., 2009a. Novel application for isothermal nucleic acid sequence-based amplification (NASBA). *J. Virol. Methods* 158, 199–201.

Bohmer, A., Schildgen, V., Lusebrink, J., Ziegler, S., Tillmann, R.L., Kleines, M., Schildgen, O., 2009b. Novel application for isothermal nucleic acid sequence-based amplification (NASBA). *J. Virol. Methods* 158, 199–201.

Bonvicini, F., Manaresi, E., Gentilomi, G.A., Di Furio, F., Zerbini, M., Musiani, M., Gallinella, G., 2011. Evidence of human bocavirus viremia in healthy blood donors. *Diagn. Microbiol. Infect. Dis.* 71, 460–462.

Bonzel, L., Tenenbaum, T., Schroten, H., Schildgen, O., Schweitzer-Krantz, S., Adams, O., 2008. Frequent detection of viral coinfection in children hospitalized with acute respiratory tract infection using a real-time polymerase chain reaction. *Pediatr. Infect. Dis. J.* 27, 589–594.

Brieu, N., Gay, B., Segondy, M., Foulongne, V., 2007. Electron microscopy observation of human bocavirus (HBoV) in nasopharyngeal samples from HBoV-infected children. *J. Clin. Microbiol.* 45, 3419–3420.

Calvo, C., Garcia-Garcia, M.L., Pozo, F., Carvajal, O., Perez-Brena, P., Casas, I., 2008. Clinical characteristics of human bocavirus infections compared with other respiratory viruses in Spanish children. *Pediatr. Infect. Dis. J.* 27, 677–680.

Campe, H., Hartberger, C., Sing, A., 2008. Role of Human Bocavirus infections in outbreaks of gastroenteritis. *J. Clin. Virol.* 43, 340–342.

Carrol, E.D., Mankhambo, L.A., Guiver, M., Banda, D.L., Group, I.P.D.S., Denis, B., Dove, W. et al. 2011. PCR improves diagnostic yield from lung aspiration in Malawian children with radiologically confirmed pneumonia. *PLoS One* 6, e21042.

Cashman, O., O'Shea, H., 2012. Detection of human bocaviruses 1, 2 and 3 in Irish children presenting with gastroenteritis. *Arch. Virol.* 157, 1767–1773.

Chen, A.Y., Cheng, F., Lou, S., Luo, Y., Liu, Z., Delwart, E., Pintel, D., Qiu, J., 2010. Characterization of the gene expression profile of human bocavirus. *Virology* 403, 145–154.

Chieochansin, T., Samransamruajkit, R., Chutinimitkul, S., Payungporn, S., Hiranras, T., Theamboonlers, A., Poovorawan, Y., 2008. Human bocavirus (HBoV) in Thailand: clinical manifestations in a hospitalized pediatric patient and molecular virus characterization. *J. Infect.* 56, 137–142.

Chorazy, M.L., Lebeck, M.G., McCarthy, T.A., Richter, S.S., Torner, J.C., Gray, G.C., 2013. Polymicrobial acute respiratory infections in a hospital-based pediatric population. *Pediatr. Infect. Dis. J* 32(5), 460–466.

Chow, B.D., Huang, Y.T., Esper, F.P., 2008. Evidence of human bocavirus circulating in children and adults, Cleveland, Ohio. *J. Clin. Virol.* 43, 302–306.

Chow, B.D., Ou, Z., Esper, F.P., 2010. Newly recognized bocaviruses (HBoV, HBoV2) in children and adults with gastrointestinal illness in the United States. *J. Clin. Virol.* 47, 143–147.

Christensen, J., Cotmore, S.F., Tattersall, P., 1995. Minute virus of mice transcriptional activator protein NS1 binds directly to the transactivation region of the viral P38 promoter in a strictly ATP-dependent manner. *J. Virol.* 69, 5422–5430.

Cotmore, S.F., Christensen, J., Nuesch, J.P., Tattersall, P., 1995. The NS1 polypeptide of the murine parvovirus minute virus of mice binds to DNA sequences containing the motif [ACCA]2–3. *J. Virol.* 69, 1652–1660.

Cotmore, S.F., Gottlieb, R.L., Tattersall, P., 2007. Replication initiator protein NS1 of the parvovirus minute virus of mice binds to modular divergent sites distributed throughout duplex viral DNA. *J. Virol.* 81, 13015–13027.

De Vos, N., Vankeerberghen, A., Vaeyens, F., Van Vaerenbergh, K., Boel, A., De Beenhouwer, H., 2009. Simultaneous detection of human bocavirus and adenovirus by multiplex real-time PCR in a Belgian paediatric population. *Eur. J. Clin. Microbiol. Infect. Dis.* 28, 1305–1310.

Deng, X., Yan, Z., Luo, Y., Xu, J., Cheng, F., Li, Y., Engelhardt, J.F., Qiu, J., 2013. *In vitro* modeling of human bocavirus 1 infection of polarized primary human airway epithelia. *J. Virol* 87(7), 4097–102.

Deng, Y., Gu, X., Zhao, X., Luo, J., Luo, Z., Wang, L., Fu, Z., Yang, X., Liu, E., 2012. High viral load of human bocavirus correlates with duration of wheezing in children with severe lower respiratory tract infection. *PLoS One* 7, e34353.

Dijkman, R., Koekkoek, S.M., Molenkamp, R., Schildgen, O., van der Hoek, L., 2009. Human bocavirus can be cultured in differentiated human airway epithelial cells. *J. Virol.* 83, 7739–7748.

Do, A.H., van Doorn, H.R., Nghiem, M.N., Bryant, J.E., Hoang, T.H., Do, Q.H., Van, T.L. et al. 2011. Viral etiologies of acute respiratory infections among hospitalized Vietnamese children in Ho Chi Minh City, 2004–2008. *PLoS One* 6, e18176.

Don, M., Soderlund-Venermo, M., Hedman, K., Ruuskanen, O., Allander, T., Korppi, M., 2011. Don't forget serum in the diagnosis of human bocavirus infection. *J. Infect. Dis.* 203, 1031–1032; author reply 1032–1033.

Don, M., Soderlund-Venermo, M., Valent, F., Lahtinen, A., Hedman, L., Canciani, M., Hedman, K., Korppi, M., 2010. Serologically verified human bocavirus pneumonia in children. *Pediatr. Pulmonol.* 45, 120–126.

Fabbiani, M., Terrosi, C., Martorelli, B., Valentini, M., Bernini, L., Cellesi, C., Cusi, M.G., 2009. Epidemiological and clinical study of viral respiratory tract infections in children from Italy. *J. Med. Virol.* 81, 750–756.

Falcone, V., Ridder, G.J., Panning, M., Bierbaum, S., Neumann-Haefelin, D., Huzly, D., 2011. Human bocavirus DNA in paranasal sinus mucosa. *Emerg. Infect. Dis.* 17, 1564–1565.

Flores, C.J., Vizcaya, A.C., Araos, B.R., Montecinos, P.L., Godoy, M.P., Valiente-Echeverria, F., Perret, P.C., Valenzuela, C.P., Hirsch, B.T., Ferres, G.M., 2011. [Human bocavirus in Chile: Clinical characteristics and epidemiological profile in children with acute respiratory tract infections]. *Rev. Chilena Infectol.* 28, 504–511.

Franz, A., Adams, O., Willems, R., Bonzel, L., Neuhausen, N., Schweizer-Krantz, S., Ruggeberg, J.U., Willers, R., Henrich, B., Schroten, H., Tenenbaum, T., 2010. Correlation of viral load of respiratory pathogens and co-infections with disease severity in children hospitalized for lower respiratory tract infection. *J. Clin. Virol.* 48, 239–245.

Garcia-Garcia, M.L., Calvo, C., Pozo, F., Perez-Brena, P., Quevedo, S., Bracamonte, T., Casas, I., 2008. Human bocavirus detection in nasopharyngeal aspirates of children without clinical symptoms of respiratory infection. Pediatr. *Infect. Dis. J.* 27, 358–360.

Ghietto, L.M., Camara, A., Camara, J., Adamo, M.P., 2012a. High frequency of human bocavirus 1 DNA in infants and adults with lower acute respiratory infection. *J. Med. Microbiol.* 61, 548–551.

Ghietto, L.M., Camara, A., Zhou, Y., Pedranti, M., Ferreyra, S., Frey, T., Camara, J., Adamo, M.P., 2012b. High prevalence of human bocavirus 1 in infants with lower acute respiratory tract disease in Argentina, 2007–2009. *Braz. J. Infect. Dis.* 16, 38–44.

Guo, L., Wang, Y., Zhou, H., Wu, C., Song, J., Li, J., Paranhos-Baccala, G., Vernet, G., Wang, J., Hung, T., 2012. Differential seroprevalence of human bocavirus species 1–4 in Beijing, China. *PLoS One* 7, e39644.

Gurda, B.L., Parent, K.N., Bladek, H., Sinkovits, R.S., DiMattia, M.A., Rence, C., Castro, A. et al. 2010. Human bocavirus capsid structure: insights into the structural repertoire of the parvoviridae. *J. Virol.* 84, 5880–5889.

Han, T.H., Kim, C.H., Park, S.H., Kim, E.J., Chung, J.Y., Hwang, E.S., 2009. Detection of human bocavirus-2 in children with acute gastroenteritis in South Korea. *Arch. Virol.* 154, 1923–1927.

Hao, R., Ni, K., Xia, Q., Peng, C., Deng, Y., Zhao, X., Fu, Z., Liu, W., Liu, E., 2013. Correlation between nucleotide mutation and viral loads of human bocavirus 1 in hospitalized children with respiratory tract infection. *J. Gen. Virol.* 94(Pt 5), 1079–1085.

Hedman, L., Soderlund-Venermo, M., Jartti, T., Ruuskanen, O., Hedman, K., 2010. Dating of human bocavirus infection with protein-denaturing IgG-avidity assays—Secondary immune activations are ubiquitous in immunocompetent adults. *J. Clin. Virol.* 48, 44–48.

Heydari, H., Mamishi, S., Khotaei, G.T., Moradi, S., 2011. Fatal type 7 adenovirus associated with human bocavirus infection in a healthy child. *J. Med. Virol.* 83, 1762–1763.

Huang, Q., Deng, X., Yan, Z., Cheng, F., Luo, Y., Shen, W., Lei-Butters, D.C. et al. 2012. Establishment of a reverse genetics system for studying human bocavirus in human airway epithelia. *PLoS Pathog.* 8, e1002899.

Hustedt, J.W., Christie, C., Hustedt, M.M., Esposito, D., Vazquez, M., 2012. Seroepidemiology of human bocavirus infection in Jamaica. *PLoS One* 7, e38206.

Jartti, T., Soderlund-Venermo, M., Allander, T., Vuorinen, T., Hedman, K., Ruuskanen, O., 2011. No efficacy of prednisolone in acute wheezing associated with human bocavirus infection. *Pediatr. Infect. Dis. J.* 30, 521–523.

Kantola, K., Hedman, L., Allander, T., Jartti, T., Lehtinen, P., Ruuskanen, O., Hedman, K., Soderlund-Venermo, M., 2008. Serodiagnosis of human bocavirus infection. *Clin. Infect. Dis.* 46, 540–546.

Kantola, K., Hedman, L., Arthur, J., Alibeto, A., Delwart, E., Jartti, T., Ruuskanen, O., Hedman, K., Soderlund-Venermo, M., 2011. Seroepidemiology of human bocaviruses 1–4. *J. Infect. Dis.* 204, 1403–1412.

Kapoor, A., Hornig, M., Asokan, A., Williams, B., Henriquez, J.A., Lipkin, W.I., 2011. Bocavirus episome in infected human tissue contains non-identical termini. *PLoS One* 6, e21362.

Kapoor, A., Simmonds, P., Slikas, E., Li, L., Bodhidatta, L., Sethabutr, O., Triki, H. et al. 2010. Human bocaviruses are highly diverse, dispersed, recombination prone, and prevalent in enteric infections. *J. Infect. Dis.* 201, 1633–1643.

Kapoor, A., Slikas, E., Simmonds, P., Chieochansin, T., Naeem, A., Shaukat, S., Alam, M.M. et al. 2009. A newly identified bocavirus species in human stool. *J. Infect. Dis.* 199, 196–200.

Khamrin, P., Malasao, R., Chaimongkol, N., Ukarapol, N., Kongsricharoern, T., Okitsu, S., Hayakawa, S., Ushijima, H., Maneekarn, N., 2012. Circulating of human bocavirus 1, 2, 3, and 4 in pediatric patients with acute gastroenteritis in Thailand. *Infect. Genet. Evol.* 12, 565–569.

Kleines, M., Scheithauer, S., Rackowitz, A., Ritter, K., Hausler, M., 2007. High prevalence of human bocavirus detected in young children with severe acute lower respiratory tract disease by use of a standard PCR protocol and a novel real-time PCR protocol. *J. Clin. Microbiol.* 45, 1032–1034.

Klinkenberg D., K., R., Schneppenheim, R., Müller, I., Blohm, M., Malecki, M., Schildgen, V., Schildgen, O., 2012. Fatal human bocavirus infection in a boy with IPEX-like syndrome and vaccine-acquired rotavirus enteritis awaiting stem cell transplantation. *Arch. Dis. Child.* 97, A274.

Korner, R.W., Soderlund-Venermo, M., van Koningsbruggen-Rietschel, S., Kaiser, R., Malecki, M., Schildgen, O., 2011. Severe human bocavirus infection, Germany. *Emerg. Infect. Dis.* 17, 2303–2305.

Korppi, M., Jartti, T., Hedman, K., Soderlund-Venermo, M., 2010. Serologic diagnosis of human bocavirus infection in children. *Pediatr. Infect. Dis. J.* 29, 387.

Koseki, N., Teramoto, S., Kaiho, M., Gomi-Endo, R., Yoshioka, M., Takahashi, Y., Nakayama, T. et al. 2012. Detection of human bocaviruses 1 to 4 from nasopharyngeal swab samples collected from patients with respiratory tract infections. *J. Clin. Microbiol.* 50, 2118–2121.

Kupfer, B., Vehreschild, J., Cornely, O., Kaiser, R., Plum, G., Viazov, S., Franzen, C. et al. 2006a. Severe pneumonia and human bocavirus in adult. *Emerg. Infect. Dis.* 12, 1614–1616.

Kupfer, B., Vehreschild, J., Cornely, O., Kaiser, R., Plum, G., Viazov, S., Franzen, C. et al. 2006b. Severe pneumonia and human bocavirus in adult. *Emerg. Infect. Dis.* 12, 1614–1616.

Lassauniere, R., Kresfelder, T., Venter, M., 2010. A novel multiplex real-time RT-PCR assay with FRET hybridization probes for the detection and quantitation of 13 respiratory viruses. *J. Virol. Methods* 165, 254–260.

Lau, S.K., Yip, C.C., Que, T.L., Lee, R.A., Au-Yeung, R.K., Zhou, B., So, L.Y. et al. 2007. Clinical and molecular epidemiology of human bocavirus in respiratory and fecal samples from children in Hong Kong. *J. Infect. Dis.* 196, 986–993.

Li, Y., Dong, Y., Jiang, J., Yang, Y., Liu, K., 2012. High prevelance of human parvovirus infection in patients with malignant tumors. *Oncol. Lett.* 3, 635–640.

Loeffelholz, M.J., Pong, D.L., Pyles, R.B., Xiong, Y., Miller, A.L., Bufton, K.K., Chonmaitree, T., 2011. Comparison of the FilmArray respiratory panel and prodesse real-time PCR assays for detection of respiratory pathogens. *J. Clin. Microbiol.* 49, 4083–4088.

Longtin, J., Bastien, M., Gilca, R., Leblanc, E., de Serres, G., Bergeron, M.G., Boivin, G., 2008a. Human bocavirus infections in hospitalized children and adults. *Emerg. Infect. Dis.* 14, 217–221.

Longtin, J., Bastien, M., Gilca, R., Leblanc, E., de Serres, G., Bergeron, M.G., Boivin, G., 2008b. Human bocavirus infections in hospitalized children and adults. *Emerg. Infect. Dis.* 14, 217–221.

Lusebrink, J., Schildgen, V., Tillmann, R.L., Wittleben, F., Bohmer, A., Muller, A., Schildgen, O., 2011. Detection of head-to-tail DNA sequences of human bocavirus in clinical samples. *PLoS One* 6, e19457.

Martin, E.T., Fairchok, M.P., Kuypers, J., Magaret, A., Zerr, D.M., Wald, A., Englund, J.A., 2010. Frequent and prolonged shedding of bocavirus in young children attending daycare. *J. Infect. Dis.* 201, 1625–1632.

Martin, E.T., Taylor, J., Kuypers, J., Magaret, A., Wald, A., Zerr, D., Englund, J.A., 2009. Detection of bocavirus in saliva of children with and without respiratory illness. *J. Clin. Microbiol.* 47, 4131–4132.

Mitui, M.T., Tabib, S.M., Matsumoto, T., Khanam, W., Ahmed, S., Mori, D., Akhter, N. et al. 2012. Detection of human bocavirus in the cerebrospinal fluid of children with encephalitis. *Clin. Infect. Dis.* 54, 964–967.

Modrow, S., Wenzel, J.J., Schimanski, S., Schwarzbeck, J., Rothe, U., Oldenburg, J., Jilg, W., Eis-Hubinger, A.M., 2011. Prevalence of nucleic acid sequences specific for human parvoviruses, hepatitis A and hepatitis E viruses in coagulation factor concentrates. *Vox Sang.* 100, 351–358.

Muller, A., Klinkenberg, D., Vehreschild, J., Cornely, O., Tillmann, R.L., Franzen, C., Simon, A., Schildgen, O., 2009. Low prevalence of human metapneumovirus and human bocavirus in adult immunocompromised high risk patients suspected to suffer from Pneumocystis pneumonia. *J. Infect.* 58, 227–231.

Nascimento-Carvalho, C.M., Cardoso, M.R., Meriluoto, M., Kemppainen, K., Kantola, K., Ruuskanen, O., Hedman, K., Soderlund-Venermo, M., 2012. Human bocavirus infection diagnosed serologically among children admitted to hospital with community-acquired pneumonia in a tropical region. *J. Med. Virol.* 84, 253–258.

Pham, N.T., Trinh, Q.D., Chan-It, W., Khamrin, P., Nishimura, S., Sugita, K., Maneekarn, N., Okitsu, S., Mizuguchi, M., Ushijima, H., 2011. Human bocavirus infection in children with acute gastroenteritis in Japan and Thailand. *J. Med. Virol.* 83, 286–290.

Pilger, D.A., Cantarelli, V.V., Amantea, S.L., Leistner-Segal, S., 2011. Detection of human bocavirus and human metapneumovirus by real-time PCR from patients with respiratory symptoms in Southern Brazil. *Mem. Inst. Oswaldo Cruz* 106, 56–60.

Salmon-Mulanovich, G., Sovero, M., Laguna-Torres, V.A., Kochel, T.J., Lescano, A.G., Chauca, G., Sanchez, J.F. et al. 2011. Frequency of human bocavirus (HBoV) infection among children with febrile respiratory symptoms in Argentina, Nicaragua and Peru. *Influenza Other Respi. Viruses* 5, 1–5.

Schildgen, O., Muller, A., Allander, T., Mackay, I.M., Volz, S., Kupfer, B., Simon, A., 2008a. Human bocavirus: Passenger or pathogen in acute respiratory tract infections? *Clin. Microbiol. Rev.* 21, 291–304.

Schildgen, O., Muller, A., Allander, T., Mackay, I.M., Volz, S., Kupfer, B., Simon, A., 2008b. Human bocavirus: Passenger or pathogen in acute respiratory tract infections? *Clin. Microbiol. Rev.* 21, 291–304, table of contents.

Schildgen, O., Qiu, J., Soderlund-Venermo, M., 2012. Genomic features of the human bocaviruses. *Future Virol.* 7, 31–39.

Schildgen, V., Malecki, M., Tillmann, R.-L., Brockmann, M., Schildgen O., 2013. The human bocavirus is associated with some lung and colorectal cancers and persists in solid tumors. *PLOS One* 8(6): e68020.

Sloots, T.P., McErlean, P., Speicher, D.J., Arden, K.E., Nissen, M.D., Mackay, I.M., 2006. Evidence of human coronavirus HKU1 and human bocavirus in Australian children. *J. Clin. Virol.* 35, 99–102.

Smuts, H., Hardie, D., 2006. Human bocavirus in hospitalized children, South Africa. *Emerg. Infect. Dis.* 12, 1457–1458.

Smuts, H., Workman, L., Zar, H.J., 2008. Role of human metapneumovirus, human coronavirus NL63 and human bocavirus in infants and young children with acute wheezing. *J. Med. Virol.* 80, 906–912.

Soderlund-Venermo, M., Lahtinen, A., Jartti, T., Hedman, L., Kemppainen, K., Lehtinen, P., Allander, T., Ruuskanen, O., Hedman, K., 2009. Clinical assessment and improved diagnosis of bocavirus-induced wheezing in children, Finland. *Emerg. Infect. Dis.* 15, 1423–1430.

Streiter, M., Malecki, M., Prokop, A., Schildgen, V., Lusebrink, J., Guggemos, A., Wisskirchen, M. et al. 2011. Does human bocavirus infection depend on helper viruses? A challenging case report. *Virol. J.* 8, 417.

Sun, Y., Chen, A.Y., Cheng, F., Guan, W., Johnson, F.B., Qiu, J., 2009. Molecular characterization of infectious clones of the minute virus of canines reveals unique features of bocaviruses. *J. Virol.* 83, 3956–3967.

Tattersall, P., Ward, D.C., 1976. Rolling hairpin model for replication of parvovirus and linear chromosomal DNA. *Nature* 263, 106–109.

Terrosi, C., Fabbiani, M., Cellesi, C., Cusi, M.G., 2007. Human bocavirus detection in an atopic child affected by pneumonia associated with wheezing. *J. Clin. Virol.* 40, 43–45.

in epithelial cells and macrophages, and a small number of epithelial cells demonstrated reactive changes. Specimens showed significant mucus. One month after the initial diagnosis, lung tissue demonstrated a lipoid pneumonia with intra-alveolar macrophages and hemosiderin-laden macrophages.[79]

30.15.2 High-Risk Populations

After MPV infection, full recovery generally occurs. Morbidity and mortality typically occur in young children, the elderly, or patients with underlying medical conditions, including those who are immunosuppressed. In a study of patients of all ages hospitalized with MPV, 35% were under the age of 5 years and 46% were over the age of 65 years. One child with acute lymphoblastic leukemia and two patients over the age of 65 years died. In patients 15–65 years old, no deaths occurred. Of the four patients requiring mechanical ventilation, two had cancer and two were under the age of 1.[13] In children, acute respiratory distress is often the cause of mortality. However, children with the highest rates of mortality from MPV are those with underlying medical problems. In one South African cohort, 87% of children with MPV had other medical conditions, including HIV, congenital heart lesions, and chronic lung disease; almost 20% of the MPV-infected patients died.[49] In addition to high mortality from MPV infection, premature infants with MPV infection in the first year of life have an elevated airway resistance noted at follow-up.[80]

In lung transplant patients, acute rejection has been associated with MPV infection, and as many as 50% of BAL specimens were positive for MPV in one study. Prolonged shedding can occur in this population, and virus has been isolated 2 months after initial diagnosis. MPV is associated with a high mortality: one-third of infected patients died.[81] In another cohort of adults with lung transplants, two of four patients with MPV died, and the remaining two developed worsened lung function.[82]

MPV can also cause significant disease in patients post-hematopoietic stem cell transplant (HSCT). Although MPV was isolated from BAL specimens in a small subset of patients, 80% of the MPV-positive patients died of respiratory failure. Pulmonary hemorrhage was a common finding. Disease occurred within the first 40 days of transplantation.[83] In a Spanish cohort of patients with hematologic malignancies, MPV was identified in 9% of adults; 73% of those infected were HSCT patients. Patients with lower respiratory tract MPV infection had a 33% mortality rate.[84] MPV is often the sole pathogen identified in fatal respiratory infections in the HSCT population.[85]

HIV-infected children were five times more likely to have MPV LRTI compared to HIV uninfected children. Children with HIV and MPV were significantly more likely to have clinical pneumonia, bacteremia, longer hospital stay, and fatal disease compared to MPV-positive, HIV-negative children.[86]

Mortality in a children's intensive care unit was independently linked to female gender and chronic medical conditions.[87] Another study noted that in hospitalized patients, risk factors for severe infection included female sex and prematurity.[88]

In a study of outpatient adults with MPV infection, only patients in the high-risk population, despite having lower incidence rates than healthy adults, required hospitalization. Additionally, the high-risk adults had a longer duration of illness (mean 16 days).[44] High-risk elderly individuals with MPV infection have higher rates of seeking medical care, hospitalization, and death compared to healthy elderly adults.[42] Elderly residents in long-term care facilities are another high-risk population. These groups can have severe disease, with mortality rates between 33% and 50% during an MPV outbreak.[89,90]

Development of asthma in school-age children has been associated with MPV bronchiolitis in infancy. In a Spanish cohort of children, MPV infection was an important risk factor for subsequent development of early childhood asthma.[91] In cohorts of children with asthma exacerbations, MPV has been identified in 5–9% of patients.[62,63] In an adult population, MPV was identified in 7% of adults presenting with an asthma exacerbation.[70] Studies of patients with cystic fibrosis demonstrate that MPV is an uncommon pathogen causing respiratory symptoms.[92,93]

While most of the mortality occurs in children with underlying medical problems, rare case reports describe children without predisposing conditions succumbing to MPV. These children may require extracorporeal membrane oxygenation (ECMO) and can develop multiorgan system failure.[94,95] In one large prospective study of MPV-infected children in the inpatient and outpatient setting, the majority did not have underlying medical conditions.[22]

30.16 IMMUNITY

The interaction between MPV and the host immune response is not fully understood. Reinfection occurs multiple times throughout childhood and later in life.

30.16.1 Innate Immunity

The G protein may play a role in inhibiting host innate responses by affecting TLR4-dependent signaling.[96] In addition, recombinant viruses lacking the G protein produce higher levels of type 1 interferon and increased transcription factors in the NF-κB and interferon regulatory factor (IRF) families. The G protein also inhibits retinoic acid-inducible gene 1 (RIG-I)-dependent gene transcription, which is often needed for interferon production in other viruses.[7] The SH protein has been postulated to interfere with NF-κB transcription and thereby decrease IL-6 and IL-8 levels.[6] Further investigation has identified that MPV induces RIG-I gene expression, and blocking RIG-I gene expression inhibits NF-κB and thus decreases IFN-β, RANTES, and IL-8 gene transcription.[97] Other studies have demonstrated that MPV induces NF-κB, IRFs, and activators of transcription (STATs).[98]

30.16.2 Adaptive Immunity

MPV induces IFN-α, TNF-α, and CCL5 in plasmacytoid dendritic cells. After MPV infection, conventional dendritic cells have decreased cytokine production. In a mouse model, they also have impaired antigen presentation and return to normal at 6 weeks post-infection.[99] MPV-infected dendritic cells cannot activate CD4+ T cells.[100] T cells are important in MPV infection, although their role is not fully understood. In a BALB/c mouse model, CD4+ cells peaked on day 6 followed by peak CD8+ T cells on day 8. Infected mice were protected against repeat infection 6 weeks later. Depletion of CD4+ T cells has been associated with decreased lung pathology. Mice depleted of CD4+ and CD8+ T cells had persistently elevated lung viral titers past the time of normal clearance. However, mice depleted of T cells at the time of infection still produced a CD8+ T cell memory response that conferred immunity upon reinfection.[76] Studies in humans demonstrate conserved cytotoxic T cell lymphocyte epitopes with responses to multiple proteins, frequently the M protein.[101] MPV causes impairment of CD8+ T cells via the PD-1/PD-L1 pathway. Upon repeat infection, the memory T cells are functionally impaired.[102] Impairment of these cells may lead to recurrent MPV infection.

Neutralizing antibody is present in mice 5–7 days after initial infection. Antibody titers further increase after repeat infection.[76] In a BALB/c mouse model, older mice had greater lung virus replication and significantly lower production of neutralizing antibody.[103] However, these animal models have also demonstrated chronic inflammation with prolonged recovery of virus, and, therefore, they may not represent human disease.[104,105] In a hamster model, infection with recombinant parainfluenza virus expressing the F, G, and SH protein demonstrated that the F protein is significantly more immunogenic and protective.[106] Soluble G protein is immunogenic but does not provide protection against challenge in animals.[107]

30.17 CYTOKINES AND CHEMOKINES

In BALB/c mouse lungs, MPV-induced lower levels of IL-1, IL-6, and TNF-α and higher levels of IFN-α and IFN-γ compared to RSV.[108] In MPV-infected infants, nasal secretions of IFN-γ and IL-4 similar to that associated with FI-RSV vaccine, with evidence of significant lung inflammation after viral challenge.[156,157] Temperature-sensitive viruses are attenuated and induce protection in hamsters.[158] However, both temperature-sensitive and formalin-inactivated viruses provided limited protection in a primate model when animals were challenged 8 weeks after vaccination.[159] Monoclonal antibodies have been effective at treating and preventing MPV disease in a mouse model,[160,161] and an epitope on the F protein has been identified.[162] Virus-like particles that display the F and G proteins on their surface protected mice upon reinfection.[163]

30.23 CONTROL

MPV RNA in nasal secretions is shed for a median of 5 days,[164] but it can be present for as long as 2 weeks.[165] In one study of an outbreak at a long-term care facility, the spread of MPV persisted for 2 weeks after institution of contact and droplet precautions.[89] Other studies have identified a 5–6-day incubation period.[166] Compulsory timed use of alcohol gel at care facilities has been shown to decrease respiratory virus outbreaks in a facility with previous MPV nosocomial outbreak.[167] Studies of MPV infectivity demonstrate that virus particles in PBS can remain infective for 7 days, thus demonstrating the importance of contact and droplet precautions in hospitals and long-term care facilities.[138] Furthermore, nosocomial spread has been identified in patients sharing rooms.[168] Epidemiologic modeling demonstrates that a significant number of nosocomial cases can be avoided by early barrier and isolation methods; however, the method of transmission is often vague, and the only contact is a shared communal room or hospital worker.[169] Thus, early recognition of an outbreak can be difficult. However, when instituted effectively, early recognition of symptoms and isolation of symptomatic patients curbed an outbreak in a long-term pediatric care facility in 16 days.[170]

30.24 CONCLUSION

MPV is a novel virus now identified to be a leading cause of respiratory tract disease in children and adults. Although full recovery generally occurs, high-risk populations can have significant morbidity and mortality. Rapid diagnostic procedures have helped to establish incidence rates of this disease, and researchers are investigating possible therapeutics and vaccine candidates.

REFERENCES

1. van den Hoogen BG, de Jong JC, Groen J et al. A newly discovered human pneumovirus isolated from young children with respiratory tract disease. *Nat Med* 2001; 7: 719–724.
2. Peret TC, Boivin G, Li Y et al. Characterization of human metapneumoviruses isolated from patients in North America. *J Infect Dis* 2002; 185: 1660–1663.
3. van den Hoogen BG, Bestebroer TM, Osterhaus AD, Fouchier RA. Analysis of the genomic sequence of a human metapneumovirus. *Virology* 2002; 295: 119–132.
4. Biacchesi S, Skiadopoulos MH, Boivin G et al. Genetic diversity between human metapneumovirus subgroups. *Virology* 2003; 315: 1–9.
5. de Graaf M, Herfst S, Aarbiou J et al. Small hydrophobic protein of human metapneumovirus does not affect virus replication and host gene expression *in vitro*. *PLoS One* 2013; 8: e58572.
6. Bao X, Kolli D, Liu T, Shan Y, Garofalo RP, Casola A. Human metapneumovirus small hydrophobic protein inhibits NF-kappaB transcriptional activity. *J Virol* 2008; 82: 8224–8229.
7. Bao X, Liu T, Shan Y, Li K, Garofalo RP, Casola A. Human metapneumovirus glycoprotein G inhibits innate immune responses. *PLoS Pathog* 2008; 4: e1000077.
8. Boivin G, Mackay I, Sloots TP et al. Global genetic diversity of human metapneumovirus fusion gene. *Emerg Infect Dis* 2004; 10: 1154–1157.
9. van den Hoogen BG, Herfst S, Sprong L et al. Antigenic and genetic variability of human metapneumoviruses. *Emerg Infect Dis* 2004; 10: 658–666.
10. Mackay IM, Bialasiewicz S, Waliuzzaman Z et al. Use of the P gene to genotype human metapneumovirus identifies 4 viral subtypes. *J Infect Dis* 2004; 190: 1913–1918.

11. de Graaf M, Osterhaus AD, Fouchier RA, Holmes EC. Evolutionary dynamics of human and avian metapneumoviruses. *J Gen Virol* 2008; 89: 2933–2942.
12. Yang CF, Wang CK, Tollefson SJ et al. Genetic diversity and evolution of human metapneumovirus fusion protein over twenty years. *Virol J* 2009; 6: 138.
13. Boivin G, Abed Y, Pelletier G et al. Virological features and clinical manifestations associated with human metapneumovirus: A new paramyxovirus responsible for acute respiratory-tract infections in all age groups. *J Infect Dis* 2002; 186: 1330–1334.
14. Tollefson SJ, Cox RG, Williams JV. Studies of culture conditions and environmental stability of human metapneumovirus. *Virus Res* 2010; 151: 54–59.
15. Schickli JH, Kaur J, Ulbrandt N, Spaete RR, Tang RS. An S101P substitution in the putative cleavage motif of the human metapneumovirus fusion protein is a major determinant for trypsin-independent growth in vero cells and does not alter tissue tropism in hamsters. *J Virol* 2005; 79: 10678–10689.
16. Schowalter RM, Smith SE, Dutch RE. Characterization of human metapneumovirus F protein-promoted membrane fusion: Critical roles for proteolytic processing and low pH. *J Virol* 2006; 80: 10931–10941.
17. Herfst S, Mas V, Ver LS et al. Low-pH-induced membrane fusion mediated by human metapneumovirus F protein is a rare, strain-dependent phenomenon. *J Virol* 2008; 82: 8891–8895.
18. Biacchesi S, Skiadopoulos MH, Yang L et al. Recombinant human Metapneumovirus lacking the small hydrophobic SH and/or attachment G glycoprotein: Deletion of G yields a promising vaccine candidate. *J Virol* 2004; 78: 12877–12887.
19. Cseke G, Maginnis MS, Cox RG et al. Integrin alphavbeta1 promotes infection by human metapneumovirus. *Proc Natl Acad Sci USA* 2009; 106: 1566–1571.
20. Cox RG, Livesay SB, Johnson M, Ohi MD, Williams JV. The human metapneumovirus fusion protein mediates entry via an interaction with RGD-binding integrins. *J Virol* 2012; 86: 12148–12160.
21. Thammawat S, Sadlon TA, Hallsworth PG, Gordon DL. Role of cellular glycosaminoglycans and charged regions of viral G protein in human metapneumovirus infection. *J Virol* 2008; 82: 11767–11774.
22. Edwards KM, Zhu Y, Griffin MR et al. Burden of human metapneumovirus infection in young children. *N Engl J Med* 2013; 368: 633–643.
23. Kim YK, Lee HJ. Human metapneumovirus-associated lower respiratory tract infections in korean infants and young children. *Pediatr Infect Dis J* 2005; 24: 1111–1112.
24. Hara M, Takao S, Fukuda S, Shimazu Y, Miyazaki K. Human metapneumovirus infection in febrile children with lower respiratory diseases in primary care settings in Hiroshima, Japan. *Jpn J Infect Dis* 2008; 61: 500–502.
25. Aberle JH, Aberle SW, Redlberger-Fritz M, Sandhofer MJ, Popow-Kraupp T. Human metapneumovirus subgroup changes and seasonality during epidemics. *Pediatr Infect Dis J* 2010; 29: 1016–1018.
26. Ludewick HP, Abed Y, van Niekerk N, Boivin G, Klugman KP, Madhi SA. Human metapneumovirus genetic variability, South Africa. *Emerg Infect Dis* 2005; 11: 1074–1078.
27. Williams JV, Harris PA, Tollefson SJ et al. Human metapneumovirus and lower respiratory tract disease in otherwise healthy infants and children. *N Engl J Med* 2004; 350: 443–450.
28. Mizuta K, Abiko C, Aoki Y et al. Seasonal patterns of respiratory syncytial virus, influenza A virus, human metapneumovirus, and parainfluenza virus type 3 infections on the basis of virus isolation data between 2004 and 2011 in Yamagata, Japan. *Jpn J Infect Dis* 2013; 66: 140–145.
29. Choi EH, Lee HJ, Kim SJ et al. The association of newly identified respiratory viruses with lower respiratory tract infections in Korean children, 2000–2005. *Clin Infect Dis* 2006; 43: 585–592.
30. Williams JV, Wang CK, Yang CF et al. The role of human metapneumovirus in upper respiratory tract infections in children: A 20-year experience. *J Infect Dis* 2006; 193: 387–395.
31. Peiris JS, Tang WH, Chan KH et al. Children with respiratory disease associated with metapneumovirus in Hong Kong. *Emerg Infect Dis* 2003; 9: 628–633.
32. Aberle SW, Aberle JH, Sandhofer MJ, Pracher E, Popow-Kraupp T. Biennial spring activity of human metapneumovirus in Austria. *Pediatr Infect Dis J* 2008; 27: 1065–1068.
33. Esper F, Martinello RA, Boucher D et al. A 1-year experience with human metapneumovirus in children aged <5 years. *J Infect Dis* 2004; 189: 1388–1396.
34. Ebihara T, Endo R, Kikuta H et al. Human metapneumovirus infection in Japanese children. *J Clin Microbiol* 2004; 42: 126–132.
35. van den Hoogen BG, van Doornum GJ, Fockens JC et al. Prevalence and clinical symptoms of human metapneumovirus infection in hospitalized patients. *J Infect Dis* 2003; 188: 1571–1577.
36. Williams JV, Edwards KM, Weinberg GA et al. Population-based incidence of human metapneumovirus infection among hospitalized children. *J Infect Dis* 2010; 201: 1890–1898.

identified.[22,23] These changes could have influenced the immune response to the virus. The observation in the Finnish study among pregnant women that the mean titers of neutralizing antibodies against EV68 (Fermon strain) declined over the years is in line with the hypothesis that the amino acid substitutions in VP1 could have had an immune modulatory effect.[17,23] Thus, the antigenic drift in the VP1 gene might explain the recent increase in incidence of EV68 infections.

In temperate regions, EV68 infections display a clear seasonality, with most cases reported through autumn and into the winter period.[20,24,25] This is in contrast to other enteroviruses, which typically circulate during the summer and early autumn. Until now, little information is available on seasonality in tropical regions.

Transmission of EV68 from one person to the other most likely occurs via the respiratory route. Similar to other viruses causing respiratory tract infections, hand contact with respiratory secretions and autoinoculation to the mouth, nose, or eyes are probably the most important routes. Also, airborne droplets may contribute to transmission of respiratory viruses in general and EV68 in particular.[26] In general, children are thought to play a prominent role in the introduction and transmission of respiratory viruses within the household.[27,28] Crowding and poor hygiene may facilitate further spread, not only in households, but also in institutions and hospitals. Nosocomial transmission has been well documented for respiratory viruses and for enteroviruses.[29–33] However, EV68-specific information on the transmission dynamics in the community and in health care-associated institutions is lacking.

The high seroprevalence of EV68 within the community and the relatively few reports of clinical illness suggest that infection with EV68 occurs very frequently, in majority associated with mild or asymptomatic disease. Which host factors contribute to the occurrence of more serious, symptomatic respiratory disease is largely unknown. Until now, most studies suggest that clinical illness caused by EV68 is most commonly found in children.[34–36] However, this could have been biased because most studies were performed in pediatric patients. In studies where patients regardless of their age were included, 20–50% of EV68 infections were detected in adults.[16,20,23] Thus, the age distribution of infections might have been blurred by the study designs and EV68 could probably be recognized as a pathogen for all age groups.

The close relationship of EV68 with human rhinovirus and their cross-reactivity in molecular diagnostic tests (also see the section on diagnosis), together with the fact that diagnostics for enteroviruses are mainly performed on fecal samples instead of respiratory specimen, further contributes to the gaps in knowledge on EV68 as a true respiratory pathogen.[37] This diagnostic bias is illustrated by the fact that several outbreaks of EV68 are reported from various parts of the world from 2010 onward: it is highly unlikely that EV68 limits its circulation to these regions and is not present elsewhere. These findings provide additional arguments that the reported burden of EV68 infections is also influenced by the diagnostic capacities of the clinical laboratories.

31.4 CLINICAL FEATURES

Until recently, reports of respiratory illness caused by EV68 have been rare. As a consequence, very limited information about the association of EV68 with clinical symptoms and disease severity was available. During the last 4 years, however, outbreaks and clusters of EV68 in different countries provided more data on EV68 as a respiratory pathogen. The clinical presentation of EV68 infections in these reports ranged from mild illness to complicated respiratory disease, for which hospitalization was necessary (Table 31.2). In a few cases, death as a consequence of EV68 infection was recorded.[19,38] All cases presented with respiratory disease, except in one, where EV68 was detected in the cerebrospinal fluid and was implicated in a fatal infection of the central nervous system.[38]

Based on observational studies, clinical presentation is dominated by signs and symptoms of acute respiratory illness like cough, fever, and shortness of breath. A study by Meijer et al. in 2012 looked retrospectively at specimens from patients with respiratory symptoms, collected as part of the surveillance of respiratory illness among general practitioners and compared patients with EV68 with patients who were EV68 negative. EV68-positive patients had significantly more shortness of

TABLE 31.2
Clinical and Demographic Features of Patients with EV68 as Reported in the Literature

Period	Study Population	EV68 (N)	Age	Sex	Symptoms	Diagnosis	Comorbidities	Hospitalization	ICU, Death	Reference
September–November 2009	Pediatric patients	10	6 mo–10 yrs	M 60%		50% bronchitis 50% asthma	80%, n.s.	100%		23
August–September 2010	Pediatric patients	7	6–18 yrs	M 39%	Cough, difficulty breathing	56% pneumonia	39%, reactive airway disease	100%	N = 1 ICU	24
2005–2010	Pediatric patients	55	5 mo–15 yrs	M:F = 1.5:1		75% URTI 15% bronchitis/bronchiolitis	NK	NK	NK	33
2006–2011	Pediatric patients	25	40% 5–12 yrs	M:F = 1:1.5	Fever, cough, dyspnea (hospitalized patients)	32% pneumonia 64% ILI	56% of hospitalized patients (40% asthma)	36%	N = 1 ICU	35
2009–2010	All ages	17	7 wks–45 yrs	M:F = 10:7		44% asthma, 38% LRTI, 19% URTI	82% (53% chronic respiratory illness)	94%	N = 8 ICU	72
2008–2009	All ages	12	1 mo–57 yrs	M:F = 1:2		50% URTI 50% LRTI	17%, transplantation	100%	NK	38
1994–2010	All ages	71	26% 50–59 yrs	NK	Dyspnea, cough	23% bronchitis, 56% ARI/ILI	NK	NK	NK	22
2009–2010	Adults	6	>20 yrs	NK	Fever, cough	NK	33% n.s.	50%	—	20
2009	Pediatric patients	28	54% 0–4 yrs	NK	NK	NK	NK	NK	N = 15 ICU	20
2010	Pediatric patients	26	4 ± 2.7 yrs	M:F = 19:7		Asthma attacks, 54% moderate, 42% severe	65% asthma	100%	NK	17
2010	All ages	15	3 mo–5 yrs	M:F = 2:1	Fever, wheezing	47% bronchitis, 20% pneumonia, 13% pharyngitis	NK	NK	NK	34

(continued)

32.3.3 Outbreaks of NiV in India/Bangladesh

Since the initial outbreak of NiV-M in 1998–1999, NiV has been involved in many other human infections in Bangladesh and India from 2001 to 2013.[2,3] Interestingly, there are clinical/pathological differences in human cases between the large NiV-M and NiV-B outbreaks. Specifically, the incubation period during the NiV-B outbreaks in Bangladesh/India is shorter compared to NiV-M outbreak in Malaysia, with an onset of clinical symptoms ranging from 6 to 11 days.[3,21]

A total of 92 patients were identified from four outbreaks of NiV-B, with a CFR of 73% ($n = 67$). An average of 62% of total patients presented cough/cold and 69% experienced respiratory difficulties. The chest radiographs showed diffuse bilateral opacities consistent with acute respiratory distress syndrome (ARDS). NiV-B viral genome was detected in eight throat swabs (53%) and four saliva samples (27%). Respiratory distress was significantly associated with death.[21]

Overall, human cases of NiV-B are associated with a higher incidence of respiratory disease and higher mortality rate.[22] However, it remains unknown whether these differences are due to the genomic variability of NiV strains, differences in medical care of patients, or modes of transmission in Bangladesh/India compared to Malaysia/Singapore.

32.4 RESERVOIR

Bats are associated with zoonoses of potentially great global public health impact and are a source of lyssaviruses, SARS-CoV and Ebola and Marburg.[23,24] Bats frequently live in very close proximity to humans, often in large numbers. They often interact closely with livestock and other domestic animals that are potential intermediate hosts for viruses that can infect humans, thus expanding the wildlife–human interface.[25] Fruit bats from the genus *Pteropus* are shown to be the natural reservoirs for NiV and HeV based on serological evidence or isolation of infectious virus from urine and saliva.[26–28]

Australian flying foxes (*Pteropus* spp, also called fruit bats) were identified as natural hosts of HeV in 1996. There are four species of *Pteropus* bats in Australia; HeV antibodies have been demonstrated in over 20% of flying foxes in Eastern Australia and the virus has been isolated from three of the four flying fox species, from fetal tissues and from blood.[28,29]

The geographic range of pteropid bats covers all known HNV outbreaks in Australia and Southeast Asia. Evidence of NiV has been demonstrated in *P. giganteus* in Bangladesh and India.[30] NiV has been isolated from Lyle's flying fox (*Pteropus lyei*) in Cambodia and viral RNA found in urine and saliva from *P. lylei* in Thailand.[29] An HNV also appears to circulate in both fruit bats and microbats in China.[31] The presence of NiV antibodies have indicated that dogs, cats, goats, and horses were infected, but only when exposed to infected pigs in Malaysia.[32]

HNV-specific antibodies and viral RNA have also been detected in *Eidolon helvum* bats in continental Africa [33,34] and in *Pteropus rufus* in Madagascar, although infectious virus has not been isolated from these animals.[35] While no outbreaks of HeV or NiV have been reported in Africa, these data suggest the presence of antigenically related viruses in bats. Recently, CedPV was isolated from pooled bat urine from a *Pteropus* population in Queensland, Australia.[4] Owing to its close relationship to HeV and NiV, it is proposed to be a new member of the genus HNV. This virus, and viruses like it, may explain the serological results observed in African species of bats.

Experimental infection of pteropid bats with either NiV or HeV does not result in clinical disease. Inoculation of HeV into *Pteropus* bats produced asymptomatic seroconversion without evidence of viral shedding in feces or urine, nor evidence of spread to in-contact bats or horses.[36] However, subsequent studies have demonstrated vertical transmission of HeV in fruit bats.[37]

The mechanisms by which these bats control HNV infection remain unknown; however, it does not seem to be dependent on interferon signaling.[38]

32.5 TRANSMISSION

The primary mode of transmission of HeV and NiV-M is believed to be contact with secretions from infected animals (horses and pigs, respectively).[18,39] For NiV-B, the main routes of transmission are believed to be consumption of contaminated date palm sap as well as human-to-human transmission.[22,40]

32.5.1 HeV Transmission

Prior to 2011, there were 14 events of spillover of HeV infection from flying foxes to horses, and subsequent transmission to humans in five of these events. All events occurred in coastal Queensland except for one in northern New South Wales.[2,41,42] In 2011, an unprecedented rise in the number of outbreaks of HeV in horses was observed, with 18 outbreaks documented between June and October. Over 60 potential human exposures occurred in association with the 2011 HeV outbreaks, although no cases of human infection have been confirmed to date.[43]

Horses are thought to be infected by ingesting food and water contaminated by urine, saliva, or birthing products of infected flying foxes. The risk of HeV transmission to horses was found to be increased during the flying fox reproductive period and at times when the colonies were undergoing nutritional stress.[44]

Similar to the human case, all equine cases of HeV infection have been associated with a respiratory disease, neurological signs, and vascular disease, resulting in localized cerebral infarction.[45] Infection in horses has been characterized by acute febrile illness with rapid, progressive respiratory system compromise and high case-fatality rates.[46] Transmission of HeV between horses appears to be more likely in horses kept in close proximity in stables; however, companion horses in padlocks also have been infected on three occasions.[44] HeV RNA was continually detected in nasal swabs and urine of experimentally infected horses over the course of the incubation period. These data indicate that nasal secretion of asymptomatic horses may pose a transmission risk during the early phase of HeV infection.[47] The only known route of HeV transmission to humans has been through direct contact with contaminated body fluids from infected horses, and no evidence for direct bat-to-human, or human-to-human transmission has been found.

32.5.2 NiV-M Transmission

Sequence comparison of viral isolates obtained from pigs, bats, and humans indicates that the Malaysian outbreak of NiV was due to a single spillover event from bats to pigs, followed by rapid spread within the pig populations and subsequent pig-to-human transmission.[48] Agricultural practices bringing flying fox foraging sites into close proximity with intensive pig farming facilities was a major factor facilitating spillover of NiV from flying foxes to pigs.[43] Oropharyngeal shedding of NiV was observed in both clinically and subclinically infected pigs experimentally, providing evidence that naturally infected pigs may have transmitted virus to humans and animals in the absence of clinical disease. The primary mode of NiV-M transmission to humans is pig to human.[39] Substantial epidemiological evidence linked occupational exposure to respiratory droplets or secretions from infected pigs or their contaminated tissues with NiV-M infection. There is currently no evidence for direct bat-to-human or human-to-human transmission of NiV-M.

32.5.3 NiV-B Transmission

In Bangladesh, where NiV-B spillover occurs almost annually, there is a temporal association between bat reproduction and potential zoonotic spillover events.[25] Interestingly, unlike outbreaks of HeV or NiV-M, no intermediate host was identified in outbreaks of NiV-B in Bangladesh and India. During

HNV infection of the CNS and the development of neurological signs are associated with the disruption of the BBB and expression of TNF-α and IL-1β in hamsters.[56] These pro-inflammatory cytokines have been shown to play a role in increasing the permeability of the BBB as well as the induction of neuronal injury and death. While the source of TNF-α and IL-1β expression in the brain is currently unknown, they can be released by microglia, which are also infected by HNV. However, it remains unclear whether disruption of the BBB is a direct cytopathic effect of virus replication in the microvasculature, or an indirect effect through expression of TNF-α and IL-1β by bystander cells such as neurons and microglia.

32.7 HNV INFECTION IN ANIMALS

Unlike other paramyxoviruses, HNV can infect a wide range of animal species. Currently, the hamster, ferret, and African green monkey (AGM) models most closely mimic the disease progression seen in human cases.

32.7.1 HeV in Animals

32.7.1.1 Horse

Similar to humans, HeV infection in horses can result in the development of severe respiratory distress and neurological disease. Gross pathological lesions in the lungs of infected animals included edema, hemorrhage, and vasculitis.[45] The histopathological lesions in the lungs are characterized by numerous alveolar macrophages, neutrophils, and lymphocytes in areas that are away from hemorrhage or edema and by small eosinophilic inclusion bodies in some cells in the alveolar walls. However, the peribronchiolar inflammation was minimal. Vascular disease was characterized by swelling of vascular walls or by cellular degeneration of the arterial walls accompanied by pyknosis. Multinucleated giant cells were observed in the endothelium of some small blood vessels.[45]

Experimental HeV infection in horses has an incubation time between 3 and 11 days, and horses presented with interstitial pneumonia, variable respiratory rates, and breathing difficulties (50%). The main gross pathological changes in the respiratory tract were edema, pulmonary hemorrhages, congestion, and edema of the bronchial and/or submandibular lymph nodes (LNs). The histopathological lesions in the lungs were characterized by vasculitis of the medium-to-small vessels, and alveolitis with immune cell infiltrates in the septa accompanied by edema and hemorrhages. Syncytial cells were visible in the endothelium of small pulmonary vessels and along alveolar walls. The bronchi were rarely affected. Viral antigen was primarily found along the alveoli walls, in some endothelial cells of pulmonary arterioles and venules including syncytial cells, and less frequently in LNs.[45]

32.7.1.2 Pig

While pigs have not been implicated in HeV outbreaks, the related NiV-M strain was shown to be highly infectious in pigs. Following an incubation period of 4–5 days, 30–50% of pigs challenged with HeV developed respiratory symptoms such as a severe respiratory distress and cough. The gross pathological changes were characterized by consolidation of the lungs, hemorrhages, and edema as well as hemorrhages in bronchial LNs and vasculitis around the affected area. Histopathological lesions found in the lungs included interstitial pneumonia and the presence of immune cells and necrotic syncytial cells in the alveoli space. The bronchiolar epithelium was also affected. The bronchial LN presented with hemorrhage, neutrophil infiltration, and numerous multinucleated cells. Viral antigen was found in the lungs and notably in the alveolar macrophages, the bronchiolar epithelial cells, as well as in syncytial cells of both areas. Viral RNA could be detected in all nasal and oral swabs as well as in all tissues from nasal turbinate and trachea, and often from the lung lobes and from the bronchial lymph nodes. Finally, infectious virus was recovered from oral and nasal swabs as well as from bronchoalveolar lavage. These data highlight the potential of pigs as spillover hosts for HeV.

32.7.1.3 Hamster

Syrian Golden Hamsters (*Mesocricetus auratus*) infected by intranasal or intraperitoneal route have an average time to death of about 3–7 days.[56] HeV infection results in respiratory symptoms such as breathing difficulties that are accompanied by blood in respiratory secretions.[56,69] Interestingly, a high dose induces a fatal respiratory disease whereas a lower dose results in a systemic spread initially characterized by respiratory disease and followed by fatal neurological disease.[56] The gross pathological changes in the lungs were characterized by edema and hemorrhages. In addition, radiographic imaging showed abnormal findings of consolidation and diffuse pulmonary interstitial infiltrates.[56] Histopathological lesions in the lungs included rhinitis,[56] bronchiolitis/peribronchiolitis with hemorrhages, and vasculitis of the small vessels.[56,69] Alveolar hemorrhages with inflammatory cell infiltrates were also observed. Viral antigen was detected in peribronchial areas, in alveolar walls, and in pulmonary vessels (endothelial cells and smooth muscle),[56,69] but not in the tracheal epithelium.[56]

32.7.1.4 Ferrets

Following oronasal challenge of ferrets (*Mustela putorius furo*) with HeV, the incubation time was 6 days prior to clinical onset that were characterized by neurological signs of disease only.[70] The gross pathological changes observed in the respiratory tract included scattered hemorrhagic foci in the parenchyma of the lungs, the submandibular and bronchial LNs. Histopathological changes in the lungs include vasculitis and necrotizing bronchoalveolitis. Viral antigen was found in pulmonary endothelial and bronchoalveolar epithelial cells.

32.7.1.5 Nonhuman Primates

HeV infection in AGMs (*Chlorocebus aethiops*) results in nasal discharge (92%) and difficulty in breathing (33%), following a 5- to 9-day incubation period.[53] Chest radiographs showed progression of the respiratory disease characterized by congestion, diffuse interstitial infiltrates, and consolidation of the lungs. Upon necropsy, the gross pathological changes were characterized by sanguineous discharge from the nares, edema, hemorrhage of the lungs, and the presence of serous fluid in the thoracic cavity.[52,53] Histopathological changes in the lungs were characterized by interstitial pneumonia, pulmonary edema, and alveolitis with hemorrhages. Vasculitis of the small vessels was also noticed and included numerous endothelial syncytial cells. Viral antigen was mainly detected in the alveoli septa and in endothelium of small vessels. Infectious virus and viral genome could be found in the trachea, bronchus, and lungs, and less frequently detected from nasal mucosa and from oro/naso pharynx tissues. Virus genome was also isolated from oral and nasal swabs at late stage of infection.[53]

32.7.2 NiV in Animals

32.7.2.1 Pig

Following natural infection of pigs with NiV, an incubation time of 7–14 days was reported. Infection resulted in respiratory signs, such as rapid breathing, breathing difficulties, and a severe nonproductive cough. A mortality rate of up to 40% was observed in pigs. Gross pathological changes in the respiratory tract included lung consolidation, petechial hemorrhages, distension of the interlobular septa, and sanguineous secretions in trachea and bronchi.[32] Histopathological lesions were characterized by bronchial and interstitial pneumonia. Hyperplasia and necrosis of the tracheal/bronchial epithelial cells were reported as well as infiltration of lymphocytes, macrophages, and neutrophils in bronchial, bronchiolar, and alveolar epithelium. Vasculitis was reported in the small vessels only. Syncytial endothelial cells were seen in small vessels and within alveolar spaces.[32,45] Viral antigen was reported in cellular exudates in the lumen of the upper respiratory tract.

Similar to natural infection, experimental NiV infection in conventional 6-week-old pigs with NiV-M resulted in respiratory symptoms characterized by mucoid nasal discharge and persistent

F

G

H

J

K

L

M

N

O

P

Q

R

S

Printed and bound by CPI Group (UK) Ltd, Croydon, CR0 4YY
24/10/2024
01778285-0011